T0202414

OXFORD MEDICAL PUBLICATIONS

Oxford Handbook of
Public Health
Practice

Published and forthcoming Oxford Handbooks

Oxford Handbook of
Public Health Practice

FOURTH EDITION

Edited by

Ichiro Kawachi, Iain Lang, and Walter Ricciardi

OXFORD
UNIVERSITY PRESS

OXFORD
UNIVERSITY PRESS

Great Clarendon Street, Oxford, OX2 6DP,
United Kingdom

Oxford University Press is a department of the University of Oxford.
It furthers the University's objective of excellence in research, scholarship,
and education by publishing worldwide. Oxford is a registered trade mark of
Oxford University Press in the UK and in certain other countries

© Oxford University Press 2020

The moral rights of the authors have been asserted

First edition published 2001
Second edition published 2006
Third edition published 2013
Fourth edition published 2020

Impression: 3

Published in the United States of America by Oxford University Press
198 Madison Avenue, New York, NY 10016, United States of America

British Library Cataloguing in Publication Data

Data available

Library of Congress Control Number: 2019957203

ISBN 978–0–19–880012–5

Printed and bound in China by
C&C Offset Printing Co., Ltd.

Foreword

Public health led the first revolution in health and healthcare in the nineteenth century. By taking a population perspective and measuring health, not only with respect to the individuals attending hospitals, the public health movement demonstrated the action that needed to be taken to prevent and control the epidemics that were sweeping the world. Implementation was of course easier in those countries that had wealth and a stable government, and different structures evolved, but the principles were the same because of the population perspective.

For the past 50 years, there has been a second revolution dominated by increasingly effective biomedical interventions delivered to individuals by well-organized and well-funded bureaucracies with the delivery being not through the population perspective but through health centres and hospitals. The modern hospital has replaced the railway station, a symbol of the first industrial revolution, as the building epitomizing the power that was most respected in society. But now a third revolution in both industry and health is underway, driven not by centralized power delivered through well-run bureaucracies but by diffuse forces that permeate the whole population through the power of the internet. All citizens now have access to knowledge that is no longer the preserve of the medical profession, and the internet allows citizens to communicate and network.

The leader of *The Lancet* of 21 July 2018 was entitled, 'Time to burst the biomedical bubble' 'and emphasized that 'the golden age of biomedical research might be over'. It is certainly vitally important to continue with biomedical research and the delivery of its fruits to individuals but, as we enter the third revolution in healthcare, the population perspective returns as the lens through which we need to look.

In prevention, too, there has been a change in focus to what is often called 'lifestyle' with the need to provide education and information about the risks of smoking or inactivity or dietary imbalance. This development has also had some beneficial effects but its limitations are obvious, particularly when we are faced with the huge gap in life expectancy—and healthy life expectancy—between the wealthiest and the most deprived subsets of populations. However, this huge gap is of course only observed if a population perspective is taken.

The second healthcare revolution has had huge benefits with chemotherapy, transplantation, joint replacement, and the diagnostic power of magnetic resonance imaging and genetics now taken for granted but, at the end of 50 years of progress, every society on earth faces three problems that can only be seen if a population perspective is taken. These problems are unwarranted variation—namely, variation that cannot be explained by variation in need, underuse of high-value care or overuse of low-value care. Thus, the public health approach to healthcare needs to be reinvented as we move from the quality paradigm focused on those patients who reach health services to the value paradigm that considers all those in a population who are in need.

In prevention, too, there is a need to strengthen the population perspective. It is essential to ensure that individuals are well informed about the risks to health and the steps that one can take to reduce that risk. However, it is equally important to take a population perspective and to accept that a problem such as inactivity is not simply a matter of lifestyle but a consequence of an environmental revolution resulting from the car, the computer, and the desk job, which means that everything from the design of cities to the pattern of work creates an environment in which activity is made more difficult to achieve and enjoy.

Of course the language needs to be right for the task and, in most countries, it is appropriate to use public health as a description of a professional discipline, in which the population perspective as well as the perspective of the individual citizen is of vital importance. Its aim is to improve the health of populations and individuals. Public health professionals need new skills, which this Handbook summarizes, because we are now in the midst of the third industrial revolution. The first industrial revolution supported the first healthcare revolution and the second healthcare revolution was part of the transformation brought about by high technology, as was the second industrial revolution, but the third healthcare and industrial revolutions are driven by three forces that cannot be controlled by powerful bureaucracies: these forces are citizens, knowledge, and the internet. Public health professionals need to develop the skills and talent to work with these forces, which are impossible to control bureaucratically but which can be influenced. This is a new era for public health professionals and this Handbook is designed to describe and define the key concepts needed for that era.

Professor Sir Muir Gray
Director of the Oxford Centre for Triple Value Healthcare

Contents

Contents

Introduction to the fourth edition

Public health practice can be a bit challenging to explain to someone you just met at a dinner party. When all is going well in the field of public health, there is no reason for the general public to be aware of what we do. There are no newspaper headlines proclaiming that tens of thousands of people *did not die* from cancer or heart disease because of the strengthening of tobacco control policies, nor that millions now live very different lives because of the near-eradication of polio through vaccination. Like air traffic controllers, public health practitioners perform essential work that mostly remains out of sight of the public. This feature of the public health profession accounts for why so many of us experience the challenge of explaining (crisply) to our dentists, neighbours, or relatives *exactly what we do* in our profession. It is in marked contrast to our colleagues in clinical practice who have little difficulty explaining what they do to the lay public. After all, most people have directly interacted with doctors, nurses, and pharmacists at some point in their lives. Yet what we do on a daily basis in public health practice is part of the basic infrastructure of a functioning society.

Another stark contrast to medicine is that in public health we tend to make a lot of enemies. We are in a profession dedicated to persuading the public to change their behaviours to improve their health. Each of these behaviors—not smoking, drinking in moderation, regular exercise, eating healthily, and getting a decent night's sleep—is associated with vested interests that stand to profit by convincing the public to do *exactly the opposite* of the advice that we dispense. In the case of tobacco, alcohol, and junk foods, the vested interests are glaringly obvious. But even the television, social media, and advertising industries have vested interests that go against public health advice to exercise and get a decent night's sleep. The more people stay on their couches to stream 'just one more' episode of a Netflix show (or stay up to check their Facebook updates before switching the light off), the more profit these industries make. Many of these vested interests have deep pockets. For instance, the budget of the Office on Smoking and Health at the US Centers for Disease Control (CDC) is roughly one-fiftieth of the advertising and promotional budget of tobacco companies. In other words, the tobacco industry spends in one week what the CDC spends in a whole year on public service announcements and anti-tobacco campaigns. Last but not least, there are issues where there is overwhelming consensus on the evidence among scientists, yet there are also vocal (often paid) commentators who reject this consensus, convincing many of the public, and often the media too, that the consensus is not based on 'sound science'—or denying that there is consensus by exhibiting individual dissenting voices as the ultimate authorities on the topic in question. The overwhelming implication of this contest is that, as public health professionals, it is not sufficient for us to be armed with the best scientific evidence—we must also become skilled in communication, advocacy, and politics.

Public health only tends to make the headlines when there has been a *failure* of our mission to protect citizens—be it a measles outbreak on college campuses, or the mass poisoning of residents from a contaminated water supply (as happened in Flint, Michigan), or a flawed response to a humanitarian crisis or disaster. Unfortunately, public health crises will continue to occur. Our failure to mitigate human-made climate change means that the frequency of disasters (hurricanes, floods, and heatwaves) will go on rising around the globe. The link between extreme weather events and crop failure will continue to generate refugee crises in vulnerable regions. In turn, the mass displacement of human populations will continue to spark social unrest and the cynical exploitation of the plight of refugees by demagogues who would use it as a wedge to divide politics and distract public attention away from the stealth transfer of wealth from the poor to the rich. And so on. Public health issues have never been more relevant in human history, and the need to apply population-level thinking to solve these issues never so urgent.

In this fourth edition of the *Oxford Handbook of Public Health Practice*, we are continuing the tradition established by our predecessors of distilling into one handy volume (literally pocket-sized) all the basic knowledge, skills, and professional competencies that are needed for the public health professional practising in the twenty-first century. It is a basic 'survival kit' for students and practitioners. Sometime in the distant future, an archaeologist chancing upon this volume (hopefully not in the rubble of a nuclear bunker) will be able to grasp what we thought and what actions we took to tackle the pressing public health concerns of our times. Some of the material will appear quaint to that archeologist—e.g. the organization of the US healthcare system, or discoveries in genomic medicine—but the organizing principles underlying the practice of public health will surely remain the same. Or that, at least, is the bet that we are willing to make as the editors.

IK, WR, and IL

Contributors

Elena Azzolini
Department of Biomedical Sciences
Humanitas University
Pieve Emanuele, Milan, Italy
Humanitas Clinical and Research Hospital IRCCS
Rozzano, Milan, Italy

Gabriele Bammer
National Centre for Epidemiology and Population Health
Australian National University
Canberra, Australia

Nicholas Banatvala
Head of Secretariat, United Nations Inter-Agency Task Force on the Prevention and Control of Non-Communicable Diseases, and Honorary Professor Humanitarian Conflict Research Institute
World Health Organization and University of Manchester
Geneva and Manchester
Switzerland and UK

Alexandra Barratt
Professor of Public Health
Sydney School of Public Health
The University of Sydney
Sydney, New South Wales, Australia

John Battersby
Public Health England
Cambridge, UK

Mefsin Bekalu
Harvard T.H. Chan School of Public Health
Boston, MA, US

Valerie Beral
Cancer Epidemiology Unit
University of Oxford
Oxford, UK

Stefania Boccia
Section of Hygiene
University Department of Health Sciences and Public Health
Università Cattolica del Sacro Cuore
Rome, Italy
Department of Woman and Child Health and Public Health—Public Health Area
Fondazione Policlinico Universitario A. Gemelli IRCCS
Rome, Italy

Paul Bolton
Center for Humanitarian Health
Department of International Health
Johns Hopkins Bloomberg School of Public Health
Baltimore, US

Peter Brambleby
Independent Public Health Consultant
North Yorkshire, UK

Anne Brice
NHS National Knowledge Service
Oxford, UK

Rachael Brock
National Cancer Registration and Analysis Service
Public Health England
London, UK
Beverley Bryant
Peel Public Health
Mississauga, ON, Canada

Frederick M. Burkle, Jr
Professor (Ret.), Senior Fellow
& Scientist
Harvard Humanitarian Initiative,
Harvard University & T.H.
Chan School of Public Health,
Senior International Public Policy
Scholar, Woodrow Wilson
International Center for Scholars
Washington, DC

Amanda Burls
Department of Primary Health
Care
University of Oxford
Oxford, UK

Hilary Burton
PHG Foundation
University of Cambridge
Cambridge, UK

Martin Caraher
Emeritus Professor of Food &
Health Policy
Centre for Food Policy
University of London
London, UK

Ben Cave
Ben Cave Associates Ltd
Leeds, UK

Charlotte Chang
University of California, Berkeley
Berkeley, CA, US

Simon Chapman
School of Public Health
The University of Sydney
Sydney, Australia

Michael S. Chin
Division of General Internal
Medicine and Public Health
Vanderbilt University School of
Medicine
Nashville, TN, US

Paul Cosford
Health Protection Agency
London, UK

Kathryn Crawford
Boston University School of
Public Health
Boston, MA, US

Diana Delnoij
Centrum Klantervaring Zorg
Utrecht, The Netherlands

Corrado De Vito
Department of Public Health
and Infectious Diseases
Sapienza University of Rome
Rome, Italy

Chiara de Waure
Department of Experimental
Medicine
University of Perugia
Perugia, Italy

Don Eugene Detmer
American Medical Informatics
Association and University of
Virginia
Charlottesville, VA, US

Margaret Douglas
Usher Institute of Population
Health Sciences and
Informatics
University of Edinburgh
Edinburgh, UK

Julian Elston
Community and Primary Care
Group
University of Plymouth
Plymouth, UK

Sian Evans
Public Health England
London, UK

Carlo Favaretti
VIHTALI, Value in Health
Technology and Academy for
Leadership and Innovation
Spin-Off of the Universita
Cattolica del Sacro Cuore
Rome, Italy

John Fien
RMIT University
Melbourne, Australia

Julian Flowers
Public Health England
London, UK

John Ford
Norwich Medical School
University of East Anglia
Norwich, UK

Becky Freeman
School of Public Health
University of Sydney
Sydney, Australia

Sharon Friel
REGNET
Australian National University
Canberra, Australia

Michael S. Frommer
School of Public Health
The University of Sydney
Sydney, Australia

Steve Gillam
Department of Public Health
and Primary Care
Institute of Public Health
Cambridge, UK

Mike Gogarty
NHS North East Essex
Colchester, UK

Lawrence Gostin
Founding O'Neill Chair in Global
Health Law
Faculty Director, O'Neill Institute
for National and Global Health
Law
Director, World Health
Organization Collaborating
Center on National & Global
Health Law

Muir J.A. Gray
Better Value Healthcare
Oxford, UK

Felix Greaves
Imperial College London
London, UK

Chris Griffiths
Barts and The London School of
Medicine and Dentistry
London, UK

Sian M. Griffiths
Emeritus Professor
School of Public Health and
Primary Care
The Chinese University of Hong
Kong
Hong Kong, China

Jeremy Grimshaw
Clinical Epidemiology
Programme
Ottawa Health Research
Institute
Ottawa, Canada

Charles Guest
Australian Capital Territory
Government Health Directorate
and Australian National
University
Canberra, Australia

Mary Harney
Global Health Diplomacy
Summer School
University of Oxford
Oxford, UK

Wendy Heiger-Bernays
Boston University School of
Public Health
Boston, MA, US

Eric Heymann
Global Brigades ASG
London, UK

Alison Hill
South East Public Health
Observatory
Oxford, UK

Richard S. Hopkins
Adjunct Professor
University of Florida
Gainesville, FL, US

Rebekah Jenkin
School of Public Health
The University of Sydney
Sydney, Australia

Edmund Jessop
National Specialist Commissioning
Advisory Group
UK Department of Health
London, UK

Christine M. Jorm
School of Public Health
The University of Sydney
Sydney, Australia

Stefanos N. Kales
Occupational Medicine
Residency Program, Harvard TH
Chan School of Public Health
Occupational Medicine Division,
Cambridge Health Alliance,
Harvard Medical School
Boston, MA, US

Marina Karanikolos
European Observatory on
Health Systems and Policies
Brussels, Belgium

Ichiro Kawachi
Harvard T.H. Chan School of
Public Health
Boston, MA, US

Aaron Kite-Powell
Health Scientist
Surveillance and Data Branch
Division of Health Informatics
and Surveillance
Center for Surveillance,
Epidemiology, and Laboratory
Services
Centers for Disease Control and
Prevention
Atlanta, GA, US

Bernadette Khoshaba
London School of Hygiene and
Tropical Medicine
London, UK

Andrew J. Kibble
Health Protection Division
Public Health Wales
Cardiff, Wales

Anita Kothari
School of Health Studies
Western University
London, ON, Canada

Mark Kroese
PHG Foundation
University of Cambridge
Cambridge, UK

Kalyanaraman Kumaran
KEM Hospital
Pune, India

Iain Lang
PenARC and IHR, University of
Exeter Medical School
Exeter, UK

Tim Lang
Professor of Food Policy
Centre for Food Policy
University of London
London, UK

David Lawrence
London School of Hygiene and
Tropical Medicine
University of London
London, UK

Sara Mallinson
Senior Consultant
Health Systems Evaluation and
Evidence
Alberta Health Sciences
Calgary, Alberta, Canada

Leonard Marcus
Harvard T.H. Chan School of
Public Health
Boston, MA, US

Rachel McCloud
Harvard T.H. Chan School of
Public Health
Boston, MA, USA

Martin McKee
London School of Hygiene and
Tropical Medicine
University of London
London, UK

Joe McManners
General Practitioner
Former Chair of Oxfordshire
Clinical Commissioning Group
Oxfordshire
Oxford, UK

Alan Maryon-Davis
Honorary Professor of Public Health
School of Population Health &
Environmental Sciences
Faculty of Life Sciences and
Medicine Kings College
London, UK

Lamberto Manzoli
Department of Medical
Sciences
University of Ferrara
Ferrara, Italy

David Melzer
Peninsula Medical School
Exeter, UK

Ruairidh Milne
University of Southampton
Southampton, UK

Rubin Minhas
British Medical Journal
Technology Assessment Group
BMJ Evidence Centre
London, UK

Meredith Minkler
School of Public Health
University of California,
Berkeley
Berkeley, CA, US

Ellen Nolte
London School of Hygiene and
Tropical Medicine
London, UK

Don Nutbeam
Professor of Public Health
Sydney School of Public Health
University of Sydney
Australia

Sarah O'Brien
Department of Public Health
and Policy
University of Liverpool
Liverpool, UK

Andrew O'Shaughnessy
Consultant in Public Health
Medicine
Public Health
Andrew O'Shaughnessy
Consulting Ltd
Halifax, West Yorkshire, UK

Virginia Pearson
NHS Devon and Devon County
Council
Exeter, UK

David Pencheon
NHS Sustainable Development
Unit
Cambridge, UK

Emily Phipps
Public Health Registrar
Public Health Medicine
Thames Valley Deanery
Oxfordshire
Oxford, UK

Jennie Popay
School of Health and Medicine
Division of Health Research
Lancaster University
Lancaster, UK

Angela Raffle
Consultant in Public Health and
Honorary Senior Lecturer
Population Health Sciences
University of Bristol Medical
School
Bristol, UK

Shoba Ramanadhan
Harvard T.H. Chan School of
Public Health
Boston, MA, US

Jem Rashbass
National Director for Disease
Reg-istration
Eastern Cancer Registry and
Information Centre
Cambridge, UK

Walter Ricciardi
Section of Hygiene
University Department of Life
Sciences and Public Health
Università Cattolica del Sacro
Cuore
Rome, Italy
Department of Woman and
Child Health and Public Health—
Public Health Area
Fondazione Policlinico
Universitario A. Gemelli IRCCS
Rome, Italy

Thomas Rice
Professor
UCLA Fielding School of Public
Health
Los Angeles, CA, US

Richard Richards
NHS Derbyshire County Primary
Care Trust
Derbyshire, UK

Sonia Roschnik
NHS Sustainable Development Unit
Cambridge, UK

AT Saunders
Research Assistant
Public Health
carolan57 Ltd
Birmingham
UK

Patrick Saunders
Visiting Professor of Public
Health
University of Staffordshire
UK

Shannon L. Sibbald
School of Health Studies
Western University
London, ON, Canada

Fiona Sim
Institute for Health Research
University of Bedfordshire
UK

Lauren Smith
FSG and Boston University
School of Medicine
Boston, MA, US

Nick Steel
Professor of Public Health
Norwich Medical School
University of East Anglia
Norwich, UK

Malcolm Steinberg
Faculty of Health Sciences
Simon Fraser University
Vancouver, Canada

Andrew Stevens
Department of Public Health
Epidemiology and Biostatistics
University of Birmingham
Birmingham, UK

Sarah Stevens
Public Health Consultant
National Disease Registration
Division at Public Health
England, UK

Barry Tennison
formerly Honorary Professor of
Public Health and Policy
London School of Hygiene and
Tropical Medicine
London, UK

Paolo Villari
Department of Public Health
and Infectious Diseases
Sapienza University of Rome
Rome, Italy

Kasisomayajula Viswanath
Harvard T.H. Chan School of
Public Health
Boston, MA, US

Jeanette Ward
Adjunct Professor
Nulungu Research Institute
University of Notre Dame
Australia

Gareth Williams
School of Social Sciences
Cardiff University
Cardiff, UK

John Wright
Epidemiology and Public Health
Bradford Teaching Hospitals
NHS Trust
Bradford, UK

Part 1

Assessment

Scoping public health problems

Gabriele Bammer

Objectives

This chapter aims to help you figure out what you can most effectively do, within the constraints of the resources you have, to address the public health problem you are concerned with.

What does scoping mean?

Scoping is the process of identifying all the aspects of the problem that are important before setting priorities for the approach that will be taken. Scoping is important because problems are almost always bigger than the resources available to tackle them.

Scoping applies when public health problems are considered as systems problems. That means that there is an extensive array of interrelationships to take into account. An important aspect of scoping is to figure out which aspects of the system will be given prominence and where the boundaries will be drawn.

Scoping is the preparatory stage of a project where systematic thought is given to what can be best done with the available time, money, and people in order to use those resources most effectively.

It involves considering the following:
- What is most important for addressing the problem?
- What needs to be done to get there?
- Who needs to be onside?
- What are the likely blocks and how can they be overcome?

The approach taken in this chapter has similarities with that taken to scoping in environmental impact assessment[1], which includes 'early application, openness to public input, engagement of key actors, adequate treatment of alternatives, a focus on key issues ... and a design orientation' (p. 40).

Why is scoping an important skill?

Scoping is particularly important because it helps:
- broaden the view of the problem beyond what those tackling it know and understand, recognizing and respecting different points of view
- determine whether a challenge to the way the problem is generally dealt with is warranted, by paying more attention to something society sees as marginal or has excluded
- identify issues of legitimacy
- set boundaries.

A central aspect of scoping is to start by broadening the view of the problem, to move those addressing it beyond their own outlooks and to help them see the problem through the eyes of others. The aim is to appreciate what various disciplines and stakeholders can contribute. The approach taken then embraces more perspectives. In this way, the problem becomes central, rather than any particular set of expertise.

This process involves recognizing and respecting different points of view, providing a rich understanding of the problem and an array of possible responses. Interestingly, in controversial areas, paying attention to the range of arguments also often smooths the path to compromise. Views may soften once people feel they have been respectfully heard. In addition, if people know that all reasonable alternatives have been considered, they will usually be more satisfied with the choice that is made. Therefore, starting off with a broad approach can help get people onside for the action that is eventually decided upon (see Box 1.1.1).

Box 1.1.1 Feasibility of a heroin trial

In the 1990s, I led a major study investigating the feasibility of trialling diamorphine (pharmaceutical heroin) prescription as a treatment for heroin dependence.[a] We took opposition to the trial proposal very seriously, investigating—*and finding ways to respond to*—concerns raised by police, ex-users, the general community, and others. To our surprise, that process turned many opponents into supporters.

a) Bammer G. (1997). The ACT heroin trial: intellectual, practical and political challenges. The 1996 Leonard Ball Oration. Drug and Alcohol Review, 16, 287–96.

In addition, by considering a range of perspectives, scoping helps in decisions about whether a fresh approach is needed to the problem, perhaps even one that challenges conventional thinking. It reviews aspects of the problem that are currently not taken into account or that are on the periphery, asking if they should be more central.

When the status quo is challenged or controversial issues tackled, issues of legitimacy often come into play. Who is funding the project? Which organizations, researchers, and stakeholders are involved? These are important in helping determine whether the project is attempting to be even-handed or is pushing a particular point of view.

The end product of scoping is to consciously set effective boundaries around how the problem will be addressed. Scoping helps get to the nub of an issue, rather than tinkering at the margins or reinventing the wheel. There is always a limit to what any project can attempt, but those tackling it can control what they undertake. They can decide what is central, what is marginalized, and what can be ignored in their work.

This is particularly important when resources are limited. It helps in planning ahead, so that the project can be finished, rather than running out of money or time halfway through. Scoping may also be able to identify a way to proceed that is most likely to lead to more resources becoming available at a later stage.

Eight questions useful for scoping

1. What is already known about the problem?
2. What can different stakeholders and academic disciplines contribute to addressing this problem?

3. Which areas are contentious?
4. What are the big-picture issues—in other words, what are the political, social, and cultural aspects of the problem?

and

5. Why is this problem on the agenda now?
6. What support and resources are likely to be available for tackling the problem?
7. Which parts of the problem are already well covered and where are the areas of greatest need?
8. Where can the most strategic interventions be made?

The first four questions help identify the dimensions of the problem, while the last four help set priorities.

Addressing the scoping questions

1. Finding out what is already known about the problem

A key issue here is to review the literature about previous research on the problem. There is growing recognition of the value of scoping reviews and how they differ from systematic reviews.[2, 3] ➲ Chapter 2.7 provides guidance for assessing evidence. To understand big-picture context, other sources of information may also be relevant, such as government White Papers, non-governmental organization position papers, and business group statements.

2. Working with stakeholders and disciplines

In terms of figuring out how existing knowledge might best be built on, liaison with a range of stakeholders and academic disciplines is critical. Key steps include:

- identifying which stakeholders and disciplines are relevant
- finding appropriate representatives
- getting their input
- rewarding them.

It is useful to cast the net widely to identify relevant players. As well as reviewing sources of existing knowledge, it is helpful to think laterally and use contacts and networks. It may be useful to identify two categories of stakeholders—those affected by the problem and those in a position to influence the problem—and to ensure that both are adequately serviced.

➲ Chapter 3.4 considers issues of representativeness and input from communities, who are usually those affected by the problem. In terms of those who can influence the problem, representativeness tends to be less of an issue. Instead, targeting the most appropriate decision makers and practitioners may be more critical. For example, there is little point involving local government officials if the decision-making power rests with the national government.

Targeting is also important in terms of disciplinary input, because any discipline is usually quite heterogeneous in terms of what it covers. Finding the right kind of expertise for the problem is therefore the challenge. For instance, a sociologist with ethnographic skills is not particularly useful if a national survey will provide the most pertinent data.

Key questions to ask before seeking input from stakeholders and disciplinary experts are as follows:

- How can they make a meaningful contribution?
- What is needed to ensure that they will be listened to respectfully?
- Will what they say actually be taken into account?

This will guide how input is solicited, and is also a critical aspect of rewarding those involved for their time and expertise. Recognition involves being included and taken seriously, as well as being kept informed about how one's input was used and, eventually, what outcomes were achieved.

3. Dealing with areas of contention

While it can be tempting to avoid areas of contention, it is generally advisable to deal with them explicitly and early. It helps greatly to be dispassionate and sincerely open to hearing all arguments, as well as to identify the basis of the controversy—for example, is it a clash of egos, a misunderstanding resulting from poor communication, a conflict of interests, or a difference in values? This helps position the approach taken to the public health issue, including whether an attempt will be made to resolve the disagreement.

There are a number of participatory methods that can help people understand why others think differently.[4] In general, people respond positively if they feel confident that their views are being heard and taken seriously. Then, even if they disagree with the final approach that is taken, they will often think it is fair.

Legitimacy particularly comes into play here (see Box 1.1.2). Taking a dispassionate stance only works if it is genuine and demonstrable.

But what if you are not disinterested but are pushing for a particular outcome? Read up on advocacy (➲ Chapter 4.5)! The issue becomes one of understanding the opposition and being able to counter it—both through being able to draw on a wide range of allies and being able to effectively frame arguments.

Box 1.1.2 Legitimacy of the World Commission on Dams

The World Commission on Dams aimed to provide a balanced assessment of how effective large dams had been in providing irrigation, electricity, flood control, and water supply, and at what cost, especially in terms of country debt burden, displacement and impoverishment of populations, and disturbance of ecosystem and fishery resources. Legitimacy came through its origins in a workshop hosted by the World Conservation Union and the World Bank, which was attended by representatives of pro- and anti-dam interests. It systematically furthered its legitimacy by striving for balance between these interests among its 12 commissioners and its 68-member stakeholder forum, as well as its broad funding base drawing on 53 public, private, and civil society organizations.[a]

a) World Commission on Dams (2000). Dams and development: a new framework for decision-making. Earthscan, London. Available at: http://pubs.iied.org/pdfs/9126IIED.pdf (accessed 24 August 2019).

4. Tackling big-picture issues

Tackling the big-picture issues is specifically linked to the stakeholders who can influence the problem. The point here is to move beyond considering the problem just in terms of individual behaviours to also take into account, for example, the influence of government policy, advertising, and business practice. Changes here can be more far-reaching and effective.

On the one hand, these perspectives should be viewed in the same way as those of any other stakeholder— i.e. they need to be respectfully taken into account. Steps include finding out who the key actors are, whether there is any formal level of coordination, and what level of authority the actors and the coordinating group carry. Attempts should be made to involve players who can represent big-picture issues. Avoid just assuming that they will not be interested: they may well be aware of the problem and welcome an opportunity to be involved in dealing with it.

On the other hand, the power imbalance must be recognized, along with the possibility that the key players may not see the problem under consideration as being of any consequence, or may not wish to legitimize activities to tackle the problem by participating in them, especially if such activities threaten their interests. Extra caution must be exercised so that these stakeholders do not hijack the agenda, bog down the process, or stymie action.

5–8. Setting priorities

The same processes of discussion with key players and lateral thinking are also relevant to setting priorities. Understanding the big-picture context of the problem is particularly useful for figuring out why the problem is on the agenda now, and the points of strategic intervention. Clarifying what is already known about the problem will point to what is well covered and give some ideas about the areas of greatest need. The latter will be enhanced by discussions with a wide range of disciplinary experts and stakeholders. Such discussions will also highlight the level of support available for tackling the problem and possibly identify additional resources.

An iterative process

An iterative, rather than a linear, process in addressing the eight scoping questions will most probably work best and reduce the danger of getting bogged down, especially when charting unfamiliar territory.

The judicious use of experts is crucial to saving time and maintaining momentum. The challenge is to discern what is needed to put together an understanding of the problem, what those tackling it know and do not know, and whom to bring in to fill the gaps. As new players are brought into the picture, their contributions may lead to revisiting understandings of what is known, or the areas of disagreement or the priorities. The scoping process must be open to this, but also needs a clear sense of direction so that it is not diverted by less relevant agendas that other players may have.

Back-to-back spirals are illustrative of the process—the outward expansion of the top spiral indicates the build-up of knowledge and perspectives, whereas the inward direction of the second shows the knowledge and perspectives being used to set priorities (see Figure 1.1.1). The loops illustrate revisiting what is known, bringing in other people who might have a useful perspective, and so on. As the figure illustrates, the starting point may be

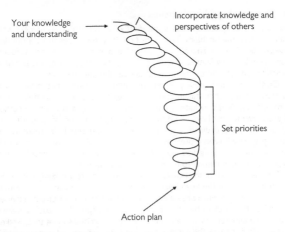

Figure 1.1.1 Broadening, aligning, and focusing perspectives.

somewhat off-centre: in other words, the initial knowledge and expertise may be limited, but the end point of scoping is an action plan that addresses central issues.

'Reality testing' can profitably be undertaken at several points. The aim is to find holes in the knowledge base or the arguments on which priorities are based and, from this, to highlight where further data gathering or consultation are required. This is where advisory and reference groups can be invaluable, because they can be asked to comment along the way.

What are the competencies needed for effective scoping?

Key competencies include:
- integrity (including being clear about whether the approach taken is dispassionate or one of advocacy)
- credibility in terms of acknowledged expertise about the problem and/or the scoping process
- ability to understand and tackle the problem as a system, when appropriate
- possession of a wide-ranging network of contacts and knowing the key players or an intermediary who can provide access to them
- skill in facilitating meetings and interactions, including encouraging open debate and the challenging of ideas, handling negotiations and conflict, and creating a positive atmosphere
- management skills
- an open mind to ideas from others

- the ability to think laterally and creatively
- understanding the 'cultures' of different stakeholders and the ability to empathize with different concerns, without being captured by them
- the ability to identify which disciplines are relevant, and enough knowledge about the disciplines to know what they can offer, to identify experts, and to involve experts in working on the problem
- understanding the relevant policies and other big-picture issues, their history, the key players, and the political sensitivities
- the ability to integrate a range of knowledge and expertise, to cut through to the essentials, and to lead a priority-setting process
- the ability to build alliances with those who need to be onside in order to move forward.

What are the potential pitfalls in the scoping process?

Potential pitfalls include the following:

- *Not having enough resources:* including time, to undertake an adequate process.
- *No real commitment:* by those in a position to act to understand and deal with the problem. For example, a process can be set in train for reasons of political expediency and the plug may be pulled as soon as the political heat dies down.
- *Not being the right person for the job:* for example, not being interested in this process, not being experienced enough to keep control, or not being able to deal with a diverse range of views respectfully.
- *Getting bogged down:* losing momentum and timeliness can be fatal. Beware of wallowing in factual detail, meetings without a clear purpose, and red herrings. Those responsible for addressing the problem should not feel that they have to be on top of all the material, but instead can rely on experts who understand the stakeholder or disciplinary perspectives.
- *Choosing inappropriate representatives of stakeholders:* involving people in a process helps legitimize their point of view and careful thought should be given to including fringe groups. If people who are not well-regarded are included in the process, respected players may pull out or not participate fully.
- *An inappropriate balance:* the problem has to be seen in perspective, so that the process involves an appropriate mix of stakeholders and academic disciplines, the powerful and the powerless, and—for a dispassionate approach to contentious issues—different points of view.
- *Avoiding the contentious issues:* ignoring particular groups in an attempt to avoid controversial issues will often backfire, with their exclusion providing them with an additional opportunity to further their cause, and even undermining the outcomes of the process.
- *Exhausting key players:* stakeholder representatives and experts from particular disciplines usually have their own jobs to do and they may get no recognition nor credit for being involved in your scoping process. Use their time wisely, sparingly, and efficiently.

- *Promoting conflict:* scoping processes that involve contentious issues usually seek to find compromise but, if the players are not chosen carefully and the process is not handled appropriately, conflict can be escalated rather than reduced.
- *Not showing leadership:* if there is no evident leadership by those in charge of the scoping process, it is open to being hijacked by the more powerful participants. This can also be a factor in the promotion of conflict.
- *Avoiding decisions:* never underestimate the temptation not to make a decision when the problem is difficult or contentious. Yield not to temptation!
- *Not being prepared to combat the wrath of the powerful:* when scoping processes involve challenging entrenched power bases, provoking a reaction could well be a measure of success. The challenge is not to be naïve and to be prepared to counter these forces.
- *Not learning from mistakes.*
- *Inexperience:* this can be overcome by finding mentors, powerful allies, and supportive colleagues.

Markers of success

Markers of success are an approach to the problem that has:
- broad-based support
- clear and implementable steps for increasing understanding and moving to a solution
- commitment from the key players and the stakeholders they represent to stay involved in seeking a solution
- respect between opponents.

For issues where a major power base has been challenged and where the power base is seeking to protect its interests, measures of success include:
- a coalition that includes people of influence, who will stand up to the power base and continue to fight for the solution
- openings for negotiation.

A successful scoping process lays a strong foundation for effectively tackling a problem, and increases the chances of developing a solution on budget and on time.

References

1 Mulvihill PR. (2003). Expanding the scoping community. *Environmental Impact Assessment Review*, 23, 39–49.
2 Levac D, Colquhoun H, O'Brien KK. (2010). Scoping studies: advancing the methodology. *Implementation Science*, 5, 69. Available at: ⅋ http://www.implementationscience.com/content/5/1/69 (accessed 30 July 2019).
3 Peters MDJ, Godfrey CM, Khalil H, et al. (2015). Guidance for conducting systematic scoping reviews. *International Journal of Evidence-Based Healthcare*, 13, 141–6.
4 McDonald D, Bammer G, Deane P. (2009). *Research integration using dialogue methods*. Australian National University Press, Canberra. Available at: ⅋ http://doi.org/10.22459/RIUDM.08.2009 (accessed 30 July 2019).

Priorities and ethics in population-based healthcare

Alan H. Griffith, Emily Phipps, and Joe McManners

This is a version of the chapter that we produced as the original
Bazian. McGuire and Davies. She are in the main edition but give too
much less at extreme portions and millions of the Phipps texts, as has
been about leaving the accurate extent employments.

Chapter 1.2

Priorities and ethics in population-based healthcare

Sian M. Griffiths, Emily Phipps, and Joe McManners

This fourth version of the chapter builds on the work of the co-authors Robyn Martin and Douglas Sinclair in the third edition, but given the changing structures, policies, and politics of the English NHS, it has been updated taking into account current arrangements.

Objectives

As a result of reading this chapter you will be able to:
• understand the language of ethics and the role ethics play in public health practice
• understand the principles of priority-setting for health and healthcare systems within a constrained budget
• appreciate how an ethical framework guides choices for population health and health policy-making, including making choices to reduce health inequalities.

Definitions

Ethics constitute a coherent and consistent system of morality, values, virtues, and responsibilities that guide issues such as who should make health decisions, how those decisions are made, and the principles that should underpin health decisions. Ethics serve as 'a beacon to warn of the danger and to show the way—as a lighthouse'.[1] In summary, ethics refers to a variety of techniques for understanding the moral life, that is, how an act is judged to be right or wrong.[2]

Public health ethics constitute the system of morality, values, virtues, and responsibilities that guides decision-makers with responsibility for the health of populations. Such a system may be implicit or explicit, but in a democracy, where legitimacy ultimately derives from the people, it may be highly desirable to codify the principles that are used to justify decisions. This allows the people to understand and possibly challenge the process by which decisions are taken.

Public health ethics recognize that there will be circumstances where the health of the wider population justifies overriding the autonomy and rights of the individual. The decision-maker with responsibility for the health of a population may be required to balance the needs of different individuals or groups within this population and to allocate resources between them, even if this disadvantages some individuals compared to others. In this way it differs from bioethics.

Priority setting can apply to health services and also to population health. For health services it describes a process by which an explicit decision is made to provide some health services, rather than other services. Such decisions may directly compare two or more services, or may evaluate one service against a set of criteria, and recommend that it be provided if it meets certain thresholds (e.g. sufficient clinical benefit for an acceptable cost). It is relatively straightforward to compare the clinical- or cost-effectiveness of two treatments that are used for the same disease. If both produce the same clinical benefit it may be sensible to provide the less expensive one. If one provides greater clinical benefit than the other, it may be necessary to compare the cost–benefit ratios for each treatment in order to recommend the more cost-effective treatment. Sometimes a health service commissioner may not be able to provide a treatment that would otherwise be regarded as cost-effective, because the overall cost would be prohibitive.

The level of priority treatments are likely to be determined by the overall budget available, but their accessibility varied according to available resources, for example, low-priority treatments may be funded in times of plenty, but in austere times the threshold for funding will go up.

Priorities for health

Ethics should underpin decisions about healthcare priorities: The distinction between the ethical responsibilities of healthcare providers and those of population health decision-makers is not always clear-cut. For example, a healthcare provider may be required to offer a scarce resource (e.g. intensive care beds) to those patients most likely to benefit from this resource, rather than to other patients. This situation is likely to arise in response to a major local or national disaster (e.g. pandemic influenza or Coronavirus) when health service capacity is overwhelmed. Judgements must then be made on which patients should or should not receive this scarce resource.

When considering population needs, choices may need to be made between preventing the need for or for providing health services. Very often the pragmatic and political factors associated with health service provision override the need for longer-term investment in preventive services.

Ethics theories are statements of principles that can be used to justify certain actions.[3] Such theories may provide a rational basis for decision-making, which is itself open to consultation and debate. Certain theories of ethics have assumed particular importance both for policy formulation and specific decision-making at various times in the history of the National Health Service (NHS). Currently, there is an intense focus on cost containment across the system, while promoting individual choice of provider.

The prevailing (and sometimes opposing) ethical theories that are used to justify particular decisions about the future of the NHS, as well as specific decisions about funding particular treatments, include:

utilitarianism[3]—making decisions that result in the greatest good for the
   greatest number
communitarianism—making decisions that arise from the values and
   traditions of local communities and populations
liberal individualism—based on rights theory (emphasizing the freedom
   of individuals to pursue their own ambitions, but recognizing that one
   person's entitlement might constitute another's obligation)
principle-based common morality theory—where the set of values shared by
   members of a society give rise to principles of obligation, for example,
   recognition of individual rights and autonomy, obligations of beneficence
   and non-maleficence and justice—the fair distribution of benefits
   and risks.

The importance of commissioning (partly planning, partly procuring) services that are responsive to the specific needs of local populations is a fundamental cornerstone to health service delivery in England. The health and social care reforms of 2012/2013 re-emphasized this.[4] Over two hundred Clinical Commissioning Groups (CCGs) were formed, made up of professional managers, general practitioners (GPs), other clinicians, and lay members are responsible for commissioning all community and most hospital services. Increasingly, this also includes primary care services. Commissioning decisions are expected to improve the health of local communities and to engage communities in decision-making processes. Nationally mandated public health interventions such as screening and immunization that are universal for all members of society remain largely under the control of Public Health England. However, by transferring public health functions of the NHS to local authorities in April 2013, it was expected that disease prevention and health promotion programmes should be procured and tailored to specific local need and to address health inequalities. By aligning public health with local authority services, it was hoped that there could be a greater emphasis on place based approaches to health communities and preventative health.

The NHS Long Term Plan (2019) articulates a direction to move away from purely commissioning organisations, towards 'Integrated Care Systems', which take a whole system approach to organising and planning healthcare. Ultimately, the universal challenge for all of these services remains the same: how can we best use our limited budget to deliver maximum health benefit for our community? Increasingly, the additional challenge is how to balance the need for investment in prevention for future benefit when resources are constrained, with greater and greater demands on hospital and social care.

Why is ethics important for population health?

Making best use of limited resources—whether it is called rationing or priority setting—is a fact of life. Limited resources need to be made to go as far as possible. This means saying 'No' to some people, while others benefit. This is not a comfortable thing to do, but one in which many people in public health are necessarily involved. This may also apply to decisions about whether it is a better use of resources to invest in education services or to provide home care to the elderly or to shorten hospital waiting times. Competition for resources may be the result of a new treatment becoming available, demand growing for treatment because of increased patient awareness, or because more people in an ageing population need the treatment. The pressures of innovation, public participation, patient expectation, person-focused care, political policies, and socioeconomic factors make priority setting a vital part of public health practice in ensuring the health of the local population.

All health services have different ways of organizing healthcare delivery and of making choices about which services will be provided within budgets set by funders—be they through taxation, insurance, or personal out-of-pocket spending. With limited resources comes the necessity to make difficult choices and the need to ensure best value for the finances available. In England at the time of writing this responsibility is devolved to CCGs. In not-for-profit organizations, contracts will be negotiated according to funders' guidelines, and in private sector organizations they may be made by boards of directors.

Whatever the mechanism for deciding priorities, funders are faced with a host of service demands and difficult decisions. Mechanisms for deciding which new investment or disinvestment decisions should be made need to be founded on ethical principles and made within a transparent policy framework that not only clinicians and managers understand but also local people agree and accept.

One aspect of rationing not usually recognized is the 'hidden' rationing, often the result of passive or default decision-making. Examples of this are long waiting times for treatment, lack of availability of beds, lack of investment in services for certain groups due to lack of knowledge of them in health services, and so on.

Ethics serve an important role in providing a framework for public health population-based policy and practice. This framework helps public health policy-makers and practitioners to make difficult decisions, but also constrains them from undertaking overzealous interventions that potentially intrude unnecessarily into private lives.

Ethics also make transparent the assumptions and values underlying health decisions so as to enable open challenge and debate of those assumptions and values. It is particularly important to address the apparent conflict between the values of clinicians (who are trained to consider the needs of individual patients without explicit reference to the competing needs of other patients) and the values of commissioners (who are responsible for planning and procuring health services for entire populations and must balance the needs of different groups of patients). In order to bring both sets of values into the decision-making process, health service commissioners have been increasingly engaging clinicians in the commissioning process (clinical engagement).

Clinical Commissioning arrangements aim to ensure that needs of local patients are addressed, but emphasizes the potential conflict between the needs of individuals and the needs of the local population. It increases the likelihood that access to services will vary across the country due to local policy-making and delegation of authority.

As with most health systems, the NHS in England is continually striving for greater efficiencies in order to better serve the public

- How can we be fair when making rationing decisions?
- How do we account for our decision?

An understanding of the ethics underpinning local decision-making when implementing the requirements of national programmes provides support to commissioning services for local populations.

Efficient health services are ones which provide the highest possible quality care with the lowest possible wastage of resources and effort. NHS England's seminal Five Year Forward View released in 2014 outlined how inefficiencies in the organization were fuelling widening gaps in care provision and health outcomes in the country.[5] In order to reverse this, the country was split into forty-four 'footprint' areas which were required to produce sustainability and transformation plans (STPs) outlining how they intended to improve the quality of care and health outcomes over the next five years, but also to close the financial gap opening up between demand for healthcare and the funding of it. These 'STPs' are evolving into Integrated Care Systems.

On a more local level, Commissioning for Quality and innovation (CQUIN) schemes are in place to help drive improvement. Introduced in

> **Box 1.2.1 Guidelines to clinicians**
> 1. If you want something outside your current fixed envelope of resource, can it be done by substituting a treatment of less value?
> 2. If demand for your service is increasing, what criteria are you using to agree to the threshold of treatment?
> 3. If you do not believe that it is possible to either draw thresholds of care or substitute treatment, then within a fixed budget which service might you give a smaller resource to in order for you to enlarge yours?

2009/10, commissioners are able to financially reward providers for accomplishing achievements against national and local quality improvement goals.[6] However, despite these drivers, inequalities in provision of care still exist. Healthcare commissioners continue to examine the imbalances in need and provision (be that under- or even over-provision) to try to determine what services should be funded routinely and which others should be of lower priority. In order for these decisions to be made in a way which is fair and transparent, commissioners and clinicians structure their discussions on agreed ethical frameworks (see Box 1.2.1).

Ethics frameworks

Legislation and professional regulation provide policy and practice frameworks, but these more rigid frameworks are not always up to date, are not always appropriate to situations where urgent decisions need to be made, and are slow to amend where new public health threats emerge.

At a local level, explicit codes of ethical practice can be applied to the process of decision-making to ensure consistency with an agreed set of values (e.g. autonomy and equity). They provide assistance in the gaps left by legislation and professional regulation and can be useful tools for helping decide which populations have the greatest need for services or which services provide the best outcomes within available resources. In addition, they can also help in articulating the decisions made (Box 1.2.2).

Ethics frameworks can be developed in consultation with communities and tested against the values of these communities. They can also be updated as necessary to reflect changes in community values or changes in the types of decision that need to be made.

As such, particularly in situations such as England where the role of local government in healthcare decision-making has grown, the use of ethics and tools (such as ethics frameworks) based on ethics principles can be a practical resource to help make consistent and transparent decisions that make sense within the context of community values. This also allows the community to assess the values underlying difficult decision-making. A decision may be judged to be reasonable if it involves an appropriate group of people reviewing an appropriate question, using a process that is itself deemed reasonable.

> **Box 1.2.2 Example of the use of an ethical framework in practice**
> (Adapted from Thames Valley Priorities Committee Ethical Framework[a])
> 1. **Equity:** people should have access to healthcare on the basis of need. Sometimes care should be given priority in order to address health inequalities.
> 2. **Need and Capacity to Benefit:** healthcare should be allocated fairly according to both need and capacity to benefit, rather than on simply a request or the fact that it is the only treatment available.
> 3. **Clinical Effectiveness:** treatments and services with the best evidence of improving the health status of patients should be prioritized.
> 4. **Cost-Effectiveness:** Treatments must provide value for money for the NHS.
> 5. **Cost of Treatment and Opportunity Costs:** Cost should be compared to the possible health benefit gained and what other investments would have to be foregone to fund it.
>
> a) https://www.england.nhs.uk/wp-content/uploads/2013/04/cp-01.pdf.

In the following section, two examples illustrate how this triumvirate of person, question, and process may operate at a national or local level.

How do ethics assist in policy and practice governing the commissioning of hospital services?

The English context

Within the English national health system, Parliament votes on departmental spending and therefore sets the overall budget for the health service. The Department of Health sets national priorities through an annual mandate and allocates money to Public Health England and NHS England, who in turn pass responsibility for spending to local authorities and CCGs. Devolved authorities such as Greater Manchester are also now using their extended powers to take greater control of health and social care budgets, and so are handling delegated responsibility for budgets previously held by NHS England. In the future we may see this trend continue if the Greater Manchester Combined Authority 'experiment', nicknamed 'DevoManc', proves successful. Whether decisions are made at national or local level, they are made in the context of a fixed amount of available resource. Investment in treatments for some groups of patients reduces the opportunity to fund treatments for other patients.

National decision-making

The National Institute for Health and Care Excellence (NICE)[6] provides evidence-based guidance and quality standards for healthcare, social care, and public health in England. Only certain NICE guidance is applicable to the devolved nations due to the legislation through which the body was established. For example, in Scotland the Scottish Intercollegiate Guidelines Network (SIGN)[7] are the primary providers of evidence-based practice guidelines but they work collaboratively with NICE to reduce duplication of effort and increase efficiency. The questions (i.e. which technologies should be considered for use in which group of patients) are initially identified by expert committees, then tested with a group of stakeholders, including patients, healthcare providers, commissioners, and manufacturers.

The finalized questions are then considered by government ministers who provide a national policy perspective. Those questions deemed by ministers to be appropriate for appraisal by NICE receive an expert assessment of the evidence and are considered in detail by appraisal committees whose members include representatives from a wide range of stakeholder groups (e.g. patients, carers, experts, professional bodies, providers, commissioners, and manufacturers). The committees hold part of their meetings in public (allowing a degree of transparency) and publish the documentation that is not deemed confidential (for commercial or academic reasons).

The appraisal committees have a defined process for considering evidence of clinical and cost effectiveness and for giving weight to certain groups of patients. There is a process for consulting the public where decisions are likely to lead to significant restrictions of the availability of a technology. There is also the opportunity for a limited set of stakeholders to appeal against NICE's recommendations. From time to time, NICE undertakes public consultations to update its procedures.[8]

Local decision-making (Box 1.2.3)

Box 1.2.3 Case study: Using a framework of ethics in making difficult choices: Historical experience from Oxford

An ethics framework was structured around three main components:

Evidence of effectiveness
- Consider:
  - Is there good evidence that the treatment is not effective?
  - Is there good evidence that the treatment is effective?
  - Is there a lack of good evidence either way?
- It is desirable to obtain good quality evidence about effectiveness, and research aimed at obtaining such evidence should be encouraged. However, when evidence is poor, then a judgement about the likely effectiveness has to be made in the knowledge that good quality evidence is not available.

Equity
The basic principle of equity (fairness) is that people with similar needs should be treated similarly. This principle should be applied consistently at different times and in different settings, with no discrimination on grounds that are irrelevant to the need for healthcare.

Box 1.2.3 *Contd.*

In developing the principles on which equity is based, two broad approaches can be taken:
- maximizing the welfare of patients within the budget available (a utilitarian approach), often expressed in terms of the cost-effectiveness of different health services
- giving priority to those in most need (a rights approach).

Patient choice

Respecting patients' wishes and enabling patients to have control over their healthcare are important values (the principle of autonomy based on liberal individualism). Within those healthcare interventions that are purchased, patients should be enabled to make their own choices about which treatment they want to receive. It is a matter of fundamental respect that patients should always be treated as much as autonomous individuals as possible. This is one of the stated reasons for the active promotion of patient choice of provider that is a feature of recent health service reforms in England.

When considering the principle of patient choice, it is important to recognize that the principle of effectiveness is usually addressed by considering the best available evidence from well-conducted published studies. These studies normally consider the effectiveness of a treatment in a large group of patients. Sometimes the evidence suggests that a treatment generally provides insufficient benefit (or is too expensive) to be provided. However, each patient is unique, and there may be a good reason to believe that a particular patient stands to gain significantly more from the treatment than most of those who formed the study group in the relevant research. Evidence that this individual patient has significantly different circumstances compared with most patients may be used to demonstrate *exceptional circumstances*. This may justify such a patient receiving treatment that is not normally provided.

This ethics framework was used in the process of making decisions to:
- Structure discussion and ensure that the important points were properly considered
- Ensure consistent decision-making, over time and with respect to decisions concerning different clinical settings
- Enable articulation of the reasons for decisions that are made.

How do ethics assist in policy and practice governing the treatment of patients in general practice?

GPs are usually independent practitioners contracted to provide NHS services to registered patients. In general, their contracts require them to provide services that they deem 'necessary and appropriate' for individual patients. These contracts do not take account of any duty to balance resources between different patient groups, but increasingly GPs are being asked to make collective decisions about prescribing drugs or commissioning services based on the needs of populations. GP training and General Medical Council guidance also emphasizes the responsibility to consider the overall health resource. This conflict between the needs of individuals and the needs of populations has become more apparent as GPs, through CCGs, take on responsibility for commissioning hospital services.[5] This brings direct conflict between the principles of autonomy (as expressed by 'patient choice') and utilitarianism, which seeks to use resources to obtain the greatest good for the population (even if this means that some individuals do not receive the best care available to them).

There is also a tension between meeting the immediate needs of the patients and preventing health problems for future patients. This is particularly interesting as a tension in investment decisions, for example, diabetes. Should we prioritize those who are already unwell or those who could be prevented from becoming unwell? What sort of balance should there be?

Answering such questions can be assisted by the use of an ethics framework if the local population and other stakeholders, particularly democratically elected local authority members, are involved in its development, adding legitimacy (by the principle of communitarianism) to the decision-making process and providing transparency (respecting the principle of autonomy).

How do ethics assist in policy and practice governing the prevention and control of communicable diseases?

Medical science has provided many solutions for the threat of communicable diseases through the development of vaccinations, antivirals, and antibiotics. However, not all diseases can be controlled by vaccination and drugs. This is particularly the case where disease carriers and contacts refuse to cooperate with medical practitioners, and where new diseases emerge for which no treatments or vaccines have yet been developed. Public health legislation often provides powers of isolation, quarantine, exclusion from public places, and in some cases compulsory screening, treatment, and vaccination (see Boxes 1.2.4 and 1.2.5). However, even when legislation provides these powers, their use relies on the judgement of the public health practitioners. Ethics assist in decisions on when to exercise such powers that while protecting the community, also potentially infringe individual autonomy and rights.

Box 1.2.4 Case A: Should you detain against their will someone with multidrug-resistant tuberculosis (MDR-TB) who refuses to remain in voluntary isolation?

There may be good public health arguments to justify long-term detention of the patient to prevent the spread of MDR-TB to others who come into contact with them. Legislation in most states provides powers to detain in these circumstances. However, a 'power' implies exercise of discretion. If there were no discretion there would be a duty to detain, rather than a power.

What ethics principles govern the exercise of this power? A utilitarian approach suggests that a coercive measure, such as detention, might be taken where the overall benefit to society resulting from detention outweighs the overall loss to society.[a] How do you measure such benefit and loss? You need to undertake a risk assessment in relation to the patient based on available scientific evidence about the disease: How infectious is this condition? How much contact does the patient have with others? How responsible is he/she in their health behaviours?

Evidence is also needed on the consequences of imposing coercive measures. Will other patients go underground to avoid detention? Will detention discourage ill persons from seeking diagnosis? What will be the economic and social consequences to the patient and the family of detention? Does detention pose the risk of discrimination, stigma, and marginalization? Are there any other alternatives to detention that might work better for the patient? Would you choose to detain other patients in the same situation or is there something about this patient that leads to you treating him/her differently?

Duties of beneficence and non-maleficence tell you that you need to do what is best for the patient and to do him no harm, so arguments that it is for the good of society to detain him will need to be convincing to override the patient's right to autonomy and private life.

The need for a professional risk assessment imposes duties on the public health community to develop an evidence base to underpin such risk assessments and a duty on individuals working in public health to keep up to date on evidence. Any such measure should only be taken where there is a demonstrable public health benefit to be achieved.

a) Coker R, Thomas M, Lock K, et al. (2007). Detention and the threat of tuberculosis: evidence, ethics, and law. *Journal of Law and Medical Ethics*, 35, 609–15.

Box 1.2.5 Case B: In case of a disease pandemic for which there are limited health resources, who should have priority access to those resources?

This is an issue unregulated by legislation and provides an example of a situation in which ethics must step in to fill the gaps left by law. There will be conflicting ethical obligations in such a case. Healthcare providers owe duties of beneficence to all patients, suggesting a duty to provide healthcare to every patient who needs health resources. Where resources are limited, however, duties of beneficence do not assist in choices between patients.

Triage principles will suggest that resources should be given to those most likely to benefit from treatment, underpinned by ethics arguments that limited resources should be used as efficiently and effectively as possible. A utilitarian approach will support the view that priority should be given to those persons who will be essential to the functioning of society during the pandemic. This would suggest that healthcare workers themselves, as well as other essential service workers should be prioritized over other patients. It may justify priority for mothers of families with small children or other carers within society. Utilitarianism will also support the view that priority should be given to the treatment that is most effective in reducing the spread of disease to others.

Other ethics theories, particularly theories of ethics of care, will support prioritizing for treatment those persons with the longest productive life years ahead of them. Opposing ethics arguments might criticize these approaches as discriminatory and suggest that a lottery for resources, or a first-come-first serve approach, would be fairer.

Ethics debate will not produce a clear and convincing answer to an ethical 'hard case' such as this. However, an ethics framework will provide language and tools for debate and demand transparency in relation to the values and virtues underpinning choices.

How do ethics assist in policy and practice governing the prevention and control of non-communicable diseases?

The ethics of public health interventions in the case of non-communicable diseases (NCDs) are more complex. Whereas communicable disease infringements of the private behaviour of individuals can be justified on the basis of prevention of the spread of disease to the wider population at a given point of time, individual behaviours and life choices play a greater role over a longer time (see Boxes 1.2.6 and 1.2.7).

Box 1.2.6 Case C: Should the state intervene to prevent an individual from smoking in a public place?

Mill's 'harm principle' states that 'the only purpose for which power can be rightfully exercised over any member of a civilized community, against his will, is to prevent harm to others. His own good, either physical or moral, is not a sufficient warrant'.[a]

The harms of first- and second-hand tobacco smoke are well documented.[b] In the case of smoking in a public place, we can begin by arguing that we are prohibiting smoking to protect other people at risk of being affected by tobacco smoke, in which case the ethics issues are similar to those in the case of communicable disease. What if all the other persons in the room are consenting adults who are themselves smoking or if the smoker is sufficiently far from any other person such that any risk is negligible? Then we will need to look for other less direct harm to justify intervention, such as the social costs to the family and friends of the smoker if he should suffer smoking harms, and the cost to society of resulting healthcare.

Our ethics arguments may also turn to the extent to which the smoker or his companions are autonomous persons making informed decisions on their own health, for Mill's harm principle is premised on the autonomy of the individual. Has the smoker made a free and non-manipulated informed choice to smoke? We can argue, using the science of behavioural psychology, that influences such as tobacco advertising, the depiction of smoking in the media, and peer pressure have distorted the smoker's ability to make a free and informed choice and caused him to put his health at risk by smoking.[c] Ethics arguments would then suggest that public health institutions have a responsibility at least to counter the malign influences so as to restore the autonomy of the individual. Similar arguments apply to the state's duty to address obesity harms by limiting advertising and misleading labelling of high fat, salt, and sugar products.

a) Mill JS. (1869/2002). *On liberty*. Dover Publications, Mineola.

b) World Health Organization (2005). *Framework Convention on Tobacco Control*. WHO, Geneva.

c) Hatsukami D, Slade J, Benowitz N, et al. (2002). Reducing tobacco harm: research challenges and issues. *Nicotine & Tobacco Research*, 4, 89–101.

Box 1.2.7 Case D: Should the state impose taxes on the purchase of alcohol to limit alcohol-related harms?

Excessive alcohol use causes health harms to individuals, and social and economic harms to family and society.[a] Evidence suggests that, because it is price sensitive, alcohol consumption can be manipulated by the pricing of alcohol.[b] Increasing alcohol taxes serves both to reduce alcohol harms and to increase government revenues to support healthcare and other public goods. This suggests the state has a public duty to use taxation as a tool to the benefit of the public's health.

However, as with smoking restrictions, alcohol taxation serves to restrict the liberty of the individual to make a lifestyle choice. We can argue that reducing alcohol levels will benefit the health of drinkers, although these arguments are not as strong as they are in relation to tobacco unless drinking is excessive. However Mill's harm principle suggests that this is not sufficient to warrant intervention. People choose to drink alcohol because it gives them pleasure even when they are aware of the risks posed to their health.

We can justify countering alcohol industry advertising with health messages to restore autonomous decision-making, but it is more difficult to justify interfering with the choice to drink alcohol. We may also justify interventions into excessive drinking, though it is arguable that even here we are interfering with autonomy. The difficulty lies in interventions that affect careful and sensible consumption of alcohol.[c]

It can also be argued that taxation of products operates in a discriminatory manner, in that an increase in alcohol prices will affect the choices of the less well off more significantly than those of the better off. Arguments that have been used to support tobacco taxation, given the inherent harmfulness of tobacco, are not as persuasive here. Nor is alcohol the only product, not harmful in itself, but only in excessive use, willingly and widely consumed.

We might argue that we should also impose high taxes on food stuffs, sweets, and snacks that, when consumed in excess, can cause dental and health harms, and which result in significant economic costs to society. Any state initiative that is not transparent and evidence-based will be contrary to ethics, regardless of the benefit of the outcome. The end does not justify the means. Hence, the ethics of alcohol taxation are complex and dependent on a solid scientific evidence base. There will always be counter-arguments. Once again, the language and theories of ethics will serve as a useful framework to facilitate transparent debate.

a) Rehm J, Mathers C, Popova S, et al. (2009). Global burden of disease and injury and economic cost attributable to alcohol use and alcohol-use disorders. *Lancet*, **373**, 2223–33.

b) Wagenaar A, Salois M, Komor K. (2009). Effects of beverage alcohol price and tax levels on drinking: a meta-analysis of 1003 estimates from 112 studies. *Addiction*, **104**, 179–90.

c) Walker T. (2010). Why we should not set a minimum price per unit of alcohol. *Public Health Ethics*, **3**, 107–14.

How do ethics assist in policy and practice governing the prevention of unintentionally harmful acts?

Legislation may be used in a number of ways to restrict the autonomy of individuals both for their benefit and for that of wider society. Ethical policy-making requires understanding of the evidence and balance of rational argument, which takes account of the respective ethics principles. For example, legislation requiring car drivers to wear seatbelts is an infringement of individual autonomy and can be viewed as paternalistic in that the state has chosen to intervene on behalf of the citizen, possibly against their wishes. However, this intervention can be justified by the reduction in fatalities and particular forms of injuries suffered by car drivers. As such, it appears that the harms and benefits affect the same people, that is, drivers. However, there are additional benefits to the rest of society in that the reduction in harm to drivers protects others in society, and is also associated with a reduction in healthcare costs to healthcare systems. Thus the restriction of drivers' autonomy can be justified by the principles of utilitarianism.

It is salutary to remember that when the compulsory seatbelt legislation was being debated, there were many opponents who not only saw this as an infringement of civil liberties, but also posed counterarguments, for example, the belief that drivers would be more likely to drive recklessly if they wore seat belts and therefore considered themselves protected.

Responding to changing policy

The model developed in Oxford (Box 1.2.3), England, was driven by the market culture of the mid-1990s, and in particular the contract culture and extra-contractual referrals. The election of a new government in 1997 brought with it changes in political philosophy as well as policy. The mode of choice and decision-making changed. However, with the election of the Coalition government in 2010, emphasis once more shifted to a more libertarian and free market philosophy, enhanced by the current Conservative government in 2017.

Resources are constrained and continually challenged by the advances in medical sciences, the increasing numbers in the elderly population who have growing needs for social as well as healthcare, and also by consumer demand. The role of public health practitioners in supporting decisions about priorities for health and healthcare for a population remains crucial, although mechanisms for providing this support are constantly changing as are health system structures, continuing to pose challenges to creating a forum in which ethical choice is transparent. While Foundation Status for hospital trusts was initially introduced with the promise of greater autonomy from government, planning guidance from NHS England introduced in 2016 puts all trusts under increasingly tight financial control. The effect this will have on limiting the influence local public health practitioners have on decision-making remains to be seen. Coupling this with planned cuts to local authority public health budgets, practitioners may find it even harder to prioritize prevention and advocate for public health and social care interventions over acute services.

Thus some key ethical questions for public health practitioners include:

- How much is local decision-making able to take into account the needs of the population not just for elective healthcare, but for prevention or long-term care?

  What values underline these decisions? For example, it is easier to calculate the cost of a quality-adjusted life year (QALY) for a new drug than for a night-sitting service in palliative care, but which is of greater value to the patient dying of cancer?

- How should one value lifestyle drugs compared with counselling in general practice?

- How can we quantify the value of social prescribing interventions such as exercise on prescription and healthy cookery classes?

Role of public health practitioners and teams

Within health economies and organizations, public health provides the support to take an overview across the community and to balance external needs of local communities. This may involve balancing issues concerning housing, employment, community safety, or domestic violence with needs specific to the health service, such as balancing competing hospital priorities.

The skills of needs assessment, critical appraisal, application of evidence-based care, and management of risk that are key to public health practice are all needed to develop this role.

Whatever changes occur to the structure of the health services, local clinicians will continue to make decisions on a patient-by-patient basis, guided by accepted good practice guidelines. The difficulty of balancing resources can be assisted by clear processes and common clearly expressed ethics values, with the development of appropriate decision-making frameworks within which trade-offs can be made. To do this requires open and mature debate.

References

1 Miké V. (2003). Evidence and the future of medicine. *Evaluation and the Health Professions*, **26**, 127.
2 Beauchamp T, Childress J. (1994). *Principles of biomedical ethics*, 4th edn. Oxford University Press, Oxford.
3 Griffiths S, Jewell T, Hope T. (2006). Setting priorities in health care. In: Pencheon D, Guest C, Melzer D, Muir Gray JA, eds, *Oxford handbook of public health practice*, 2nd edn, pp. 404–10. Oxford University Press, Oxford.
4 Mill J. (1969). Utilitarianism. In: *Collected works of John Stuart Mill*, Vol. 10. University of Toronto Press, Toronto.
5 https://www.gov.uk/government/publications/health-and-social-care-act-2012-fact-sheets
6 https://www.england.nhs.uk/publication/next-steps-on-the-nhs-five-year-forward-view/
7 https://www.england.nhs.uk/nhs-standard-contract/cquin/cquin-17-19/
8 nice.org.uk

Assessing the health of populations

Julian Flowers and Sian Evans

Objectives

Assessing population health is a fundamental element of most public health activity. We cannot improve health and measure success without being able to conduct health assessments. These may be components of, for example:
- measuring burden of disease
- needs assessment
- assessing health equity and health inequality
- resource allocation
- planning
- health impact assessment (HIA)
- service evaluation.

This chapter is intended to identify key principles involved in assessing the health of a defined population rather than individual health status. It should help identify some techniques and approaches that can be applied in practice. Good health assessments require skills in epidemiology and information management and analysis; synthesis of information and opinion from a range of sources; leadership, political and partnership working, and persistence. A successful health assessment should influence decision making—something should change as a result, for example:
- a service should be commissioned
- further work could be undertaken
- a decision to undertake a health policy or programme should be informed.

A typology of health assessments

There are a range of approaches to health assessment depending on the objective. Health assessments often have both quantitative and qualitative elements. They synthesize a range of information and views from a range of sources. A few common approaches are listed below:
- *Health needs assessment* (see Chapter 1.4): starts with a population and identifies key health issues to aid prioritization, development of health programmes, and commissioning of services.
- *HIA* (see Chapter 1.5): starts with a policy or programme and tries to identify and weigh the health benefits or disbenefits, which might accrue. It has been defined as 'a combination of procedures, methods and tools by which a policy, program or project may be judged as to its potential effects on the health of a population, and the distribution of those effects within the population'.[1]
- *Health equity audit*: starts with defined sub-populations and tries to identify health inequalities and inequities of service provision.[2]
- *Health care needs assessment*: starts with a defined population at risk of receiving an intervention and attempts to quantify the number who might benefit and the magnitude of that benefit.
- Other types of health assessment include health economic evaluation, environmental impact assessment, and health technology assessment.

Key steps of health assessment

Health assessment is an iterative process (Figure 1.3.1)

Key steps include:
- Being clear about why you are conducting the assessment, who it is intended for, and what you hope to achieve.
- *Defining your population clearly:* for example, the adult population (aged 18 and over) in such and such area. Patients on general practice register with chronic obstructive pulmonary disease.
- *Population health relative to whom:* assessments usually include a comparative element. The choice of comparator may depend on the audience, for example:
  - a regional health officer may be interested in comparison with other regions and also variation within their region
  - a national policy maker may be more interested in international comparison and a local practitioner may be more interested in peer comparison of similar organizations
  - the choice of comparator can be political, as well as scientific, and may affect acceptance of the assessment.
- *What aspects of health are you considering?* Specificity is generally helpful.
- *Who needs to be involved?* There is often a 'desk-based' element to health assessments which can be done in isolation, but usually assessments are joint efforts and partnership working is important. For example, in England a joint strategic needs assessment (JSNA) process has been introduced (see Box 1.3.1). Working out who you

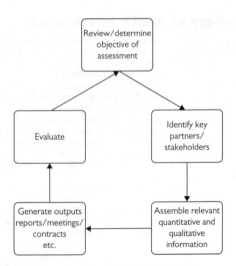

Figure 1.3.1 Health assessment is a cyclical, iterative processes.

Box 1.3.1 Joint strategic needs assessment

JSNA was first introduced as a statutory needs assessment in England in 2007 and was retained under the Health and Social Care Act 2012. The 2012 Act requires local Health and Wellbeing Boards (HWBs), comprising local authorities, Clinical Commissioning Groups, and other local partners, to undertake JSNA as a way of assessing the current and future health and social care needs of the local community. The JSNA should draw together quantitative and qualitative information on health needs and outcomes for the local population, taking into account specific groups or geographical areas. The JSNA are intended to inform local Joint Health and Well-being Strategies (JHWS) which set out the HWBs plans for addressing the health needs identified in the JSNA. There is no template for how JSNA should be carried out, although guidance and data tools are available to support the local analysis required. National guidance highlights the importance of partnership working to produce a rounded view of local health needs. Some areas have adopted innovative ways of presenting the JSNA as a way of engaging local people in the process.[3] A key indicator of the effectiveness of JSNA is the extent to which they inform JHWS. A thematic analysis of a random sample JHWS in 2013–14 showed that most, but not all, used the JSNA to inform strategy.[4]

Further information

Department of Health (2011) Joint Strategic Needs Assessment and joint health and wellbeing strategies explained. @Crown Copyright. Available at: ℳ https://www.gov.uk/government/publications/joint-strategic-needs-assessment-and-joint-health-and-wellbeing-strategies-explained. Accessed January 2020.

Department of Health (2013) Statutory guidance on joint strategic needs assessment and joint health and wellbeing strategies. @Crown Copyright. Available at: ℳ https://www.gov.uk/government/publications/jsnas-and-jhws-statutory-guidance. Accessed January 2020.

need to involve is a key step which will depend on the objective of the assessment. For example, if you are trying to determine key health priorities for a community, it will be important to involve key informants or the public directly through surveys or focus groups. If the assessment relates to a health care intervention, clinicians, and patient representative groups maybe important.

- *Perspectives on health:* professionals, the public and their representatives, and policy makers often have different perspectives on health and health priorities.

- *Identify and assemble data, facts, and other information:* can you use what is routinely available or do you need to collect data especially for the assessment?
- *Appraise and synthesis the information gathered:* do you understand the reasons for any differences between your population and the comparator? Could the differences between due to chance or differences in how the data were collected, or do they represent real differences in health status?
- How will you communicate the results of your assessment?
- How will you evaluate success?

Assembling relevant information

The essence of all assessment is to:
- assemble relevant information on a particular issue
- determine if there is a problem and if so the priority and magnitude of that problem(s)

and
- determine what (if anything) to do about it.

Some general principles for assembling data

- *Be systematic:* there is usually more than one source of data or potential set of health indicators (summary measures of health)
- *Have a framework:* the data needed for the assessment may vary according to whether the assessment is focusing on people with particular disease or health condition or is a broader assessment of the health needs of a community or population group. Common groups of data are shown in Table 1.3.1. Not all of these data will be available to inform, or be applicable to, all health assessments.
- *Consider time, place, person:* a useful approach for most health assessments is to consider how the data vary with time, between different population groups, or between geographical areas.
- *Consider health inequalities:* health status measures may differ between subsections of populations such as ethnic or racial groups, socioeconomic groups, or age and sex. Some vulnerable groups may have greater or differing needs to others in the population.

Frameworks such as the Dahlgren and Whitehead model[5] and the life course approach of the Fair Society, Healthy Lives report on inequalities in health (the Marmot Review) can be used to help with indicator identification and grouping.[6]

Table 1.3.1 Typical types of data to consider when assembling data for a population health assessment

Domains	Examples of data or indicators
Population	Current population, age and sex, ethnicity, birth rate, projected future population size
Socioeconomic factors	Income, social class, deprivation
Behavioural risk factors / wider determinants of health	Smoking status, alcohol use, housing, employment, transport
Burden of disease	Disease prevalence and incidence from registers or surveys
Service use: Community Primary, Secondary, Tertiary health care, social care	General Practice appointments, prescribed medications, Accident and Emergency attendance, emergency or planned admissions
Summary measures of population health	Life expectancy and healthy life expectancy
Broad health status or quality of life	Patient reported outcomes, surveys of quality of life, days missed from school or work
Mortality	Age standardised death rates by cause, premature mortality, place of death

Measuring health status and summary measures of population health

Health is difficult to measure directly: we often therefore make inferences about population health status from other metrics such as mortality and morbidity. There is good evidence that asking people to rate their health on a simple scale from excellent to bad is predictive of mortality and health services utilization.[7, 8]

Increasingly, measures of health or disability are being combined with life expectancy to produce summary measures of population health. There are two variants:

• health expectancies
• health gaps.

Figure 1.3.2 attempts to illustrate this. It shows population survivorship against age. The overall area of the figure illustrates an idealized lifespan of 100 years lived in perfect health until a sudden death at age 100.

Curve C represents actual survivorship, and curve A that which is lived in good health. Area A represents a measure of health expectancy, whereas area B, which is the difference between idealized and actual health, is a health gap.

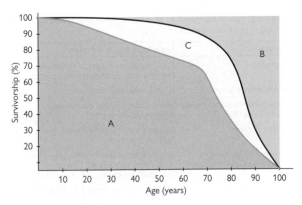

Figure 1.3.2 Summary measures of population health.[9]

Examples of each in routine use include:
- *Health expectances:* healthy life expectancy, disability-free life expectancy, health active life expectancy.
- *Health gaps:* years of life lost, disability-adjusted life years (DALYs), healthy life years.

While these measures have a strong appeal in assessing health, they have several drawbacks:
- *Availability of data:* all these measures rely on some population estimates of health or disability which can be difficult to obtain, particularly subnationally. DALYs rely on estimates of disease prevalence and duration and severity of disability which are rarely available.
- *Uses:* although in countries with well-developed systems for monitoring mortality it may be possible to monitor death rates and life expectancy, lack of systematic measurement of relevant morbidity measures reduces the usefulness of summary measures of public health in monitoring health over time although they are useful in comparative health assessment.
- Complexity of calculation.
- Reliability of self-reported health status.

Estimating future health status

Despite caveats, using the Global Burden of Disease (GBD) framework is now an essential step in population health assessments. It provides a comprehensive, comparative assessment framework.[10]

The GBD programme now provides burden of disease estimates as summarized by DALYs for a wide range of diseases and risks at country and in some cases subnational level. For England, for example, data is available at NUTS 3 level and for populations stratified by a measure of socio-economic disadvantage (quantiles of the score of the Index of Multiple Deprivation).

The GBD data are publicly available and can be obtained and viewed at https://vizhub.healthdata.org/gbd-compare/.

Sources of data

There is a wealth of data available for population health assessments. One of the challenges for today's public health practitioner is being able to navigate the wide range of population health data available and identify the data sources of most relevance to the population or health issue under investigation. Data is published for a range of issues and geographies. Increasingly, sophisticated online data tools are being developed, which incorporate statistical analysis and data visualization with the intention of making it easier to access and interpret health data.

Useful data sources include:

- *Global:* country wide from WHO, Gapminder, GBD
- *European:* WHO European Health Information Gateway; EUROSTAT
- *National*: government bodies, national data repositories, and health observatories
- *Local*: local government or administrative bodies, local health observatories.

Although there is a considerable range of health data routinely available, there may be a need for dedicated data collection if routine data sources do not address the population or issue being assessed. There may also be a need to consider bespoke data analysis if data is routinely collected but not routinely analysed and published for the desired population subgroup, geography or time period. Bespoke data collection and analysis has the advantage of greater control over the quality and type of data collected but is time-consuming and can be resource intensive.

There will be occasions when no routine data are available and bespoke data collection or analysis is not feasible. In these circumstances, it may be possible to make inferences using data from other populations, for example, a national average or estimates from the published scientific literature. Sociodemographic data on how the assessment population compares to elsewhere will help in assessing the validity of such estimates. Other options include using proxy measures, for example, contacts with health services in place of the population prevalence of a health disorder; or drawing on expert opinion.

The data cube and diagram in Figure 1.3.3 provide a useful framework for thinking about the kinds of data that can be helpful.

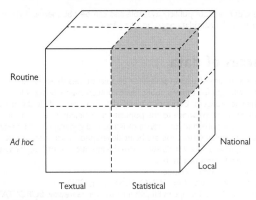

Figure 1.3.3 The data cube (after Stevens and Gillam, 1998).[11]

Selecting data

With a plethora of data and limited resources for conducting assessments, it is important to select data and indicators that provide useful insight on the health status of the population. Guidance is available to help assess the value and quality of health indicators,[12] although some of the evaluation criteria may be of more use to those developing and publishing indicators. A key place to look when reviewing health indicators is the data definition or 'metadata' (literally 'data about data'). This should provide information on:

• why the indicator was created and what it is intended to measure
• which data sources were used
• the method used to create the indicator
• any statistical tests that have been applied
• issues with the underlying data quality.

The GATHER guidelines provide a useful checklist to help evaluate the quality of a dataset or indicator.[12]

Understanding how an indicator was created is important when interpreting what it tells us about a population. Changes over time or differences to comparators may indicate true differences in the health of the population but could also be due to chance or to changes or differences in methods of data collection and coding.

It is also important to consider the range and type of health data and indicators used to describe the population's health. Ultimately, what matters most to people is the outcome of a policy, programme, or intervention. Health outcomes might be a change in people's perception of their own health, an increase in the number of people who take regular exercise or a reduction in the number of people requiring emergency admission to hospital. However, as population health outcomes are influenced by a range of factors, it can be difficult to assign a change in health outcome to a particular intervention or policy. Using measures of health processes as well as outcome make it easier to monitor the impact of services on population health. For example, the proportion of pregnant women who smoke is an important measure of maternal and child health. Monitoring the number of women who were smokers in early pregnancy, the proportion who were referred to smoking cessation services, and the proportion who had stopped smoking by the time of delivery provides a richer insight on the impact of services on the health status of pregnant women.

Presenting data

Health assessments should lead to change by informing subsequent action to address the health issues identified. The results of the assessment should be presented to decision-makers in an accessible format. Weighty reports full of dense, technical data outputs risk having limited impact. Videos of the much missed Hans Rosling from the Gapminder Foundation are an excellent demonstration of how to tell the story behind the data to ensure that health data makes an impact (https://www.gapminder.org/).

Methods of visualizing data are continually improving, making it easier to present relatively large amounts of data in accessible summary formats. For example, Figure 1.3.4 shows a 'spine chart', originally developed by the former Public Health Observatories and now widely used in a range of health profiles throughout the United Kingdom. These present health indicators in 'spine chart' format that compares for an area, each indicator against the national average. It also scales and shows the overall distribution of each indicator and includes a measure of statistical significance represented by the colour of the 'blobs', which show the indicator value for that area. In this example (Figure 1.3.4), we show an area with a range of health problems relating to child health (relative to England)—including more children in low income families and higher family homelessness, lower levels of educational attainment, higher rates of infant and child mortality, and higher levels of obesity and dental decay.

There is also a growing awareness of, and evidence base for, the use of knowledge translation approaches which attempt to bridge the 'know-do gap' between evidence and policy[13]. Knowledge translation approaches stress the importance of understanding and addressing decision-makers' needs. Social marketing techniques which use segmentation to match the communication methods and channels with the audience can help to ensure that evidence is presented in a way that decision-makers find compelling.

Figure 1.3.4 A spine chart presentation of a population health profile.[14]

Domain	Indicator	Local No Per Year	Local Value	Eng Avg	Eng Worst	England Range	Eng Best
Our communities	1 Deprivation	37812	23.2	19.9	89.2		0.0
	2 Children in poverty	9267	27.1	22.4	66.5		6.0
	3 Statutory homelessness	413	5.93	2.48	9.84		0.00
	4 GCSE achieved (5A*-C inc.Eng & Maths)	929	40.6	50.9	32.1		76.1
	5 Violent crime	3576	29	16.4	36.6		4.8
	6 Carbon emissions	1316	8.1	6.8	14.4		4.1
Children's and young people's health	7 Smoking in pregnancy	434	15.7	14.6	33.5		3.8
	8 Breast feeding initiation	1980	71.6	72.5	39.7		92.7
	9 Physically active children	15767	58.4	49.6	24.6		79.1
	10 Obese children	199	9.2	9.6	14.7		4.7
	11 Tooth decay in children aged 5 years	n/a	1.6	1.1	2.5		0.2
	12 Teenage pregnancy (under 18)	171	53.0	40.9	74.8		14.9
Adult's health and lifestyle	13 Adults who smoke	n/a	27.0	22.2	35.2		10.2
	14 Binge drinking adults	n/a	19.7	20.1	33.2		4.6
	15 Healthy eating adults	n/a	30.0	28.7	18.3		48.1
	16 Physically active adults	n/a	8.3	11.2	5.4		16.6
	17 Obese adults	n/a	24.1	24.2	32.8		13.2
Disease and poor health	18 Incidence of malignant melanoma	17	10.8	12.6	27.3		3.7
	19 Incapacity benefits for mental illness	2800	27.5	27.6	58.5		9.0
	20 Hospital stays for alcohol related ham	3502	1970	1580	2860		784
	21 Drug misuse						
	22 People diagnosed with diabetes	7115	4.34	4.30	6.72		2.69
	23 New cases of tuberculosis	37	23	15	110		0
	24 Hip fracture in over-65s	156	517.7	479.2	843.		273.6
Life expectancy and causes of death	25 Excess winter deaths	82	18.4	15.6	26.3		2.3
	26 Life expectancy - male	n/a	76.8	77.9	73.6		84.3
	27 Life expectancy - female	n/a	81.0	82.0	78.8		88.9
	28 Infant deaths	15	5.26	4.84	8.67		1.08
	29 Deaths from smoking	232	218.5	206.8	360.3		118.7
	30 Early deaths: heart disease & stroke	144	89.9	74.8	125.0		40.1
	31 Early deaths: cancer	176	110.2	114.0	164.3		70.5
	30 Road injuries and deaths	103	63.1	51.3	167.0		14.6

Legend:
- Significantly worse than England average
- Not significantly different from England average
- Significantly better than England average
- No significance can be calculated

England Worst — Regional average+ — England Average — England Best — 25th Percentile — 75th Percentile

+In the South East Region this represents the Strategic Health Authority average

Data sharing, open data, and transparency

Organizations that use data from an individual have responsibilities or duties both to protect confidentiality, and to publish and share results and outputs of that data, provided it does not breach individual confidence.

In England, a 2013 review led by Dame Fiona Caldicott established seven key principles for how data about patients should be handled (see Box 1.3.2).[15] Improving the way we share information should support future assessments of population health. A complete picture of population health is likely to require data from a range of organizations. Safe sharing of information will also allow linkage of records to provide a much richer picture of population health.

Box 1.3.2 Caldicott Principles revised 2013[9]
- Justify the purpose(s) for using confidential information
- Don't use personal confidential data unless it is absolutely necessary
- Use the minimum necessary personal confidential data
- Access to personal confidential data should be on a strict need-to-know basis
- Everyone with access to personal confidential data should be aware of their responsibilities
- Comply with the law
- The duty to share information can be as important as the duty to protect patient confidentiality.

Further resources

Pencheon D. (2008). The Good Indicators Guide: understanding how to use and choose indicators. Available at: ℘ https://fingertips.phe.org.uk/profile/guidance. Accessed January 2020

Public Health England. Health Equity. Available at: ℘ https://www.gov.uk/government/collections/health-equity. Accessed January 2020

WHO Health Equity Assessment Toolkit. Available at: ℘ https://www.who.int/gho/health_equity/assessment_toolkit/en/. Accessed January 2020

WHO. Health Impact Assessment. Available at: ℘ https://www.who.int/hia/en/. Accessed January 2020

Data sources

European Commission Statistical Office EUROSTAT. Available at: https://ec.europa.eu/eurostat/web/main/home. Accessed January 2020

Gapminder Foundation. Gapmider: Available at: www.gapminder.com. Accessed January 2020

Institute of Health Metrics and Evaluation (IHME), University of Washington. Global Health Data Exchange. Available at: ℘ http://ghdx.healthdata.org/. Accessed January 2020

OECD. OECD data. Available at: ℘ https://data.oecd.org/. Accessed January 2020

Public Health England. Public Health Profiles. © Crown copyright 2020. Available at: ℘ https://fingertips.phe.org.uk. Accessed January 2020

United Nations Statistics Available at: ℘ https://unstats.un.org/home/. Accessed January 2020.

WHO European Health Information Gateway. Available at: ℘ https://gateway.euro.who.int/en/. Accessed January 2020

WHO Health Statistics and Information Systems. Available at: ℘ https://www.who.int/healthinfo/en/. Accessed January 2020

References

1 Mindell J. (2003). A glossary for health impact assessment Journal of Epidemiology Community Health, 57(9), 647–51. Available at: ℘ https://jech.bmj.com/content/57/9/647. Accessed January 2020.

2 WHO Health Equity Impact Assessment. Available at: ℘ http://www.euro.who.int/en/health-topics/health-determinants/social-determinants/activities/putting-a-social-determinants-of-health-focus-into-public-health/health-equity-impact-assessment. Accessed January 2020.

3 Healthy Suffolk, Suffolk Public Health. Joint Strategic Needs Assessment @Suffolk County Council 2020 Available at: ℘ https://www.healthysuffolk.org.uk/JSNA Accessed January 2020.

4 Beenstock J et al (2014). Are health and well-being strategies in England fit for purpose? A thematic content analysis. J Public Health (Oxf). 2015 Sep;37(3):461-9. Available at: ℘ https://academic.oup.com/jpubhealth/article/37/3/461/2362725. Accessed January 2020.

5 Dahlgren, G & Whitehead M (2007) Policies and strategies to promote social equity in health Background document to WHO—Strategy paper for Europe. Institute for Future Studies. Available at: ℘ https://core.ac.uk/download/pdf/6472456.pdf Accessed January 2020.

6 Marmot M et al Fair Society, Healthy Lives (The Marmot Review) Strategic Review of Health inequalities in England post-2010. The Marmot Review. Available at ℘ http://www.instituteofhealthequity.org/resources-reports/fair-society-healthy-lives-the-marmot-review Accessed January 2020.

7 Kyffin RGE, Goldacre MJ, Gill M. (2004). Mortality rates and self reported health: database analysis by English local authority area. British Medical Journal, 329, 887–8.

8 Miilunpalo S, Vuori I, Oja P, Pasanen M, Urponen H. (1997). Self-rated health status as a health measure: the predictive value of self-reported health status on the use of physician services and on mortality in the working-age population. Journal of Clinical Epidemiology, 50, 517–28. Available at: ℘ https://www.jclinepi.com/article/S0895-4356(97)00045-0/fulltext Accessed January 2020.

9 Murray, CJL, Salomon JA, and Mathers C Chapter 1.2 A critical examination of summary measures of population health. In: Murray, Christoper J.L, Salomon, Joshua A, Mathers, Colin D, Lopex, Alan & World Health Organisation (2002). Summary measures of population health: concepts, ethics, measurement and applications. Edited by Christopher J.L, Murray....[et al]. World Health Organisation. Available at: ℘ https://apps.who.int/iris/handle/10665/42439 Accessed January 2020.

10 Global Burden of Disease, The Lancet Available at: ℘ https://www.thelancet.com/gbd Accessed January 2020.

11 Stevens A, Gillam S. (1998). Needs assessment: from theory to practice, BMJ series 3 316: 1448–51. Available at: ℘ http://www.bmj.com/content/316/7142/1448 Accessed January 2020.

12 Guidelines for Accurate and Transparent Health Reporting (GATHER). Available at: ℘ http://gather-statement.org/ Accessed January 2020.

13 Bennet G and Jessani N (2001) The knowledge translation toolkit. Sage Publications India Pvt Ltd. Available at: ℘ https://idl-bnc-idrc.dspacedirect.org/bitstream/handle/10625/46152/IDL-46152.pdf?sequence=1&isAllowed=y Accessed January 2020.

14 Public Health England Child and Maternal Health Profiles Public Health Profiles. © Crown copyright 2020. Available at: ℘ https://fingertips.phe.org.uk. Accessed January 2020.

15 National Data Guardian (2013) Information: To share or not to share? The Information Governance Review. Produced by William Lea for the Department of Health Available at: ℘ https://www.gov.uk/government/publications/the-information-governance-review Accessed January 2020

Assessing health needs

Andrew O'Shaughnessy, John Wright, and Ben Cave

Objectives

HNA (health needs assessment) is a systematic method of identifying the unmet health and healthcare needs of a population and recommending changes to meet these unmet needs. It is used to improve health and other service planning, priority setting, and policy development. HNA is an example of public health working outside the formal health sector and presenting back to colleagues. Successful HNAs will also ensure that non-health agencies benefit from their findings.

This chapter will describe why HNA is important and what it means in practice. Professional training and clinical experience teach that a health professional must systematically assess a patient before administering any treatment that is believed to be effective. This systematic approach is often omitted when assessing the health needs of populations.

Box 1.4.1 shows what can happen when an HNA is conducted systematically—both health outcome and service delivery were improved.

Box 1.4.1 Tuberculosis service in a rural African hospital[a]

- *Setting:* a rural district hospital in South Africa.
- *Problem:* increasing overcrowding in the hospital due to the rising incidence of tuberculosis (TB) resulting from human immunodeficiency virus (HIV)/acquired immune deficiency syndrome (AIDS). Concerns by staff about high levels of treatment failure.
- *Methods:* review of TB register information on detection rates and outcomes. Review of current clinical practices. Interviews with health professional and patients to determine views of TB care.
- *Results:* case detection rate of TB had increased by 90% over a period of four years. Patients were admitted to hospital for the 2-month intensive phase of treatment creating major problems of overcrowding. Haphazard follow-up in any local clinic led to poor data on outcomes. Outcome data indicated that only 27% ($n = 66$) of patients were cured or completed treatment and 43% ($n = 160$) were lost to follow-up. Major gaps in patients' understanding about TB and its relationship to HIV/AIDS were identified.
- *Action:* new guidelines were developed for the region to allow home-based treatment. A community-based treatment service was established using village health workers to support treatment in patients' own homes. An outreach team was set up to coordinate care, promote community awareness, and train and support village and clinic health workers. Within 12 months, care and completion rates had improved to 86% with patients having to stay for days, rather than months in hospital.

a) Wright J, Walley J, Philip A, et al. (2004). Direct observation for tuberculosis: a randomised controlled trial of community health workers versus family members. Tropical Medicine & International Health, 9, 559–65.

Defining need

Need, in the sense used in this chapter, implies the capacity to benefit from an intervention. 'To speak of a need is to imply a goal, a measurable deficiency from the goal and a means of achieving the goal.'[1]

HNA is *not* the same as population health status assessment (see ⊃ Chapter 1.3). HNA incorporates the concept of a capacity to benefit from an intervention. It therefore introduces an assessment of the effectiveness of relevant interventions to supplement the identification of health problems. Thus, the researcher does not start with a blank sheet but with a theory to test or a technology to apply—HNA is not a value-free examination of a population, but starts from a specific point. HNA should also make explicit what benefits are being pursued by identifying particular interventions.

The capacity to benefit is always greater than available resources and so HNA should incorporate questions of priority setting through considering the cost-effectiveness of the available interventions (see ⊃ Chapters 1.2 and 1.6).[2]

Thus, at different times, HNA is used to define:

- the goal (improved health outcomes and improved health equity)
- the deficiency (poor health outcomes, inequities in health)
- the means of achieving the goal (effective intervention).

Approaches to needs assessment

A number of approaches to needs assessment have been suggested,[3] including:

- *'Epidemiologically based'*: combining epidemiological approaches (specific health status assessments) with assessment of the effectiveness and possibly the cost-effectiveness of the potential interventions
- *Comparative*: comparing levels of service receipt between different populations
- *Corporate*: canvassing the demands and wishes of professionals, patients, politicians, and other interested parties.

In this chapter, an epidemiological approach to determining priorities is explored. This incorporates clinical effectiveness, cost-effectiveness, and patients' perspectives.[4] It incorporates qualitative and quantitative information. While comparisons of health service usage are commonly used as indicators of need, population-based usage rates typically vary markedly between areas, often for unexplained reasons. In addition, the link between usage rates and improved health outcomes is often hard to demonstrate.

The distinction between individual needs and community needs is important to consider. Some needs will be shared across communities, while others will be specific to smaller subsets or to individuals. HNA should be sensitive to these differences.

HNA involves the active, explicit, and systematic identification of needs, rather than a passive, ad hoc, implicit response to demand. The assessment of health needs can be clarified by differentiating between needs, demands, and supply (see Box 1.4.2) and by remembering that health needs are not

Box 1.4.2 Different aspects of health needs[a]

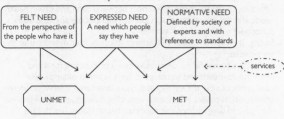

This figure does not engage with the relationship between the different types of need. A need is shown as a claim for service.

Health and social care services cater for normative needs. By definition, they do not cater for unmet normative needs. Health needs assessment (HNA) should ensure that normative needs, met and unmet, are catered for. The HNA process should ensure that normative needs adequately reflect felt and expressed needs, and the best scientific evidence.

a) Definitions of need are adapted from Spicker P. *Social need*. Available at: ℜ www2.rgu.ac.uk/publicpolicy/introduction/needf.htm (accessed 30 July 2019).

necessarily restricted to healthcare needs. Ideally, HNA will identify both met and unmet need. Health needs include wider social and environmental determinants of health, such as deprivation, housing, diet, education, and employment. Health needs should ideally be appropriately addressed ('met'), but these needs are too often unmet (e.g. poor housing, poor access to primary care, health illiteracy, undiagnosed hypertension, ignored moderate depression) or 'over met' (e.g. prescribing antibiotics for sore throats).

HNA provides the opportunity for:

- profiling/examining the population's health status, and describing the patterns of disease in the local population and the differences from district, regional, or national disease patterns
- learning more about the needs and priorities of patients, and the local population
- highlighting areas of unmet need and providing a clear set of objectives to work towards meeting these needs
- deciding rationally how to use resources to improve the health of the local population in the most effective and efficient way
- influencing policy, interagency collaboration, or research and development priorities.

Importantly, it also provides a method of monitoring and promoting equity in the provision and use of health services and addressing inequalities in health (see Box 1.4.3 for the case of addressing the health needs of older people after an earthquake and Box 1.4.4 for the case of health services needs assessment among patients with coronary heart disease).[5]

Box 1.4.3 Health needs of older people after earthquake[a]

- *Objective:* to compare the differences between rural and urban health needs and the utilization of services of older people after the 2005 (October) earthquake in Kashmir.
- *Setting:* the Neelum Valley of Kashmir, Pakistan, four months after the earthquake.
- *Methods:* a comparative, descriptive study to examine rural and urban health needs and to compare ways in which older people used services after the earthquake. Semi-structured interviews were conducted to collect information regarding demographic background, medical and drug history, self-reported health status, health care access and utilization, and social/financial concerns. Clinical records were reviewed. Physical indicators for older patients also were collected on site.
- *Results:* the health profile, access to healthcare, service availability, and prevalence of non-communicable diseases were found to differ between urban and rural settings. The greatest gap, at all sites, was that non-communicable disease management was inadequate during non-acute, post-earthquake medical care. Health service utilization varied by gender: in conservative rural areas, older, traditional women were less likely to receive medical services while older, traditional men were less likely to access psychological services in all sites.
- *Conclusion:* findings highlight specific health needs and issues related to long-term, chronic disease management. It is important to strengthen capacity to respond appropriately to medical disasters, which includes preparedness for treating the health needs of older people.[7]

a) Chan EY, Griffiths S. (2009). Comparison of health needs of older people between affected rural and urban areas after the 2005 Kashmir, Pakistan earthquake. Prehospital and Disaster Medicine, 24, 365–71.

Box 1.4.4 Epidemiologic health needs assessment—coronary heart disease[a, b]

- *Objective:* to assess whether the use of health services by people with coronary heart disease reflected need.
- *Setting:* a health district in the UK with a population of 530,000.
- *Methods:* the prevalence of angina was determined by a validated postal questionnaire. Routine health data was collected on standardized mortality ratios, admission rates for coronary heart disease, and operation rates for angiography, angioplasty, and coronary heart disease. Census data was used to calculate Townsend scores to describe deprivation for electoral wards. The prevalence of angina and use of services were then compared with deprivation scores for each ward.
- *Results:* angina and mortality from heart disease were more common in wards with high deprivation scores. However, treatment by revascularization procedures was more common in more affluent wards that had low deprivation scores.
- *Conclusion:* the use of revascularization services was not commensurate with need. Steps should be taken to ensure that health care is targeted to those who most need it.

a) Jacobson B. (2002). Delaying tactics. Health Service Journal, 112, 22.

b) Payne N, Saul C. (1997). Variations in use of cardiology services in a health authority: comparison of coronary artery revascularisation rates with prevalence of angina and coronary mortality. British Medical Journal, 314, 256–61.

A framework for assessing the health needs of a population

Box 1.4.5 summarizes the questions or steps involved in a formal HNA process. This seldom follows a simple linear progression through the steps—needs assessments often develop from several steps concurrently. HNA can be approached in much the same way as doing a jigsaw, so that different pieces are put together to give a full picture of local health requirements and potential interventions.

Needs assessment requires careful preparation

Undertaking needs assessment involves identifying the right issue, using the right technical methods, and managing the process effectively. Start with attention to defining the problem. Objectives should be clarified, and as simple and focused as possible. Care should be taken not to raise unrealistic expectations. The right team should be convened, with all relevant stakeholders, including (as relevant to the issue) the service funders, the clinicians, and the users (public involvement) (see ➲ Chapters 3.4 and 6.6).

> **Box 1.4.5 Questions to be answered in a formal HNA process**
>
> - *What is the problem?* Identify the health problem to be addressed in the defined population.
> - *What is the size and nature of the problem?* Carry out a health status assessment for the population, covering the relevant areas of ill health and/or potential health gain.
> - *What are the current services?* Identify the existing services and interventions being delivered, focusing where relevant on quality, effectiveness, and efficiency.
> - *What interventions do patients, professionals and other stakeholders want?* Consult with these groups.
> - *What interventions does scientific knowledge recommend?* Identify interventions by reviewing the scientific knowledge. What are the most appropriate and cost-effective solutions? Find and appraise.
> - *What are the resource implications?* Choose between competing ways of meeting needs (competing interventions) and decide on competing priorities—resources are always limited.
> - *What are the recommendations and the plan for implementation?* What agencies need to take action and by when?
> - *Is assessing need likely to lead to appropriate change?* Identify expected health gains and how the effect of subsequent actions can be monitored.

Leadership is important (see ➲ Chapter 6.1), as is clear and effective communication during the process, especially if there is multi-agency involvement. Access to relevant information and informants should be sought at an early stage.

What is the health problem?

The focus of the needs assessment exercise should be clearly identified. A health problem may come to attention from many sources, including the results of a population health status assessment, input from patients or stakeholders, government priority setting, or the scientific and professional literature.

An initial clarification of the issues can be valuable. A first step in clarifying the definition of the problem is a search of the health and social science databases for the topic. A review of the published health literature will provide a national and international perspective about the health topic, and methods and results (e.g. case definitions, disease incidence and prevalence, current provision of health services) that may be applicable to the local population.[3, 5] When access to journals is limited, then search engines such as PubMed, Google, and Google Scholar can provide useful evidence. A search of grey literature sources (e.g. public health professional bodies and government health department databases) can provide models and information.

After initial clarification, it should become apparent whether the problem justifies a full and systematic needs assessment.

What is the size and nature of the problem?

With a working definition of the health problems in mind, relevant health status data can then be collected. This should aim to establish:

- the number of people in the studied population who are likely to be suffering from the target condition or conditions
- their characteristics
- the extent to which they are already receiving appropriate interventions.

Accurately estimating how many people would benefit from each of the potential interventions is desirable but often difficult. Graham[6] challenges public health to look to the future: populations and health needs change, especially in the context of a changing climate, whereas health status data is usually historical. HNAs should identify a timescale. Previous chapters provide a guide to sources of information.

What are the current services?

There are several sources of data on healthcare in a locality. Hospital activity data can provide information on hospital admissions, diagnoses, length of stay, operations performed, and patient characteristics. Clinical indicators can provide information on the comparative performance of hospitals and health authorities.

Health care provision (e.g. numbers of family doctors per capita, number of operations per capita) is often compared with national or international norms, although there is rarely evidence of a link between provision and health outcome.

What do professionals, patients, and other stakeholders want?

Consult a wide range of stakeholders to describe local health needs. Local health professionals in primary and secondary care will have valuable contributions to make about the health needs of their local community. Other stakeholders, such as health authorities, local government agencies, and voluntary groups are also important contributors, not only for their knowledge and beliefs, but also so as to engage them in the assessment, and encourage ownership and eventual implementation of the results.

Consult users, carers, and the public (see ➜ Chapters 3.4 and 6.6). Historically, health services have been weak at involving users and the public in decision making about local health care. Best practice now recognizes the importance of obtaining greater public involvement: various methods for ensuring public input to health service planning are summarized below.[7]

- *Citizens' juries*: local people, representative of the population, who are selected to sit on a jury for a specified period of time. Members are presented with information from different experts on health topics and debate the issues surrounding them.
- *Health panels*: standing panels of local people representative of the population. These can be large (more than 1,000 people) panels, which are surveyed at regular intervals about key health issues, or smaller panels where the members meet and discuss different topics. Members are replaced at regular intervals.

- *Focus groups*: groups of 6–12 participants with a facilitator who encourages discussion about health topics, which is recorded on tape or by an observer.
- *Interviews*: interviews with randomly or purposefully selected individuals to canvass their views and opinions. Users, carers, or other stakeholders (e.g. community leaders) can all be valuable contributors.
- *Questionnaires*: these allow structured information to be collected from a large sample of local people on one or more health topics. Such surveys can provide information on user satisfaction, perceived needs, and use of health services. Other generic health measures such as quality of life scores,[8] or disease-specific measures can also be included.
- *Specific planning methodologies*: for example, meta-planning, 'Planning for Real', 'open space' events. These are all approaches to planning that use specific techniques to promote the involvement of local communities and stakeholders.

What are the most appropriate and cost-effective interventions?

An essential part of an HNA is the review of the clinical effectiveness and cost-effectiveness of interventions that can address the identified health needs. Evidence about the effectiveness of health interventions or services can be found in databases of good-quality systematic reviews such as the Cochrane Library,[9] or publications such as the *Effective Health Care Bulletins*.[10] The United States' Agency for Healthcare Research and Quality[11] and the UK's National Institute for Health and Care Excellence[12] can also be good sources of information on effectiveness and on professional consensus on treatment. When there is limited evidence of effectiveness of interventions, then professional consensus about best practice may have to be relied on.

What are the resource implications?

Economic appraisal, including cost-effectiveness, should be considered if health needs are to be met optimally with limited resources. At a practical level this involves:[13]

- determining how resources are currently spent (programme budgeting—see ➌ Chapter 7.2)
- defining options for change (marginal analysis) by specifying alternatives:
  - (a) Identify potential services requiring additional resources.
  - (b) Identify services that could be provided at the same level of effectiveness, but at reduced cost, releasing resources for (a).
  - (c) Identify services that are less cost-effective than those identified in (a).
- assessing the costs and benefits of the principal options
- decide on the best option, aiming to increase investment in (a) and reduce investment in services identified in (b) and (c).

The third example in this chapter (see Box 1.4.6) shows how the needs assessment process can help plan services, using generalizable research and local surveys involving users.

Box 1.4.6 Health needs assessment in an English prison[a]

- *Objective:* to quantify the need for alcohol interventions in a prison population and to make recommendations.
- *Setting:* a large prison in the south of England.
- *Methods:* epidemiological data from national prison surveys was applied to the prison population, taking into account age, gender, ethnicity, and sentence/remand status. Expected incidence and prevalence of alcohol problems were compared with data from prison records of alcohol interventions. Semi-structured interviews were carried out with a sample of prison staff, service providers, and some prisoners. Information on national policy, the impact of alcohol and evidence of effectiveness was also used to highlight issues for attention.
- *Results:* dependent drinkers were very likely to be identified and treated appropriately. However, there were substantial gaps in services for people with less severe problems (particularly identification and brief advice as recommended nationally). Alcohol services provided relatively little monitoring data and there were questions about the value for money of some interventions. Recommendations for improvement were made.
- *Conclusion:* prison staff were keen to make improvements and recognized that, despite the damage it causes, alcohol misuse receives little attention when compared with drug services. The project helped to quantify service requirements and opened a dialogue about the re-alignment of alcohol services.

a) Brotherton P, Withers M. (2010). Health needs assessment in an English prison. Unpublished case study prepared for Oxford University Press.

Implementation

The information collected in the needs assessment must be clearly collated, analysed, and presented. This will usually be in a written report. A summary of key findings is useful in communicating the results to the decision makers and those who will be affected by the decisions.

Reporting the results, however, is not the end of the process. The HNA should develop a plan for action. Building agreement to a practical implementation plan for meeting the unmet needs is an essential part of needs assessment.

Does assessing need create change?

Factors that will increase the likelihood of needs assessment leading to change are:

- consideration of the potential resource implications of the assessment from the beginning (discussion between commissioners and assessors)
- methodological rigour to ensure that the results are valid and believed
- ownership of the project by relevant stakeholders from the start and effective involvement during the work
- effective dissemination of the results (see ➲ Chapters 6.4 and 6.5) and the existence of a practical plan for implementing the necessary actions to partly or fully meet the identified unmet needs.

HNA starts from the health of a defined population and results in proposals (for policy, programmes, strategy, plans, or other developments). Health impact assessments (HIAs) (see ➲ Chapter 1.5) start from proposals and compare how they may affect population health and health inequity. Table 1.4.1 shows the similarities between these two approaches. HNAs can be useful inputs to HIAs.

Table 1.4.1 Comparison of HNA with HIA

	HNA	HIA
Starting point	Population	Proposal (policy, plan, programme or project) within or outside the health sector
Primary output	Inform decisions about strategies, service priorities, commissioning, and local delivery plans, and inform future HIAs	Recommendations to maximize beneficial, and minimize adverse, effects on health; these are made with reference to a specific proposal and are made to inform decision making
Does each approach take account of inequalities and aim to improve health?	Yes: describe health needs and health assets of different groups in local population	Yes: identify how proposals may affect the most vulnerable groups in population
Involve stakeholders	Ideally (dependent on resources)	Ideally (dependent on resources)
Involve sectors outside health sector	Sometime	Always
Based on determinants of health	Sometime	Always
Use best available evidence	Always	Always

Conclusion

HNAs should, ideally, be an expression and analysis of community need. Care should be taken over the dissemination and storage of these reports. They will contain valuable information about local communities and so confidentiality may be an issue. They will also be of great use to local communities and to other services, and so the results should be shared. It must also be acknowledged that health needs are not static: assessments provide snapshots of the needs of the local population. Health needs, and the health and social care services that try to address them, are always changing. It is important to ensure that the assessment work is reviewed and updated and that service delivery is in line with current and projected health needs for all groups and individuals within any given community.

Further resources

Hooper J, Longworth P. (2002). *Health needs assessment workbook*, Health Development Agency, London.

Murray SA. (1999). Experiences with 'rapid appraisal' in primary care: involving the public in assessing health needs, orientating staff, and educating medical students. *British Medical Journal*, **3**, 440–4.

National Health Service Management Executive (1991). *Assessing health care need*. Department of Health, London.

Wright J. (1998). *Health needs assessment in practice*. BMJ Books, London.

References

1 Wilkin D, Hallam L, Dogget M. (1992). *Measures of need and outcomes in primary health care*. Oxford Medical Publications, Oxford.

2 Donaldson C, Mooney G. (1991). Needs assessment, priority setting, and contracts for healthcare: an economic view. *British Medical Journal*, **303**, 1529–30.

3 Stevens A, Raftery J. (eds). (1997). *Health care needs assessment*, series 2. Radcliffe Medical Press, Oxford.

4 Wright J, Williams DRR, Wilkinson J. (1998). The development of health needs assessment. In: Wright J, ed., *Health needs assessment in practice*, pp. 1–11. BMJ Books, London.

5 Rawaf S, Bahl V. (1998). *Assessing health needs of people from minority ethnic groups*. Royal College of Physicians, London.

6 Graham H. (2010). Where is the future in public health? *Milbank Quarterly*, **88(2)**, 149–68.

7 Jordan J, Dowswell T, Harrison S, et al. (1998). Whose priorities? Listening to users and the public. *British Medical Journal*, **316**, 1668–70.

8 Bowling A. (1997). *Measuring health: a review of quality of life measurement scales*, 2nd edn. Open University Press, Buckingham.

9 Cochrane Library summaries. Available at: ℬ http://www.cochrane.org/evidence (accessed 30 July 2019).

10 Royal Society of Medicine Press. *Effective health care bulletins*. Available at: ℬ http://www.york.ac.uk/inst/crd (accessed 7 August 2019). [Effective health care bulletins are bi-monthly publications for decision makers, which examine the effectiveness of a variety of healthcare interventions. They are based on a systematic review and synthesis of research on the clinical effectiveness, cost-effectiveness, and acceptability of health service interventions. This is carried out by a research team using established methodological guidelines, with advice from expert consultants for each topic. The bulletins are subject to extensive and rigorous peer review.]

11 The Agency for Healthcare Research and Quality. Available at: ℬ http://www.ahrq.gov (accessed 30 June 2005).

12 The National Institute for Health and Care Excellence. Available at: ℬ http://www.nice.org.uk (accessed 14 January 2006).

13 Scott A, Donaldson C. (1998). Clinical and cost effectiveness issues in health needs assessment. In: Wright J. ed., *Health needs assessment in practice*, pp. 84–94. BMJ Books, London.

Assessing health impacts

Margaret Douglas and Ben Cave

Objectives

By reading this chapter, you will become familiar with:
- the definition and purpose of health impact assessment (HIA)
- concepts and values that underpin HIA
- the stages of an HIA process
- methods used in HIA
- experiences of HIA.

What is health impact assessment?

HIA is defined as 'a combination of procedures, methods and tools that systematically judges the potential, and sometimes unintended, effects of a policy, program or project on the health of a population, and the distribution of those effects within the population. HIA identifies appropriate actions to manage those effects.'[1, 2]

HIA is part of a 'family' of impact assessments that seek to identify, and to inform policy makers about, the implications of any given policy, plan, programme, or (PPPP).[3] PPPPs represent the different levels of policy making, from national and international to the very local. The relationship of an HIA to other assessments is considered below. Impact assessment is conducted while the PPPP is being developed and designed, and before it has approval to proceed. It is for this reason that, in this chapter, the PPPPs that are the subjects of an HIA, or another form of assessment, are collectively called 'proposals'.

An HIA may be completed at any level, from a national policy on alcohol, to a regional transport strategy, to more specific and local projects such as a housing development or infrastructure for energy, road, rail, air, etc. An HIA may assess national, regional, local government, or private sector proposals.

HIA is prospective, before a proposal is implemented, and it is iterative so that it takes into account any changes in the proposal or the relevant social and economic context. The final outputs of an HIA include evidence-based recommendations to ensure that population health is protected and, where possible, improved, and to minimize any potential adverse effects on health inequalities. These recommendations can be voluntary or may be enforced through conditions that are attached to the proposal to enable it to proceed. The HIA may also set out a monitoring and evaluation framework.

The context for health impact assessment

The Adelaide Statement on Health in All Policies (HiAP) identifies impact assessments as one of the tools and instruments that have been shown to be useful at different stages of the policy cycle.[4] HiAP is increasingly being promoted as a way to improve health by engaging with policy makers in other sectors that influence health. HiAP has been defined as 'a collaborative approach to improving the health of all people by incorporating health considerations into decision making across sectors and policy areas'.[5] HIA offers a systematic, structured way to identify potential impacts and make recommendations to improve them. This can be a useful way to engage with and influence other sectors within an HiAP approach.[6, 7]

As noted earlier, HIA and health within environmental assessment have been added to the suite of assessments that considers potential environmental impacts. For example, the European Union directives on strategic environmental assessment[8] and environmental impact assessment (EIA)[9] explicitly require human health to be considered. There are institutional and technical challenges for the assessment teams and the regulatory authorities to ensure that they cover an appropriate range of potential health impacts.[10, 11]

Major drivers of global change (e.g. population growth and urbanization, growing pressure on natural resources and climate change) inordinately affect low- and medium- human development index (HDI) countries but in such countries HIA is rare.[12] In low-HDI countries, HIA is missing from programme and policy development except when required by an external project driver such as an international financial institution. EIA regulations may also provide a mechanism to consider health protection as a core aspect in the approval of projects.[13] For example, recent work recommends assessing health impacts within integrated EIA of mining projects in sub-Saharan Africa to help prepare for, and respond to, emerging infectious diseases.[14]

HIAs may be done in-house by the organization developing the proposal if there is relevant health expertise available. They may also be externally commissioned or undertaken in partnership with a local public health department.

HIA should take place early enough in the development of a proposal to permit constructive changes to be made before implementation, but late enough to have a clear idea about its nature and content.

Values in health impact assessment

Both the World Health Organization (WHO)[1] and the International Association for Impact Assessment[2] have defined values that should underpin HIA.[1,2] These are as follows.

Equity

Most proposals benefit some groups of people more than others, so may have a positive or negative impact on health equity. Thus a challenging but important role of HIA is to raise the issue of current and future inequities. All HIAs can consider equity impacts by:
- identifying different populations that will be affected in different ways, and the distribution of impacts across populations
- seeking to involve at all stages of the HIA people at high risk of poor health whose views are otherwise least likely to be heard
- ensuring that recommendations aim to maximize benefits, and mitigate risks, to populations at highest risk of poor health.[15]

Democracy

HIA should involve affected people and support transparent decision making.

Sustainability

HIA should consider long-term as well as short-term impacts.

Ethical use of evidence

HIA should use the best available evidence from different relevant disciplines, interpret it robustly, and declare assumptions and uncertainties in the analysis. An HIA should be impartial and not set out to support a predetermined position.

Comprehensive approach to health

HIA should take a systematic approach to consider the wide range of potential determinants of health that a proposal might have an impact on.

Benefits of health impact assessment

HIA has a number of benefits. It:
* promotes equity, sustainability, and healthy public policy making
* improves decision making by highlighting health issues
* promotes social and environmental justice by highlighting differential impacts
* uses a multidisciplinary, mixed-method approach
* offers a flexible process that can be adapted to suit the scale and nature of the proposal
* supports public participation
* facilitates public scrutiny of decision making
* demonstrates that health is far broader than healthcare.

The health impact assessment process

An HIA may range from a rapid tabletop exercise with a small group of stakeholders to a comprehensive assessment that analyses a large volume of evidence. In any HIA, the scale of the assessment, evidence, and methods should be appropriate to the scale and scope of the proposal and the nature of potential impacts. Guidance documents for HIA[16–22] set out broadly similar processes and stages for the assessment (as shown in Figure 1.5.1). These stages are, in turn, similar to the stages used in other forms of impact assessment.

Screening

Screening means deciding whether it would be useful to carry out an HIA. In practice, this means considering the following:
* Is the proposal likely to affect health?
* Is there an opportunity to influence the proposal?
* Is an HIA likely to provide useful information to influence decisions?
* Are there resources for an HIA?

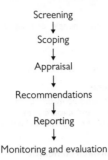

Screening
↓
Scoping
↓
Appraisal
↓
Recommendations
↓
Reporting
↓
Monitoring and evaluation

Figure 1.5.1 Stages in the HIA process.

It may seem difficult to determine whether a proposal will affect health before completing an HIA. It is often useful to use a health impact checklist like that in Table 1.5.1 to identify the determinants of health that the proposal may influence.

Scoping

Scoping involves setting terms of reference (TOR) for the assessment and establishing, or commissioning, an HIA team with the relevant expertise to do the work.

Usually a steering group is set up to agree the TOR and the HIA team will report to this steering group. The steering group should include people who will be in a position to agree and take forward the recommendations after the HIA is completed.

The TOR may include:
- the aim of the HIA
- the scope of the proposal including any alternative options
- the boundaries of the HIA in time and space
- populations to consider and stakeholders to consult
- impacts to assess
- methods and evidence to be used and expertise required
- the decision-making framework for the proposal with timescales
- reporting and deadlines for the HIA.

Appraisal

This is the stage in which the HIA team collects, analyses, interprets and presents different sources of evidence. Both qualitative and quantitative evidence may be used. Methods commonly used in HIA are described further below. The purpose is not simply to identify and describe health impacts but to inform recommendations to improve the impacts of the proposal. The questions to ask may include the following:
- What are the pathways by which impacts will arise?
- Is there research evidence to support the predicted steps in the pathways?
- How do affected people perceive the potential impacts?
- How many people, in which populations, will be affected by impacts?

Table 1.5.1 Populations and determinants to consider

Issues to consider	How might the proposal impact on:
Populations	Different groups of people by age, sex, disability, ethnicity, sexual orientation, geography, employment status, socio-economic status
Equality between groups	Equality of opportunity, discrimination, relations between groups
Health-related behaviour	Nutrition, physical activity, substance use, sexual health, learning and skills
Social environment	Social status, employment (paid or unpaid), income and income inequality, crime and fear of crime, family support, social networks, stress, resilience, community assets, participation, social interaction, influence and sense of control, identity and belonging
Physical environment	Living conditions, working conditions, natural space, pollution—air, water, soil, climate change, waste, energy, resource use, transport patterns, unintentional injuries, public safety, transmission of infectious disease
Access to and quality of services	Healthcare, transport and connections, social services, housing quality, housing mix, education provision, culture, leisure and play provision

Source: adapted from Douglas M. (2019). Health impact assessment guidance for practitioners. Scottish Health and Inequalities Impact Assessment Network. Available at: ℗ https://www.scotphn.net/wp-content/uploads/2019/07/Health-Impact-Assessment-Guidance-for-Practitioners-SHIIAN-updated-2019.docx (accessed 29th October 2019)

Recommendations

The recommendations of an HIA aim to mitigate adverse impacts and/or enhance beneficial impacts. Some HIAs make recommendations broader than the proposal being assessed—for example, an HIA of a transport policy may make recommendations about land use policy. Recommendations should be negotiated with and owned by the steering group for the HIA. Recommendations should:

- aim to maximize health gain and minimize health loss
- relate clearly to the identified impacts
- be clearly specified and identify the lead agency for each
- be practical, realistic, and acceptable
- focus on affected groups at risk of poorer health
- not extend beyond the technical expertise of the HIA team
- be capable of being monitored and evaluated.

Reporting

An HIA report should give enough information to enable it to be appraised by others and to justify the recommendations. It is important to communicate findings with stakeholders who may be responsible for implementing the recommendations. It is good practice to include a short version and consider other ways to disseminate the information to affected populations.

Sometimes an HIA feeds into a formal process in which a nominated senior officer is required to give evidence, and it is essential to ensure that they have sufficient information to present a case.

Monitoring

An HIA may include a plan for monitoring the recommendations and/or monitoring the impacts of the proposal on health after implementation. Ideally, this should be incorporated into other routine monitoring processes. In most cases, it is better to monitor changes in determinants rather than changes in health outcome because often it would be difficult to attribute any changes in health outcome solely to the proposal.

Evaluation

Evaluation of an HIA may include both process and/or impact evaluation.[23] Process evaluation considers whether the HIA:

- met the terms of reference
- identified impacts systematically
- engaged stakeholders appropriately
- analysed the evidence robustly
- made practical recommendations that are appropriate to the impacts.

Impact evaluation considers whether the HIA effectively influenced the decision and whether the recommendations were implemented.

Guidance is available with standards for evaluation of HIA reports.[24, 25]

Methods used in health impact assessment

A range of methods may be used in the appraisal stage of an HIA to identify and assess impacts. HIA does not require new methods but uses the public health skills and methods that are appropriate to the proposal being assessed. These will depend on the nature and complexity of the proposal but may include:

- policy analysis
- preparing a community profile
- identifying health impacts
- involving stakeholders
- reviewing literature
- valuing health impacts
- summarizing and presenting health impacts.

Policy analysis

HIAs of policies will require initial policy analysis to determine key aspects that the HIA will need to address. This may build on or use material already available from earlier policy development work.[5] Key features to describe may include:

- content and dimensions of the policy
- policy objectives, priorities, and intended outputs
- socio-political context and links to other policies
- constraints and trade-offs.

Community profile

A profile of the areas and populations likely to be affected by the proposal is compiled using available socio-demographic and health data and information from key informants. The profile should identify the different groups whose health could be enhanced or placed at risk by the proposal, including those who are particularly vulnerable or disadvantaged. It should also identify relevant features of the locality that might affect the impacts.

Identifying potential health impacts

Most HIAs use a socio-environmental model of health with a causal model of health impact in which a proposal may cause changes in health determinants that then lead to changes in health outcomes. Impacts may arise indirectly, at different stages of a causal pathway. The HIA team needs to use a systematic approach to identify potential impacts. This often involves using a checklist like the one in Table 1.5.1 at a stakeholder workshop, using other qualitative methods to involve stakeholders and/or reviewing HIA reports or evidence on health impacts of similar proposals.

Participation in health impact assessments

Participation throughout the HIA is essential for several reasons. Stakeholders hold much of the evidence needed for the assessment—such as information about the locality and what value people place on different impacts. Involving affected communities also helps to ensure that local concerns are addressed. Stakeholders and key informants to involve include:

- people likely to be directly affected by the proposal
- people involved at all levels in the proposal
- people with knowledge of the local context
- local or outside experts with relevant expertise
- interest groups.

Methods to involve stakeholders include interviews, focus groups, meetings, surveys, workshops, and participatory prioritization methods. It is important to consider how representative informants are, and to make special efforts to speak to people who are less confident to raise their concerns.

Literature review

Most HIAs include a literature review that explores evidence for each link in the hypothesized pathways between the proposal, health determinants, and health outcomes. It will include health literature and also literature on the policy area of the proposal. The research evidence from the literature needs to be integrated with evidence about the local context to determine how transferable it is to the specific proposal.

Assessing and valuing health impacts

There are different ways to value and prioritize health impacts. It is difficult to quantify predicted health outcomes, and not always necessary if this will not help to inform or support recommendations.[26] Some HIAs quantify the changes in health determinants, and/or the number of people expected to be affected by these changes. In some cases, it is possible to use modelling techniques to quantify the resultant change in health outcomes. There is no standard model that can be used routinely in HIAs to quantify impacts.[27, 28]

Models designed for other purposes—such as the WHO HEAT tool to assess the health impact of changes in transport behaviour[29]—are sometimes used. When summary quantitative measures are produced, it is important also to highlight the susceptible populations that are most likely to be affected.

Some HIAs ask stakeholders to prioritize the most important impacts using methods such as Delphi surveys. Criteria to prioritize impacts may include, for example, each impact's anticipated probability and frequency of occurrence and its severity or importance.

HIAs may identify impacts that are deemed to be 'significant' because they:

- have severe or irreversible adverse impacts
- affect a large number of people
- affect people who already suffer poor health
- have positive impacts with large potential for benefit.

Summarizing and presenting health impacts

HIAs should show clearly the pathways through which the proposal is expected to have an impact on health determinants and thereby on health. This should also help to identify potential points in the pathway where changes could improve health impacts. This may be done by using a diagram mapping the causal pathways, by outlining the pathways in text, and/or by presenting a summary matrix like the one in Table 1.5.2.

Experience of health impact assessment

While coverage in low- and middle-income countries is not extensive, HIA has been used in the context of development projects since the 1980s[30] and in the UK since the early 1990s.[31, 32] HIA can be used as a technical approach focusing on environmental determinants and quantification of risks, and/or as a way to engage stakeholders and promote HIaP. The World Health Organization (WHO) has promoted and supported both these approaches over the years. International interest in HIA increased following the WHO European Centre for Health Policy conference on HIA held in Gothenburg in 1999.[33] There have been international HIA conferences and textbooks are now available.[34–38] In the USA alone, over 300 HIAs have been completed since 2010, many of which were supported by philanthropic grant funding.[39]

There is evidence of the effectiveness of HIA. A study of 17 European case studies documented examples of positive impacts of HIAs.[40] Similarly, a study of 55 Australasian HIAs found that most influenced decision making directly or indirectly.[41] Studies commonly report that HIA has produced unpredicted benefits such as improved partnership working, raising the profile of health issues, reducing social exclusion, and empowering and engaging local communities, as well as informing decision making.

HIA uses public health skills, methods, and approaches to engage meaningfully with other sectors and with communities. It should not be viewed as a specialist technical area but as part of core public health work.

Table 1.5.2 Matrix of health impacts

Health impact	Pathways	Positive/ negative	Affected populations	Likelihood	Severity	Approx. no. people
IMPACT 1						
IMPACT 2, etc.						

References

1 World Health Organization European Centre for Health Policy (1999). *Health impact assessment: main concepts and suggested approach*, Gothenburg consensus paper. ECHP, Brussels. Available at: ℘ http://www.impactsante.ch/pdf/HIA_Gothenburg_consensus_paper_1999 (accessed 28th October 2019).

2 Quigley R, den Broeder L, Furu P, et al. (2006). *Health impact assessment: international best practice principles*. Special Publication Series No. 5, International Association for Impact Assessment: Fargo, USA. Available at: ℘ http://www.iaia.org/uploads/pdf/SP5_3.pdf (accessed 18 October 2019).

3 Fehr R, Viliani F, Nowacki J, et al. (eds), (2014). *Health in impact assessments: opportunities not to be missed*. World Health Organization Regional Office for Europe. Available at: ℘ www.euro.who.int/en/health-topics/environment-and-health/health-impact-assessment/publications/2014/health-in-impact-assessments-opportunities-not-to-be-missed (accessed 18 October 2019).

4 World Health Organization (2010). *Adelaide statement on health in all policies: moving towards a shared governance for health and well-being*. WHO and Government of South Australia. Adelaide, South Australia. Available at: ℘ www.who.int/social_determinants/hiap_statement_who_sa_final.pdf (accessed 18 October 2019).

5 Rudolph L, Caplan J, Ben-Moshe K, et al. (2013). *Health in All Policies: a guide for state and local governments*. American Public Health Association and Public Health Institute. Washington, DC and Oakland, CA. Available at: ℘ http://www.phi.org/uploads/application/files/udt4vq0y712qpb1o4p62dexjlgxlnogpq15gr8pti3y7ckzysi.pdf (accessed 18 October 2019).

6 Collins J, Koplan JP. (2009). Health impact assessment: a step towards Health in All Policies. *Journal of the American Medical Association*, **302**, 315–7.

7 Delany T, Harris P, Williams C, et al. (2014). Health impact assessment in New South Wales and Health in All Policies in South Australia: differences, similarities and connections. *BMC Public Health*, **14**, 699.

8 Directive 2001/42/EC of the European Parliament and of the Council on the assessment of the effects of certain plans and programmes on the environment. (2001). *Official Journal of the European Communities*, **L197**, 30–7.

9 Directive 2014/52/EU of the European Parliament and of the Council amending Directive 2011/92/EU on the assessment of the effects of certain public and private projects on the environment. (2014). *Official Journal of the European Communities*, **L124**, 1–18.

10 Cave B, Fothergill J, Pyper R, et al. (2017). *Health and environmental impact assessment: a briefing for public health teams in England*. Public Health England, London. Available at: ℘ www.gov.uk/government/publications/health-and-environmental-impact-assessment-guide-for-local-teams (accessed 18 October 2019).

11 Cave B, Fothergill J, Pyper R, et al. (2017). Health in environmental impact assessment: a primer for a proportionate approach. Ben Cave Associates, IEMA and the Faculty of Public Health, Lincoln. Available at: ℘ www.iema.net/assets/newbuild/documents/IEMA%20Primer%20on%20Health%20in%20UK%20EIA%20Doc%20V11.pdf (accessed 18 October 2019).

12 Winkler MS, Krieger GR, Divall MJ, et al. (2017). Untapped potential of health impact assessment. *Bulletin of the World Health Organization*, **91**(4), 237–312. Available at: ℘ https://dx.doi.org/10.2471/BLT.12.112318 (accessed 18 October 2019).

13 Harris P, Viliani F, Spickett J. (2015). Assessing health impacts within environmental impact assessments: an opportunity for public health globally which must not remain missed. *International*

Journal of Environmental Research and Public Health, **12**(1), 1044–9. Available at: ℜ https://dx.doi.org/10.3390/ijerph120101044 (accessed 18 October 2019).

14 Viliani F, Edelstein M, Buckley E, et al. (2016). Mining and emerging infectious diseases: results of the infectious disease risk assessment and management (IDRAM) initiative pilot. *Extractive Industries and Society*. Available at: ℜ http://dx.doi.org/10.1016/j.exis.2016.08.009 (accessed 18 October 2019).

15 Heller J, Malekafzali S, Todman LC, et al. (2013). Promoting equity through the practice of health impact assessment. *Policy Link*. Available at: ℜ http://www.policylink.org/sites/default/files/PROMOTINGEQUITYHIA_FINAL.PDF (accessed 18 October 2019).

16 Scott-Samuel A, Birley M, Ardern K. (2001). The Merseyside guidelines for health impact assessment, 2nd edn. ISBN 1 874038 56 International Health Impact Assessment Consortium. Available at: ℜ http://www.precaution.org/lib/06/mersey_hia_guide_2nd_edn.010601.pdf (accessed 28th October 2019).

17 Harris P, Harris-Roxas B, Harris E, et al. (2007). Health impact assessment: a practical guide. Centre for Health Equity Training, Research and Evaluation (CHETRE), Sydney. Part of the UNSW Research Centre for Primary Health Care and Equity, UNSW. Available at: ℜ http://hiaconnect.edu.au/wp-content/uploads/2012/05/Health_Impact_Assessment_A_Practical_Guide.pdf (accessed 18 October 2019).

18 Public Health Advisory Committee (2005). *A guide to health impact assessment: a policy tool for New Zealand*. Public Health Advisory Committee, National Advisory Committee on Health and Disability, Wellington. Available at: ℜ http://www.moh.govt.nz/NoteBook/nbbooks.nsf/0/D540E1D80F7DB72CCC2578670072F996/$file/guidetohia.pdf (accessed 18 October 2019).

19 Douglas M. (2019). Health impact assessment guidance for practitioners. Scottish Health and Inequalities Impact Assessment Network. Available at: ℜ https://www.scotphn.net/wp-content/uploads/2019/07/Health-Impact-Assessment-Guidance-for-Practitioners-SHIIAN-updated-2019.docx (accessed 28th October 2019).

20 Welsh Health Impact Assessment Support Unit (2012). Health Impact Assessment: a practical guide. Available at: ℜ http://www.wales.nhs.uk/sites3/Documents/522/Whiasu%20Guidance%20Report%20%28English%29%20V2%20WEB.pdf (accessed 18 October 2019).

21 International Petroleum Industry Environmental Conservation Association, International Association of Oil and Gas Producers (2016). *Health impact assessments: a guide for the oil and gas industry*. IPIECA, IAOGP. Available at: ℜ www.ipieca.org/resources/good-practice/health-impact-assessment-a-guide-for-the-oil-and-gas-industry/ (accessed 18 October 2019).

22 International Council on Mining & Metals (2010). Good practice guidance on Health Impact Assessment. ICMM, London. Available at: ℜ www.icmm.com/en-gb/publications/health-and-safety/good-practice-guidance-on-health-impact-assessment (accessed 18 October 2019).

23 Parry JM, Kemm J. (2005). Criteria for use in the evaluation of health impact assessments: recommendations from an European workshop. *Public Health*, **119**, 1122–9.

24 Fredsgaard MW, Cave B, Bond A. (2009). *A review package for health impact assessment reports of development projects*. Ben Cave Associates Ltd, Leeds.

25 Bhatia R, Farhang L, Heller J, et al. (2014). Minimum elements and practice standards for health impact assessment, Version 3. Society of Practitioners of Health Impact Assessment (SOPHIA). Available at: ℜ https://hiasociety.org/resources/Documents/HIA-Practice-Standards-September-2014.pdf (accessed 28th October 2019).

26 Mindell J, Hansell A, Morrison D, et al. (2001). What do we need for robust, quantitative health impact assessment? *Journal of Public Health Medicine*, **23**, 173–8.

27 Veerman JL, Barendregt JJ, Mackenbach JP. (2005). Quantitative health impact assessment: current practice and future directions. *Journal of Epidemiology and Community Health*, **59**, 659–62.

28 Lhachimi SK, Nusselder WJ, Boshuizen HC, et al. (2010). Standard tool for quantification in health impact assessment. *American Journal of Preventative Medicine*, **38**(1), 78–84.

29 World Health Organization/Europe (2019). Health economic assessment tool (HEAT) for walking and cycling. Available at: ℜ http://www.heatwalkingcycling.org/ (accessed 18 October 2019).

30 Birley MH. (1995). *The health impact assessment of development projects*. HMSO, London.

31 Will S, Ardern K, Spencely M, et al. (1994). *A prospective health impact assessment of the proposed development of a second runway at Manchester International Airport*, written submission to the public inquiry. Manchester and Stockport Health Commissions, Manchester.

32 Scott-Samuel A. (1996). Health impact assessment—an idea whose time has come. *British Medical Journal*, **313**, 183–4.

33 Diwan V, Douglas M, Karlberg I, et al. (2000). *Health impact assessment: from theory to practice.* Report on the Leo Kaprio Workshop, Goteborg, 28-30 October 1999. Nordic School of Public Health report 9.

34 Ross CL, Orenstein M. (2014). *Health impact assessment in the United States.* Springer, New York.

35 Birley M. (2011). *Health impact assessment principles and practice.* Earthscan, New York.

36 O'Mullane M. (ed.). (2013). *Integrating health impact assessment into the policy process: lessons and experience from around the world.* Oxford University Press, Oxford.

37 Kemm J. (ed.). (2013). *Health impact assessment past achievement, current understanding and future progress.* Oxford University Press, Oxford.

38 Jackson RJ, Bear D, Bhatia R, et al. (2011). Improving health in the United States: the role of health impact assessment. Washington DC. Committee on Health Impact Assessment. Board on Environmental Studies and Toxicology, Division on Earth and Life Studies, National Research Council of the National Academies. Available at: ⌖ www.nap.edu/catalog.php?record_id=13229 (accessed 18 October 2019).

39 Bourcier E, Charbonneau D, Cahill C, et al. (2015). An evaluation of health impact assessments in the United States, 2011–2014. *Preventing Chronic Disease*, **12**, 40376. Available at: ⌖ http://dx.doi.org/10.5888/pcd12.140376 (accessed 18 October 2019).

40 Wismar M. Blau J. Ernst K, et al. (eds). (2007). *The effectiveness of. health impact assessment.* European Observatory on Health Systems and Policies, World Health Organization, Copenhagen.

41 Haigh F, Baum F, Dannenberg AL, et al. (2013). The effectiveness of health impact assessment in influencing decision making in Australia and New Zealand 2005–2009. *BMC Public Health*, **13**, 1188.

Chapter 1.6

Economic assessment

Peter Brambleby

Objectives

This chapter will help the reader to:

- understand the tools, techniques, and approaches of health economics
- apply a health economics way of framing a discussion when the need arises in management situations
- pose better questions when important choices are apparent and when the help of a professional health economist is involved.

What is health economics?

Health economics is concerned with managing scarcity, supporting decisions, and evaluating results when resources are deployed in health and healthcare (see Box 1.6.1).

> **Box 1.6.1 Health economics**
> Health economics is a discipline that brings a systematic approach to the management of issues of scarcity and choice in healthcare.

All professional healthcare activity involves making choices. This can be particularly challenging in promoting health, preventing disease, and treating ill health because:

- the outcome may be attributable to multiple interventions
- the outcome may not be evident for several years
- resources are insufficient to meet every need (ability to benefit from an intervention) and demand (what patients or the caring professions ask for)
- the evidence base on outcomes and resources is often incomplete.

The practitioner often has to make, or advise others on making, choices such as:

- deciding whether or not to introduce a new intervention or service
- deciding how one could go about comparing many bids for new money when only a few of the bids could be funded
- deciding the best way to find how to take money out of a service.

Whether one is involved with the planning or the delivery of healthcare, the job involves many complex choices. In predominantly publicly funded systems (such as the UK's National Health Service ([NHS]), or public/private mixed economies (such as in most of continental Europe), there is the added dimension of having to be publicly accountable for stewardship of scarce resources. The techniques of health economics help to expose the trade-offs between the options, and make the decision-taking process open to scrutiny and participation.

Despite its name, economics is not primarily about 'making economies' nor even about money. Money is just one type of resource. Other resources include people, time, and buildings. Costs can be tangible and easy to ascribe a monetary value to (such as medicines, staff, or journeys to hospital) or they can be intangible (such as pain and disability). All types of cost are potentially relevant, although some are set aside in particular applications. Economic appraisal is about relating costs to outputs and outcomes. It is about return on investment in health and healthcare. It is therefore just as concerned with evidence of effectiveness as it is with resources.

The steps of economic appraisal often follow this sequence:
- What are we trying to achieve?
- What are the different ways of achieving this (the options)?
- How do these options compare with each other, taking adverse effects into account as well as benefits?
- What costs are involved for each option, taking not only healthcare factors and intangible costs into consideration, but also other factors such as costs to social services or to the patient?

Similarly, if a service might be stopped, the considerations are:
- What are we trying to achieve?
- What are the different ways of achieving this (the options)?
- What benefits will be lost with each option?
- What resources will be released with each option?
- If resources might be redeployed, what is the net gain and net cost (or saving)?

Health economics provides a means of handling these decisions. It can be regarded as a way of framing the discussion (a shared perspective on problem solving that decision makers find useful), and as a particular set of tools and techniques to articulate the costs, benefits, and trade-offs.

Health economics as a way of thinking

Health economics is not a substitute for thought but a way of organizing it.[1] It is not a technical fix that tells you precisely what to do.[2-7] The approach is *utilitarian*—trying to get the greatest good for the greatest number, and concerned with *efficiency*—getting the greatest outcome from a fixed amount of resource.

Although these are the health economist's starting points, they need not necessarily be adopted as the deciding criteria when decisions are taken. The gulf between what is possible and what can be afforded (by the individual or the state), and the inevitability of having to choose, is the starting point for economic appraisal. Health economics recognizes the existence of trade-offs inherent in any system. Choice involves sacrifice. It is perfectly legitimate to trade-off some efficiency for the sake of other considerations, such as equity. Equity can be described as the willingness to give a protected 'fair share' to a particular group in society in need, even if that does not maximize total outcomes from the available resources for the population as a whole. It serves to emphasize that choices are not free—there is an *opportunity cost* (benefit foregone) once resources are committed. In other words, once resources have been committed, the real cost is not the monetary value but the best alternative use to which that resource could have been put. Just like many other disciplines that contribute to the practice of public health (e.g. epidemiology and sociology) economic appraisal is concerned with whole populations and not just individuals.

Economic evaluations

Economic evaluations deal with the relationships between costs and outcomes when choices have to be made between competing options. Sometimes the outcomes are the same and the issue is simply 'which option consumes least resources, taking all costs into consideration?' In this situation, the appropriate tool is *cost-minimization analysis*.

More often the costs and outcomes are both different, but the units in which the outcomes are measured are the same (e.g. years of life added for choices between cancer treatments; peak expiratory flow rates for choices between asthma treatments; or successful live births in choices between infertility treatments). In such cases, the appropriate tool is *cost-effectiveness analysis*.

Sometimes the choice is between very different types of outcome, measured in very different units and with very different costs. An example would be deciding whether to put some additional resources into cancer care, orthopaedics, or diabetes. The issue is one of finding a common set of units such as quality-adjusted life years (QALYs) to allow a 'cost per QALY' comparison on a like-for-like basis. The term given to appraisals that convert different sorts of outcome into these common 'utility' units is *cost–utility analysis*. The great advantage of this approach, despite the limitations of ascribing QALY units, is that it allows comparisons between very different interventions, and that is helpful to policy makers in pursuit of allocative efficiency.

Sometimes it is simply a question of weighing up whether the costs of a new intervention outweigh the benefits or not, and whether it should go ahead at all. Costs and benefits are both ascribed a monetary value in order to make the comparison. This is *cost–benefit analysis*. (Note that 'cost–benefit analysis' has a precise meaning and is not a blanket term for all comparisons of costs and outcomes—a better phrase to describe these techniques collectively is *economic appraisal*.)

The tools for addressing these situations are shown in Box 1.6.2.

Box 1.6.2 Forms of economic evaluation
- *Cost-minimization analysis:* when the outcomes (benefits) of alternative interventions are the same in terms of volume and type, the cheapest programme should be chosen on the grounds of efficiency—for example, choosing between a branded and a generic antibiotic to treat a streptococcal infection.
- *Cost-effectiveness analysis:* when both the costs and outcomes of alternative interventions are *different*, then the efficient choice is the intervention that costs least to produce a unit of outcome (such as a life saved)—for example, choosing between two interventions of different cost and effectiveness that both lower blood pressure in people with hypertension.
- *Cost–utility analysis:* when the outcomes from alternate interventions are *not* the same, then a 'common outcome currency' (such as a QALY) is used as a measure of benefit and to enable comparisons to be made between interventions. Choice of intervention will then depend on the cost of producing a unit of the chosen currency (e.g. the cost per QALY)—for example, choosing between hip replacements, coronary artery bypass grafts, and haemodialysis for the next year's investment.
- *Cost–benefit analysis:* the preceding evaluative methods all leave the outcome/benefit side of the equation in 'natural' units (clearing infection, lowering blood pressure, QALYs, etc.). Cost–benefit analysis places monetary values on these benefits (to enable direct comparison between the inputs and the outcomes). This analysis can help to decide whether to do something at all or not (e.g. if the value of the input is greater than the output, it might be better not to do it), or when choosing between options to assess which gives the greatest ratio of outcome to input. An illustration of this application might be whether or not to invest in installing crash barriers along a 10-mile stretch of road to avoid road traffic deaths and injuries (when deaths and injuries are ascribed a monetary value).

Additional concepts

The appraisal tools described above are a simplification of the decision-guiding process. A health economist will also apply an annual percentage *discounting* to costs and benefits that fall at some time in the future to give them all a present-day value (this could be of the order of, for instance, 6% per annum). A benefit in the future is valued less highly than a benefit today (hence, the value of a benefit only available at some time in the future is 'discounted').

A *sensitivity analysis* would also be done to several values, rather than single point estimates, because data on costs and outcomes is seldom precise. This yields a range of estimates to assist decision makers.

Priority setting through programme budgeting and marginal analysis

A pioneer of programme budgeting and marginal analysis (PBMA) was Professor Alain Enthoven, who took it from its application to the American armed forces and applied it to healthcare planning (or purchasing) at the population level. He endorsed its use in the UK NHS in his 1999 Rock Carling Fellowship review.[8]

An entire issue of *Health Policy*[9] was devoted to articles on this topic. Table 1.6.1 gives an outline of PBMA.

The UK Department of Health, with parallels in other parts of the UK NHS, has been exploring PBMA. This was promised by the 1997 Labour government in its first major policy document on health, *The New NHS: Modern, Dependable* (London, 1997):

- Para 6.22: 'Partnerships between secondary and primary care physicians and with social services will provide the necessary basis for the establishment of "programmes of care", which will allow planning and resource management across organisational boundaries.'
- Para 9.18: 'Efficient use of resources will be critical to delivering the best for patients. It is important that managers and clinicians alike have a proper understanding of the costs of local services, so that they can make appropriate local decisions on the best use of resources.'

Another significant strand of policy was the creation of the National Institute for Health and Care Excellence (NICE), now emulated in many other countries around the world, which appraises evidence of effectiveness and cost-effectiveness and publishes technology appraisals and clinical guidance (see ➲ Further resources).

Is *health* economics different from conventional economics?

From the conventional point of view of economics, health care is unusual.[10] Standard economic ideas of supply and demand are often difficult to square with the reality of how healthcare systems actually function. In virtually all countries, demand for healthcare is mediated through a medical professional—consumers are not sovereign as in a typical market model. Patients need the help of a clinician to identify what their state of health really is, what their healthcare needs are, and what interventions are appropriate to address them. This is known as the *agency role* of the health professions.

Both supply and demand for healthcare, especially secondary healthcare, are heavily regulated and managed. Complex insurance markets—run by the state, the independent sector, or a mixture of the two—have grown up in response to the inherent uncertainties of illness and the costs of treatment. Governments can play a significant part in healthcare regulation, from setting rules about practitioner qualifications through to resource allocation, standard setting, and direct control of provision.

Table 1.6.1 Programme budgeting and marginal analysis

Action	Comments
Define healthcare programmes	Break down the priority-setting process into more manageable and meaningful programmes (e.g. client groups, specialties, disease groups), and define healthcare objectives and outputs for each.
Establish programme management groups	Management groups (clinicians, managers, user representatives) are responsible for priority setting within their programmes.
Understand the chosen programmes	Identify current spending on, and broad outputs from, each programme.
Define subprogrammes of care (if it helps)	Identify further breakdowns in programmes, with estimates of spending and defined objectives.
Focus on marginal change	Most priority setting concerns changes to existing services (i.e. changes at the margin). Therefore, most attention can be paid to changes *within*, rather than *between*, programmes. However, do not be afraid to look across programmes for a population, perhaps spread across several providers, and examine marginal changes between programmes. Just bear in mind that the management challenge of shifting resources between programmes is considerable and needs agreement in principle at the outset.
Identify incremental 'wish lists' (and decremental 'hit lists')	Given extra (or fewer) resources, what services should be expanded (or reduced) to deliver a closer fit with the programme's stated objectives?
Make proposals based on relative benefits generated by changes in spending	What would be implemented from the wish lists if specific amounts of money were made available or taken away?
Consider equity and policy implications	The steps above focus on efficiency—getting more healthcare/healthiness for each unit of resource—but check against other considerations such as 'fair shares', local strategy, and national policy.
Consult	Out of necessity, 'point estimates' of cost and outcome are used in PBMA. If you can, conduct a sensitivity analysis. Do not let the veneer of scientific precision blind you to the underlying value judgements. PBMA helps clarify and organize thought. It is imperative to check the assumptions with those most affected.
Choose where to invest and where to disinvest; evaluate results and share the learning	Having identified new patterns of spending based on clinical and economic evidence, decisions need to be taken to implement changes and then evaluate them. Share the learning by disseminating your experience.

The importance of the margin

Another important concept in health economics is that of the *margin*—the cost of the *next* (or one additional) unit of input, or the benefit of the *next* unit of output. The importance of this is that in healthcare many choices are made about relatively small incremental changes in service (either to increase or decrease), rather than wholesale strategic shifts. The issue is often described thus: 'What is the extra cost over and above what we pay now, and what is the extra benefit?' (The reverse applies for disinvestment decisions: 'What resources do we release and what benefits do we lose?')

A related concept is the *stepped cost*.

Examples

Suppose a cardiac surgery unit is built, staffed, and equipped to deal with 900 patients a year and funded accordingly. This would mean all the costs—'fixed costs' (like buildings), 'semi-fixed costs' (like staff salaries), and 'variable costs' (like medicines)—were covered. Suppose that, with this complement of buildings, the staff and equipment could actually cope with a further 50 patients. The additional (marginal) cost of each extra patient up to 50 would be relatively small and chiefly reflect the 'variable costs'. However, a point would come when, to accommodate just one more patient, extra staff would have to be taken on or a new ward built—that would be a substantial 'stepped cost'.

To see the relevance of this, imagine you are a healthcare purchaser with 200 extra patients requiring cardiac surgery and three cardiac centres within reasonable travelling distance for your population. It would be in everyone's interest to try and spread that additional workload between all three centres if that would enable them all to work closer to capacity, but, if that were not possible, then it might be better to make a single strategic investment (stepped development) at just one.

The same applies to benefits. Suppose an immunization programme reaches only 80% of the child population. An additional £50,000 might enable a further 10% to be reached, but the addition of a yet another £50,000 on top of that might only enable a further 5% to be reached. In common parlance, this is 'the law of diminishing returns'. To the economist, it is known as 'diminishing marginal benefit'.

The important points to remember are that *average* cost and benefit (*total* cost divided by *total* benefit) can differ substantially from *marginal* cost and benefit. Marginal cost and marginal benefit do not increase (or decrease) in a smooth linear fashion: they tend to go in steps.

A further important point is that harm arising from unintended consequences and known adverse effects of powerful therapeutic interventions tend to rise in linear fashion or accelerate, rather than diminish. There may come a time when increasing inputs lead to net added harm and pass the point of *optimal* health investment.

Ethics and equity

The ethical stance of health economics is sometimes questioned by clinicians because the utilitarian approach can seem to be at odds with the 'Hippocratic' ethic of doing the very best for the individual in a trusting doctor–patient relationship. (Economics is not known as the 'dismal science' for nothing!) However, an economist would justify the pursuit of efficiency on the grounds that the true cost of inefficiency is borne in terms of pain, disability, and premature death by those waiting for treatment. In a publicly funded healthcare system, where policy making, funding, and provision are all controlled largely by the state, the primary objective of trying to ensure the greatest good for the greatest number is legitimate. One could extend this and argue that it is better to have a system where everyone gets access to a service that meets basic standards, even if those are not the very best possible, if the alternative means that some should go without altogether.

Efficiency (allocative versus technical)

In general terms, healthcare policy makers and those who 'commission' are primarily concerned with *allocative efficiency*—trying to maximize the population health gain from a fixed allocation of resources. (One is trying to reach a position where no one waiting for treatment has a greater ability to benefit than anyone who is already being treated.)

Healthcare 'providers' are more often concerned with *technical efficiency*—achieving a desired objective at the least cost. Many of the objectives are set for them: numbers to be treated, waiting times, and so on. Allocative efficiency is about doing the right things. Technical efficiency is about doing things right.

Since the 1990s, in an attempt to address both types of efficiency, the NHS in England has experimented with a market model whereby the funds are held by 'commissioners' and devolved, ostensibly according to population need, to 'providers' who deliver the care. This was an attempt to harness 'market forces' to drive up quality and drive out inefficiency. Although introduced by a Conservative administration, the Labour administration that followed it in 1997 perpetuated many elements of the model, especially the separation of purchasing and providing roles. For a lucid analysis of the strengths and weaknesses of the market models in the NHS see Enthoven.[8]

Conclusions

Everyone concerned with healthcare can benefit from a familiarity with health economists' ways of thinking, language, and some of the tools in the toolkit. Health economics gives a structured approach to decision making in healthcare where resources are always scarce, need appears almost limitless, and choices are inevitable. It is not a formulaic approach that bypasses critical appraisal, but it can greatly improve the rigour and transparency of the decision-making process.

Further resources

Brambleby P, Jackson, A, Knight K. Programme Budgeting and Marginal Analysis. HealthKnowledge (video course). Available at: ℗ www.healthknowledge.org.uk/interactivelearning/index_margins.asp (accessed 24 August 2019).

Donaldson C, Bate A, Brambleby P, Waldner H. (2008). Moving forward on rationing: an economic view. *British Medical Journal*, **307**, 905–6.

Mitton C, Donaldson D. (2001). Twenty-five years of programme budgeting and marginal analysis in the health sector, 1974–1999. *Journal of Health Service Research Policy*, **6**, 239–48.

National Institute for Health and Care Excellence. Available at: ℗ http://www.nice.org.uk/ (accessed 24 August 2019).

Ruta D, Mitton C, Bate A, Donaldson C. (2005). Programme budgeting and marginal analysis: bridging the divide between doctors and managers. *British Medical Journal*, **330**, 1501–3.

References

1 Drummond MF, O'Brien BJ, Stoddard GL, et al. (1997). *Methods for the economic evaluation of health care programmes*, 2nd edn. Oxford University Press, Oxford.

2 Robinson R. (1993). Economic evaluation and health care (a series of six articles in the BMJ). What does it mean? *British Medical Journal*, **307**, 670–3.

3 Robinson R. (1993). Costs and cost minimisation analysis. *British Medical Journal*, **307**, 726–8.

4 Robinson R. (1993). Cost effectiveness analysis. *British Medical Journal*, **307**, 793–5.

5 Robinson R. (1993). Cost utility analysis. *British Medical Journal*, **307**, 859–62.

6 Robinson R. (1993). Cost benefit analysis. *British Medical Journal*, **307**, 924–6.

7 Robinson R. (1993). The policy context. *British Medical Journal*, **307**, 994–6.

8 Enthoven A. (1999). *Rock Carling Fellowship 1999. In pursuit of an improving National Health Service*. Nuffield Trust, London.

9 Health Policy (1995). Special issue devoted to programme budgeting and marginal analysis, **33**.

10 McGuire A, Henderson J, Mooney G. (1988). *The economics of health care: an introductory text*. Routledge, London.

Part 2

Data and information

Chapter 2.1

Understanding data, information, and knowledge

Barry Tennison and Lamberto Manzoli

Objectives

The aim of this chapter is to help the public health practitioner to:
- appreciate the subtleties of the varied forms of information about the health of a population and related matters
- develop a toolkit for thinking about the complexity of information, its interpretation and uses
- orientate positively towards the decisions and actions needed, applying wisely the information and knowledge available.

In addition, the classification (taxonomy) of types of information given in this chapter should support the public health practitioner to:
- assess the relevance, timeliness, accuracy, and completeness of available information
- decide which types of information are most appropriate for a particular public health task
- make optimal use of information that is not ideal, and assess the effects of its departure from perfection.

The use of the words 'data' and 'information'

Some people are purists. They use the word 'data' (singular or plural) for raw numbers or other measures, reserving the word 'information' for what emerges when data is processed, analysed, interpreted, and presented. This has the virtue of making clear the sequence of steps that are involved in turning observations about the world into a form that is useful to decision makers. This always involves the use of judgement in assessing the information as a source of evidence, and combining this judiciously with accepted best practice to arrive at usable knowledge. This process is summarized in Figure 2.1.1.

In practice, most people use 'data' and 'information' more or less interchangeably, perhaps on the grounds of the greyness of some of these distinctions and steps. However, in assessing the value of what emerges as information from these steps, the practitioner must bear in mind the fundamental issues that affect the quality of the data:

- *Validity*: is the data capturing the concept or quantity the practitioner intends? Are the definitions and methods of data collection explicit and clear? Validity is a main concept, referred to in many steps of a study from test validity (accuracy: the degree to which it measures what it is supposed to measure, that is not to be confused with reliability—how consistent are the results of the test—and that is further subclassified into content, construct, and face validity), to internal and external validity (respectively, an inductive estimate of the degree to which conclusions about causal relationships can be made, based on the whole research design, and the extent to which internally valid results can be held to be true for other cases, e.g. to different people).

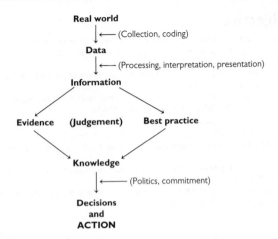

Figure 2.1.1 From reality to action.

- *Selection bias:* when the data misleads because the sample is not representative of the population being considered—for example, because of poor sampling.
- *Classification bias:* when there is a non-random effect on putting data into groupings. Misclassification can occur for any reason on both an exposure (classifying a man as a non-smoker when he actually smokes) and an outcome (classifying a patient as healthy when they are sick), and it may lead to bias when we have a different amount of misclassification in the groups being compared, or when it is so large as to produce an underestimation of an association.
- *Statistical significance:* when, although differences seem apparent, the analysis shows that they may have occurred by chance (see, e.g. Marshall and Spiegelhalter[1]).
- *Precision:* is the sample size sufficient to estimate the prevalence of disease (say) with precision? Similar to political polls, all epidemiological studies need to infer the results of the sample to the general population, computing the margin of error, which is expressed in the form of confidence intervals (95% safe). Thus, if we have a 7.5% incidence of a disease in our sample, how wide are the confidence intervals surrounding the estimate? If the interval is narrow, such as 7%–8%, our study has been able to provide precise estimates of what would reasonably be the incidence in the general population (between the two values), but, if the 95% confidence interval is wide (e.g. 2%–13%), uncertainty remains and the contribution of the study is minimal.

What kinds of data sources are there?

In most countries, there are many different sources of information on the health of the population.[2] Different types of information vary in their 'CART': Completeness, Accuracy, Relevance (and/or Representativeness), Timeliness.

Data sources also vary in the ease with which a 'base population' can be identified, for use in the denominator or for calculating rates. Typical data sources for local areas are summarized in Table 2.1.1.

Table 2.1.1 Data sources

Source	Strengths	Weaknesses
1. Routine data sources		
Population estimates. Census or population registers (demographic information, residence)	Usually reasonably accurate, especially if complemented by local authority or other government data	May be problems with small area estimates, especially between censuses
Birth and abortion notifications	Reasonably accurate— often several possible data sources	No complete data on spontaneous abortions. Sometimes non-standard coding used
Mortality records	Most reliable health data as death tend to be unequivocal. Total mortality reliable	Insensitive measure of health. Physician's cause of death specification often inaccurate or incomplete. Non-fatal disease not reflected in mortality figures
Health services data: access and supply, utilization, activity, costs. The main routinely collected datasets are hospital discharge data, pharmaceutical prescriptions, and ambulatory services	Extremely useful, especially if condition almost always results in healthcare use, e.g. fractured femur	Data quality, especially for outpatients services, may be suboptimal. May be difficult to obtain. All data coded, and the handling of several millions of repeated information (such a pharmaceutical prescriptions) can be challenging
Morbidity measures: infectious disease notifications (see ➜ Chapter 2.4)	Certain diseases notifiable (mandatory)	Often incomplete, especially for less severe diseases (e.g. chickenpox), sometimes inconsistently incomplete
Morbidity measures: other disease (e.g. cancer) registers (see ➜ Chapter 2.7)	Key group identified. Often do not cover whole country	May miss people due to no contact or non-identification. Validated information often 3–4 years old
Impairment, disability and handicap	Functional status sometimes more relevant than disease status	Usually available from surveys only (expensive)

Table 2.1.1 (*Contd.*)

Source	Strengths	Weaknesses
Data from other agencies—social care, housing, environmental exposure, etc.	Sometimes essential (e.g. assessment of the environmental risks)	May be poor quality and incomplete. Environmental exposure difficult to assess over time
2. Surveys (see ➔ Chapter 2.8)		
National surveys, or surveys from other countries	**Available.** May be authoritative and highly relevant	Require 'modelling' to local population characteristic. May not be generalizable to local population. Quality variable
Previous local surveys	Relevant and usually appeal to a local audience	Quality variable, difficult to find (grey literature)
Local surveys to be commissioned	Can be tailor-made	Often expensive
3. Qualitative data		
Local descriptive accounts of environmental or social factors	May give a good understanding or stimulate research	The scale of health impact of identified problems is typically difficult to assess
People's perceptions of how health problems affect them	May give a good understanding of what really affects people	Qualitative data can need careful handling, because details of context, background, and question wording can result in unstable responses

A 'population health information' system can help in assembling data sources on a population. Such systems often involve a partnership between different agencies involved with a population, and can allow linkage of data sources and coordination of health information activities. A comprehensive population health information system would ideally record both the following:

- *Personal health events:* both health-related occurrences (e.g. diseases) and states pertaining to an identified person (e.g. an exposure to a certain risk factor—smoking, or lifestyle behaviour).
- *Population health factors:* health-related features or occurrences that apply to an entire population defined by some combination of person, time, and place (examples are exposure of a defined population to a health risk like a toxic spill or prevalence of smoking in teenage girls in a specified locality, derived from a survey).

Such a system would also allow both routine and ad hoc analyses in such a way that both events and potential risk factors are linked.

What does the information describe?

Information about the health of a population can cover the following:

- *Demography:* the basic characteristics of the population, such as age, sex, geographic distribution, and mobility.
- *Health-related characteristics or risk factors:* such as measures of deprivation, living conditions, employment, housing, or more medical factors or physiologic measurements (e.g. blood glucose levels).
- *Health need data:* such as the distribution of the indications for an intervention such as hip replacement[3] or the distribution of different thresholds for intervention.
- *Mortality:* the death experience of the population, including causes of death and variation according to the dimensions of person, place, and time.
- *Morbidity:* the health or illness experience of the population, including prevalence and incidence of diseases.
- *Health service use data:* such as diagnoses, interventions, procedures, and health outcomes of interventions. It may be useful to distinguish patient interactions with *agents*, such as nurses or doctors, from their *settings*, such as hospital, day hospital, health centre, or home, in using the health service.
- *Health economic data:* often concerning the costs of interventions and the distribution of activity and costs at marginal or average levels.

Clarity and judgement are needed about when one of these types of data is being used as a *proxy* for another. For example, when mortality data is firm and morbidity data poor in quality, with care, mortality may be seen as a good proxy for morbidity. This might work well for certain kinds of heart disease or cancer, but very poorly for most mental health problems. Similarly, care is needed in moving from burden of disease (mortality, morbidity, or, even more carefully, health service use) to health *need*.

In terms of how it is collected, assembled, and made available, information can be one of the following:

- *Routine:* collected, assembled, and made available repeatedly, according to well-defined protocols and standards. Such data is usually part of a *system of data collection by which information is*:
  - made available at regular intervals
  - intended to allow tracking over time
  - codified according to national or international standards (e.g. as made in most hospitals, using the standardized codes of the international classification of diseases—icd[4]—to define a patient's diseases or interventions).
- *Specially collected:* for a particular purpose, without the intention of regular repetition or adherence to standards (other than those needed for the specific study or task). Such data is usually:
  - aimed at a specific, time-limited study or task
  - codified according to the task in hand and the wishes of the investigators (sometimes differently from suitable standard codes and methods that are available; an in-depth literature search should be made before performing any data collection)
  - difficult to compare (between times, places, and people) with routine data and other specially collected data.

Table 2.1.2 shows important examples of information according to these dimensions. Note that these are only *examples*, but the table may help to show where an existing, new, or proposed data source sits, and the corresponding opportunities and drawbacks.

Table 2.1.2 Information collected according to the dimensions 'routine' and 'specially collected'

	Routine data	Specially collected data
Demography	Census counts, birth registration	Survey of homeless, roofless, and rough sleepers
Risk factors	Census details, such as housing conditions. General practitioners' records (although often incomplete)	Survey of ethnicity and coronary risk factors. Local survey of tobacco or alcohol use
Mortality	Death registration, coroners' records, medical examiners' records	Cohort studies that search for deaths probably due to suicide, using multiple sources
Health service use	Use of in-patient beds. Attendances at out-patient department, emergency room, or physician's office.	Observational study of use of a hospital department. Follow-up study of outcomes of hip replacement
Morbidity	National health surveys (such as the Health Survey for England[a] or the National Health Interview Survey in the USA[b]). Disease notifications and registers. Health service utilization data where information on diseases diagnosed and interventions made during the stay can be used as proxies of morbidity (typically from hospital discharge abstracts)	Case finding for an outbreak. Survey to establish prevalence of a specific disease
Health need	As above, mainly estimated from health service utilization data: hospital diagnoses or pharmaceutical prescriptions can be used as proxies of health need	Survey of prevalence of indications for specific intervention, such as hip re-placement
Economic	Accounts of health service organizations. Cost and price tables[c, d]	Costing of an existing or proposed service

a) Department of Health. Health Survey for England. Available at: ॐ https://www.gov.uk/government/statistics/health-survey-for-england-health-survey-for-england-2015 (accessed 5 May 2017).

b) National Center for Health Statistics. National Health Interview Survey (NHIS). Available at: ॐ https://www.cdc.gov/nchs/nhis/ (accessed 5 May 2017).

c) Department of Health. NHS reference costs. Available at: ॐ https://www.gov.uk/government/collections/nhs-reference-costs (accessed 5 May 2017).

d) Centers for Medicare & Medicaid Services. Cost reports. Available at: ॐ https://www.cms.gov/Research-Statistics-Data-and-Systems/Downloadable-Public-Use-Files/Cost-Reports/ (accessed 5 May 2017).

Classification of intrinsic types of data

It is often useful to categorize data as 'hard' or 'soft' (Table 2.1.3). In fact, there is a spectrum from hard to soft data: data is never completely hard or soft.

Harder data tends to be:
- precise (or intended to be precise)
- numerical; if not, then coded according to a firm protocol
- reproducible and likely to be similar even if the data collectors or individuals studied are varied.

Softer data tends to be:
- qualitative, attempting to capture some of the subtlety of human experience
- narrative or textual in form, at least as they are collected
- imbued with some subjectivity, due to the complexity of the personalities of the data collectors and the individuals studied.

Table 2.1.3 Examples of data considered to be harder or softer

	Harder	Softer
Demography	Age and gender of an individual. Ethnic breakdown of a population according to a given ethnic classification. Proportion of houses with a specific amenity (e.g. a bath)	Narrative account of nature and composition of a neighbourhood
Risk factors	Blood pressure, proportion of smokers, non-smokers, and ex-smokers (according to precise definitions)	Patient experience of symptoms. Smoking 'careers' of teenagers
Mortality	Numbers dying of a specific disease. Survival data after specific interventions	Impact of deaths on survivors
Morbidity	Prevalence of disease in a population at a moment in time. Numbers of admissions to a particular hospital	Reasons why a family doctor refers patients to hospital. Reported quality of treatment given by a particular hospital

(Note that some people will use the term 'soft' when they wish to imply that the data has inherent tendencies to imprecision, even if they are 'hard' in the sense of being numeric or strongly coded.)

Also, note that the terms 'soft' or 'hard' are here applied only to data and not to disease outcomes or end points. The latter are often defined as 'soft' when they measure an intermediate parameter that is linked to the disease—e.g. decrease in blood pressure—or 'hard' when they measure the occurrence of the real disease—e.g. myocardial infarction or stroke)

Neither hard nor soft data is intrinsically better than the other. The utility of the information (in terms of better decision making) often comes from combining the two:

- Harder data usually allows more precise analysis and comparisons, but may fail to capture subtleties of human experience and preferences.
- Softer data usually captures more of the 'truth' about the world, but often at the expense of emphasizing the uniqueness of circumstances, rather than aiding comparisons and conclusions.

The important thing to assess is *fitness for purpose*: is the existing or proposed data fit for the purpose for which it is intended, the conclusion to be drawn, the decision to be made, or the action to be taken? For example, for deciding the allocation of resources, one requires relatively hard data to obtain a degree of precision and transparency, so that the judgements involved are explicit. On the other hand, soft data may be useful in deciding on a change in the pattern of services provided—for example, when a client population (such as teenagers) seems to make poor use of current services, a well-designed qualitative survey may reveal some of the reasons, and a potential service configuration response. Softer data is also essential when capturing patient preference[5] or professional experiences.[6]

Absolute and comparative information

Often data about one single location, one time, or one population is difficult to interpret in isolation—or, worse, seem to beg obvious conclusions when, in fact, *comparison* with similar data elsewhere, previously, or in another population suggests a different conclusion or decision.

Comparative data is essential and is available on a local, regional, national,[7–9] and international[10] level. The WHO publishes comparative data between countries, for example on comparative performance of health systems.[11]

Big Data

The term 'Big Data' refers to extremely large sets of complex, linkable information that require specialized computational tools to enable their analysis and interpretation. Beyond genomics and other 'omic' fields, Big Data includes medical, environmental, financial, geographic, and social media information, most of which was unavailable a decade ago and which will continue to grow, recorded by sources that are currently unimaginable.[12]

The potential health benefits are large: Big Data may improve health by providing insights into the causes and outcomes of disease, drug targets for precision medicine, and disease prediction and prevention. From simple cases, such as heart rate monitoring through wearable devices to prevent stroke among patients with arrhythmias, to complex artificial intelligence algorithms able to diagnose a rare form of leukaemia cross-referencing patient's genetic data with millions of scientific papers and datasets.[13]

Although there is growing enthusiasm for the notion of Big Data, the collection of more information has so far rarely translated into the generation of more actionable insights into the best ways of treating patients.[14] In fact, several issues remain to be addressed before healthcare systems might be able to make full use of Big Data, the first of which being data acquisition. Some data sources, such as sensor networks, can produce astonishing amounts of raw data, and frequently the information collected is not in a format ready for analysis. Given the underuse of existing uniform data standards for electronic medical records, we need analytic approaches that embrace the data turmoil by relying less on standardized data items and having the capacity to process data in any format.[14, 15] Also, much available information currently resides in separated silos with restricted access (e.g. genetic information stored in research databases separately from medical records): a lack of linkage that is frequently attributable not to technical difficulties but to privacy concerns.[16, 17] Indeed, privacy and data protection are further major challenges. Because medical data is considered among the most private of all information, when it comes to sharing such data, even the slightest risk of identifiability is deemed unacceptable. Yet, completely anonymizing data is a non-trivial endeavour.

A third main issue pertains to Big Data analysis interpretation. Although it may be rational to assume that Big Data are most commonly leading us to true findings, this may be far from reality. In fact, there are many possible sources of error: computer systems can have bugs, models almost always have assumptions, and results can be based on erroneous data.[17] Moreover, Big Data are observational in nature and fraught with many biases such as selection, confounding variables, and lack of generalizability.[12] And even when associations between variables are correct, there is potential for many false alarms triggered by large-scale examination of putative associations with disease outcomes. Somewhat paradoxically, the proportion of false alarms among all proposed 'findings' increases when more information can be measured, and spurious correlations and ecological fallacies may multiply. It must be kept in mind that Big Data strength is in finding associations, not in showing whether these associations have meaning, and finding a signal is only the first step.[12]

Big Data is a hypothesis-generating machine, but the pillars of evidence-based medicine still apply. Even after robust associations are established, evidence of health-related utility is needed, as well as replication of study findings and testing of emerging treatments and preventive tools.[12] As correctly acknowledged by the Very Large Data Bases Endowment organization, and as witnessed by the White House Big Data R&D Initiative[18] and the dedicated task forces created by the Heads of Medicines Agencies[19], there are multiple steps to the data analysis pipeline, whether the data is big or small, and at each step there is work to be done.[17] Big Data linkage and analyses are currently made with huge successes in several other fields of science, and it cannot be accepted any more that in medicine, an utmost priority for the human being, Big Data's vast potential benefits are neither achieved nor sufficiently pursued.

Assessing the appropriateness and usefulness of particular information

Experience shows the truth of the adage that the information you think you want is seldom the information you actually need; and the information you have seldom matches either need or want (often attributed to Finagle: in full, Finagle's law is often quoted thus: 'The information you have is not what you want; the information you want is not what you need; the information you need is not what you can get; the information you can get costs more than you want to pay.')

The pragmatic public health practitioner must learn to cope with what is possible, not to set impossible standards, and to make the appropriate allowances, professionally, for the shortcomings of the available information. Above all, public health practitioners must not allow themselves or others to despair and to declare tasks impossible without the necessary information (which is, in fact, unavailable or unfeasible).

This concept is far less obvious than it may seem, and in real practice public health professionals regularly deal with compromises on data. Box 2.1.1 is a checklist of issues to consider when assessing data or a data source for fitness for purpose. None of these issues is absolute, and the balance of advantage and disadvantage must be assessed using judgement.

Box 2.1.1 Checklist for assessing appropriateness and usefulness of data and data sources

Technical issues
- Are the definitions sufficiently clear and appropriate?
- Are the target and study populations sufficiently clear?
- Are the data collection methods sufficiently clear and sound?
- How complete, accurate, relevant, and timely is the data? How much does this matter?
- Do any differences that appear reach statistical significance, and what are the confidence limits or intervals?

Issues relating to the conclusion or decision involved
- Is the study population sufficiently representative of the target population for the purpose of the decision or proposed action?
- Do we need absolute or relative estimates to make the best decision?
- What precision is needed for the decision (taking into account confounding factors, random variation, and the influence of external factors such as resource availability, professional opinion, economic influences, and politics)?
- Would a simpler or existing data source suffice—for example, by using comparative data; by extrapolating or interpolating, with care; or by transferring data from a similar or analogous situation?
- Would qualitative information suffice (or be better), when habit automatically suggests quantitative data?

Conclusion

All too often, when faced with a decision, there is a call for more information (or, worse, a new information system). More frequently than it seems
at first view, either the available data is in fact, with care and interpretation, fit for the purpose for the decision needed, or the costs (including
money, skills, burden of effort, and delay) of the new information or system
is not commensurable with the problem faced. The above checklist, and this
chapter, should help the practitioner to find a pragmatic but wise balance
between what is needed and what is feasible and adequate.

Further resources

Reddy CK, Aggarwal CC. (eds) (2015). *Healthcare data analytics.* CRC Press, Taylor & Francis Group,
New York.

Rigby M. (ed.) (2004). *Vision and value in health information.* Radcliffe Medical Press, Oxford.

US Department of Health & Human Services. Available at: ℘ https://www.hhs.gov (accessed 5
May 2017).

World Bank Data. Health. Available at: ℘ http://data.worldbank.org/topic/health (accessed 5
May 2017).

References

1 Marshall EC, Spiegelhalter DJ. (1998). Reliability of league tables of in vitro fertilization
clinics: retrospective analysis of live birth rates. *British Medical Journal,* **316,** 1701–5.

2 Detels R, McEwen J, Beaglehole R, Tanaka H. (eds) (2002). *Oxford textbook of public health.*
Oxford University Press, New York.

3 Frankel S, Eachus J, Pearson N, et al. (1999). Population requirement for primary hip-replacement
surgery: a cross-sectional study. *Lancet,* **353,** 1304–9.

4 World Health Organization. *The WHO family of international classifications.* Available at: ℘
http://www.who.int/classifications/en/ (accessed 5 May 2017).

5 Silvestri G, Pritchard R, Welch HG. (1998). Preferences for chemotherapy in patients with advanced non-small cell lung cancer: descriptive study based on scripted interviews. *British Medical
Journal,* **317,** 771–5.

6 Jain A, Ogden J. (1999). General practitioners' experiences of patients' complaints: qualitative
study. *British Medical Journal,* **318,** 1596–9.

7 UK Office for National Statistics. Available at: ℘ https://www.ons.gov.uk (accessed 5
May 2017).

8 Statistics Canada. Available at: ℘ http://www.statcan.gc.ca/eng/start (accessed 5 May 2017).

9 CDC National Center for Health Statistics, USA. Available at: ℘ https://www.cdc.gov/nchs
(accessed 5 May 2017).

10 WHO Statistical Information System (WHOSIS). Available at: ℘ http://www.who.int/whosis/
en (accessed 5 May 2017).

11 WHO Health Systems. Available at: ℘ http://www.who.int/topics/health_systems/en (accessed 5 May 2017).

12 Khoury MJ, Ioannidis JP. (2014). Medicine. Big data meets public health. *Science,* **346,** 1054–5.

13 Otake T. (2016). IBM big data used for rapid diagnosis of rare leukemia case in Japan. *The
Japan Times.* Available at: ℘ http://www.japantimes.co.jp/news/2016/08/11/national/
science-health/ibm-big-data-used-for-rapid-diagnosis-of-rare-leukemia-case-in-japan/
#.WQirNmgVxnw (accessed 5 May 2017).

14 Schneeweiss S. (2014). Learning from big health care data. *New England Journal of Medicine,* **370,**
2161–3.

15 Park RW. (2017). Sharing Clinical Big Data While Protecting Confidentiality and
Security: Observational Health Data Sciences and Informatics. *Healthcare Informatics and
Research,* **23,** 1–3.

16 Faden RR, Kass NE, Goodman SN, et al. (2013). An ethics framework for a learning health care
system: a departure from traditional research ethics and clinical ethics. *The Hastings Center Report,*
Special number, S16–S27.

17 Labrinidis A, Jagadish HV. (2012). Challenges and opportunities with big data. *Proceedings of the VLDB Endowment*, 5(12).
18 Office of Science and Technology Policy, White House (2012). Obama Administration unveils 'Big Data' Initiative: announces $200 million in new R&D investments. Available at: ℘ https://obamawhitehouse.archives.gov/the-press-office/2015/11/19/release-obama-administration-unveils-big-data-initiative-announces-200 (accessed 5 May 2017).
19 European Medicines Agency (2017). HMA/EMA Joint Big Data Task Force. Available at: ℘ http://www.ema.europa.eu/docs/en_GB/document_library/Other/2017/03/WC500224262.pdf (accessed 5 May 2017).

Chapter 2.2

Information technology and informatics

Don Detmer

Objectives

After reading this chapter, you should be able to:

- identify the emerging sub-disciplines within biomedical and health informatics that are critical to the skilful use of health information and communications technology in the health sciences
- appreciate how informatics is applied to public health, clinical medicine, and research, and that its roles are in rapid evolution
- consider clinical informatics as a professional career choice regardless of your health discipline.

Introduction

Informatics relating to health encompasses significant applications in public health, clinical care, and biomedical research. Despite the relative youth of the scientific discipline, biomedical and health informatics are recognized widely as essential to competent practice as a health professional (see Box 2.2.1). This is due primarily to the limits of human cognition and the growth in the knowledge base of medicine. The limitations of natural human memory cannot match the capacity of relevant knowledge managed through computer systems. This is as true for public health and population health management as it is for 'just in time' patient-specific decision support at the point of care. Indeed, with the addition of genomics and proteomics, all patients acquire the equivalent of orphan diseases because each has unique biology and differing life experiences. Plus, the explosive growth of information and communications technology allows an infrastructure capable of supporting this trend. It is anticipated that continued evolution of learning health care systems consisting of adaptive evidence-based decision support systems will assure far greater efficiency, effectiveness, quality, safety, and integration of new knowledge resulting in better outcomes for individuals and populations. *Data analytics, augmented intelligence, and artificial intelligence are the newest emerging areas of development and application. These draw on machine learning, 'big data', and data science from within computer science.*

The field will expand to include informatics applications to traditional care plus primary prevention, health education, and computer-based therapies, including robotic surgery and self-administered programmes for cognitive psychological therapy. Models for all these dimensions exist today. Development of computer-based public health and population's records has lagged behind patient and personal health records in many nations, but this is likely to change dramatically over the next decade as the repositories of person-specific health data become more and more accessible to health system managers, clinicians, and researchers. *Computer-based patient records deserve renewed attention, especially to improve ease of use and to incorporate patient narratives.*

Box 2.2.1   Informatics

Informatics is an integrating scientific field that draws upon the information sciences and related technology to enhance the use of the knowledge base of the health sciences to improve healthcare, biomedical and clinical research, education, management, and policy.

Definition

While there is no formally accepted nomenclature or taxonomy for informatics relating to health today, one can identify seven overlapping yet somewhat distinct domains:

- *Translational bioinformatics:* computing for genomics, proteomics, epigenetics, and management of the knowledge bases these fields generate.
- *Clinical informatics, or informatics for use in patient care:* electronic medical records of three types: patient, personal, and population.
- *Public health informatics* or informatics relating to the health of populations, including populations with special needs.
- *Computer methods*, semantics, and ontologies for health applications, as well as natural language processing, data analytics, data science, 'big data', machine learning, augmented intelligence and artificial intelligence.
- *Consumer health*, or e-health informatics: including links to patients and professional caregivers.
- *Health information policy.*
- *Health information networks:* local, regional, national, and global.
- *Knowledge management:* utilizing structured databases such as results of randomized clinical drug trials.
- *Adaptive evidence-based decision support systems:* computer-based software that offers expert advice as guidelines and protocols, and the capacity to determine whether or not the advice proves to be good for a patient's health status or a population of generally similar people.

Some fields that integrate with informatics are as follows:

- Computer science, information and telecommunication science, cognitive science, statistics, decision science, and management/organizational science.
- Library science.
- Bioscience and biomedicine.
- Knowledge management, decision support.
- Evidence-based medicine, knowledge bases such as PubMed.
- Public and populations health sciences—biostatistics, epidemiology, health services research.
- Health policy and management, organization behaviour, risk management, quality and safety.
- Health values and bioethics.[1]

Using informatics in healthcare

Early use focused disproportionately on primary care settings in Europe and administrative functions and laboratory results reporting in North America, but attention was also given to improving decision making through clinical alerts and diagnostic supports. Widespread adoption of electronic medical record systems has been slower than desired because of a number of factors among which are perverse financial incentives, clinician resistance, awkward user interfaces, and legal and cultural barriers.[2] Recently, public investment has greatly improved widespread availability of electronic health records (EHRs) in the USA.

Robust systems are of necessity complex and they require a mixture of hardware, software, and maintenance. Relevant legal and policy infrastructures are essential to handle such issues as authentication, security, and confidentiality. Further, evolutionary standards are essential to enhance interoperability, refinement, and utility of data emerging from biomedical, clinical, and public health care, and research into relevant knowledge banks. Recently, a number of developed economies have embarked on national health information infrastructures and global efforts to collaborate on standards are underway.[3]

Once consistent inputs are made into EHRs, an era of precision care can begin. Meanwhile, genomics and proteomics reflecting the individual's make-up are beginning to introduce personalized medicine or precision medicine into care. The rise of the internet linked to the above components may in time dramatically change the practice of health care. For example, personal health records that allow a patient to interact with their clinicians and the patient's own medical record, whenever and wherever they wish, offer the potential to greatly improve performance and outcomes of a variety of chronic illnesses including home monitoring.[4] De-identified data from these records and other sources can then be used for a host of public health investigations including biosurveillance and community health.[5] Public policy relating to privacy can conflict with the need for access to person-specific data for a variety of types of biomedical and public health research.[6]

Implementation of computer systems into clinical environments typically involves substantial change in work processes, change management and an understanding of organizational behaviour as well as ongoing tailoring of software programmes to local circumstances.

Substantial creative efforts are needed to improve ease of use of patient records as well as to include patient narratives. Leadership is essential and complex adaptive systems theory is particularly useful in supporting implementation and gaining major improvements in performance, particularly for safety and quality of care.[7]

Evidence on IT systems improving care processes and outcome

A growing body of evidence reveals that computer-based health records systems (incorporating decision support) can improve the safety of care, particularly with respect to medications.[8]

Research is still needed, but there is evidence that EHRs, IT systems and communication technology can result in better care, better outcomes, and more informed patients.[9, 10] *Augmented intelligence coming from a combination of data analytics, neural networks, and deep learning techniques are beginning to improve clinical performance in selected areas such as management of sepsis.* Meanwhile, the impact of artificial intelligence on clinical care through the use of such methods as large datasets and machine learning techniques is just beginning and a wide range of issues are relevant.[11, 12, 13, 14, 15] Evidence of the usefulness of health information and communications technology for public health is needed. While more research would be helpful, the bulk of evidence today reveals that better-informed patients are less anxious, begin treatment earlier, are more satisfied with their care, follow advice better, opt for lower-risk interventions, and reduce health care costs through greater self-management and a more efficient use of resources.

IT and public health

Global epidemics such as HIV/AIDS or SARS offer real evidence that IT systems can be extremely important in determining the spread of a disease, analysing patient care data for clusters of symptoms to help understand the nature of the disease, and evaluating programmes that seek to manage the disease effectively. As the population health record matures during this decade, benefits are likely to become more impressive with ongoing surveillance critical for wellness programmes, community health, environmental risks, disease control, and potentially bioterrorism.[5]

Clinical informatics as a formal health professional discipline

Clinical informatics is a recognized clinical discipline in the USA, globally, and is emerging as such in the United Kingdom.[15] In 2011, clinical informatics was approved by the American Board of Medical Specialties as a medical subspecialty and certification examinations for informally trained informaticians began in 2013. By 2019, 1,868 physicians who already possess at least one specialty certificate are now also certified in clinical informatics. The USA Accreditation Council for Graduate Medical Education (ACGME) began formally accrediting Fellowship training programmes in 2014. By 2019, 34 programmes had ACGME approval. AMIA, the organization that serves as the professional home for health-related informaticians seeks to offer certification in advanced clinical informatics for all health professionals including non-boarded physicians who meet the entry criteria.[16] Globally, the International Medical Informatics Association has formed an International Academy of Health Sciences Informatics.

In the UK, the NHS has formed a Digital Academy for training chief information officers (CIOs) and chief clinical information officers (CCIOs). Additionally, The UK Faculty of Clinical Informatics was established in 2017 to give professional leadership to clinicians working in informatics in health or care who are registered with the UK councils that regulate health-related professions. Over 350 are now members. It approves clinical competencies required in informatics, accredits individuals, training programmes and course curricula, oversees appraisal and revalidation, and promotes career structures and opportunities in the discipline. It has established informatics as a safe, recognizable, respected and influential professional discipline in health and care in the UK.

An IT system that will deliver better quality and outcomes?

Capabilities in IT systems that are likely to improve patient safety, quality, and outcomes include electronic prescribing, continuity of care records that offer a concise summary of key patient data and can be accessed from a variety of clinical settings, decision support for medications that incorporate such capabilities as clinical alerts, reminders for preventive care, dosage calculation support, 'just-in-time' knowledge service, integrated evidence-based clinical pathways that allow for over-riding by the clinician, and personal health records that capture records added by the patient that include alternative medications not typically listed by patients in ordinary paper-based settings, and the capacity to aggregate performance data on clinical practice for both clinician and statistical analysis.

If one is 'shopping' to purchase a clinical IT system for use in either a primary care or institutional setting, it is important to visit sites that are actively using the system to determine its functionality in real-world terms. The more complex the system, the more important it is for a team to visit to assure that all key users' needs will be met. The capacity of systems to interoperate with other systems outside the core setting is of increasing importance. Ease of implementation, cost, and built-in decision support are other factors worthy of evaluation.[14]

A key challenge for complex institutions is assuring that the entire enterprise can cross-communicate. Dedicated systems for individual specialties may keep one set of consultants happy but greatly limit the capacity to achieve major gains in productivity across the institution.

Public health informaticians have recently generated a list of competencies for this discipline (see ⊃ Educational infrastructure below). Readers interested in a personal assessment of their informatics capabilities should find it helpful.

Further resources

There are far too many websites available to do justice to the issues raised here, but what follows will give the reader some sense of the scope of issues involved.

Medical knowledge bases

Clinical Trials are biomedical research databanks relating to clinical trials of medications. Available at: ℘ https://clinicaltrials.gov (accessed 18 August 2019).

UK Biobank is a major international health resource. Available at: ℘ https://www.ukbiobank.ac.uk (accessed 18 August 2019).

All of Us is a somewhat parallel effort in the USA. Available at: ℘ https://allofus.nih.gov/ (accessed 18 August 2019).

GenBank is a biomedical research databank at the National Center for Biotechnology Information (National Library of Medicine, National Institutes of Health) Available at: ℘ https://ncbi.nlm.nih.gov/genbank (accessed 18 August 2019).

Medline Plus is a website with range of consumer health information. Available at: ℘ https://medlineplus.gov (accessed 18 August 2019).

Public Library of Science. Available at: ℘ http://www.plos.org (accessed 18 August 2019).

PubMed Central® is a free continually updated source for access to the medical literature at the US National Library of Medicine. Available at: ℘ http://www.ncbi.nlm.nih.gov/pmc (accessed 18 August 2019).

Unbound Medicine. Available at: ℘ https://www.unboundmedicine.com (accessed 18 August 2019), Map of Medicine. Available at: ℘ https://medical-dictionary.thefreedictionary.com/Map+of+Medicine (accessed 18 August 2019).

Up-to-Date offers PDA and computer-based knowledge support for busy clinicians. Available at: ℘ https://www.uptodate.com/contents/search (accessed 18 August 2019).

Standards, vocabulary, and terminology

CDISC allows clinical research to work smarter. Available at: ℘ https://www.cdisc.org (accessed 18 August 2019).

Health Level 7 is a major standards development group. Available at: ℘ https://www.hl7.org (accessed 18 August 2019).

REDCap is a web application for standards compliant online surveys and databases. Available at: ℘ https://www.project-redcap.org (accessed 18 August 2019).

SNOMED-CT is a systematized nomenclature of medicine (SNOMED) that incorporates universal health care terminology. Available at: ℘ https://www.snomed.org (accessed 18 August 2019).

Unified Medical Language System® is a compendium of knowledge sources for medicine. Available at: ℘ http://www.nlm.nih.gov/research/umls (accessed 18 August 2019).

National health information infrastructures

Australia: My Health Record. Available at: ℘ https://www.myhealthrecord.gov.au (accessed 18 August 2019).

Canada: Health Infoway. Available at: ℘ https://www.infoway-inforoute.ca/en (accessed 18 August 2019).

UK: NHS England. Available at: ℘ https://www.england.nhs.uk/digitaltechnology (accessed 18 August 2019).

USA: The Office of the National Coordinator for Health Information Technology (ONC) Available at: ℘ https://www.healthit.gov (accessed 18 August 2019).

USA: National Committee on Vital and Health Statistics (NCVHS). Available at: ℘ http://ncvhs.hhs.gov/ (accessed 18 August 2019).

Educational infrastructure

NHS Digital Academy. Available at: ℘ https://www.england.nhs.uk/digitaltechnology/nhs-digital-academy/ (accessed 18 August 2019).

AMIA Academic Forum. Available at: ℘ https://amia.org/membership/academic-forum (accessed 18 August 2019).

Public health informatics training. Available at: ℘ http://www.cdc.gov/InformaticsCompetencies (accessed 18 August 2019).

References

1 Shortliffe EH, Cimino JJ. (2006). *Medical informatics: computer applications in health care and bio-medicine*, 3nd edn. Springer, New York.

2 Berner ES, Detmer DE, Simborg D. (2005). Will the wave finally break? A brief view of the adoption of electronic medical records in the United States. *Journal of the American Medical Informatics Association*, **12**, 3–7.

3 Detmer DE. (2003). Building the national health information infrastructure for personal health, health care services, public health, and research. *BMC Medical Informatics and Decision-Making*, **3**, 1–40.

4 Detmer DE, Bloomrosen M, Raymond B, et al. (2008). Integrated personal health records: Transformative tools for consumer-centric care. *BMC Medical Informatics and Decision-Making*, **8**, 45–72.

5 Friedman DJ, Parrish RG. 2nd (2010). The population health record: concepts, definition, design, and implementation. *Journal of the American Medical Informatics Association*, **17**, 359–66.

6 Nass SJ, Levit LA, Gostin LO. (2009). Beyond the HIPAA privacy rule: enhancing privacy, improving health through research. National Academy Press, Washington, DC.

7 Institute of Medicine (2001). Crossing the quality chasm: a new health system for the 21st century. National Academy Press, Washington, DC.

8 Bates DW, Gawande AA. (2003). Improving safety with information technology. *New England Journal of Medicine*, **348**, 25–34.

9 Chaudhry BD, Wang JD, Wu SD. (2006). Systematic review: impact of health information technology on quality, efficiency, and costs of medical care. *Annals of Internal Medicine*, **144**, 742–52.

10 Black AD, Car J, Pagliari C, et al. (2011). The impact of eHealth on the quality and safety of health care: a systematic overview. *PLoS Medicine*, **8**, e1000387. doi:10.1371/journal.pmed.1000387

11 Fairchild KD, Lake DE, Kattwinkel J, et al. (2011). Vital signs and their cross-correlation in sepsis and NEC: a study of 1,065 very low weight birth weight infants in two NICUs. *Pediatric Research*, **2**, 315–21.

12 Academy of Medical Royal Colleges. (2011). Artificial intelligence in healthcare. Available at: ℘ https://www.aomrc.org.uk/wp-content/uploads/2019/01/Artificial_intelligence_in_healthcare_0119.pdf (accessed 18 August 2019).

13. The National Academies of Sciences, Engineering, Medicine. (2016). Continuing innovation in information technology. Workshop report. National Academies Press. Available at: ℘ http://nap.edu/23393 (accessed 18 August 2019).

14 Blue Ridge Academic Health Group. (2018/19). *Separating fact from fiction: recommendations for academic health centers on artificial and augmented intelligence*. Report 23, winter. Emory University. Available at: ℘ http://www.whsc.emory.edu/blueridge (accessed 18 August 2019).

15 Detmer D, Shortliffe E. (2014). Clinical informatics: prospects for a new medical subspecialty. *JAMA*, **311**(20), 2067–8.

16 Gadd CS, Williamson JJ, Steen EB, et al. (2016). Creating advanced health informatics certification. *Journal of the American Medical Informatics Association*, **23**(4), 848–50.

17 Lorenzi NM, Kouroubali A, Detmer DE, et al. (2009). How to successfully select and implement electronic health records (EHR) in small ambulatory practice settings. *BMC Medical Informatics and Decision-Making*, **23**, 9–15.

Chapter 2.3

Questions, design, and analysis in qualitative research

Sara Mallinson, Jennie Popay, and Gareth Williams

Objectives

Our chapter provides a concise introduction to qualitative research methods and explains how a qualitative approach contributes to the public health evidence base and public health practice. After reading it, you will be able to:

- understand the key principles and features of qualitative research
- decide when a qualitative approach is most appropriate
- identify different study designs and methods and their strengths and weaknesses
- understand the main steps in analysis and how to reporting findings from qualitative research.

What is qualitative research?

Qualitative research refers to a range of design, data collection, and analysis strategies that are used to explore and build a better understanding of social phenomena. While there are many different approaches to qualitative inquiry, most have roots in interpretivist philosophy. This means the researcher starts from an assumption that social phenomena are created through processes of interpretation and construction by people experiencing them: rather than being fixed and 'objective'. If you have questions about people's perspectives or experiences, want to understand social structures and phenomena, or maybe aim to explain the complex way that structure and individual agency intertwine to lead to different outcomes, qualitative research is appropriate.

Qualitative research generates data in many different forms. Familiar formats include interview or focus group recordings and transcripts, diaries, observations or visual data such as video. For the many different approaches to collecting data, there are corresponding strategies for managing and analysing data. What most qualitative data analysis strategies share is sensitivity to the constructed nature of data. Qualitative researchers try not to treat their data as an objective 'slice of reality' because it is the product of contextually bounded 'meaning-making' between the researcher and the researched. Paying attention to the constructed nature of data, sometimes called 'reflexivity', is important in all the stages of qualitative research. The researcher (their interests, background, and theories), the study design (the sampling, the data collection method, and the analysis), and the context (where and how the study is conducted and with whom) will affect the outcome of the research. Instead of trying to control all these factors (which is impossible in naturally occurring settings), the researchers attempt to account for all possible influences. This 'transparency' at all stages of the research process *should* improve quality by surfacing the strengths and weaknesses of a piece of work. Unfortunately, qualitative research is not always done well, so an awareness of quality markers is important for those doing and using qualitative research.[1]

When to use a qualitative approach

Although qualitative health research has been used to address a wide range of questions, it is possible to group these into four broad types concerned with (i) the meanings different social groups attach to particular phenomena and how these interact with agency; (ii) perceptions about the needs of different social groups and how these needs can be met; (iii) barriers to and enablers of effective implementation and/or uptake of new policies/interventions/practices; and (iv) how understandings of subjective experience and meanings can help to explain results of larger quantitative studies.

In describing the type of knowledge produced by qualitative research addressing these questions and the general approaches used, we draw on examples of research involving people living in disadvantaged circumstances because of the significance of this work to public health practice. However, it is important to recognize that qualitative research has also been used to illuminate the social, cultural, and organizational factors shaping the behaviour of professional groups such as doctors and public health practitioners.[2]

The meanings different social groups attach to particular experiences and behaviours

Questions about the meanings individuals attach to phenomena and how these shape human 'agency' in the context of social structures are the core concern of qualitative research and underpin all the other types of questions. However, much of this research is primarily concerned to increase empirical and/or theoretical understanding about social life rather than explicitly to inform policy and/or practice, although the results can have important implications for both. These studies are often standalone, but some are linked with larger quantitative studies. Many use a single method of data collection, typically semi- or un-structured interviews. Others use multiple methods combining individual and group interviews or including observations.

This body of research includes studies of the meanings attaching to health-damaging behaviour (see Box 2.3.1) and of the experience of living in disadvantaged places (see Box 2.3.2). These studies highlight the need to contextualize risk factors, such as smoking, diet, alcohol, lack of exercise, and drug taking, by reference to the wider material and environmental conditions in which risks are embedded. They also reveal that 'lay knowledge' about the causes of ill health and health inequalities is complex and multi-faceted. This type of research can contribute to the planning and delivery of more appropriate interventions. Box 2.3.3 similarly focuses on research on lived experiences of inequalities but also illustrates how new multidisciplinary approaches to qualitative research are combining social science and arts-based approaches to co-produce research. Without the understanding studies such as these offer, public health practice may inadvertently reduce disadvantaged groups to unthinking bearers of various assets, deficits, and risks.

Box 2.3.1 Smoking and coping with poverty

Hilary Graham's study of smoking among women in the UK included secondary analysis of existing quantitative data on smoking prevalence among different groups and a qualitative study based on semi-structured interviews with a small sample of poor white mothers bringing up young children in poverty. In her analysis of the qualitative data, Graham developed the concept of smoking as a coping mechanism demonstrating how women caring for children while living in poverty relied on a cigarette to help them manage very stressful situations. Later research suggested that this relationship did not hold for mothers from South Asian and African Caribbean backgrounds.[a]

a) Graham H (1993). When life's a drag: women, smoking and disadvantage. HMSO, London.

Box 2.3.2 Understanding people, place, and health inequalities

A mixed-method study in four contrasting urban areas consisted of analysis of routine health data at local authority ward level, a household survey of perceptions of place and subjective health status in smaller neighbourhoods in these wards, and a longitudinal qualitative study using in-depth interviews with a small sample of adults drawn from the household survey. The findings of the qualitative study highlighted multiple pathways between the material, social, and psychological dimensions of place, health-related behaviours and health outcomes. People living in difficult circumstances acknowledged the differential impact of social and economic conditions on health but also emphasised 'strength of character' as a way of coping with these. The researchers argued that this was a form of resistance to the moral judgements made about poor people's failure to cope and their unhealthy behaviours.[a]

a) Graham H. (1994). Surviving by smoking. In: Wilkinson S, Kitzinger C, eds, Women and health: feminist perspectives. Taylor and Francis, London.

Subjective perceptions about the needs of different social groups and how these needs can be met

Qualitative health research addressing this type of question aims to contribute to the development of more appropriate or effective ways of preventing ill health and/or promoting health. One approach is to undertake a stand-alone qualitative study and then use the findings to develop a more appropriate intervention and evaluate it (see Box 2.3.3). Another is to embed qualitative research into a *health impact assessment* (HIA). HIA can be particularly useful to inform decisions in contested circumstances where official and community views could be in conflict (see Box 2.3.4). These studies provide a more holistic picture of the phenomenon under investigation by incorporating the perspectives of different stakeholders and combining different types of knowledge and evidence. HIAs may also use participative qualitative approaches involving the group targeted by a proposed intervention in the design and conduct of the research.

Box 2.3.3 Using visual arts and theatre to debate research findings on everyday life, health, and well-being

Against a background of negative reporting by various media, particular places become tarnished with 'territorial stigma' in discourses that seek to blame people for the poverty-related troubles they face.[a, b] This study uses traditional social science methods alongside arts-based approaches to explore and challenge media and related policy representations and to create spaces where policy issues, such as health and well-being, can be discussed and research co-produced in the context of everyday local concerns.[c, d] The project used a multi-generational approach to data collection, working with participants ranging from primary school pupils to older adults. Data was generated using interviews and group discussion, photography, songs, digital stories, and poetry. The findings related to the physical environment, housing, volunteering, the job centre, benefits sanctions, drug misuse, vandalism, social and informal support, networks, community spirit, future aspirations, and pride. The climax was a piece of theatre, *The People's Platform*[e], derived from the data that aimed to create a sensory form of 'locational narratives'[f] and a space for dialogue and understanding between community members and decision-makers. The purpose of drama was to relate the findings to current policy debates on well-being, co-creating a powerful drama while maintaining the integrity of the data. To make this connection between the micro-social and policy, we linked the event to the Well-being of Future Generations (Wales) Act 2015.

a) Tyler I. (2013). Revolting subjects: social abjection and resistance in neoliberal Britain. Zed Books. London.

b) Wacquant, L. (2007). Territorial stigmatization in the age of advanced marginality. Thesis Eleven, 91(1), 66–77.

c) Byrne E, Elliott E, Williams, G. (2015). Poor places, powerful people: co-producing cultural counter-representations of place, Visual Methodologies, 3(2), 77–85.

d) Byrne E, Elliott E, Williams, G. (2016). Performing the micro-social: using theatre to debate research findings on everyday life, health and well-being, Sociological Review, 64(4), 715–33.

e) A film about the response to the People's Platform. Available at: ♫ https://www.youtube.com/watch?v=fH2JwZRdMnU (accessed 9 August 2019).

f) Paton K. (2013). Housing in 'hard times': marginality, inequality and class. Housing, Theory and Society, 30, 84–100.

Box 2.3.4 Health impact assessments

A recent HIA of plans to demolish sub-standard housing in a South Wales community included a qualitative study (involving individual in-depth interviews and focus groups) alongside public meetings and secondary analysis of existing data about the locality. Although in theory the plan could be seen to be positive with clear health benefits, the qualitative findings revealed that, despite recognising housing problems, residents and local professionals were ambivalent and uncertain about the developments because of the potential disruption to social and family networks.[a]

a) Mukoma W, Flisher AJ. (2004). Evaluations of health promoting schools: a review of nine studies, Health Promotion International, 19(3), 357–68.

Barriers to, and enablers of, effective implementation and/or uptake of interventions and/or services

Qualitative research is a common element of process evaluations that aim to understand the strengths and weaknesses of new policies, interventions, or practices, and to identify the factors that impinge on successful implementation. Process evaluations are typically mixed method and the qualitative element is usually not an identifiable separate study. They may focus on a single 'case' or involve a series of case studies as with the process evaluations of healthy school initiatives.[3] Process evaluations involving integrated qualitative elements or separate qualitative studies can also be embedded in impact evaluations using experimental or quasi-experimental designs (See Box 2.3.5).

Box 2.3.5 Qualitative research and process evaluations

A trial aimed at reducing smoking in early teenage years through a 'peer-led' intervention used qualitative methods as part of a process evaluation that aimed to understand the strengths and weaknesses of the intervention design.[a]

A randomized controlled trial of the installation and use of domestic smoke alarms included an embedded qualitative study that used semi-structured interviews to explore people's perceptions of the risk of fire, and barriers and enablers to the installation and maintenance of domestic smoke alarms.[b]

a) Roberts H, Curtis K, Liabo K, et al. (2004). Putting public health evidence into practice: increasing the prevalence of working smoke alarms in disadvantaged inner city housing, Journal of Epidemiology and Community Health, 58(4), 280–5.

b) Noyes, J, Popay, J. (2007). Directly observed therapy and tuberculosis: how can a systematic review of qualitative research contribute to improving services? A qualitative meta-synthesis, Journal of Advanced Nursing, 57(3), 227–43.

Understanding subjective experience and meaning to explain results of larger quantitative studies

The findings of the process evaluations described in Box 2.3.5 were used to understand the results of the randomized controlled trials in which they were embedded. For example, the qualitative study of smoke alarm use found that people disabled alarms because they went off when they were cooking. Qualitative research conducted independently of a larger quantitative study can also be used in this way. For example, Noyes and Popay[4] conducted a systematic review of qualitative research on help-seeking behaviour in an effort to explain the diverse results of multiple trials of tuberculosis treatment interventions.

Qualitative study designs and methods

There are a range of study designs used in qualitative research (sometimes referred to as 'methodology') and within these designs different methods of data collection can be used. A study design should be tailored to answer a particular research question. Choices about scope, ethics and access, feasibility and timing, sample size, sampling strategy, data collection method and analysis technique should all be addressed at the stage of planning a research project. Qualitative research can be unexpectedly time-consuming. A poorly planned project will usually produce poor-quality results. Below, the most common types of design are briefly described. More details can be found in the texts listed in the bibliography.

Study designs

Ethnography

- Studies of communities or groups of people in their naturally occurring settings using a range of methods.

The focus is on developing a holistic, in-depth understanding of the social context and 'way of life' of the community or group through immersion in and understanding of its social milieu. Participant observation is a key element of most ethnographies, alongside other data collection methods. A classic ethnography in the health field is Goffman's[5] 1961 study of a single mental hospital for which he posed as a member of staff for over a year. This work has had a profound impact on mental health policy and practice around the world.

Case study

Generally case study designs involve the systematic study of an individual, a group, or an event with a view to understanding why something happens in a particular context. There is less emphasis on members' tacit knowledge than in ethnography, although the study can incorporate a similar range of data, collected from different sources.

Action research

A combination of action and research (usually in cycles) in which the researcher and participants perform an action, reflect upon it, and then use this knowledge to perform the next action. The emphasis is on the development of practices.

Grounded theory

- A methodology where data collection and analysis are conducted at the same time in an iterative process with the one informing the other.

Data analysis produces theoretical insights and these are used to collect new data through theoretical sampling to 'test' the theoretical ideas further. This process continues until categories and relationships are 'saturated' (i.e. new data does not lead to new developments in the theory developed in the analysis). Thus the theory generated is 'grounded' in the data.

Data collection methods

While ethnographies and case studies will often use more than one type of data collection to get different perspectives, it is also acceptable to use just one method to collect data. Some common methods are as follows.

Observation

Researchers attempt to immerse themselves in a study context to watch 'everyday' activities and practices in their natural context. Observers may be participant (fully active members of the context) or non-participant (maintaining distance from the context by not having a formal role in the activities there). The ethical challenges of being an observer have been a source of debate (covert observation, of the kind commonly used in journalism, is particularly delicate and not often undertaken). The legitimacy of non-participant observation has been questioned as researcher presence may change the context under investigation. Most observation studies use field diaries to record data. Occasionally, video and audio recording may be used.

Interviews

Individual in-depth interviews are a commonly used approach in qualitative research. They usually involve the identification of a particular sample of people who have experience or knowledge about the topic of interest (e.g. a health condition, an intervention, a place). Many studies use a purposive/purposeful sampling strategy to identify and recruit people for interview. This sometimes involves an intensity sample (targeting people who are very similar—for example, females, under-25s, using service X) or a diversity sample (people selected to represent different dimensions such as age, sex, social class, urban living or rural, etc.) Sample sizes can vary, but typically include 20–30 interviewees to achieve data 'saturation' (that means reaching the point where no new concepts or ideas are emerging). Interviews can be unstructured and allow an interviewee to speak freely (e.g. oral history or life history) or use a topic guide to semi-structure the talk and ensure a shared set of topics are discussed with each interviewee. Topic guides and similar tools used in qualitative interviews always have open-ended questions and allow people to express ideas and talk about experiences in their own words. The interviews are usually recorded and transcribed for analysis.

Focus group discussion

A small number of subjects are brought together to discuss the topic of interest (ideally 6–8 people). Care is taken with the composition of the group to ensure that members do not feel intimidated but can express opinions freely. A topic guide is usually used to focus the discussion and the researcher moderates the group to ensure that group dynamics are managed and that a range of aspects of the topic are explored. The discussion is frequently tape-recorded and transcribed for analysis.

Diaries/autobiographies

Participants keep a diary for a set period focusing on key events they judge to be memorable. The method is particularly good for longitudinal data collection where recall may be a challenge and where repeated interviews are not feasible. Diaries may be more or less structured and may be paper-based, computer-based, or online blogs. The data is likely to be analysed in the same way as an interview transcript.

Analysing and reporting qualitative data

Qualitative analysis is the point at which data and theory are examined together to try and generate new understandings and explanations of social phenomena. Done well, it is a time-consuming and intellectually challenging process and new researchers will frequently underestimate the time required for an analysis phase. Two elements in the analysis process can be distinguished: the purpose (what is being sought) and the practice (how it is done). These are briefly discussed below and more details can be found in the resources listed at the end of the chapter.

The purpose of data analysis

As we have already said, the purpose of a research project (defined by the research questions) should shape the study design and methods for data collection (e.g. whether interviews or observations have been conducted). This purposeful data collection should also shape how questions are asked and the extent to which something like an interview, for example, is guided by the researcher (as in a traditional topic-guided interview) or left to run with as little intervention as possible (e.g. in life-history work). How data are analysed will be driven by these interests. For example, one might perform a narrative, life-history, discourse, or conversation analysis (CA) on the same extract from an interview. Hence the importance of surfacing the researcher standpoint and the theory driving a particular piece of research. Some examples of different approaches to analysis are summarised below.

Narrative analysis

Looks at the way a person constructs a 'story' in the light of the audience and their purpose for giving the account. There is a focus on language, imagery, metaphor, and rhetorical purpose in the story being told.

Content analysis

Looks at the way themes and issues arise across texts (including interview transcriptions). Analysis may focus on the context, frequency, and/or how themes are patterned by, for example, gender or ethnicity. This is a descriptive level of analysis.

Conversation analysis

Focuses on the structure of communication and conversation management such as turn taking, grounding, pause with the aim of revealing how *meaning* is constructed in interaction. CA is a very specialized form of analysis, and marks both words spoken and how conversation proceeds (e.g. intonation).

Discourse analysis

Explores the way knowledge is produced in particular contexts through the use of specialised language or theories and through performances, interaction, and rhetorical devices used to persuade. A range of texts can be analysed (e.g. interview transcripts, video, letters, policy documents).

The practice of data analysis

There are different approaches to qualitative data analysis (QDA) underpinned by different theories but some common elements can be identified. In the broadest terms, QDA involves identification of themes, concepts, and categories in order to develop ideas or 'theories' about the data and relationships within it.

Most researchers begin by getting to know their data—for example, by mapping instances of events and themes before moving on to more abstracted and theoretical analysis. However, if grounded theory is being used, rudimentary and emergent theoretical categories would be introduced at a much earlier stage to inform further data collection.

Thematic analysis involves sifting and reducing raw data to an accessible summary of 'themes' identified in the data about the nature of whatever topic is being researched—whether it is living through urban regeneration, experiencing depression, doing public health work, or being incontinent. One approach to thematic analysis is to use a 'code and retrieve' system. This involves devising a system of codes and applying these across the whole dataset (e.g. all interview transcripts) to maximise opportunities for exploring emerging themes and areas of difference or non-conformity. This is a useful process of immersion, although it can be time-consuming. While manually indexing transcripts is feasible, many qualitative researchers use computer-aided qualitative data analysis software (CAQDAS) to facilitate the process. Whether done manually or with software, the system for thematic analysis should be as follows:

- Order and sort raw data into a manageable form.
- Ensure that analysis is rigorous and transparent.
- Allow within- and across-case searching to identify recurring categories and typologies.
- Allow easy movement from categories and themes back to raw data to check that the link between analysis and data is maintained during abstraction.
- Allow for revision and additions to be made as ideas are 'tested'.

While computer software can help with various stages of analysis, it will not perform analysis. The intellectual work of devising coding schemes and developing theories about the data is the responsibility of the researcher. Software is simply a tool that can help with the systematic sorting of data, if appropriately applied.

Conclusion

This chapter aims to introduce the reader to some of the most common approaches to qualitative work, the importance of ensuring that qualitative research remains sensitive to the constraints of data and context, and the value of qualitative research for public health practice. Issues around ethical research practice and governance are important features of good-quality qualitative research and all research must be planned and executed with appropriate protection for the participants involved (public or professionals). We acknowledge that this is a brief review and only touches lightly on a range of complex issues. The references below provide more detailed discussion of qualitative methods, analysis, and study appraisal. While training and excellent books and papers on qualitative methods are available to those wishing to explore qualitative research, seeking out qualitative expertise for research teams is essential. Fully embracing the contribution of qualitative data and qualitative thinking in a field like public health, which is dominated by quantitative approaches, requires an openness of perspective, but bringing together qualitative and quantitative research will enhance the public health evidence base. Science cannot develop if it remains trapped within dualisms that cut it off from the insights and understandings provided by qualitative forms of social science.[6]

Further reading

Bourgault I, Dingwall R, de Vries R. (eds). (2010). *Qualitative methods in health research*, Sage, London.
Creswell JW, Poth CN. (2017). Qualitative inquiry and research design, 4th edn, Sage, London.
Denzin KN, Lincoln YS. (2005) *The Sage handbook of qualitative research*, 3rd edn, Sage, London.
Hammersley M, Atkinson D. (1983). *Ethnography: principles in practice*. Tavistock, London.
Morgan D. (1996). *Focus groups as qualitative research*. Sage, London.
Pope C, Mays N. (2006). *Qualitative research and health care*, Blackwell Publishing, Oxford.
Ritchie J, Lewis J. (2003). *Qualitative research practice*. Sage, London.
Ruben, H. Ruben I. (2005). *Qualitative interviewing: the art of hearing data*. Sage, London.
Silverman D. (2006). *Interpreting qualitative data*, 3rd edn. Sage, London.
Yin RK. (2008). *Case Study Research: Design and methods*. Sage, London.

References

1 Seale C. (1999). *The quality of qualitative research*. Sage, London.
2 Mallinson S, Popay J, Kowarzik U. (2006). Developing the public workforce: a 'communities of practice' perspective. *Policy and Politics*, **34**(2), 265–85.
3 Campbell R, Starkey F, Holliday J, et al. (2008). An informal school-based peer-led intervention for smoking prevention in adolescence (ASSIST); a cluster randomized trial. *Lancet*, **371**, 1595–602.
4 Noyes, J, Popay, J. (2007). Directly observed therapy and tuberculosis: how can a systematic review of qualitative research contribute to improving services? A qualitative meta-synthesis, Journal of Advanced Nursing, 57(3), 227–43.
5 Goffman E. (1961). *Asylums: essays on the social situation of mental patients and other inmates*. Doubleday/Anchor, New York.
6 Midgley M. (2001). *Science and poetry*. Routledge, London.

Epidemiological approach and design

Walter Ricciardi and Stefania Boccia

Objectives

- Understand epidemiological thinking and approaches in a public health context.
- Use the most appropriate measures of disease occurrence.
- Measure the association between an exposure and a health event by using a two-by-two table (consider Table 2.4.1 in Box 2.4.1).
- Measure the impact of a certain disease at the population level.
- Identify the main epidemiological studies.

For more detailed discussion on epidemiologic understanding, refer to a standard textbook.[1]

Thinking epidemiology

Epidemiology is the core science of public health, and may be defined as 'the study of the occurrence and distribution of health-related states or events in specified populations, including the study of the determinants influencing such states, and the application of this knowledge to control the health problems'.[2] One of the first examples of an epidemiological approach within a public health context comes from London, 1854, when John Snow first proposed the mechanism for the transmission of cholera. He did this by systematically collecting data regarding the affected individuals. In doing so, he discovered an association between cholera diffusion and a local public water pump. Prior to the discovery of bacteria, Snow pushed the local health authorities to close the water pump, eventually resulting in the end of the epidemic.

Modern epidemiology starts in late 1940s, with a more systematized body of principles for the design and evaluation of epidemiological studies. The largest formal human experiment ever conducted was the Salk vaccine field trial in 1954, the results of which laid the foundation for the prevention of paralytic poliomyelitis. In recent years, epidemiologic research has steadily attracted public attention, with the news media boosted by increasing social concern about health issues. Examples are H1N1 influenza, hormone replacement therapy and heart disease, the effectiveness of mammography screening in the prevention of breast cancer, and many others.

Measuring disease occurrence

Three key measures of disease occurrence are *risk*, *incidence rate*, and *prevalence* (see Box 2.4.1).

Risk or incidence proportion

This is calculated as the proportion of individuals developing a certain disease or event during a time period divided by the number of subjects at risk to develop the same disease at the beginning of the study. It can be interpreted as the probability that a person will develop a certain disease in the time period considered. Calculation of risks implies that the entire denominator does not change during the study period. However, unless the

Box 2.4.1 The 2 × 2 table, with details of occurrence, associations, and impact according to the study design

Table 2.4.1. Two-by-two table

		Disease		
		Present	Absent	Total
Exposure	Present	a	b	a+b
	Absent	c	d	c+d
	Total	a+c	b+d	N

Cross-sectional studies
- Prevalence of disease = $a+c/N$
- Prevalence of disease in exposed = $a/a+b$
- Prevalence of disease in unexposed = $c/c+d$

Cohort studies
- Risk of disease in exposed (R_1) = $a/a+b$*
- Risk of disease in unexposed (R_0) = $c/c+d$*
- Relative risk or risk ratio = R_1/R_0
* denominators change if person-time (PT) can be calculated
- Incidence rate of disease in exposed (IR_1) = a/PT_1,
- Incidence rate of disease in unexposed (IR_0) = a/PT_0
- Rate ratio = IR_1/IR_0.

Measures of impact
- Attributable Fraction = $(R_1-R_0)/R_1 = 1-(1/RR) = (RR-1)/RR$
  Attributable Fraction in the population = $(R-R_0)/R$, where R is the risk of disease in the entire population under study (= $a+c/N$).

Case-control studies
- Odds of disease among exposed = a/b
- Odds of disease among unexposed = c/d
- Odds ratio = $a/b/c/d = a×d/b×c$

time is very short, populations usually change over time. As such, it is always advisable to use the incidence rate.

Incidence rate

This is the rate at which new events occur in a population. The numerator is the number of new events that occur in a defined period or other physical span. The denominator is the population at risk of experiencing the event during this period, sometimes expressed as person-time (PT).

Prevalence proportion

Prevalence proportion is a measure of disease status in a population, as such it is a measure of disease burden. It is calculated by dividing the total number of individuals who have an attribute or disease at a particular time by the population at risk of having the same attribute or disease at that time.

In a steady state, prevalence depends on the incidence and the duration of the disease (Prevalence = Incidence × Duration).

Prevalence data is used to plan health services and allocate resources. Prevalence proportion is commonly used in cross-sectional studies (see Box 2.4.1).

Risk and incidence rates, on the other hand, are useful for predicting the risk of a disease, to identify causes and treatment of the disease, to *describe trends* over time, and for evaluating the efficacy or effectiveness of preventive programmes.

Practical examples are shown in Box 2.4.2.

Other occurrence measures commonly used in healthcare are:

- *attack rate* = the proportion of a group that experiences the outcome under study over a given period (e.g. the period of an epidemic)
- *death rate* = an estimate of the proportion of a population that dies during a specified period.

Box 2.4.2 Measures of occurrence, impact, and association

- *Risk:* assume you wish to measure the annual occurrence of an hypothetical disease in a population of 100,000 individuals. During the year study period, 1,400 cases were detected, so that the annual risk (R) of disease is 1,400/100,000 = 0.014 (or 1.4%) (see Table 2.4.2)
- *Incidence rate:* suppose that from Table 2.4.2, during the 12-months study period, 100 of 100,000 individuals initially at risk died and that 200 individuals left the study and were no longer traceable. All these 300 people left the study 6 months after the study commenced: that is, 300 individuals contributed only 6 months of follow-up, with the loss of 150 person-years. Suppose again that all the 500 cases of the hypothethical disease arise after 5 month, so that these 1,400 cases contribute each to 5 month person-time at risk. Therefore, the remaining 7 months for each of the 1,400 cases cannot be considered as time at risk in the denominator, and should be removed: 1,400 persons × 7 months = 9,800 person-months = 816.6 person-years. Therefore, the denominator for the incidence rate is 100,000 − 150 − 816.6 = 99,033.4 person-years. Thus, incidence rate = 1,400 cases/ 99,033.4 person-years = 0.0141 cases/person-years, or 1.41 cases for 100 person-years.
- *Prevalence proportion:* the prevalence of disease among exposed from the Table 2.4.2 is 500/90,000 = 0.0055 = 0.55%.
- *Measures of association:* From the study in Table 2.4.2 we can calculate the risk ratio = [(a/a+b)/(c/c+d)] = (500/10,000)/(900/ 90,000) = 5.0. Alternatively, if the same data were from a case-control study, the appropriate measure of association would be the

Box 2.4.2 (*Contd.*)
odds ratio = (axd/bxc) = 5.21. These similar results show that there is an excess of risk of disease associated with the exposure.
- *Attributable Fraction* (AF): from the study reported in Table 2.4.2, the AF% = $R_1 - R_0 / R_1$ = (500/10,000) – (900/90,000)/(500/10,000) = 0.80.
- *Interpretation*: the exposure appears to account for 80% of the disease that occurs among exposed people during the 1-year period.
  - *Attributable Fraction* (AFp) in the population: using the same data from Table 2.4.2, the AFp would be = $R - R_0 / R$ = (1,400/100,000) – (900/90,000)/ (1,400/100,000) = 0.286. *Interpretation*: 28.6% of the disease that occurs among the entire population during the 1-year period are attributable to the exposure.

Table 2.4.2 Hypothetical Data giving 1-year disease risk for exposed and unexposed people

		Disease		
		Present	Absent	Total
Exposure	Present	500	9500	10,000
	Absent	900	89,100	90,000
	Total	1,400	98,600	100,000

Measures of association

Measuring the effect of a certain exposure or intervention on health status is a key objective of epidemiologic research. There are several approaches to measure associations depending on the type of study design adopted. Consider the two-by-two table (see Box 2.4.1), reporting the absolute number of individuals according to the two main dichotomous characteristics under investigation: disease and exposure.

Two main different measures of association are commonly used, according to the study design that generates the data. These are the *relative risk* (RR) and the *odds ratio* (OR) (formulas in Box 2.4.1, example in Box 2.4.2):
- RR is the ratio of the risk of an event among the exposed to the risk among the unexposed. This usage is synonymous with risk ratio. It can be calculated only in cohort studies.
- OR estimates the RR when this cannot be calculated directly. What we compare are not risks but *Odds* of disease among exposed and unexposed, where the Odds are the ratio of the probability of occurrence of an event to that of non-occurrence. This can be calculated in both cohort and case-control studies.

How to interpret a relative risk (and odds ratio)?

Relative risk is equal to 1 when the exposure does not affect the disease's onset, while it is higher than 1 if the exposure increases the risk for the studied disease, or lower than 1 if the exposure decreases the risk for that disease. An RR can vary between 0 and ∞. The RR indicates the *relative effect* of the exposure against the non-exposure. If the relative effect is = R_1 − R_0 (also called *risk difference* [RD]) divided by R_0, this can easily be re-written as RR − 1. For example, if we have an RR of 2.50, the relative effect of the exposure is to increase the risk of disease by 150%. Compared with those unexposed. If an effect is described as a 10% increase in risk, it will correspond to an RR of 1.10. A protective exposure (e.g. vaccination) may lead to an RR of 0.80, a reduction in risk among the exposed of 20%.

Measures of impact

When we measure the association between a certain exposure and a disease/event within a cohort study design, we may also wish to take into account the burden of that disease at the population level. These further measures are 'Attributable Fraction' and 'Attributable Fraction for the population' (see Box 2.4.1):

- The *Attributable Fraction* (AF) (or 'attributable proportion') is the proportion of disease burden among exposed people that is caused by the exposure. It is estimated by subtracting the risk of the outcome among the unexposed from the risk among the exposed individuals, divided by the risk in the exposed (see Box 2.4.1–2).
- The *Attributable Fraction in the population* (AFp) quantifies the proportion of disease burden in the population that is caused by the exposure. It is estimated by subtracting the risk of the outcome in the entire population from the risk among the unexposed individuals, divided by the risk in the entire population (see Boxes 2.4.1–2).

Epidemiological study designs

The simplest studies estimate a risk and an incidence rate or a prevalence, while 'analytical' studies examine putative causal relationships. Epidemiological studies may be classified as in Figure 2.4.1.

In *experimental studies* (intervention studies), the investigator intentionally alters one or more factors, and controls the other study conditions in order to analyse the effects of so doing. A key issue in experimental studies is the comparability of the groups under treatment, which is obtained by a randomization process (see Chapter 2.5).

These include:

- *randomized controlled trials* (RCTs): epidemiological experiments in which subjects in a population are randomly allocated into groups, usually called 'intervention' and 'control' groups, to receive or not to receive an experimental preventive or therapeutic procedure or intervention (e.g. efficacy of statins versus placebo in preventing cardiovascular diseases among hypercholesterolemic patients).

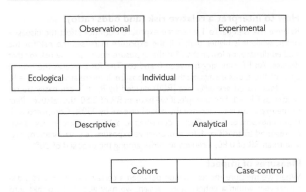

Figure 2.4.1 Types of epidemiological study.

- other trials such as *field trials*, conducted in the general population, or in primary care setting among non-diseased subjects [e.g. efficacy of vaccination with hepatitis B virus [HBV] in a certain high-risk population for the prevention of HBV infection]; *community intervention trials* in which the unit of allocation to receive a preventive, therapeutic, or social intervention is an entire community or political subdivision (e.g. efficacy of fluoridation of potable waters for the prevention of dental caries).
- *observational studies*, which do not involve intervention (experimental or otherwise) on the part of the investigator.

Among them we have:

- *Ecological studies*, in which the units of analysis are populations or groups of people rather than individuals. Usually data comes from updated current statistics—for example, mortality rate data from national bodies or tumour incidence data from registers. With respect to the individual studies, ecological studies have the strengths of being economic and easy to perform using routinely collected data. Sometimes it is the only approach that can investigate environmental determinants of health: the studies allow the researcher to explore associations that cannot easily be done at the individual level (e.g. the relationship between mortality and income[3]) and, finally, they allow the study of the effect of exposures that vary strongly between populations but little within populations. Ecological studies are useful to generate hypotheses on a certain relation between an exposure and a disease, which is usually tested later using individual data.
- *Individual studies* can be classified into *descriptive studies* and *analytical studies*, depending on whether the study aims to simply describe the distribution of a disease in a population according to some covariate(s), or to study the association between a disease and a postulated risk factor, respectively.

- *Descriptive studies* (*cross-sectional studies* or *prevalence studies*) are concerned with and designed only to describe the existing distribution of variables without much regard to causal relationships or other hypotheses. These studies find broad applications in public health—for example, investigating the lifestyle habits in the population (e.g. smoking habits among elderly people[4]) or the knowledge of the population of a certain health problem in order to better tailor educational programmes (e.g. knowledge of cervical cancer risk factors in the population[5]) and to quantify a certain health condition in a subgroup of population to plan screening programmes (e.g. prevalence of extrapancreatic malignancies among high-risk groups[6]). In *cross-sectional studies*, a critical issue is sampling in a population that is truly representative of the entire population that we wish to describe.
- *Analytical studies* allow causal inference, so are also often called 'aetiological studies'. They do not require that the sample under investigation is representative of the entire population source because the critical issue here is the biological meaning and insights based on scientific knowledge, rather than the statistical representativeness of the actual study participants.
- *Cohort studies* measure the occurrence of disease or health related event in individuals (grouped in one or more cohorts) followed over time. Typically, we have two groups, one exposed to a certain risk factor, the other not exposed. They allow calculating risks/incidence rates and RR and can be prospective or retrospective depending on whether the disease has already occurred or not when the study begins. Examples are:
  - *the Framingham Heart Study*[7]—the first to investigate the role of lifestyle and related factors in the risk of cardiovascular disease (CVD). At its inception in 1948, thousands of citizens without CVD from Framingham (a small US city) were enrolled and data from extensive physical examinations and lifestyle interviews were collected. Subjects were then followed for many years to study CVD incidence.
  - *for investigating diseases with short induction*—e.g. food-borne infections. Individuals who ate foods at one or more meals over a short period are identified as a cohort. Among them, some might have eaten certain contaminated foods and some not. In these studies, the risk of infection among those exposed to particular foods, compared with those who did not eat those foods.[8]
  - *occupational health studies*—where employees exposed to a certain risk factor (e.g. asbestos) are followed over time (prospective or retrospective) to trace the incidence of disease (e.g. mesothelioma[9]), and then compared with cohorts of unexposed subjects (e.g. employees from the same company with different duties, or another company).
  - *prognostic studies* which aim to investigate the association between certain exposure (also called "predictors") that can be also individual characteristics including age, gender, stage of a certain disease, on overall survival, or disease recurrence.[10]

- *Case-control studies* aim to achieve the same goal as cohort studies but more efficiently, using sampling, frequently adopted when the disease is not common. In order to measure the association between a postulated risk factor and a disease (e.g. folate intake and head and neck cancer), we compare the experience of all diseased subjects recruited over a defined time period, with control individuals, defined as subjects who are free from the disease at the time of enrolment and that are sampled from the sace case-source population.[11] Case-control studies do not allow the direct calculation of risk because there is no follow-up of the studied population. The OR, however, should be a good estimate of the RR.

References

1 Rothman KJ, Greenland S, Lash TL. (2008). *Modern epidemiology*, 3rd edn. Lippincott, Williams, & Wilkins, Philadelphia.

2 Porta M, Last JM. (2008). *Dictionary of epidemiology*, 5th edn. Oxford University Press, Oxford.

3 Auger N, Zang G, Daniel M. (2009). Community-level income inequality and mortality in Québec, Canada. *Public Health*, **123**, 438–43.

4 Lugo A, La Vecchia C, Boccia S, et al. (2013). Patterns of smoking prevalence among the elderly in Europe. *International Journal of Environmental Research and Public Health*, **10**(9), 418–31.

5 De Vito C, Angeloni C, De Feo E, et al. (2014). A large cross-sectional survey investigating the knowledge of cervical cancer risk aetiology and the predictors of the adherence to cervical cancer screening related to mass media campaign. *BioMed Research International*, Article ID 304602.

6 Larghi A, Panic N, Capurso G, et al. (2013). Prevalence and risk factors of extrapancreatic malignancies in a large cohort of patients with intraductal papillary mucinous neoplasm (IPMN) of the pancreas. *Annals of Oncology*, **24**(7), 1907–11.

7 Mahmood, SS, Levy D, Vasan, RS, et al. (2014). The Framingham Heart Study and the epidemiology of cardiovascular disease: a historical perspective. *The Lancet*, 15 March, 383(9921), 999–1008. doi: 10.1016/S0140-6736(13)61752-3. Epub 29 September 2013. Available at: ℘ https://www.framinghamheartstudy.org/Lancet (accessed 25 August 2019).

8 Schmid D, Schandl S, Pichler AM, et al. (2005). *Salmonella enteritidis* phage type 21 outbreak in Austria. *European Surveillance*, **11**, 67–9.

9 Hansen J, de Klerk NH, Eccles JL, et al. (1993). Malignant mesothelioma after environmental exposure to blue asbestos. *International Journal of Cancer*, **54**, 578–81.

10 Leoncini E, Vukovic V, Cadoni G, et al. (2018). Tumour stage and gender predict recurrence and second primary malignancies in head and neck cancer: a multicentre study within the INHANCE consortium. *European Journal of Epidemiology*, **33**(12), 1205–18.

11 Galeone C, Edefonti V, Parpinel M, et al. (2015). Folate intake and the risk of oral cavity and pharyngeal cancer: a pooled analysis within the International Head and Neck Cancer Epidemiology Consortium. *Int J Cancer*, **136**(4), 904–914.

Statistical understanding

Kalyanaraman Kumaran and Iain Lang

Objectives

In public health practice, you are likely to use statistics for two purposes as follows:
- To summarize information about populations (descriptive statistics).
- To make inferences from data derived from research or other analysis (inferential statistics).

The objective of this chapter is to help you (a) understand when statistical analysis would be useful, and (b) interpret correctly the statistics you encounter. It also contains an outline of how to use standardization to compare two populations.

Why is this an important public health skill?

Statistics are important to public health practice but most public health practitioners are not statisticians. Because statistics are widely used in public health to present and summarize information, you need to be confident in interpreting what they mean.

We use statistics to get away from the vagueness of words ('very common', 'quite risky', 'highly unlikely', and so on) in place of which we use numbers: proportions (such as percentages), ways of comparing risks (such as odds ratios), and so on. You will typically want to achieve the best estimate of a value or effect size while having an eye to the extent to which your estimate is likely to approximate the truth. An important part of understanding statistics is recognizing when you need to use statistics (see Box 2.5.1).

Box 2.5.1 When do you need to use statistics?
- To summarize, in numbers or in graphical form, quantitative information using *descriptive statistics*. Terms you may come across are averages (mean, median, and mode) and deviation (variance and standard deviation); range, interquartile range, and outlier; histograms, bar charts, and scatterplots.[1]
- To infer general rules or relationships based on observed or gathered data using *inferential statistics*. When you use inferential statistics in public health practice, you will often be doing one of two things: estimating a value (such as a proportion or a risk) and quantifying the uncertainty around that value (e.g. by using confidence intervals). Some of the practical, conceptual, and epistemological details of being able to draw appropriate inferences are discussed in ➔ Chapter 2.6.

When should you consult a statistician?

The short answer is that you should consult a statistician whenever you are in doubt about using statistics. Public health practice covers a lot of ground and few public health practitioners would claim a high level of expertise in all areas. As a result, you will need to consult experts on particular topics when you do not have the skills needed to tackle a particular problem. Statistics is a highly technical discipline and in certain situations there are right and wrong ways to approach your data. If in doubt, approach a statistician for advice earlier rather than later. This avoids the situation statisticians encounter all too often: a dataset with poor measures or uncontrolled confounding or inappropriate sample size and the question 'What can I do now?'—when the real question is 'What should I have done at the start?' Even worse, it avoids having your final findings questioned by someone who points out statistical errors, casting doubt on the whole project. Befriend a statistician, or group of statisticians, and enrol their help whenever you can. They will often add value in unexpected ways!

Probability

If you read about probability in elementary statistics textbooks, you will typically find it introduced using simple examples with simple answers: What are the chances that a coin will land heads, rather than tails, if you flip it once? What are the chances of getting two 6s if you throw two 6-sided dice? However, when faced with complex real-world situations in public health, both the questions and the answers will be complex and may relate, for example, to the expected number of cases of a disease in a population, the likelihood a particular exposure has led to an observed health outcome, or the assessment of your organization's performance when benchmarked against similar organizations. To describe and deal with probability—which we may come across in relation to risk (see ➲ Chapter 6.5)—it is useful to know some of the statistical ways in which it is conceptualized: in terms of distributions, and using *P* values and confidence intervals.

Distributions

Distributions have to do with the way in which the values of something that has been measured (a 'variable') are distributed in a population.

For example, are they all the same (everybody has one head), split into two groups (most people think of themselves as either male or female), or do they come with a broad range of values (people are of different heights)? The most commonly referred to is the normal distribution—this has a 'bell-shaped curve' when plotted, indicating that there are many cases with values in the middle of the range and then a decreasing number with values farther away from the middle.

This distribution often occurs in physiological measurement (such as blood pressure) or in standardized tests (such as IQ tests). Figure 2.5.1 shows an example of approximately normally distributed data—in this case, the data represented in the histogram are body mass index scores, based on self-reported weights and heights, of women in India who responded to

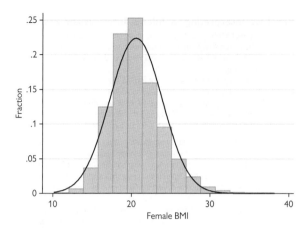

Figure 2.5.1 Normal distribution.

the World Health Organization's World Health Survey. The smooth line shows the normal distribution—you will see that the actual values correspond closely, though not exactly, to this distribution.

Like all statistical distributions—and there are many—the normal distribution has specific statistical characteristics (which you can look up for yourself if you are interested).

P values
Short for 'probability value', a P value is helpful in assessing whether a given value (or difference) is likely to have arisen by chance. In simple terms, the lower the P value, the less likely it is the thing you are interested in happened by chance. The cut-off value for statistical significance is conventionally set at P = 0.05 (although lower values are sometimes used), meaning that P values of less than this are considered statistically significant: meaning that the probability that the effects observed could be due to chance alone is 1 in 20 (or less) if they occurred purely randomly. The smaller the P value, the less likely your results are due to chance alone. Bear in mind, however, that 1 in 20 is an arbitrary figure used by the scientific community to indicate statistical significance.

Confidence intervals
Confidence intervals (CIs) are the ranges within which you can be confident, to a specified level, that the true value you are estimating lies. In this way, they provide a measure of the robustness of results. The most commonly used CI is 95% and you will see something like '28.3 (95% CI 27.1–29.5)', which means an estimated value (point estimate) of 28.3 and a 95% likelihood that the true value is somewhere between 27.1 and 29.5. Another way to think about it is to assume that, if you repeat the same study 100

Box 2.5.2 Interpreting confidence intervals and *P* values

Imagine you want to compare the effects of two interventions, Ash-it and Butt-out, that each aim to help people quit smoking. You have gathered some data and ask a statistician to help you analyse the results. She tells you the following:

- The successful quit rate with Ash-it is 71.5%.
- The successful quit rate with Butt-out 61.5%.
- The difference in quit rates between Ash-it and Butt-out is 10% (this is the 'mean' difference in effect) and the 95% confidence interval (CI) for this difference is 8 to 12, with a *P* value of 0.003.

What do these numbers mean? In this case, the CI is the range of values between which the mean difference would lie on 95 occasions if the study was done 100 times. Put another way, you can be 95% confident that the true difference at population level is between 8% and 12% (i.e. Ash-it may be as much as 12% more effective than Butt-out or as little as 8% more effective).

The *P* value is the probability that a result of this magnitude would occur by chance alone if there were really no difference in effect between the two treatments (i.e. the likelihood of such a result occurring due to chance alone is only 3 in a 1,000.

In this case, it seems likely that Ash-it is more effective than Butt-out and that the difference is about 10%.

times, the results would lie within the estimated confidence intervals 95 times out of the 100.

You should bear in mind that uncertainty in estimates is mostly determined by sample size—the larger the sample, the greater the likelihood that the sample value is closer to the true population value. It also follows that a narrow confidence interval indicates a large sample and therefore a more precise estimate of the true population value. Box 2.5.2 contains an example of how to interpret confidence intervals and *P* values.

Standardization

You will often want to compare mortality or disease incidence between two or more populations—for example, between your region and a neighbouring one, or between your local population and the national average. The comparison of *crude* mortality or incidence rates can be misleading if the populations differ in terms of basic characteristics such as age and gender (which are potential confounders—see ➲ Chapter 2.6). Standardization is a technique used to account for potential confounding variables when comparing two or more population groups, and is most commonly used to adjust for differences in age structure between populations.

Two main techniques are used, direct standardization and indirect standardization, and it is important you understand the differences between them.

- In *direct standardization*, the age-specific rates in the populations of interest are applied to age-specific bands in a reference population, thereby allowing direct comparison of the two populations. The main advantage of this approach is that it can be used to compare rates across various geographical areas and time, and that it allows comparison of the relative burden of different diseases and causes of death within a population. Its main disadvantages are that age-specific rates may not be available for the population of interest, as well as not being very reliable or stable for a small number of events.
- In *indirect standardization*, the observed pattern is compared with what would be expected if the population had the same age-specific rates as in a defined reference population (i.e. the number of actual events is compared with the number of expected events). This produces a ratio called a 'standardized ratio' (e.g. SMR or 'standardized mortality ratio'; SIR or 'standardized incidence ratio'). The standardized ratio for a reference population is always 100. Therefore, a value of less than 100 indicates lower rates than the reference population and a value of greater than 100 indicates a higher rate than the reference population. Box 2.5.3 contains a worked example of how to use both forms of standardization.

Box 2.5.3 Direct and indirect standardization

Imagine you are interested in comparing mortality rates in two regions, A and B. Table 2.5.1 shows the number of deaths occurring in each age band in the two populations, the number of people in each band and the calculated death rate in each age band (for simplicity, only four age bands have been used).

Table 2.5.1 Number of deaths and death rate by age band in two regions

Age band	Region A			Region B		
	Number of deaths	Population	Rate (per 100,000)	Number of deaths	Population	Rate (per 100,000)
0–14	2	100,000	2.0	3	110,000	2.72
15–44	19	150,000	12.66	18	130,000	13.84
45–74	196	140,000	140.0	330	250,000	132.0
75+	1,480	110,000	1345.45	3,560	260,000	1,369.23
Total	1,697	500,000		3,911	750,000	

The crude death rate (number of deaths divided by population) in Region A is 339.4 and in Region B is 521.5 so it appears that Region B has a higher death rate than A. There are, however, differences in the age structure of the two populations—in Region B, more than two thirds of the population are aged 45 or over, but in Region A less than half the people are that age—and most deaths happen in older age groups.

Box 2.5.3 (*Contd.*)

You can compare the two regions by direct standardization using a standard reference population. Assume the standard population here has 150,000 people aged 0–14, 300,000 aged 15–44, 400,000 aged 45–75, and 250,000 aged 75+ (Table 2.5.2).

Table 2.5.2 Expected number of deaths by age band in two regions based on direct standardization

| Age band | County A | | | County B | | |
	Rate (per 100000)	Population	Expected number of deaths	Rate (per 100000)	Population	Expected number of deaths
0–14	2.0	150,000	3	2.72	150,000	4
15–44	12.66	300,000	38	13.84	300,000	42
45–74	140.0	400,000	560	132.0	400,000	528
75+	1345.45	250,000	3364	1,369.23	250,000	3,423
Total		1,100,000	3965		1,100,000	3,997

If you apply the age-specific rate in each region to the standard population, the age-standardized death rates—360.5 in Region A, 363.4 in Region B—are very similar, suggesting that the difference in crude death rates is due to the differences in the age distributions.

You can compare the death rates in the two populations using indirect standardization (i.e. applying the age-specific death rates in a standard or reference population to the two regions). Assume the age-specific death rates in the standard reference population are 3 in people aged 0–14, 13 in people aged 15–44, 135 in people aged 45–74, and 1,350 in people aged 75+. You can apply these rates to the age bands in the two regions (Table 2.5.3).

Table 2.5.3 Expected number of deaths by age band in two regions based on indirect standardization

| Age band | Region A | | | Region B | | |
	Rate (per 100000)	Population	Expected number of deaths	Rate (per 100000)	Population	Expected number of deaths
0–14	3	100,000	3	3	110,000	3
15–44	13	150,000	20	13	130,000	17
45–74	135	140,000	189	135	250,000	338
75+	1,350	110,000	1,485	1350	260,000	3,510
Total		500,000	1,687		750,000	3,868

Standardized mortality ratio (SMR) = observed events × (100/expected events)

SMR (Region A): 87.73   SMR (Region B): 101.11

If the mortality rates in the two populations were similar to that of the reference population, their SMRs would be 100. These figures suggest that Region A has a lower rate than Region B, but further examination is needed to determine if this is a real difference or just due to chance.

Potential pitfalls

Statistics are tools and, like any tools, can be misused.

- *Using arbitrary cut-points:* cut-points at 0.05 for P values and 95% for CIs present the problem that 1 in 20 times they will be wrong: that is, 1 in 20 times, the true value being estimated will fall outside the bounds of a 95% CI, and 1 in 20 times a P value of more than 0.05 will be assigned to a difference that is, in fact, statistically significant. The use of 0.05 and 95% is conventional and other values can be used. It is unclear what the difference is, for example, between a difference with a P value of 0.049 and one with a P value of 0.051: in conventional terms, one is statistically significant and the other is not, but in practice there is little difference between them.

- *Drawing faulty conclusions from results that are not statistically significant:* when a P value is above 0.05, you cannot conclude that there is no difference—just that you have not found one. This may occur for a number of reasons—often because the sample size is too small. Remember that absence of evidence is not evidence of absence!

- *Prioritizing statistical over practical significance:* establishing statistical significance is useful, but people can become too attached to it and you must always consider clinical or other practical significance. For example, a study reports that a new intervention reduces systolic blood pressure by 0.2mmHg and that the reduction is statistically significant ($P < 0.001$). Great—but what does that mean in practice? A change in blood pressure of that size is unlikely to make a difference to any individual patient and even on a population level is not likely to be discernible. It would be easy, if reviewing the evidence, to seize on the low P value and clear statistical significance of this finding and to ignore the practical significance, but it is important you always consider statistics in context and use your professional judgement to interpret what is going on.

- *Forgetting the limitations of statistics in summarizing:* a useful demonstration of this is known as 'Anscombe's quartet'.[2] This shows graphs of four different datasets, each with different x and y values and a different overall shape, which nevertheless share key descriptive statistics (see Figure 2.5.2) In each of the datasets, the following values are all identical or very close: the number of observations (11), the mean of the x's (9.00), the variance of the x's (11.00), the mean of the y's (7.50), the variance of the y's (4.1), the correlation between x and y (0.816), and the linear regression line ($y = 3 + 0.5x$). Despite these similarities, the distribution of the values is obviously different in each case. This example highlights the value of graphing data as well as the importance of identifying outliers. More generally, it should remind us to be cautious in assuming that we know everything that is happening in a situation based solely on the use of some summary statistics.

- *Relying on frequentist approaches:* the way of dealing with statistics described here is called a 'frequentist approach' and many statisticians feel this is inferior to a Bayesian approach.[3] It is beyond the scope of this chapter to deal with this but, briefly, the difference relates to how you use existing information about a situation and how you modify this in light of new information received.

- *Thinking you know too much:* it is possible to go wrong with statistics, particularly because the rules that apply in one situation may not apply in others. You should seek the input of a dedicated statistician when in doubt, and do so earlier rather than later—see p. 124.

Anscombe's quartet								
I		II		III		IV		
x	y	x	y	x	y	x	y	
10	8.04	10	9.14	10	7.46	8	6.58	
8	6.95	8	8.14	8	6.77	8	5.76	
13	7.58	13	8.74	13	12.74	8	7.71	
9	8.81	9	8.77	9	7.11	8	8.84	
11	8.33	11	9.26	11	7.81	8	8.47	0.38345
14	9.96	14	8.1	14	8.84	8	7.04	
6	7.24	6	6.13	6	6.08	8	5.25	
4	4.26	4	3.1	4	5.39	19	12.5	
12	10.84	12	9.13	12	8.15	8	5.56	
7	4.82	7	7.26	7	6.42	8	7.91	
5	5.68	5	4.74	5	5.73	8	6.89	

Figure 2.5.2 Anscombe's quartet.

How will you know when/if you have been successful?

You will know that you have a good grasp of statistics and their application in public health practice when you find other people approaching you for help with their statistical problems!

Further resources

Bland M. (2015). *An introduction to medical statistics,* 4th edn. Oxford University Press: Oxford.
Harris M, Taylor G. (2014). *Medical statistics made easy,* 3rd edn. Scion Publishing, London.
Kirkwood BR, Sterne JAC. (2019). *Essential medical statistics,* 3rd edn. Wiley-Blackwell, Harlow.
Rothman KJ. (2019). *Modern epidemiology,* 4th edn. Lippincott Williams & Wilkins, London.
Tufte ER. (1983). *The visual display of quantitative information.* Graphics Press, Cheshire.

References

1 Porta M. (2014). *Dictionary of epidemiology,* 6th edn. Oxford University Press, Oxford.
2 Anscombe FJ. (1973). Graphs in statistical analysis. *American Statistician,* **27,** 17–21.
3 Spiegelhalter DJ, Abrams KR, Myles JP. (2004). *Bayesian approaches to clinical trials and health-care evaluation (Statistics in practice).* Wiley Hoboken, New York.

Inference, causality, and interpretation

Iain Lang

Felix qui potuit rerum cognoscere causas

(Fortunate is the person who can understand the causes of things)[1]

Objectives

Understanding causality and interpreting evidence in public health practice can be challenging. This chapter describes some of the key concepts involved, including association, causation, bias, confounding, and error. Although understanding the causes of things is a key public health skill, just as important are being aware of the limits to our understanding of what causes things, being able to communicate these limits to other people, and being able to make decisions even when the information we have is incomplete or inconclusive. This chapter will introduce you to some of the main concepts in this area, help you understand how the inferences we can draw from data are shaped, and give you some insight into the limits of the conclusions we can draw from the available evidence. You may find it useful to read this chapter alongside ➔ Chapters 2.1, 2.4, 2.5, 2.7, and 6.5.

Why is this an important public health skill?

Being able to assess evidence and understand what it represents in terms of cause and effect, or what it might represent, or what it definitely does not represent, is crucial to public health practice. If you lack the skills and understanding to do this, you could find yourself adrift in a sea of claim and counter-claim, unable to differentiate association from causation, confounding from true effect, or important information from fake news.

When it comes to understanding the causes of things, the 'things' we are concerned with in public health are usually diseases or other harmful conditions (the causes of which we want to identify in order to reduce or prevent them) or positive outcomes (the causes of which we want to identify in order to stimulate or reproduce them).

We may need to understand the causes of things in relation to a piece of formal evidence, such as a critical appraisal of a peer-reviewed study, or in a range of other settings: an article in a newspaper, a letter or email from a concerned individual or group, or a public challenge in a meeting.

Definitions

- *Inference*: the process of passing from observations and axioms to generalizations. Making causal inferences from observational data is an important aspect of epidemiology and public health practice.[2] When we make inferences, we are typically concerned with the interpretation of evidence in light of our prior understandings to reach conclusions about what has occurred (or what will occur).

- *Causation:* the act of causing something. *Causality* is the relationship between cause and effect. As *The Dictionary of Epidemiology* notes, most 'clinical, epidemiological, and public health research concerns causality'.[2] *Association* between two things means that they co-occur, or that a change in one has been observed to happen alongside a change in the other. In statistics, association means dependence between two or more events or characteristics.[2]

- *A mechanism:* the way a particular event or outcome occurs, and often described in terms of agents or steps involved.[2] Although the name suggests a physical or mechanical understanding of how things work, in public health a mechanism may be biological, social, cultural, or of some other type or combination of types.

- *Causes* are sometimes referred to as *necessary* or *sufficient:* if a cause is necessary for an outcome, then the outcome will not arise unless that cause is present. If a cause is sufficient for an outcome, then the outcome can arise if that cause is present and no other cause is needed. If a cause is both necessary and sufficient for an outcome, then the cause by itself can bring about the outcome and the outcome cannot occur without the cause. If a cause is neither necessary nor sufficient for an outcome, then the outcome can occur without the cause: the cause by itself is not enough to bring about the outcome and other factors are needed. In public health, we rarely come across causes that are both necessary and sufficient—that is, single causes with single outcomes. An individual cause is typically neither necessary nor sufficient and we have to consider combinations of causes as well as the importance of context (see later).

- *Confounding* or *confounding bias:* distortion of the measure of the effect of an exposure on an outcome because of the association of both the exposure and the outcome with another factor or factors.[2]

- *Error:* a false or mistaken result. There are two types: sub-bullets

  - *Random error*—refers to variation in measurements or results with no apparent connection to other measurements or variables, and thought of as being due to chance.

  - *Systematic error* or *bias*—refers to variation in measurements or results that is consistently wrong in a particular direction, often because of an identifiable source.[2]

Association versus causation

The difference between association and causation is important and you may hear the warning 'association does not equate to causation'. Two things may occur closely together (in time or in space) and be described as associated, but this does not necessarily mean that one caused the other: they may both be consequences of some third event or there may be no relationship between them.

For example, on a population level, we might observe an association between having grey hair and cancer: the more grey hair a person has, the more likely they are to receive a cancer diagnosis. These two things are associated, but this does not mean that one causes the other: having grey hair does not make you more likely to have cancer and having cancer does not make your hair turn grey. In this case, association does not imply causation. (A more reasonable explanation is that both grey hair and likelihood of cancer diagnosis are related to age, although even here the causal relationship is not straightforward and we would not say age causes cancer.)

A noteworthy text on causation in public health contains 'the Bradford Hill criteria[3]' and presents them as a series of viewpoints 'we should especially consider' when thinking about whether an observed association involves causation. The nine points are summarized in Box 2.6.1.

Some epidemiologists have pointed out that Hill did not use the word 'criteria' and that these points are not suitable as a checklist to differentiate association from causation.[4]

You will soon realize that it is hard, in a public health context, to talk about 'causes'. Does smoking cause lung cancer? Yes, in a sense, but there are plenty of people who smoke and never develop lung cancer, and of course people who develop lung cancer who have never smoked. Often it is easier to talk about risks and say, for example, that smoking increases the risk of lung cancer (see also ➔ Chapter 6.5). There is also a line of argument that points out that the mechanisms of disease aetiology and of prevention differ, and that we may be sent in the wrong direction by mistakenly focusing on the former.[5]

Box 2.6.1 Austin Bradford Hill's criteria for identifying an association likely to involve causation

- *Strength of association:* how strong is the relationship?
- *Consistency:* is the cause always followed by the supposed outcome, or only sometimes?
- *Specificity:* does the outcome only follow this cause or does it occur in other ways too?
- *Temporal relationship:* does the cause precede the outcome?
- *Biological gradient:* is there a dose-response relationship—that is, does more of the cause lead to more of the outcome?
- *Plausibility:* does it make sense that the outcome and the cause are related, biologically or otherwise?
- *Coherence:* does the apparent relationship between cause and outcome make sense in relation to what we already know on this or related topics?
- *Experiment:* is there evidence from experiments or quasi-experiments to support the relationship?
- *Analogy:* are there comparable relationships that would support the idea that this association is a causal one?

See also Hill AB. (1965). The environment and disease: association or causation? *Proceedings of the Royal Society of Medicine*, **58**, 295–300.

Confounding and other complications

For something to be classed as a confounder, it must satisfy three conditions:

- It must be associated with the suspected cause.
- It must be associated with the outcome.
- It must not be on the causal pathway between the two—so, if a causes b and b causes c, then we would not call b a confounder.

Some examples may help here. If we noticed that lung cancer was more common in people who consumed alcohol than those who did not, we might infer that alcohol causes lung cancer. However, this would be an incorrect inference and the confounder here is smoking. Those who drink alcohol are more likely to smoke, smokers are more likely to get lung cancer, and it is not the case that alcohol consumption causes smoking causes lung cancer. All three conditions are satisfied so we can identify smoking as a potential confounder of the relationship between alcohol and lung cancer.

To take another example, if we found heart attacks were more common in obese people, we might infer that obesity causes myocardial infarctions (heart attacks). A factor that is *not* a confounder in this case is high blood pressure. Obesity is associated with high blood pressure and high blood pressure with myocardial infarctions, so the first two conditions are satisfied, but people who are obese are more likely to have high blood pressure and those with high blood pressure are more likely to experience a myocardial infarction. High blood pressure is not a confounder, in this case, because it is on the causal pathway between obesity and myocardial infarction. (There may, of course, be other confounders present.)

In epidemiological studies, confounding can be controlled to some extent through study design (by using matching or randomization) or through statistical analysis (through stratification or modelling), but these approaches depend on being able to identify confounders.[6] A big problem relates to unidentified confounding—that is, those situations in which we fail to recognize the presence of one or more confounders. Even in peer-reviewed epidemiological studies, the significance of confounding is often not fully addressed but it is an important threat to study validity.[7] In the example of alcohol, smoking, and lung cancer, if we did not realize smoking was playing a role (i.e. failed to identify it as a confounder) we might wrongly conclude alcohol causes lung cancer.

Another complication relates to interaction, which occurs when the combined effects of two or more exposures on an outcome are different from the effects we would expect from each when considered separately. This may reduce or increase the magnitude or likelihood of an outcome. A well-known example relates to the combined effects of smoking and asbestos exposure on lung cancer: the chances of developing lung cancer in those who both smoke and are exposed to asbestos are greater than we would expect based on the chances of developing lung cancer associated with each exposure by itself. We may also see gene-environment interactions: for example, the apolipoprotein E (APOE) gene is a predictor of late-onset Alzheimer's disease, and various lifestyle factors increase the risk of Alzheimer's disease, but those who have both specific alleles of *APOE* and risky lifestyle behaviours have a magnified risk of dementia.[8] (See also ➲ Chapter 3.7.)

Random and systematic error

All measurements are imprecise on some level—measurements to the nearest kilometre are imprecise in terms of metres, measures to the nearest metre are imprecise in terms of centimetres, and so on—so random error is present in any measurement. In public health information, one possible source of random error relates to sampling from populations. No single sample, random or otherwise, is fully representative of the population from which it is taken. This means that, for example, the mean of a sample will differ from the mean of the population from which the sample has been drawn. Ways of reducing the random error include drawing a larger sample or drawing multiple samples from the same population.[9]

The important difference between random error and bias is the 'systematic' element of bias such that measured values not only differ from true values but do so as the result of an underlying factor or factors that affect all the differences in a specific way. As an analogy, think of two archers aiming at a target. One of them is not a good aim and tends not to hit the bullseye but to scatter their shots around the target. The other always aims too far to the left and so their shots always land to the left of the target. If the target was removed after they had fired, but you could see where the arrows had landed, you might be able to guess where the first archer had been aiming by picking somewhere in the middle of the holes. This tactic would not work with the second archer and you would tend to misidentify where the target had been—unless you knew they always aimed to the left. In the same way, with random error present, we can infer approximately where the true value lies, but with systematic error we risk making an incorrect inference unless we are aware of the type and size of the bias.

Many forms of bias have been described and some of the more common ones are set out in Table 2.6.1. Biases can be addressed, although not necessarily fully, in either the design or the analysis of a study. Randomized controlled trials (RCTs) involving random allocation and blinding represent one of the best ways of minimizing bias but they do not remove it entirely.[10] A well-designed RCT is likely to contain the strongest evidence we can obtain from a single study, but we still need to consider the extent to which its results may be generalized (see ➡ Chapter 2.4).

Table 2.6.1 Common types of bias

Type of bias	Source of bias	Example
Selection	Systematic differences between individuals participating in a study and those who do not. This can arise because of self-selection or other aspects of the study selection procedure.	People in households with higher socio-economic status were more likely to allow measurements of magnetic fields in the home to be taken, but less likely to live close to sources of magnetic fields than those in lower socio-economic status households.[a]
Reporting	People may be selective about the way they report information. Certain types of information are particularly likely to be withheld or misreported (e.g. drug abuse or sexual history).	Women who have experienced abortions may be uncomfortable telling researchers about them, leading to systematic under-reporting[b]
Recall	Individuals wrongly remember and report information about past events, for example because certain events or experiences are particularly memorable.	In retrospective studies, mothers' reports of gestational age at birth differ depending on whether the delivery was at term or preterm.[c]
Detection	Different assessment or diagnostic techniques tend to be better or worse at detecting particular conditions, or to be applied differently in different settings.	In randomized controlled trials, knowledge of the arm to which a participant has been assigned can influence assessment of outcome.[d]

a) Mezei G, Kheifets L. (2006). Selection bias and its implications for case-control studies: a case study of magnetic field exposure and childhood leukaemia. International Journal of Epidemiology, 35, 397–406.

b) Jones EF, Forrest JD. (1992). Underreporting of abortion in surveys of U.S. women: 1976 to 1988. Demography, 29, 113–26.

c) Yawn BP, Suman VJ, Jacobsen SJ. (1998). Maternal recall of distant pregnancy events. Journal of Clinical Epidemiology, 51, 399–405.

d) Noseworthy JH, Ebers GC, Vandervoort MK, (1994). The impact of blinding on the results of a randomized, placebo-controlled multiple sclerosis clinical trial. Neurology, 44, 16–20.

What do we do when the evidence is not good enough?

These considerations—of causation versus association, of causes and confounders, of bias and error—are central to the formal critical appraisal of study findings. As a public health practitioner keen to ensure that your practice is appropriately evidence-based and that you achieve the outcomes we want (and avoid those you do not), you may wonder how we can achieve anything, and make any decisions, when there are so many caveats about causes and inferences and the information you have in front of you is, almost inevitably, less than conclusive. What do you do when the evidence is not good enough?

You might begin by reflecting on the fact that the evidence is never good enough—or, at least, not often. For some core public health activities, like vaccination, the evidence available is strong, but for others, like eating five pieces of fruit and vegetables a day, it is less compelling than you might imagine. On some topics, RCTs are impractical or unethical and in these situations we are reliant on observational studies. This means that on issues, such as the health effects of exposure to environmental toxins and the long-term consequences of health-related behaviours, we must rely on data that is suggestive, rather than conclusive.

In the end, you will have to make decisions and recommendations, and simply declaring that the existing evidence is inconclusive is not likely to be helpful (unless you are making the case for conducting research or evaluation). A useful theoretical orientation on this is provided by work on realistic evaluation[11, 12] and evidence-based policy making.[13] This approach to evidence and decision making, in contrast to the standard focus on weight of evidence, depends instead on the basic realist formula of causation:

context + mechanism = outcome

In this understanding, causes (or mechanisms) do not exist in a vacuum but operate, and must be understood, in complex social and organizational environments. This implies that what works in one setting will not always work in another, and is one reason to be cautious about assuming that what has been shown to work in an RCT, for example, will produce the same outcomes when put in place elsewhere. The context of a trial is probably different from the 'real' contexts in which we each work so, even if the mechanism is the same, the outcome may be different. Approaches to evaluation that identify it as a social practice, rather than as scientific testing, can also usefully inform our understanding of how evidence is created and interpreted—all these things occur in complex social and organizational environments.[14]

Once you have realized that the evidence is typically not going to be as strong as you would like it to be, you will probably proceed on a pragmatic basis—making the best decision you can based on the best evidence that is available, what you know about the local situation, your prior experience of related issues, and the advice and input of colleagues or partners. In such contexts, the more inclusive notion of knowledge-based practice may be more useful than thinking in terms of pure evidence-based practice[15] and in fact a lot of decisions, including clinical ones, are made on this basis.[16]

Conclusion

Being able to appraise the strengths and weaknesses of evidence is crucial to effective public health practice. Knowing what is meant by inference, association, causation, bias, and confounding is crucial to shaping our understanding of what can and cannot be inferred from the information available to us. In practice, our decisions and actions will be shaped by combining this understanding with our knowledge of complex local factors and politics.

Further resources

Bonita R, Beaglehole R, Kjellström T. (2007). *Basic Epidemiology*, 2nd edn, pp. 83–97. World Health Organization, Geneva. Available at: ℜ http://libdoc.who.int/publications/2006/9241547073_eng.pdf (accessed 19 August 2019).

References

1 Virgil, *Georgics*, no 2, l,490 quoted in Wilson J. (2008). *Inverting the pyramid*. Orion, London.

2 Porta M. (ed.) (2014). *A dictionary of epidemiology*, 6th edn. Oxford University Press, Oxford.

3 Hill AB. (1965). The environment and disease: association or causation? *Proceedings of the Royal Society of Medicine*, **58**, 295–300.

4 Rothman KJ. (2012). *Epidemiology: an introduction*. 2nd edn. Oxford University Press, Oxford.

5 Kelly MP, Russo F. (2017). Causal narratives in public health: the difference between mechanisms of aetiology and mechanisms of prevention in non-communicable diseases. *Sociology of Health & Illness* **40(1)**, 82–99. Available at: ℜ https://doi.org/10.1111/1467-9566.12621 (accessed 10 August 2019).

6 Rothman KJ, Greenland S, Poole C, et al. (2012). Causation and causal inference. In: Rothman KJ, Greenland S, Lash TJ, eds, *Modern epidemiology*, 3rd edn, pp. 5–31. Lippincott Williams & Wilkins, Philadelphia.

7 Hemkens LG, Ewald H, Naudet F, et al. (2018). Interpretation of epidemiologic studies very often lacked adequate consideration of confounding. *Journal of Clinical Epidemiology*, **93**, 94–102. Available at: ℜ https://doi.org/10.1016/j.jclinepi.2017.09.013 (accessed 10 August 2019).

8 Kivipelto M, Rovio S, Ngandu T, et al. (2008). Apolipoprotein E ε4 magnifies lifestyle risks for dementia: a population-based study. *Journal of Cellular and Molecular Medicine*, **12**, 2762–71.

9 Levy PS, Lemeshow S. (2013). *Sampling of populations: methods and applications*. Wiley Series in Survey Methodology, 4th edn. Wiley, Hoboken.

10 Jüni P, Altman DG, Egger M. (2001). Systematic reviews in health care: assessing the quality of controlled clinical trials. *British Medical Journal*, **323**, 42–6.

11 Pawson R, Tilley N. (1997). *Realistic evaluation*. Sage Publications, London.

12 Pawson R. (2013). *The science of evaluation: a realist manifesto*. Sage Publications, London.

13 Pawson R. (2006). *Evidence-based policy: a realist perspective*. Sage Publications, London.

14 Greenhalgh T, Russell J. (2010). Why do evaluations of eHealth programs fail? An alternative set of guiding principles. *PLoS Medicine*, **7**, e1000360.

15 Glasby J. (ed.) (2011). *Evidence, policy and practice: critical perspectives in health and social care*. Policy Press, Bristol.

16 Gabbay J, le May A. Evidence based guidelines or collectively constructed "mindlines?" Ethnographic study of knowledge management in primary care. (2004). *British Medical Journal*, **329(7473)**, 1013. Available at: ℜ https://doi.org/10.1136/bmj.329.7473.1013 (accessed 10 August 2019).

Chapter 2.7

Finding and appraising evidence

Anne Brice, Amanda Burls, and Alison Hill

Objectives

Making good public health decisions requires integrating relevant local knowledge about your population with national guidance and best research evidence. However, public health research evidence is more diverse than clinical research and needs to be sought in a much wider range of information sources. Furthermore, evidence comes from a range of different study types, which adds a further challenge when assessing the quality of the research. This chapter has two aims. The first is to help you find research evidence efficiently, so that you can access the best, most relevant research evidence for your research query. The second is to help you make sense of research through the technique of critical appraisal, which is the systematic assessment of research evidence. Finding and appraising evidence is an essential skill in the process of improving the health of the population.

Finding research evidence

Constructing a focused question

To build an effective search strategy, you need to formulate a focused question, so that you are clear about what you are looking for. To facilitate this, there are different frameworks available[1], which are described in Table 2.7.1.

Table 2.7.1 Different frameworks to devise a focused question

Framework	Definition	Area of interest
PICO	Patient/problem/population, intervention, comparison, outcome	Clinical interventions
PECOT	Patient/problem/opulation, exposure, comparison, outcome, time	Causation or prognosis
SPICE	Setting, perspective/population, intervention, comparison, evaluation	Project, service or intervention evaluation
SPIDER	Sample, phenomenon of interest, design, evaluation, research type	Qualitative or mixed methods
ECLIPSE	Expectation, client group, location, impact, professionals, service	Service evaluation

Use the framework that best suits your question, and fit the key terms from your focused question to the headings. Underneath those key terms, add synonyms, relevant terms on which to base your search and to build the blocks of your search strategy.

What type of evidence do you need?

Before searching for evidence, you need to know what type of evidence to look for. Table 2.7.2 briefly describes study designs that are relevant to public health questions. If an appropriate study design has not been used, then the study is unlikely to provide information of value to your decision.

Table 2.7.2 Best primary research design for different questions

Type of question	Study design
Aetiology and risk factors	Cohort and case-control studies
Incidence and prevalence	Cohort or cross-sectional
Harm	Cohort and case-control studies
Prognosis	Inception cohort/survival studies
Value for money	Economic evaluation (e.g. cost-effectiveness study or cost–benefit study)
Effectiveness	Randomized controlled trial
Diagnosis	Diagnostic test study (or randomized controlled trial)
Patient experience (e.g. of illness, treatment or service)	Qualitative studies (e.g. questionnaires, focus groups, or interviews)

If available, a good-quality, up-to-date systematic review of studies of the appropriate design will give the best overview.

Finding the evidence

Research evidence can be found in a wide range of sources, particularly for public health topics. In 2014, 28,200 scholarly peer-reviewed journals were identified as being active[2], with more than 3,000 biomedical articles being published every day[3, 4]. Therefore, you need a clearly defined question and knowledge of which sources to search. However, it is also important to be systematic in your searching so that you do not miss any relevant papers or waste time searching through lots of irrelevant papers.

Searching techniques need to be *sensitive* (to get as much of the information you do need as possible) and *specific* (to minimize the amount of retrieved information that you do not need). It is important not to limit or narrow the search too quickly, because this may exclude vital evidence from your search results.

Searching for scientific literature is not a linear process. Search strategies may need to be refined in the light of citations retrieved to improve the identification of relevant papers—often called 'iterative searching', whereby additional search terms are identified during the original search and integrated into a refined search strategy.

Sources of information

Many people use internet search engines to find information, particularly if they need it quickly. However, information retrieved from search engines can be more biased and there are fewer quality controls in place compared with other sources.

If you are aiming to do a quick search (*specific* but not *sensitive*), there are some freely available sources you can go to that filter for higher-quality information. The TRIP database and the National Institute for Health and Care Excellence (NICE) Evidence search are two such information sources that are as quick as more general search engines but retrieve more relevant content from publishers, such as peer-reviewed journals, guideline producers, and professional colleges (see Table 2.7.3).

Table 2.7.3 Suggested sources of information for different levels of public health evidence

Level	Type of information	Information source
Systems	Decision support systems	For example: National Library of Medicine disaster apps. Available at: ⬯ https://disaster.nlm.nih.gov/dimrc/disasterapps.html
Summaries	Guidelines, evidence summaries	Epistemonikos. Available at: ⬯ https://www.epistemonikos.org
		National Guideline Clearinghouse. Available at: ⬯ https://www.ahrq.gov/gam/index.html
		NICE Evidence search. Available at: ⬯ http://www.evidence.nhs.uk
		TRIP database Available at: ⬯ http://www.tripdatabase.com
Synopses of syntheses	Summaries of critically appraised research, such as systematic reviews	BestBETs. Available at: ⬯ http://bestbets.org/database/browse-bets.php
		Cochrane evidence summaries. Available at: ⬯ http://www.cochrane.org/evidence
		EPC evidence-based reports. Available at: ⬯ https://www.ahrq.gov/research/findings/evidence-based-reports/index.html
Syntheses	Systematic reviews	Campbell Collaboration. Available at: ⬯ https://www.campbellcollaboration.org/library.html
		Cochrane Library. Available at: ⬯ http://www.cochranelibrary.com
		EPPI-Centre. Available at: ⬯ https://eppi.ioe.ac.uk/cms/Default.aspx?tabid=185
		Health Evidence. Available at: ⬯ http://www.healthevidence.org/search.aspx
		Joanna Briggs Institute database of systematic reviews and implementation reports. Available at: ⬯ http://journals.lww.com/jbisrir/Pages/default.aspx
		PubMed clinical queries. Available at: ⬯ https://www.ncbi.nlm.nih.gov/pubmed/clinical
Synopses of single studies	Summaries of individual, high-quality studies	ACP Journal Club. Available at: ⬯ http://annals.org/aim/journal-club
		Epistemonikos. Available at: ⬯ https://www.epistemonikos.org
		BMJ evidence-based medicine. Available at: ⬯ http://ebm.bmj.com
		BMJ evidence-based nursing. Available at: ⬯ http://ebn.bmj.com
		National Institute for Health Research signals. Available at: ⬯ https://discover.dc.nihr.ac.uk/portal/search/signals
		TRIP database. Available at: ⬯ http://www.tripdatabase.com

Table 2.7.3 (*Contd.*)

Level	Type of information	Information source
Single studies	Primary, pre-appraised research	Epistemonikos. Available at: 🔗 https://www.epistemonikos.org
		Global Index Medicus. Available at: 🔗 http://www.globalhealthlibrary.net/php/index.php
		PubMed. Available at: 🔗 https://www.ncbi.nlm.nih.gov/pubmed
		TRIP database Available at: 🔗 http://www.tripdatabase.com

For more comprehensive searches (*sensitive* and *specific*), it is necessary to search bibliographic databases, such as PubMed or Embase.

Selecting sources

Deciding which sources to search and the nature of your search will depend on many factors, including the purpose of your search, time available, and the sources you have access too.

Using a protocol can help you plan your approach and ensure that the search is reproducible. A sample protocol is included in Table 2.7.3, based on the 6S Pyramid[5]. The 6S Pyramid is a model that sets out a hierarchy of evidence to guide decision making, with the top of the pyramid being systems, where research knowledge is embedded into clinical and public health systems to aid decision making, and the bottom being single studies. The search for evidence should begin in the upper range. The table suggests information sources that are pertinent to different levels of public health evidence. Links to more information about these resources are available at the end of the chapter.

Doing the search

When searching a database, it is important to search one term and one database at a time. Start by looking for the term in the database thesaurus (in some databases, this is known as 'MeSH' or 'Medical Subject Headings'). Each reference that is added to a database is assigned a set of thesaurus/MeSH terms that reflect the content of the paper. Therefore, by searching the thesaurus, you will find papers that are specifically about the subject you are looking for. Within the thesaurus, there is the option to explode a term, which means it will search for that term, but also any narrower terms beneath it. This broadens the search options, which is best practice, because you will narrow your search down later by adding additional terms from the other concepts in your search framework. Another option is to choose subheadings, although best practice includes all the subheadings, because otherwise there is a risk of excluding key papers from your search. It is important to combine the thesaurus search with a free-text/text word search: it takes time for thesaurus terms to be assigned to new records, so, if you rely on the thesaurus terms, you may miss the latest evidence on your topic.

Truncation and wildcards

With free-text/text word searches, you can use symbols to help broaden your search. For example, *behavi?or* will search for 'behaviour' or 'behavior', while *obes** will search for obesity or obese, and *nurs** will retrieve papers on nurse, nurses, nursing, and nursery. The asterisk (*) and the question mark (?) are the most common symbols used in databases, but some databases may use other symbols, so, when in doubt, check the 'Help' features on the individual databases.

Combining search terms

Within each search concept, terms can be combined with OR, which can result in many results, but, once all the terms have been combined within their concepts, then you can combine each concept with AND (see Figure 2.7.1). We give an example of a search strategy in Table 2.7.4.

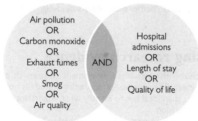

Figure 2.7.1 Combining search terms.

Table 2.7.4 Example of a database search strategy

Search no.	Search terms	Search type
1	exp air pollution/	MeSH
2	exp carbon monoxide/	MeSH
3	exhaust fumes.tw.	Free text
4	smog.tw.	Free text
5	air quality.tw.	Free text
6	1 or 2 or 3 or 4 or 5	OR
7	exp hospital admission/	MeSH
8	patient admission*.tw.	Free text
9	exp "length of stay"/	MeSH
10	exp "quality of life"/	MeSH
11	7 or 8 or 9 or 10	OR
12	6 and 11	AND

Applying search filters

Search filters are tried and tested search strategies that provide a more effective way of refining your search to find high-quality evidence appropriate to your type of question. Some of the larger databases, such as PubMed/Medline and Embase, have a selection of in-built search filters for different study types. They can be applied at the end of your search, when you apply other limits, such as language and/or date restrictions.

Search strategies should be explicit and reproducible. Start with a broad search, and then narrow the results down by using quality filters. Remember to match the search strategy to the question and that searching is an iterative process. While database interfaces may differ in appearance, they all apply similar techniques for information retrieval. Remember the 'Help' features, which often contain useful search tips and tutorials, or contact a librarian for support.

For more information about search filters, go to ISSG Search Filters Resource, available at: ℘ https://sites.google.com/a/york.ac.uk/issg-search-filters-resource/home/search-filters-by-design (accessed 10 August 2019).

Appraising research evidence

Critical appraisal is the systematic assessment of research evidence. No research is perfect. The purpose of appraising a study is not to find fault because it is less than ideal but to identify what, if anything, is of value for informing your decision.

When critically appraising any study, you need to be able to tell:
- what question the researchers set out to answer (concise, answerable question in full)
- whether they used an appropriate study design (see Table 2.7.2)
- what they did (the right methods done correctly)
- what they found (results in numbers and words)
- the implications for practice of the findings in your context (relevance, so what?).

Screening questions for *any* study

Given the vast number of potential studies available, you need to triage papers for their potential usefulness. Thus, the first question to ask is, 'Is a clear question being addressed?' You need to ensure here that you can identify all the components of the question, as described at the start of this chapter. If the answer is no, or you cannot tell, then the paper is unlikely to be useful (in fact, it is likely to be positively unhelpful).

The next question is, 'Did the researchers use an appropriate study design for the question they were asking?' Remember it is usually only worth appraising a study in more depth if it has a clear question and appropriate study design.

Appraising the validity of studies of different designs

We use studies to inform our decision making. Thus, we need to know to what extent a study's findings are likely to reflect the 'truth'. For example, if a study finds the death rate in those treated with a new treatment is half that in patients given the standard treatment, we would like to be convinced that this is because the new treatment actually halves the death rate and was not simply due to the way study was done (such as people in the new treatment group being not as ill as those in the comparison group). Systematic deviation of results from the truth because of the way a study is conducted is known as *bias*.

An important element of critical appraisal is to check that potential biases were both identified and minimized. Because different study designs are prone to different biases, there are specific questions you need to focus on to check their validity. Boxes 2.7.1–2.7.6 provide checklists as an *aide-mémoire* for the important biases you need to check for when appraising studies of different designs.

Learning critical appraisal skills requires practice and experience. Therefore, resources that can help with further learning are provided at the end of the chapter.

Box 2.7.1 Randomized controlled trials

- Was the allocation of patients to treatments randomized?
- Was this allocation concealed?
- Were the groups similar at the start of the trial in terms of factors that might affect the outcome, such as age, sex, and social class?
- Were patients, health workers, and study personnel 'blind' to treatment?
- Apart from the experimental intervention, were the groups treated equally?
- Were all the patients who entered the trial properly accounted for at its conclusion?
- Were patients analysed in the groups to which they were randomized? (See also the validated scale for assessing the quality of an randomized controlled trial.)[a]

a) Jadad A, Moore R, Carroll D, et al. (1996). Assessing the quality of reports of randomized clinical trials: is blinding necessary? Controlled Clinical Trials, 17(1), 1–12.

Box 2.7.2 Systematic reviews and meta-analyses

To be valid, a review should systematically identify and evaluate all appropriately designed studies that address the question being considered and, when appropriate, combine their results. If this is not done properly, there is the potential for bias and the results will not be trustworthy even when the included papers were well conducted.

- Did the reviewers do enough to identify all relevant studies?
- Did the reviewers assess the quality of the included studies?
- If the results of the studies have been combined, was it reasonable to do so?

Box 2.7.3 Cohort and case-control studies

- Was the cohort recruited in an acceptable way?
- Was the exposure accurately measured to minimize bias?
- Was the outcome accurately measured to minimize bias?
- Have the authors identified all important confounding factors?
- Have the authors taken account of the confounding factors in the design and/or analysis?
- Was the follow-up of subjects complete enough?
- Was the follow-up of subjects long enough?

Box 2.7.4 Economic evaluations

- Was a comprehensive description of the competing alternatives given (i.e. can you tell who did what to whom, where, and how often)?
- Was there evidence that the programme's effectiveness had been established?
- Were all important and relevant consequences and costs for each alternative identified?
- Were consequences and costs measured accurately in appropriate units (e.g. hours of nursing time, number of physician visits, years of life gained) prior to valuation?
- Were consequences and costs valued credibly?
- Were consequences and costs adjusted for differential timings (discounting)?
- Was an incremental analysis of the consequences and costs of alternatives performed?
- Was a sensitivity analysis performed?

Box 2.7.5 Diagnostic tests

- Did all patients get the diagnostic test and the reference standard?
- Could the results of the test of interest have been influenced by the results of the reference standard or vice versa?
- Is the disease status of the tested population clearly established?
- Were the methods for performing the test described in sufficient detail?

Box 2.7.6 Qualitative studies

- Was the recruitment strategy appropriate to the aims of the research?
- Was the data collected in a way that addresses the research issue?
- Has the relationship between researchers and participants been adequately considered?
- Have ethical issues been taken into consideration?
- Was the data analysis sufficiently rigorous?

Making sense of results

One should not waste time looking at the 'results' of a study when the methods lack sufficient validity because it will not be possible to know if an apparent finding is a real effect or simply due to bias because of the way the study was conducted. However, even if the study methods are trustworthy, it is important to consider the results, and the way they are expressed, critically. The way the results are expressed is important because this can influence the reader's interpretation and subsequent decision making.

What are the results?

- How were the outcomes expressed (e.g. odds ratios, risk ratios, risk differences, numbers needed to treat [NNTs], or, in a diagnostic test study, likelihood ratios)?
- If these results are only expressed as a relative risk, such as the risk ratio or odds ratio, is there sufficient information to calculate the absolute risk (such as a risk difference or NNT)? (Relative risks, such as odds ratios and risk ratios, tend to over-influence our decisions.)
- What was the bottom line or estimate for each outcome?

Could they have occurred by chance?

- How likely is it that a result occurred simply by chance? (The *P* value estimates how frequently a result, or a more extreme result, would be seen by chance if there were no true effect in an unbiased study.)
- Confidence intervals (CIs) also indicate how much uncertainty due to chance surrounds an estimate. (This is known as 'precision'.) In an unbiased study, the CIs can be interpreted as telling you the range in which the true effect lies with a certain degree of confidence (conventionally 95%). If the 95% CIs of an estimate of relative risk do not cross 1, or the 95% CIs of an estimate of risk difference do not cross 0, then the result is 'statistically significant'.

What do they mean?

- How important is this result for the patient or policy decisions? It is important to consider other ways of expressing the results because the way in which results are expressed can influence how important they appear. Try to calculate the NNT if results are reported as relative risks (see Box 2.7.7) or, in diagnostic test studies, the likelihood ratios where

---

Box 2.7.7 Example of the impact of expressing the same evidence in different ways

Consider the following result. If nicotine replacement therapy increases the 6-month quit rate from 10% to 17%, there are at least two ways of communicating this result. On the one hand, if it is expressed as a relative risk, one could say it nearly doubles the quit rate. Alternatively it can be expressed as an absolute risk (an extra 7% of people stopped smoking) or as an NNT of 14 (i.e. 1/0.17-0.1), an absolute risk. An NNT of 14 means that, for every 14 people who take nicotine replacement therapy, only one extra person will quit. Thirteen of them gain no additional benefit (approximately two out of 14 quit, but one would have quit anyway).

results are expressed as sensitivity and specificity (LR=sensitivity/ (1-specificity). See ➜ Chapter 3.6: Assuring screening programmes.
• Were all important outcomes considered? (E.g. did the study explicitly consider adverse events?).

Can the results be applied to the local population?
You need to consider whether there are any important differences between the local population or setting and the study population or setting that would mean that the results would be likely to be different locally.

Are the benefits worth the harms and costs?
This is usually not explicitly considered in individual studies. However, the bottom line is that the probable benefits of a decision need to outweigh the probable harms and costs. To make this judgement, public health practitioners will usually need to draw on their wider experience and background knowledge. Bear in mind that, when making policy decisions, this usually requires a consideration of the opportunity costs as well.

If you know the NNT, you can do a quick cost/consequence analysis yourself by multiplying the cost per treatment by the NNT. Using the example in Box 2.7.7, if the cost of nicotine replacement therapy is £100, then it costs £1,400 for each person who stops smoking (14 x £100).

Further reading

Breckon J. (2016). *Using research evidence: A practice guide.* Nesta/Alliance for Useful Evidence, London. Available at: ℛ https://www.nesta.org.uk/toolkit/using-research-evidence-practice-guide (accessed 10 August 2019).

Ciliska D, Thomas H, Buffett C. (2010). *An introduction to evidence-informed public health and a compendium of critical appraisal tools for public health practice.* National Collaborating Centre for Methods and Tools, Canada. Available at: ℛ www.nccmt.ca/uploads/media/media/0001/01/b331668f85bc6357f262944f0aca38c14c89c5a4.pdf (accessed 10 August 2019).

De Brún C, Pearce-Smith, N. (2014). *Searching skills toolkit: finding the evidence*, 2nd edn. Wiley-Blackwell, Chichester.

European Centre for Disease Prevention and Control (2011). *Evidence-based methodologies for public health: how to assess the best available evidence when time is limited and there is lack of sound evidence.* ECDC, Stockholm. Available at: ℛ ecdc.europa.eu/en/publications/Publications/1109_TER_evidence_based_methods_for_public_health.pdf (accessed 10 August 2019).

Glasziou P, Del Mar C, Salisbury J. (2008). *Evidence-based medicine workbook: bridging the gap between health care research and practice,* 2nd edn. BMJ Books, London.

Gray JAM. (2009). *Evidence-based health care and public health: how to make decisions about health services and public health,* 3rd edn. Churchill Livingstone Elsevier, London.

Greenhalgh T. (2014). *How to read a paper: the basics of evidence-based medicine,* 5th edn. Blackwell Publishing, Oxford.

Guyatt G, Rennie D, Meade M, Cook D. (2008). *Users' guides to the medical literature: essentials of evidence-based clinical practice,* 3rd edn. JAMA & Archives Journals, Chicago.

National Collaborating Centre for Methods and Tools (2012) *A model for evidence-informed decision making in public health.* National Collaborating Centre for Methods and Tools, Canada. Available at: ℛ www.nccmt.ca/uploads/media/media/0001/01/9e2175871f00e790a936193e98f4607313a58c84.pdf (accessed 10 August 2019).

Rychetnik L, Hawe P, Waters E, et al. (2004). *A glossary for evidence based public health. Journal of Epidemiology and Community Health,* **58**(7), 538–45. Available at: ℛ jech.bmj.com/content/jech/58/7/538.full.pdf (accessed 10 August 2019).

Straus S, Glasziou P, Richardson S, et al. (2011). *Evidence-based medicine: how to practice and teach EBM,* 4th edn. Churchill Livingstone Elsevier, London.

Tools and techniques

Centre for Evidence-Based Medicine (2014) Tools: The five stages of evidence-based medicine. Available at: ℰ www.cebm.net/category/ebm-resources/tools (accessed 10 August 2019).

Critical Appraisal Skills Programme (2017). CASP checklists. Available at: ℰ www.casp-uk.net/checklists (accessed 10 August 2019).

U.S. National Library of Medicine (2017). PubMed® online training. Available at: ℰ learn.nlm.nih.gov/rest/training-packets/T0042010P.html (accessed 10 August 2019).

References

1 Davies K. (2011). Formulating the evidence based practice question: a review of the frameworks. *Evidence Based Library and Information Practice*, **6**(2). Available at: ℰ https://journals.library.ualberta.ca/eblip/index.php/EBLIP/article/viewFile/9741/8144 (accessed 10 August 2019).

2 Ware M, Mabe M. (2015). *The STM report: an overview of scientific and scholarly journal publishing*. STM: International Association of Scientific, Technical and Medical Publishers. The Hague, Netherlands.

3 Huang C-C, Lu Z. (2016). Community challenges in biomedical text mining over 10 years: success, failure and the future. *Briefings in Bioinformatics*, **17**(1), 132–44.

4 Vardakas K, Tsopanakis G, Poulopoulou A, et al. (2015). An analysis of factors contributing to PubMed's growth. *Journal of Informetrics*, **9**(3).

5 Haynes R. (2009). Resources for evidence-based practice: the 6S Pyramid. McMaster University, Ontario, Canada. Available at: ℰ http://hsl.mcmaster.libguides.com/ebm (accessed 10 August 2019).

6 Jadad A, Moore R, Carroll D, et al. (1996). Assessing the quality of reports of randomized clinical trials: is blinding necessary? *Controlled Clinical Trials*, **17**(1), 1–12.

Monitoring disease and risk factors: surveillance

Richard Hopkins and Aaron Kite-Powell

Disclaimer: The findings and conclusions in this report are those of the authors and do not necessarily represent the official position of the Centers for Disease Control and Prevention.

What is surveillance?

Public health surveillance is 'the ongoing, systematic collection, analysis, interpretation, and dissemination of data about a health-related event for use in public health action to reduce morbidity and mortality and to improve health. Data disseminated by a public health surveillance system can be used for immediate public health action, program planning and evaluation, and formulating research hypotheses.'[1]

Examples of health-related events or conditions that may be put under surveillance include episodes of illness or injury, diagnoses of chronic conditions, risk behaviours for adverse health outcomes (e.g. tobacco use or non-use of seatbelts), or completion of a healthcare procedure (e.g. Pap smear or measles immunization). The principles of public health surveillance are the same for infectious and non-infectious diseases.

Historically, infectious disease surveillance and some forms of non-infectious disease surveillance have depended upon legally mandated disease reporting by healthcare providers, laboratories, hospitals and healthcare systems. Increasingly, surveillance for both infectious and non-infectious disease events relies on surveys and on data originally collected for other purposes (e.g. administrative data, electronic medical records, vital registration). The European Centre for Disease Prevention and Control espouses a comprehensive model of surveillance referred to as 'Epidemic Intelligence', which combines traditional surveillance methods with expanded methodologies in order to identify and characterize emerging threats.[2] The World Health Organization has issued interim guidance[3] for the strengthening of national and subnational systems for early detection, assessment, and response to acute public health events, so that countries may effectively meet their obligations under the 2005 International Health Regulations[4]. The recommended multifaceted approach includes using a combination of disease-specific indicator-based surveillance, syndromic surveillance, and event-based surveillance (using multiple types of unstructured data) to identify and monitor events.

Why conduct surveillance?

Public health surveillance can be used to support interventions in response to individual cases; detect and monitor outbreaks; understand the natural history of a disease or injury; support treatment guidance, policy development, or programme planning and evaluation; conduct exploratory research; and identify research needs. These purposes of surveillance systems can be classified into three main categories: case detection and management, outbreak detection and management, and programme planning and evaluation.

Individual cases of diseases of public health interest (e.g. tuberculosis or infectious syphilis) are routinely reported to public health authorities to ensure proper case management and response for both the individual and the community (e.g. investigation to locate and treat exposed contacts to an infectious disease or toxin). Public health authorities use surveillance data to detect, track the course and extent of, and manage outbreaks or clusters (e.g. of foodborne diarrhoea and haemolytic uremic syndrome due to toxigenic *Escherichia coli*, of birth defects due to introduction of a new medication, or of injuries or cancers due to a new occupational hazard). They also use surveillance data for the planning and continuous evaluation necessary to ensure that programmes to prevent and control disease at the community level are effective (e.g. immunizations to prevent infectious diseases, educational campaigns about sleep position and bedding to prevent sudden unexplained infant deaths, or interventions to improve quality of clinical care).

Surveillance opportunities

Electronic management of clinical data and its submission to public health agencies afford the possibility of instantaneous identification, reporting, and review of disease, injury, and health indicator data, including laboratory results, very close to the time they are recorded by the provider, at all levels of the public health system. Effective use of such near real-time health data is transforming the practice of surveillance.[5]

Syndromic surveillance is an example of an approach to surveillance that is facilitated by availability of health-related data stored in an electronic form. Health department staff, assisted by automated data acquisition and generation of statistical signals, monitor disease indicators continually to detect and investigate possible outbreaks of disease earlier and more completely than might otherwise be possible, to rapidly characterize outbreaks, and to monitor the magnitude, geographic extent, and risk groups of outbreaks as they unfold.[6] These methods have demonstrated benefit for monitoring trends, such as the course and impact of the 2009 pandemic of influenza A (H1N1), as much as or more than for outbreak detection.[7] It is a useful source of near real-time surveillance data in situations where the public health event of interest is not otherwise reportable.[8]

Disease-specific surveillance has also been enhanced in many countries by implementation of electronic reporting of relevant findings by laboratories to public health agencies, and in the near future will increasingly be enhanced by automated recognition and reporting of likely cases of reportable diseases that meet certain criteria in electronic health record systems.[9]

When multiple streams of data can be examined in the same analytic environment, the public health analyst's capabilities for detection and characterization of important events are improved. Such data may include cases of reportable diseases, emergency department visits for various syndromes, death registration data, and environmental data such as weather. Even if surveillance data supporting different programme areas is collected and stored in different ways, modern information technology tools allows it to be displayed in a common format and with common query tools. Analysts should in future be able to enhance their ability to combine information from multiple sources using statistical methods.

Molecular and genetic fingerprinting are increasingly used to separate isolates of pathogenic organisms from ill people into smaller genetically related categories. This approach can greatly facilitate the detection and assessment of common-source outbreaks due to a single strain of an organism. Serogrouping and serotyping of isolates of Salmonella species and of influenza viruses have long been standard tools for recognition of related human (and animal) cases of disease, for confirming the environmental source of human infections, and for recognition of new outbreak threats. Newer technologies are faster and can be applied to a much wider range of pathogens, but also require extensive data management infrastructure. These approaches can be used to recognize outbreaks—when several or many apparently unrelated or sporadic cases of a disease can be shown to be due to identical strains and thus a search for a common source is initiated—and also to determine which cases of a disease are and are not part of a recognized outbreak. These technologies are most effective when all known isolates of pathogens of interest are tested in a single laboratory with these fingerprinting capabilities. The utility of these approaches is threatened by widespread use of non-culture technologies for making etiologic diagnoses in clinical practice.

Effective surveillance can be and is still carried out through organized use of non-computerized information, and through intermediate technologies—for example, those based on mobile telephones and text messaging. Even highly computerized systems still depend ultimately on timely and accurate manual documentation of information at a local level. All surveillance systems, whatever their degree of technological sophistication, need to be operated consistently and in accordance with the principles outlined below.

In event-based surveillance[10], diverse sources of unstructured data, mostly from the internet (e.g. news, blogs, and social media), are collected prospectively and analysed for emerging infectious disease events. These data may include timely information about outbreaks or clusters that have not otherwise been reported officially, and may not have been validated at the time of reporting. Other related non-health data may also be included (e.g. travel patterns or weather information). Integration of these data with other indicator-based or syndromic data sources may provide more timely and complete situational awareness to public health practice than any of these types of data considered alone.

Designing a surveillance system

The first step in designing a surveillance system is to state its purpose clearly. The relative importance of many system attributes depends on the purpose (Table 2.8.1). For example:
- A system that is designed to support programme planning with a several-year time horizon will likely not be sufficiently timely for outbreak recognition or immediate control measures.
- For diseases where each individual case reflects a possible epidemic with risk of mortality and an urgent public health intervention is needed (such as botulism, meningococcal disease or infectious syphilis), high sensitivity for case detection may take priority over positive predictive value (PPV).

Table 2.8.1 Relative importance (5-point scale) of surveillance system performance attributes that vary by purpose of surveillance

Attribute	Purpose of surveillance		
	Case detection and management	Outbreak detection and management	Program planning and evaluation
Timeliness	****	*****	*
Sensitivity	****	****	***
Positive predictive value	****	***	****
Negative predictive value	N/A	*****	***
Data quality	*****	***	****
Representativeness	**	**	****
Flexibility	***	****	*
Stability	****	*****	***

- When resources are scarce, an automated alarm system for outbreak detection may need to be set with low sensitivity and high PPV (the probability that a system signal identifies an outbreak of the type being sought.) This may mean that some small outbreaks are missed or detected later than desired.
- If reassurance that an outbreak is not occurring when there is no signal is important to the system, a high negative predictive value (NPV) for outbreaks is important. NPV reflects the probability that no signal from the system correctly indicates that no outbreak is occurring.
- Data quality needs to be particularly high when medical treatment decisions will be made on the basis of data in the system. When surveillance is used as a screening tool to detect events that may require further investigation, lower data quality may be tolerated. When investments in prevention programmes are costly, high-quality data are needed for planning and evaluation purposes.
- Flexibility reflects the ability of a system to change diseases under surveillance, case definitions, or data sources as needs change. Outbreak detection systems particularly require flexibility to adapt to changing threats and levels of risk over time.
- At the same time, stability, reflected by consistency in fundamental operations over long periods of time, producing a stable baseline, is also important for outbreak detection.

System characteristics also vary with the primary purpose of the system (see Table 2.8.2).

There are typically more different kinds of data available for programme management and fewer for case management (where individual treatment and case management decisions require a follow-up with personal identifiers). Outbreak detection can often be done with data that do not contain

Table 2.8.2 Surveillance system design characteristics by purpose of surveillance

System design characteristic	Case detection and management	Outbreak detection and management	Programme planning and evaluation
Data sources	Case reports from clinicians, healthcare facilities, schools, or laboratories, both manual and electronically generated.	Case reports; electronic health records; administrative healthcare data; results of molecular subtyping of isolates); reports from community members who have observed an apparent outbreak; news and other internet reports; environmental and workplace monitoring for hazards and exposures; poison centre consultations; sales of over-the-counter or prescription medicines; calls to nurse hotlines; mentions of syndromes or diagnoses on social media; web searches for terms indicating illness or concern.	All previous plus: repeated population-based surveys; vital registration; Census data; social services data; public safety data; disease registries.
Collection method	Reports by mail, phone, fax, email, website, electronic lab reporting (ELR), electronic case reporting.	Case reports; direct electronic acquisition or web entry of records coded by ICD10-CM, chief complaint, or other early diagnostic information; ELR; supply of medical treatments.	All previous; personal report; observation (e.g. seat belt use).
Collection frequency	Reported on a set interval after a case is identified at a reporting source (e.g. 24 hours or 1 week)	Case reports as they occur, or batch reporting on a frequent (e.g. daily) or continuous (real-time) basis	Extended periodic interval (e.g. annually)
Data processing	Limited (tabulation and sorting for case investigation and follow-up)	Automated steps for organizing and detecting aberrations	Extensive cleaning and updating of data
Statistical and epidemiologic analysis	Line lists and histograms; simple measures of central tendency and time plots; direct action case by case.	Inspection of routinely collected data by time, place and person; analytic routines for pattern recognition; stratified analysis for risk groups; combination of data from multiple sources; modelling for forecasting.	Routine tables and more advanced modelling or projections (e.g. time series, complex stratified and cluster models).
Audiences for reporting and dissemination	Case managers (public health); clinicians; case reporters.	Public health and medical practitioners at local, state, federal levels; emergency responders; business; news media; public	Programme managers; policy makers; news media; public

personal identifiers, yet timely investigation of cases that may be part of an outbreak requires that identifiers be accessible on request. Cultural norms and governmental rules for use and protection of personal data for public health purposes vary by jurisdiction. For example, in the United States, the Privacy Rule of the Health Information Portability and Accountability Act[11] is the controlling authority while, in the United Kingdom, Section 251 of the National Health Service Act 2006, as implemented in Health Service (Control of Patient Information) Regulations 2002, fills this role.[12]

The following outbreak detection principles should be considered:

- At any time when personally identified data are collected for public health purposes, utmost care must be taken to meet applicable ethical and legal standards and to ensure privacy and confidentiality of the data. This is one of several reasons why one should not collect data that are not needed.

- Data collection may be manual or electronic. The point in a collection system at which it makes sense to switch from manual data entry and data management to automated processes will depend on the level of technology and of trained staff realistically available, as well as on the volume of reports and the timeliness needed. In most settings, surveillance data are collected manually at the most local level in the system and gradually aggregated as they are passed up the chain to surveillance units responsible for larger areas (e.g. county, district, province, or country). When the data source for surveillance is inherently centralized (e.g. a national survey), data may be collected in a central office and be made available promptly to local public health units.

- Analysis of surveillance data should be appropriate to the task at hand and can be quite simple. Localized acute disease surveillance may need no more than line lists of cases, cases plotted over time (i.e. epidemic curves, time series analysis), and simple mapping. Effective use of data in support of programme planning or evaluation may require more complex analysis. Systems with multiple streams of data and many data elements (e.g. disease indicators, symptoms, diagnoses, and age, race, sex, ethnicity, occupation, and geographic unit of people with cases) may benefit from automated aberration detection and from more complex visualizations.

- Increased availability of highly detailed molecular subtyping of organisms causing disease (e.g. PulseNet) also creates a need for software to identify similar isolates and apparent time or space clustering among a multitude of cases.

- Descriptive and analytic epidemiology (e.g. calculations of rates by subgroups and time intervals, mapping of cases and rates, age adjustment to support geographic comparisons, and calculation of relative risks) are especially useful in support of programme planning and evaluation.

- Surveillance data, summaries, analyses, and recommendations should be disseminated regularly to suppliers of data, those with a need to know for clinical and public health purposes, and the general public. Doing this well is a challenge even for experienced applied epidemiologists and must be customized to the environment in which the surveillance is being carried out.

- There will be increased opportunities to provide relevant just-in-time information to clinicians who are entering information into an electronic health record about a case of disease that may be part of an outbreak.

Public health informatics

Public health informatics[13] is 'an interdisciplinary profession that applies mathematics, engineering, information science, and related social sciences (e.g. decision analysis) to important public health problems and processes'.[14] Modern surveillance systems increasingly acquire electronic data and rely on information and computer science to optimize the collection, storage, and use of these data. As more clinical records are computerized using standardized electronic health records, and vocabulary standards (e.g. LOINC and SnoMED), rapid and complete transfer of such data using standardized messages (e.g. HL-7) into surveillance systems is becoming the norm in developed and many middle-income countries. Informatics expertise should be engaged early in the design of surveillance systems.

Evaluating a surveillance system

Surveillance systems should be evaluated regularly and modified promptly as needed. Evaluations of all types of surveillance systems can be guided by Centers for Disease Control and Prevention's 'Updated guidelines for evaluating public health surveillance systems'[1], or by more recent European Centre for Disease Prevention and Control recommendations[15] that identify triggers for periodic assessments and for formal evaluations. Evaluations should always be undertaken in close consultation with system stakeholders, to whom results should also be disseminated.

Table 2.8.1 shows performance attributes assessed in surveillance system evaluation that are likely to vary by purpose. Additional attributes that are common to all surveillance systems are also important, such as acceptability, the willingness and authority of participants to contribute to data collection, analysis, and use. Cost is always important, but thresholds for acceptable costs will differ based on the condition, local circumstances, and the purpose or intended use of the data. Ultimately, the performance of a surveillance system depends on whether it accomplishes its stated purpose. To the extent possible, usefulness should be assessed by whether prevention and control actions are taken as a result of receipt of case reports or analysis and interpretation of data from the system.

General principles for effective surveillance systems

The key contributions of public health professionals to establishing, running, and quality assurance of surveillance systems are to understand the strengths and limitations of the data for the intended purpose of the system, and to analyse the data frequently so that utility and quality can be assured. The following principles should be diligently applied:

- Have clear objectives and design the system to meet those objectives.
- Collect only the data needed to meet the explicit objectives.

- Evaluate the performance of the system against its objectives on a regular basis and as needed.
- Reassess objectives periodically to reflect experience with the system and changing programme needs.
- Value and build personal relationships, as well as laws, rules, and technology.
- Demonstrate the public health uses of the data to participants (e.g. clinicians and laboratories).
- Provide authoritative consultation to those who supply the data, because this can enhance active cooperation with the surveillance system.
- Identify and remove barriers to rapid reporting of cases or other data.
- Build redundancies to minimize the impact of reporting gaps.
- Analyse and interpret data by time, place, and person routinely and frequently.
- Integrate the analysis and interpretation of data across all the systems your organization manages.
- Convey confidence about the value of surveillance, epidemiology, and public health practice.

Further resources

Lee LM, Teutsch SM, Thacker SB, et al. (eds). (2010). Principles and practice of public health surveillance, 3rd edn. Oxford University Press, New York.

References

1 Centers for Disease Control and Prevention (2001). Updated guidelines for evaluating public health surveillance systems: recommendations from the guidelines working group. *Morbidity and Mortality Weekly Report*, **50**(RR-13), 1–35. Available at: ℛ http://www.cdc.gov/mmwr/preview/mmwrhtml/rr5013a1.htm (accessed 21 June 2010).

2 Paquet C, Coulombier D, Kaiser R, et al. (2006). Epidemic intelligence: a new framework for strengthening disease surveillance in Europe. *Eurosurveillance*, **11**(120), ii–665. Available at: ℛ http://www.eurosurveillance.org/ViewArticle.aspx?ArticleId=665 (accessed 30 April 2017).

3 World Health Organization. Early detection, assessment and response to acute public health events: implementation of early warning and response with a focus on event-based surveillance. Interim version. WHO/HSE/GCR/LYO/2014.4 Available at: ℛ http://apps.who.int/iris/bitstream/10665/112667/1/WHO_HSE_GCR_LYO_2014.4_eng.pdf?ua=1 (accessed 6 April 2017).

4 World Health Organization. *International health regulations (2005)*. Available at: ℛ http://www.who.int/topics/international_health_regulations/en (accessed 21 August 2019).

5 Brownstein JS, Clark C, Freifeld CC, et al. (2009). Digital disease detection—harnessing the web for public health surveillance. New England Journal of Medicine, **360**, 2153–7. doi: 10.1056/NEJMp0900702

6 Centers for Disease Control and Prevention. National Syndromic Surveillance Program (NSSP): syndromic surveillance data in action. Available at: ℛ https://www.cdc.gov/nssp/biosense/index.html (accessed 21 August 2019).

7 Chu A, Savage R, Willison D, et al. (2012). The use of syndromic surveillance for decision-making during the H1N1 pandemic: a qualitative study. BMC Public Health, **12**, 929.

8 Yoon, P. W., Ising, A. I., & Gunn, J. E. (2017). Using syndromic surveillance for all-hazards public health surveillance: successes, challenges, and the future. Public Health Rep, **132**(suppl I), 3S–6S.

9 Lazarus R, Klompas M, Campion FX, et al. (2009). Electronic support for public health: validated case finding and reporting for notifiable diseases using electronic medical data. *Journal of the American Medical Informatics Association*, **16**(1), 18–24. doi: https://doi.org/10.1197/jamia.M2848

10 Hartley D, Nelson N, Walters R, et al. (2010). The landscape of international event-based biosurveillance. *Emerging Health Threats Journal*, **3**(1), doi: 10.3402/ehtj.v3i0.709

11 United States Department of Health and Human Services. Summary of the HIPAA Privacy Rule. Available at: ✍ https://www.hhs.gov/hipaa/for-professionals/privacy/laws-regulations/index. html. (accessed 11 August 2019).

12 National Health Service Health Research Authority. What is Section 251? Available at: ✍ http:// www.hra.nhs.uk/about-the-hra/our-committees/section-251/what-is-section-251 (accessed 30 April 2017).

13 Magnusson JA, Fu PC, eds. (2014). *Public health informatics and information systems*, 2nd edn. Springer-Verlag, New York.

14 Savel TG, Foldy S. (2012). The role of public health informatics in enhancing public health surveillance. *Morbidity and Mortality Weekly Report*, **61**(3), 20–4.

15 European Centre for Disease Prevention and Control (2014). *Data quality monitoring and surveillance system evaluation – a handbook of methods and applications*. ECDC, Stockholm.

Investigating alleged clusters

Patrick Saunders, Andrew J. Kibble, Amanda Burls, and AT Saunders

Objectives

This chapter aims to:
- describe the methodological and communication challenges in investigating allegations of environmentally related disease clusters
- provide public health practitioners with a structured and systematic approach to preparing for, and responding effectively and appropriately to, such allegations.

Introduction

This chapter describes methods conventionally used to investigate alleged clusters of disease and a number of contemporary methodological developments, and makes recommendations for an effective public health response. While the Chemical Abstracts Service has recorded over 127 million unique naturally occurring and synthesized chemical substances[1] all of which have the potential to cause harm to human health, there is scant information on the toxicology of the majority of chemicals.[2]

Major chemical releases receive considerable publicity and several countries have formal mechanisms for the surveillance of, and response to, such events, reducing their potential for public health impact.[3, 4] However, much less is known about the effects of community exposure to low levels of chemicals. While a dramatic effect on public health is unlikely, the potential for exposure is real as is the toxicity of many of the chemicals involved and the genuine nature of the concerns of local populations.

Community suspicions about unusual diseases or prevalence of disease can be easily raised. A person with a disease may be looking for a cause and focus on a local environmental issue. This understandable reaction can lead to a campaign raising awareness and recruiting further cases that may be entirely unrelated. These campaigns can be extremely difficult to respond to effectively. Community concerns must be taken seriously and treated professionally. Not only could the campaigners be right, but, as Centers for Disease Control (CDC) has noted, 'From a public health perspective, the perception of a cluster in a community may be as important as, or more important than, an actual cluster'.[5] However, clusters of disease will occur purely by chance. Cancer, for example, is a common condition and clustering is inevitable.[6] As populations age and cancer survival rates improve, people are increasingly aware of cases within their communities leading to a perception of a remarkable pattern[7] and expectations that an epidemiological investigation will be undertaken[8]. However, such studies rarely demonstrate a clear association with an environmental contaminant and there is a real risk of simply identifying a false positive.[9] Reviews of over 500 US investigations found only one that could be linked to a clear cause and that was occupationally related.[10] While advances in statistical methods, data quality, and the power and utility of geographical information systems have all facilitated the analysis of clusters, such studies will continue to be challenging despite the emergence of innovative methods including genomic technologies and biomarkers.[8] Investigations will mostly fail to resolve community anxieties and may even exacerbate them[7]. A refusal to carry out a detailed study though can heighten concerns, and allaying these without seeming to avoid the issue is a major challenge. That is not to say, however, that there should be no investigation. Indeed, a professional, informed, and sympathetic assessment of the facts and allegations should be the first stage of every response and is an opportunity to both address community apprehensions and potentially provide an important health education intervention[11] without recourse to an expensive, unnecessary, and time-consuming epidemiological and environmental study. This is probably the most important element in a successful response. Unless it is done rationally, investigations may be carried out unnecessarily or be refused inappropriately. Doing nothing is not an option. It is important that public health practitioners have the confidence to employ the correct method at the right time, and the confidence and justification, when appropriate, not to conduct a study.

Several agencies have produced guidance addressing some of these issues, but none specifically deals with them all.[8, 12–17] All these guidelines share some common themes, including endorsing an incremental approach—i.e. begin with relatively simple but robust methods, and only proceed to more sophisticated analyses if positive results are obtained that justify further study.

Before the investigation

Intelligence on potential sources of environmental contamination

There has been a significant shift in the approach of environmental law from one of response to an incident to one of prior control and approval. In many countries, data on existing and historical sources of potential environmental contamination can be accessed through prior authorization of industries, local air quality review and assessment, chemical incident surveillance systems, inventories of contaminated land, and site emergency plans, etc. Such information can provide useful background information to any site-specific investigations (e.g. identifying potential environmental confounders) and can provide an indication of the sort of hazards that exist and the appropriate resources necessary to respond to them.

Point of contact/responsible individual

There should ideally be nominated individuals acting as a first point of contact. These staff must have appropriate training in dealing with the public and be supported by a system that ensures the recording of appropriate details. This can be achieved through the use of standardized pro forma which should be retained for audit purposes. The first contact should also be used to make an initial assessment of the level and direction of concern.

Review committee

A review committee should be developed to act as an expert forum for investigations. Access to an expert group to offer advice in difficult cases (perhaps even arbitration in disputes) is essential. Placing this responsibility outside the remit of any one particular agency will also add credibility to the decision and will incorporate some degree of both validation (important scientifically) and independence (important in dealing with the media and public) to the investigation.

Initial response (stage 1)

Reported health problem

When an agency is alerted to a community concern by individual member(s) of the public, it is important that as much relevant information as possible is obtained on first contact. This will enable an early assessment and ensure that the response is treated professionally. The symptoms reported must be clearly and consistently documented—for example, are people reporting the same type of symptoms; are conditions self-reported or clinically confirmed? Allegations from individuals do not necessarily mean that the whole community is worried about potential health effects of contamination. Self-appointed pressure groups do not necessarily represent the views of the community. Unfounded concern can lead to property blight and the wider community may actually want an agency to reassure others that there is no public health concern.

Plausibility

This stage requires assessing whether the reported relationship makes sense given what is known about the mechanisms of health and disease, and the temporal and spatial relationships between the disease and the putative source. Is there any evidence that the alleged exposure will result in the effect reported? There is little point initiating a study if the pollutant under investigation cannot cause the effect reported. However, for most diseases, environmental risk factors are poorly understood and in many cases the concerns will be about disease(s) in general rather than specific disease/exposure linkages. For many diseases, there is a latency period between the point of first exposure and the development of clinical disease. For some cancers, this could be decades. Therefore, the address on diagnosis is not necessarily the address at the time of exposure and the investigator must decide whether the effect reported is plausible in terms of the likely period and extent of exposure. Some basic assessment of the geographic relationship between cases and alleged source can also be made at this stage of the process.

Exposure verification

There is a range of information sources that can be assessed for any evidence of a real or potential exposure. A preliminary investigation of the putative source can reveal whether it has been the subject of previous complaints, regulatory action, or could be the source of relevant environmental pollution. However, such a judgement can be extremely difficult to make—for example, reported symptoms will often be generalized and may not provide any meaningful information on the plausibility of chemical exposure. It is important to establish the number, characteristics, distribution, and timing of complaints. The latency of diseases such as cancer means that the exposure assessment may include potential exposures that occurred many years before. Such data may be poorly characterized, limited, of variable quality, or simply unavailable. Further assessment of the source is not warranted at this stage.

Environmental hazard

The existence of viable source–pathway–receptor relationships should be considered. Each component needs to be identified and evaluated in order to assess risk. A toxic substance has to be present and there has to be a viable exposure pathway(s) to a target or receptor. If no pathway exists, the contamination may well be a hazard (i.e. there could be an intrinsic toxicity) but it will not present a risk (e.g. the chemical cannot come into contact with a vulnerable target). This is particularly important when specific chemical/disease relationships are being alleged. Again the issue of biological and temporal plausibility will need to be considered. When dealing with historical clusters, care is also required to avoid introducing potential bias by exposure misclassification through the inevitable speculation about (historical) potential sources of exposure.

Apparent excess of cases

If the plausibility criteria are met, it may be possible at this stage to ascertain whether the number of cases reported is excessive. For example, region-wide rates of various diseases can be used as an initial screening tool.

Scoping review

At this early stage, an initial scoping literature search will provide useful background information on the nature of the process, toxicological mechanisms, biologic plausibility, and the volume and quality of the literature, and help refine the potential research question.

The decision to continue

By now it should be possible to make some initial judgements. If the referral is clearly unfounded or even malicious in nature, then it would be appropriate to stop any further investigation and document the concern for future reference. If a health-based or environmental standard has been exceeded at the site of interest, the appropriate regulator should take action. In the case of no apparent disease excess and no environmental standard being exceeded, the investigation should stop. If there is an apparent excess of cases (as reported by the complainant) and a plausible link with an environmental hazard, then it would be appropriate to move to stage 2. However, in many cases, there will be few, if any, environmental data available. In these cases, if the type of site means that contamination was, or is, feasible, then the investigation should proceed to stage 2 particularly if there are concerns that the alleged exposures occurred some time ago. If there is no possibility of prior exposure and data indicate that there is no relevant environmental contamination, the investigation can stop. For example, there would be little need to continue if the only possible source/hazard is a landfill site known to contain inert materials. In this case, the investigator should stop and report back to the community. In the event of no plausible exposure, but a potential excess of disease, the issue should be considered by the agency and, if necessary, referred to the review committee.

Verification of cases and potential excess (stage 2)

Introduction

The aim of this stage is to determine whether a detailed environmental and epidemiological assessment is justified. Appropriate spatial and temporal boundaries should be developed. This will require consideration of factors including meteorological conditions, operational conditions, emissions, land use change, possible period of exposure, and latency periods. Detailed environmental monitoring or modelling is not required at this stage, but the investigator should obtain sufficient information to decide whether the source of the contamination is biologically, spatially, and temporally plausible given the health problems reported. Whenever possible, multi-site studies should be considered.

Verification of cases

Case details including any evidence of exposure should be obtained and diagnoses confirmed. The latter may need the input of primary care, hospital departments, and routine data sources such as cancer registration systems.

This is particularly important when dealing with investigations carried out by pressure groups or concerned individuals that purport to show an excess of disease. An active surveillance system for potentially environmentally related diseases would provide valuable intelligence. This is the basis of environmental public health tracking and there are established mechanisms already available.[18]

Literature review refined

The literature search should now be refined and papers obtained. This should be carried out in a systematic way focusing on the peer-reviewed literature, but may also include good-quality grey literature. The review committee should be able to provide support.

Test for excess cases

Statistical power can be a serious issue with single-site studies because of relatively low numbers of cases, and may preclude a plausible analysis. An observed/expected (O/E) analysis using a suitable reference population is appropriate at this stage. The simplest method of analysis is to identify a study area and compare the observed number of cases in that area with the number of cases that would be expected if the area had the same incidence rate as a larger reference area or population. This analysis, while relatively simple, still requires good-quality data and there are methodological issues that need to be considered when interpreting the results. Two methods are commonly used—indirect and direct standardization—although indirect has become the standard methodology. An O/E comparison might show an apparent excess but, if the prevalence of the condition is related to age or deprivation, this could be due to large numbers of elderly or deprived people in that population. Analysis should take account of such factors as age and gender, and, when necessary, other factors that may (but not always) need controlling—for example, deprivation. It is important to recognize the risk of over-adjustment for social class (any association with environmental factors may be 'adjusted away', because deprived people also are typically more exposed to environmental hazards). A clear explanation of the computation of the expected number is given in a number of reference works.[19] Another potentially useful method is the statistical control chart that will identify those areas with levels of disease outside expected variability. This method has been used for decades as a quality control tool in industry, and has increasingly been applied to public health research.[20]

Problems and limitations

People living in areas in the vicinity of a source of pollution (e.g. a factory) can identify themselves as being at risk and it may be tempting to initiate studies in order to clarify the cause of these apparent risks. By their very nature, these studies are *post hoc* since they were prompted by complaints of apparent 'clusters' of ill health. *Post hoc* hypotheses may lead to bias by focusing on narrow time bands and spatial areas where an excess risk has been observed. The theoretical basis of standard statistical analyses has been questioned, given the effect of silent multiple comparisons inevitable in these studies, and accordingly Bayesian methods[21] and a greater emphasis on exposure assessment have been advocated.[9] Other potential weaknesses include small numbers, inadequate control for confounders, and, almost invariably, absence of exposure measures. If an association is suggested, the investigation can move to stage 3. Otherwise stop, document, and report back to the community.

Environmental and exposure assessment (stage 3)

Monitoring and analysis

Direct measurements of exposure are ideal but can be of poor quality, incomplete or unavailable at an individual level.[22] This can present a major issue as a reliable measure of exposure is a key requirement for drawing conclusions of causality from epidemiological investigations. Furthermore, current environmental monitoring is unlikely to be representative of past exposure. If the population under consideration is still being exposed to a pollutant(s) of interest, it would be highly desirable to have a direct measure of individual exposure. Personal or biological monitoring may be helpful in establishing current levels of exposure or estimating dose levels. Personal air monitors that can be worn during normal day-to-day activities are almost never used to measure environmental exposure in epidemiological studies, despite the fact that they can provide actual data on individual exposure. Biological monitoring may be helpful in establishing exposure or estimating dose levels. Biomarkers can help demonstrate that exposure has occurred and can be used to identify exposed populations for investigation (e.g. urinary thioether assays can be used as biomarkers for chemicals such as polycyclic aromatic hydrocarbons). They can also provide an estimate of past exposure provided the pollutant under investigation has a long half-life in the body and is relatively easy to detect (e.g. dioxins). In the absence of biological measurements or personal air monitoring, exposure has to be indirectly estimated through some other method. Typically, these are through the use of proximity to the potential source as an indicator of exposure, environmental measurements such as ambient air monitoring, or through the use of computer models such as atmospheric dispersion modelling. The use of distance from the source is a common and easy-to-use approach. However, this takes no consideration of the influence of meteorological conditions or process characteristics such as stack height, efflux velocity, plume temperature, etc. Exposure zones may often be several kilometres beyond the site or point of release, introducing considerable exposure misclassification and possibilities for confounding co-exposures from other sources. It is inevitable that these zones will include a large degree of variability of exposure and may include people who are not exposed at all. This may dilute an effect and might result in a true greater effect downwind of the point source being missed. Individuals will also move within and outside these zones, and many people will not reside within the zone for most of the day. A direct measurement of exposure is more robust. If an active industrial site is being investigated as a source, emission data may provide an indirect measure of exposure and can be extremely useful in identifying the pollutants emitted. Such data will be readily available as industrial releases are required to meet mandatory limits. However, they are of limited value in terms of a direct measure of exposure because most point sources will release pollutants at a considerable height above ground level.

In many countries, environmental data are routinely collected for regulatory purposes by environment agencies and local authorities. For example, in the UK, ambient air is monitored in networks such as the Automatic Urban and Rural Network and London Air. Such networks can provide useful data on background levels of air pollution and 'hotspot' monitoring at urban roadsides and, occasionally, around point sources. However, monitoring sites may not be located near the area or source under investigation, or may not measure the specific pollutants of concern. As a result, it may be necessary to commission environmental monitoring to help identify exposed communities. For example, analysis of soil and vegetation downwind of a point source can often prove to be a good indication of exposure. Following the release of a large quantity of dioxin from an accident at a pesticide plant in Seveso, Italy, the extent and level of dioxin contamination in soil in the prevailing wind direction was used to identify the most exposed populations.[23] Subsequent analysis of dioxin levels in the plasma of people from those affected areas showed that body burden was closely correlated with levels of environmental contamination. If monitoring reveals that the concentrations of pollutants are below a recognized standard, the nature of the investigation should be reconsidered. This does not necessarily mean it should be stopped, because some controlled chemicals may be non-threshold toxins and there are very few chemicals that have been fully evaluated for their health risk. A toxicological input will be particularly important in the interpretation of the environmental data.

Another approach is to use modelling to predict exposure. Air dispersion models are a widely accepted method for regulating emissions to atmosphere from major industry, and many commercially available models can predict the worst case ground-level concentration over the short- and long-term around industrial sources. However, the accuracy of any model is heavily dependent on the quality of the input data. Most studies tend to use a combination of proximity and environmental measurements. In a review of exposure assessment methods in 41 epidemiological studies of incinerators, all used residence as a proxy for exposure, although more recent studies also used more refined methods such as dispersion modelling and environmental monitoring to improve exposure assessment.[24]

A site visit can be helpful to confirm details of potential sources and the plausibility of an exposure pathway. Detailed exposure assessment should not be undertaken unless the health concerns are properly defined and there is biological plausibility.

The decision to continue

If there is evidence of a potentially significant chemical exposure (chemical, level, pathway, spatial, and temporal plausibility) and the health effect is plausible, proceed to stage 4. Otherwise consider referral to the review committee or stop and document.

Epidemiological assessment (stage 4)

Boundaries

It is useful to engage the concerned community in confirming the most appropriate spatial and temporal boundaries. This can help engender a real sense of being involved in the design of the study. It can also provide the researchers with pre-defined boundaries. The areas of concern may not necessarily reflect the realities of exposure assessment. The investigators should consider how meteorological, operational, and technical factors may affect exposure and whether additional environmental sampling and modelling are required to refine the area of exposure. The area of interest may also be manipulated to assess whether there is a risk from proximity (e.g. examining areas at different distances from a putative source).

Identifying all cases within the spatial and temporal boundaries

Appropriate case-finding techniques should be employed. If the study is relying on routine datasets, the investigators must assure themselves of the data quality and be aware of the limitations of each data source used. This may have significance in determining the spatial boundaries of the study (e.g. cancer registration may only be available for a specific period).

Agree an appropriate method

If there are no resources available, such as academic units, to assist in developing an appropriate method, the review committee should provide advice. At its simplest, this may be a refinement of the O/E analysis performed in stage 2 and/or the use of a dispersal model to identify exposed populations more accurately. There are several methods available[25] and it may be more appropriate to use a more refined analysis such as Bayesian modelling or link the study to a larger multisite study. A number of new innovative methods are being developed and deployed such as the intrinsic conditional autoregressive model[26], kernel density contouring[27], and methods that account for residential history.[28, 29] If this stage still shows an apparent excess of disease, the issue should be referred to the review committee to assess the quality of the study and to determine the need and method for more sophisticated epidemiological or other research studies. Biomarkers of exposure may also be considered appropriate in some circumstances.

Communication strategy

The statutory agencies should seek the involvement of the affected or concerned communities. It is not enough to simply make information available for use by the public. Traditional approaches have undervalued 'active listening' and ignored the human needs of a population in a suspected cluster investigation.[10] Involving the community must be an integral part of the process and should be planned for recognising that laypeople can interpret facts about disease clusters differently from 'experts'.[30] Worry and concern can lead to stress or anxiety, which can exacerbate existing conditions or result in an increase in the reporting of symptoms including those that do not have a toxicological basis. Openness with the community can alleviate community and individual concerns and help generate a more positive working relationship with the community reflected in CDC's revised guidelines, which emphasize transparency, engagement, and active listening to its members' concerns.[7] The oral histories of the community are critical in establishing a full understanding of the issue, empowering residents and demonstrating that the agencies value their perspectives and experiences.[10]

References

1 CAS Registry. The gold standard for chemical substance information. Available at: ℘ https://www.cas.org/content/chemical-substances (accessed 21 August 2019).

2 Baker D, Karalliedde L, Murray V, et al. (eds). (2012). *Essentials of toxicology for health protection. A handbook for field professionals*, 2nd edn. Oxford University Press, Oxford.

3 Agency for Toxic Substances and Disease Registry (2010). National Toxic Substances Incidents Program (NTSIP). Available at: ℘ http://www.atsdr.cdc.gov/ntsip/index.html (accessed 21 August 2019).

4 Health Protection Agency Chemical surveillance reports. Available at: ℘ http://webarchive.nationalarchives.gov.uk/20140629102627/http://www.hpa.org.uk/Publications/ChemicalsPoisons/ChemicalsSurveillanceReports/ (accessed 21 August 2019).

5 Centers for Disease Control (1990). Guidelines for investigating clusters of health events. *Morbidity and Mortality Weekly Report*, 39(RR-11), 1–23.

6 Thun MJ, Sinks T. (2004). Understanding cancer clusters. *CA: A Cancer Journal for Clinicians*, 54 (5), 273–80.

7 Centers for Disease Control (2013). Investigating suspected cancer clusters and responding to community concerns: guidelines from CDC and the Council of State and Territorial Epidemiologists. *Morbidity and Mortality Weekly Report*, 62(RR08), 1–14.

8 Goodman M, LaKind JS, Fagliano JA, et al. (2014). Cancer cluster investigations: review of the past and proposals for the future. *International Journal of Environmental Research and Public Health*, 11(2), 1479–99.

9 Coory MD, Jordan S. (2013). Assessment of chance should be removed from protocols for investigating cancer clusters. *International Journal of Epidemiology*, 42(2), 440–7. doi:10.1093/ije/dys205

10 Simpson BW, Truant P, Resnick BA. (2014). Stop and listen to the people: an enhanced approach to cancer cluster investigations. *American Journal of Public Health*, 104(7), 1204–8.

11 Trumbo CW. (2000). Public requests for cancer cluster investigations: a survey of state health departments. *American Journal of Public Health*, 90(8), 1300–2.

12 Alexander FE, Cuzick J. (1996). Methods for the assessment of disease clusters. In: Eliott P, Cuzick J, English D, et al., eds, *Geographical and environmental epidemiology methods for small-area studies*, pp. 238–50. Oxford University Press, Oxford.

13 Alexander FE, Boyle P. (1996). *Methods for investigating localized clustering of disease*. IARC Scientific Publication No. 135. International Agency for Research on Cancer, Lyon.

14 Department of Health (2000). *Good practice guidelines for investigating the health impact of local industrial emissions*. Department of Health, London.

15 Leukaemia Research Fund (1997). *Handbook and guide to the investigation of clusters of disease*. Leukaemia Research Fund Centre for Clinical Epidemiology, University of Leeds.

16 Rothenberg RB, Thacker SB. (1996). Guidelines for the investigation of clusters of adverse health events. In: Eliott P, Cuzick J, English D, et al., eds, *Geographical and environmental epidemiology methods for small-area studies*, pp. 264–77. Oxford University Press, Oxford.

17 Kingsley BS, Schmeichel KL, Rubin CH. (2007). An update on cancer cluster activities at the Centers for Disease Control and Prevention. *Environmental Health Perspectives*, **115**(1), 165–71.

18 Saunders PJ, Middleton JD, Rudge G. (2016). Environmental public health tracking: a cost-effective system for characterizing the sources, distribution and public health impacts of environmental hazards. *Journal of Public Health*, doi:10.1093/pubmed/fdw130

19 Kirkwood BR, Sterne JAC. (2003). *Essentials of medical statistics*, 2nd edn. Blackwell Scientific Publications, Oxford.

20 Mohammed MA. (2004) Using statistical process control to improve the quality of health care. *Quality & Safety in Health Care*, **13**(4), 243–5.

21 Coory MD, Wills RA, Barnett AG. (2009) Bayesian versus frequentist statistical inference for investigating a one-off cancer cluster reported to a health department. *BMC Medical Research Methodology*, 11(9), 30.

22 Kibble A, Harrison R. (2005) Point sources of air pollution. *Occupational Medicine*, **55**(6), 425–31.

23 Bertazzi PA, Consonni D, Bachetti S, et al. (2001) Health effects of dioxin exposure: a 20-year mortality study. *American Journal of Epidemiology*, **153**(11), 1031–44.

24 Cordioli M, Ranzi A, De Leo GA, et al. (2013) A review of exposure assessment methods in epidemiological studies on incinerators. *Journal of Environmental and Public Health*. doi:10.1155/2013/129470

25 Robertson C, Nelson TA, MacNab YC, et al. (2010) Review of methods for space–time disease surveillance. *Spatial and Spatio-temporal Epidemiology*. 1(2–3), 105–16.

26 Thompson JA, Bissett WT, Sweeny AM. (2014) Evaluating geostatistical modeling of exceedance probability as the first step in disease cluster investigations: very low birth weights near toxic Texas sites. *Environmental Health*. doi:10.1186/1476-069X-13-47

27 James L, Matthews I, Nix B. (2004) Spatial contouring of risk: a tool for environmental epidemiology. *Epidemiology*, 15(3), 287–92.

28 Cook AJ, Gold DR, Li Y. (2009) Spatial cluster detection for repeatedly measured outcomes while accounting for residential history. *Biometrical Journal*, 51(5), 801–18.

29 Vieira V, Webster T, Weinberg J, et al. (2009). Spatial analysis of bladder, kidney, and pancreatic cancer on upper Cape Cod: an application of generalized additive models to case-control data. *Environmental Health*, **10**(8), 3.

30 Levy AG, Weinstein N, Kidney E, et al. (2008). Lay and expert interpretations of cancer cluster evidence. *Risk Analysis*, **28**, 1531–8.

Assessing longer-term health trends: disease registers

Rachael Brock, Sarah Stevens, and Jem Rashbass

Objectives

The objectives of this chapter are to:
- describe different types of disease register
- explain the principles and requirements of disease registration
- explore two examples of disease registration: cancer registration, and the English National Congenital Anomaly and Rare Disease Registration Service (NCARDRS)
- enable you to use disease registers effectively, with an awareness of their strengths and limitations.

Introduction

Disease registers

A disease register is a record of all cases of a particular disease or health condition, limited to a defined population.[1] Data collected varies widely between registers, but often includes personal identifiers, socio-demographic information, disease status (including stage or severity), details of treatments and other interventions, and eventual outcomes. Population-level registers have traditionally been used in public health as a source of data to support epidemiology and surveillance. Data collection has focused on small, high-quality longitudinal datasets for one or more diseases while the continuous follow-up and accretion of information on registered cases has been limited. In general, users request snapshots of data from the register to perform analyses on a cohort. Time series analysis usually involves sequential snapshots. The restricted breadth of datasets and the relative tardiness[2] of data collection results in registers that, although useful in identifying cases, mean that the collection of additional data items to answer specific detailed or clinical questions, or pursue high-resolution studies, is almost always necessary.

There are several different types of disease register, each with a different primary purpose and associated uses. Epidemiological registers are based on a disease or risk factor, such as a specific exposure, intervention, or treatment, within a defined population. Registers designed to support service provision, such as 'at risk' registers for children, can be used to ensure adequate protection for such children. Clinical researchers, pharmaceutical companies, patient groups, and charities often maintain registers of patients with a specific disease or condition who are keen to participate in research. Generally, registers that are not population-based are more useful for technology assessment and quality improvement than for epidemiological purposes because the denominator is often unknown and ascertainment may be biased.[3] However, they can operate as a support network, providing patients with a link to the community and information directly relevant to their condition.

Disease registration services

In the past five years, with a rapidly increasing recognition of the value of large-scale, detailed population-level healthcare data, there has been a move toward national disease registration services. Unlike a disease register, a disease registration service aims to collect data along the whole care pathway in near real-time, collecting and linking individual clinical event data from multiple sources to build a comprehensive resource. For example, a tumour may be correctly staged at diagnosis in a variety of ways. So, a cancer registration service will record several different staging data items for one tumour, recording whether each is based on imaging, pathology, clinical assessment, or other parameters. Similarly, no single date may be defined as the date of diagnosis: rather, dates of all relevant episodes on the patient pathway will be recorded. The interpretation of the collected data then forms an integral part of future analyses.

Requirements of a disease registry

A registry must establish processes and systems to:
- collect data: maintain reliable notification or identification of cases within the defined population to ensure high case ascertainment
- process data: ensure comparability of inclusion criteria on to the register; for a diagnosis, strict rules are needed to identify the studied condition, within an agreed, ideally internationally recognised, classification
- quality assure data: ensure that duplication of cases within the register does not occur
- follow up cases: keep the register updated to ensure completeness of outcomes—tracking those who have recovered, died, or moved out of the area
- Report findings: collate and analyse the data.

Patient consent

Most registers require patient consent to collect and hold their data. However, in England, legislation has allowed selected disease registers to collect identifiable patient information without prior informed consent (section 251, NHS Act 2006), in recognition of the important public health function these registers play. This important caveat is currently subject to annual review by the Confidentiality Advisory Group in England and Wales. Any research use of registry data can only occur with appropriate ethical approval and either patient consent or a valid legal basis, especially if identifiable data is requested.

Why are registers important?

If case ascertainment is high and a register is population-based, prevalence and incidence rates can be calculated. Analysis of risks and aetiology can be explored, using individual as well as area characteristics. With follow-up data, outcomes can be measured (e.g. survival rates for cancer). If registers are maintained over time, they can produce evidence of change in, for example, epidemics or the effectiveness of interventions.

Registers can be used to assist in the management of disease in clinical settings, triggering follow-up care for people with, for example, diabetes or asthma within a primary care practice. Registers can also form the basis for clinical audit and quality improvement efforts.

Example 1: Cancer registration

The cancer registration system is a unique worldwide resource: there are more than 700 cancer registries worldwide.[4] Many European cancer registries, including those in the UK and Scandinavia, provide national coverage of all diagnosed cancers. Other countries, such as Germany, Italy, and France, comprise a network of regional registries.[5] Further afield, Canada maintains a national cancer registry, while the USA runs a network of state-based registries under the auspices of the North American Association of Central Cancer Registries (NAACCR).

Cancer registries in Europe work together through the European Network of Cancer Registries (ENCR) to define data standards and align cancer registration practices. Worldwide, the International Association of Cancer Registries (IACR) promotes the development and application of standardized methods for cancer registries, and supports the analysis and publication of their data.

What data is collected?

Most cancer registries are population-based, providing a denominator for numbers of tumours in relation to the population of which the patients are members. It is important to remember that registries only contain records of diagnosed cancers: they do not contain information on the small proportion of tumours that remain undiagnosed at the time of death.

Individual records start at the point of diagnosis and record details of the patient and tumour at that time. Increasingly, information is available on treatment and events post-diagnosis. Data items recorded may differ slightly between registries, but minimum content is often nationally defined. In the UK, for example, all cancer registries record:

- patient details: name, address, postcode, date of birth, sex, unique patient identifier
- tumour characteristics: site, histological type, grade, and stage at diagnosis
- date of diagnosis
- treatment received during the first six months after diagnosis
- date and cause of death.

Many registries collect and record extra data on each patient and tumour, and links between multiple tumours in the same patient will be recorded. Consistent use of a unique patient identifier enables linkage to other datasets using this identifier: in England, the NHS number is used to link tumour records to national healthcare datasets such as Hospital Episode Statistics (HES) to provide valuable information about a patient's inpatient, outpatient, and emergency hospital attendances.

What can the data be used for?

Traditionally, use of cancer registry data has been the preserve of the epidemiologist: most registries have a distinguished history of publishing regular reports on incidence rates, survival, and stage (for selected tumours),[6] including assessments of historical trends and, with sufficient longevity of data, robust future projections.

Increasingly, registry data is being used to drive wider healthcare system aims: as a data source for clinical audits; as real-world evidence for pharmaceutical trials and research; to assess adherence to national clinical guidelines; to evaluate cancer screening programmes; and to evaluate treatment effectiveness in defined patient populations. The power of cancer registry data in supporting these activities increases markedly when linked to other healthcare and national datasets: for example, linkage with socioeconomic data enables in-depth assessment of healthcare inequalities. The advent of big data, machine learning, and artificial intelligence has the potential to fuel explosive growth in this wider arena.

Example 2: The National Congenital Anomaly and Rare Disease Registration Service for England

Public Health England established the National Congenital Anomaly and Rare Disease Registration Service (NCARDRS) in 2015, in response to the national requirements for high-quality public health disease surveillance identified by the Chief Medical Officer. The creation of the NCARDRS is part of the UK Strategy for Rare Diseases and the Department of Health's 2020 Vision on Rare Diseases.[7]

What data is collected?

Data is collected from a number of different sources: maternity units, neonatal units, paediatrics, specialist clinics, diagnostic departments (clinical genetics, testing laboratories, antenatal ultrasound, fetal medicine, and pathology), child health systems, and disease-specific registers. Data relating to the same case is drawn from multiple independent sources to maximise the level of detail available. This multiple-source capture enables NCARDRS to achieve the highest possible ascertainment and completeness of cases in the population.

Data is collected on all suspected and confirmed congenital anomalies and rare diseases identified in utero, at birth, in childhood, or as an adult. NCARDRS collects information about both mother and child, including postcode of residence, mother's age, pregnancy length, pregnancy outcome, when and how the condition was identified, and the details of each diagnosis. Identifiable information is collected only insofar as it is needed to avoid duplicate registrations and for the validation of cases, ensuring accurate matching between antenatally diagnosed cases and postnatal notifications.

NCARDRS reports to the European Surveillance of Congenital Anomalies (EUROCAT) and has been designed to be interoperable with other national and international rare disease registries and repositories.

What can the data be used for?

Similar to cancer registration, NCARDRS aims to be a valuable resource for clinicians and patients, service delivery, commissioning, and public health. It works to:

- provide a resource for clinicians to support high-quality clinical practice
- support and empower patients and their carers by providing information relevant to their disease or disorder
- improve epidemiology and monitoring of the frequency, nature, cause, and outcomes of these disorders
- support research into congenital anomalies, rare diseases, and precision medicine including basic science, cause, prevention, diagnostics, treatment, and management
- inform the planning and commissioning of public health and health and social care provision
- provide a resource to monitor, evaluate, and audit health and social care services, including the efficacy and outcomes of screening programmes.

Accessing data

As outlined above, most registries publish regular reports based on their data so, if your enquiry is simple, these may provide you with the information you need. If your enquiry is more complex, or if you are not quite sure what you need, the registry will be able to advise you. All registries employ statisticians or epidemiologists, and part of their job is to advise on the use and the limitations of the data. Before contacting the registry, make sure you have considered:

- which disease or condition you are interested in
- which cohort of patients you are interested in: age, sex, area of residence, year of diagnosis.

Registries have clear policies that govern the release of data. For cancer registries, these are developed in line with IACR recommendations, which state that clinicians should be given access to data needed for management of their patients, in accordance with national law.[8] For research and healthcare planning purposes, most registries are willing to release aggregate or anonymised data that does not directly identify patients. However, even anonymised data may be potentially disclosive: for example, the identity of a patient who has a rare disease, or is a member of a small population, may be inferred if age or area of residence is known. The release of such data is governed by strict ethical and confidentiality requirements, including the demonstration of a genuine need for data at this level of detail.

Limitations of disease registers

Often, notification to a registry is not a mandatory requirement—it requires the goodwill of notifiers. Electronic records have improved accessibility and timeliness of data and patients can be better identified in countries where a unique patient identifier is in routine use. However, collating information from disparate electronic systems is a challenge. Despite the wealth of data available, the ability to investigate and pursue local hard-to-find data is essential for comprehensive registration. Experience indicates that data quality is enhanced when registration staff develop a good working relationship with hospital trusts, health professionals, and clinicians.

A register is only as good as the data that is available. The data is never entirely complete: occasionally, data may appear many years after diagnosis. If the diagnosis or the death certificate is wrong, then even a complete dataset will be flawed. Be sceptical and question all your data sources—even disease registers!

Further resources

European Network of Cancer Registries (n.d.). Available at: ℘ http://www.encr.eu (accessed 21 August 2019).

European Surveillance of Congenital Anomalies (n.d.). Available at: ℘ http://www.eurocat-network.eu (accessed 21 August 2019).

International Association of Cancer Registries (2017). Available at: ℘ http://www.iacr.com.fr (accessed 21 August 2019).

International Agency for Research on Cancer (2017). Available at: ℘ http://www.iarc.fr (accessed 21 August 2019).

References

1 Rankin J, Best K. (2014). Disease registers in England. *Paediatrics and Child Health*, **24(8)**, 337–42.

2 Zanetti R, Schmidtmann I, Sacchetto L, et al. (2015). Completeness and timeliness: cancer registries could/should improve their performance. *European Journal of Cancer*, **51(9)**, 1091–8.

3 Rankin J, Best K. (2014). Disease registers in England. *Paediatrics and Child Health*, **24(8)**, 337–42.

4 Forman D, Bray F, Brewster DH, et al. (2013). Cancer incidence in five continents, Vol. X (electronic version). IARC, Lyon.

5 Siesling S, Louwman WJ, Kwast A, et al. (2015). Uses of cancer registries for public health and clinical research in Europe: results of the European Network of Cancer Registries survey among 161 population-based cancer registries during 2010–2012. *European Journal of Cancer*, **51(9)**, 1039–49.

6 Siesling S, Louwman WJ, Kwast A, et al. (2015). Uses of cancer registries for public health and clinical research in Europe: results of the European Network of Cancer Registries survey among 161 population-based cancer registries during 2010–2012. *European Journal of Cancer*, **51(9)**, 1039–49.

7 The UK Strategy for Rare Diseases (2013). Available at: ℘ https://www.gov.uk/government/uploads/system/uploads/attachment_data/file/260562/UK_Strategy_for_Rare_Diseases.pdf (accessed 21 August 2019).

8 Tyczynski JE, Démaret D, Parkin DM (2003). Standards and guidelines for cancer registration in Europe: the ENCR recommendations. European Network of Cancer Registries, International Agency for Research on Cancer.

Part 3

Direct action

Communicable disease epidemics

Sarah O'Brien

Objectives

After reading this chapter you should be able to:
- define the terms 'communicable disease', 'epidemic', and 'outbreak'
- explain the principles of preventing communicable disease
- explain the key features of different types of outbreaks or epidemics
- understand the key steps in investigating an outbreak or epidemic.

Definitions

A *communicable* (or *infectious*) *disease* is an illness due to the transmission of a specific infectious agent (or its toxic products) from an infected person, animal, or inanimate source to a susceptible host, either directly or indirectly.[1]

A commonly used definition of an *epidemic* is that of Abram Benenson, who defined it as 'the occurrence in a community or region of cases of illness (or an outbreak) with a frequency clearly in excess of normal expectancy'. The meaning of the term 'epidemic' is broad. It encompasses both communicable diseases (e.g. meningitis) and non-communicable diseases (e.g. obesity). In this chapter, however, we will concentrate on communicable diseases. The numbers of cases, geographic extent, and time period need to be specified to be able to describe an epidemic.

The term *outbreak* is often used to describe any of the following:
- *Two or more related (i.e. epidemiologically linked) cases of a similar disease:* acute food poisoning after a wedding breakfast may present like this.
- *An increase in the observed incidence of cases over the expected incidence within a given time period:* this way of detecting outbreaks, through routine surveillance, implies a less acute onset but, paradoxically, may be more serious than the previous example. This is because the problem was detected later, there is no immediate indication as to source, and many more cases may be pending.
- *A single case of a serious disease:* a single case of botulism or smallpox constitutes a public health emergency and should trigger a very detailed investigation.

Why does preventing epidemics matter?

Severe acute respiratory syndrome (SARS), the first new severe disease of the twenty-first century, reminded us that new diseases emerge in human/microorganism interactions. Similarly, old diseases, like tuberculosis, re-emerge, this time with antimicrobial resistance. People's susceptibility and/or exposure to microorganisms also changes so that communicable diseases pose a constant threat to global security either naturally or, potentially, through bioterrorism.

Communicable diseases lead to around 12 million deaths worldwide (21% of global mortality) (Table 3.1.1). Furthermore, they cause approximately 23% of cancers in the developing world and 7% of cancers in the industrialized world (Table 3.1.2).[2] So reducing mortality and morbidity means tackling these preventable infections.

Table 3.1.1 World Health Organization estimates of global mortality from infectious diseases, 2015

Infectious disease	Deaths (millions)
Respiratory infections	3.2
Diarrhoeal disease	1.4
Tuberculosis	1.4
Acquired immunodeficiency syndrome	1.1
Malaria	0.4
Total due to all infectious causes	5.7

Source: Global Health Estimates 2015: Deaths by Cause, Age, Sex, by Country and by Region, 2000–2015. Geneva, World Health Organization, 2016.

Table 3.1.2 Selected infection/cancer combinations, 2012

Infectious agent	Cancer	% of cancers due to infection	No. of cases globally/yr
Helicobacter pylori	Non-cardio gastric adenocarcinoma	89	73,000
			13,000
	MALT lymphoma	74	
Hepatitis B virus and Hepatitis C virus	Liver	73	570,000
Human papilloma virus	Cervix	100	530,000

Source: data from Plummer M, de Martel C, Vignat J, et al. (2016) Global burden of cancers attributable to infections in 2012: a synthetic analysis. *Lancet Global Health*, 4(9), e609–16.

How can we prevent epidemics?

Classically, prevention is described as primary, secondary, or tertiary.

Primary prevention: preventing disease onset

In the context of communicable diseases, various options include the following:

- Eliminating the organism:
  - controlling organisms in their natural reservoir (e.g. maintaining Brucella-free cattle herds to prevent human brucellosis).
- Environmental protection:
  - ensuring a safe drinking water supply, with proper separation of sewage from drinking water (taken for granted in high- and some middle-income countries)
  - safeguarding the food supply.
- Interrupting the chain of transmission:
  - controlling the insect vector for arthropod-borne diseases (e.g. West Nile Virus—an emerging cause of encephalitis in North America)
  - controlling the rodent vector for diseases like leptospirosis

- modifying behaviour (e.g. practising safe sex or avoiding injecting drug use, to prevent the spread of sexually transmitted diseases and blood-borne viruses like hepatitis B, hepatitis C, and HIV)
- personal hygiene—a simple yet effective means of control.
- *Reducing susceptibility in the host:*
  - reversing malnutrition and micronutrient deficiency to boost people's immunity in low-income countries helps to prevent the spread of, for example, tuberculosis
  - vaccination—perhaps the most successful example of primary prevention, leading to global eradication of smallpox and to a sustained reduction in the incidence and consequences of childhood diseases. Childhood vaccination schedules vary by country, but an up-to-date list is posted on the World Health Organization's website (see ➔ Further resources). This is very useful for assessing whether children moving into the community from overseas are likely to have completed their courses of vaccinations.
- *Health education and community participation:*
  - promoting vector control programmes, in particular the use of personal protection like insect repellents and mosquito nets
  - supporting personal hygiene and food hygiene measures in preventing gastroenteritis
  - endorsing vaccination campaigns.

Secondary prevention: arresting the progression of established disease

The options here include the following:
- *Screening:* when there is an asymptomatic or pre-symptomatic period in the infection process, screening programmes are useful.
- Outbreak/epidemic investigation.

The main aims of epidemic/outbreak investigation are to:
- identify the causative agent(s), route(s) of transmission, and risk factors for the outbreak
- develop and implement control and prevention strategies and provide advice to prevent a similar event in the future.

Tertiary prevention: limiting the consequences of established disease

One example of this is providing artificial limbs for a child who has needed amputations following severe meningococcal septicaemia.

What are the key tasks?

Epidemic/outbreak investigation needs to be systematic, thorough, and rapid.
Conventionally, investigating and managing outbreaks/epidemics is divided into stages, although in practice these often run in parallel. The technical stages (Box 3.1.1) are as follows.

> **Box 3.1.1 Key elements of outbreak/epidemic investigation and management**
> - Establish that there really is an outbreak.
> - Confirm the diagnosis.
> - Create a case definition.
> - Find and count cases.
> - Draw an epidemic curve.
> - Determine who is at risk.
> - Generate and test hypotheses for exposure.
> - Consider what additional evidence is needed.
> - Implement control measures.
> - Write up your findings.

Establish that there really is an outbreak

Look at your local surveillance data and combine this with your local knowledge to help you determine whether or not an epidemic/outbreak is occurring. Consider artefactual reasons why an epidemic/outbreak might appear to have occurred, including:
- changes in reporting practice
- introduction of new microbiological methods
- increasing awareness of an infection in the community leading to increased reports
- a laboratory contamination incident.

Confirm the diagnosis

Arrange for appropriate specimens to be obtained and examined. The types of specimens needed depend on the precise circumstances so seek the advice of an expert in microbiology. If nothing else, warn laboratory staff of an impending influx of specimens so that they can organize their work, prioritizing outbreak samples. Agree with laboratory staff how to identify outbreak-related samples. Because laboratory diagnosis takes time and must not delay investigations, look for a degree of commonality of symptoms to form a case definition.

Create a case definition

Construct a case definition comprising clinical criteria, which should be simple and objective, with limitations on time, place, and person. Sometimes you will need different levels of case definition—probable (patients with similar symptoms) and confirmed (where a laboratory diagnosis is added to the definition for a probable case).

Count cases (case finding)

Where an outbreak is focused on an event or discrete location (e.g. a hotel or hall of residence), contacting everyone who might have been exposed and finding out if they have symptoms is relatively easy. When the extent of the outbreak is less well defined, trawl through laboratory returns or approach primary care physicians to find additional cases. Whatever method you choose, the case definition should be applied without bias. Typically, information is recorded in a questionnaire:

- *Personal demographic data:* name, address, date of birth, gender, and occupation.
- *Clinical details:* date of illness onset, a listing of symptoms so that the case can select those affecting them, duration of illness, days off work, need for admission to hospital, and outcome of illness.
- *Data items determined by the nature of the outbreak:* for example, travel history, immunization history, exposure to possible causal sources (such as food, water, recreational, environmental), places visited, shopping habits, contacts with ill people or animals, all depending on circumstances.

Draw an epidemic curve

Plot the number of cases over time on a graph. The shape of the epidemic curve provides clues to the nature of the outbreak. A point-source epidemic curve, where exposure has been limited in time, usually shows a sharp upswing and a fairly rapid tail-off (Figure 3.1.1). A propagated, or continuing, source epidemic curve tends to be flatter in shape and continues over a much longer time (Figure 3.1.2). In an outbreak transmitted from person to person, epidemic waves can be seen. The epidemic curve should be updated on a daily basis. In an outbreak of Legionnaires' disease, plotting cases on a map can also yield helpful clues to potential sources of contamination.

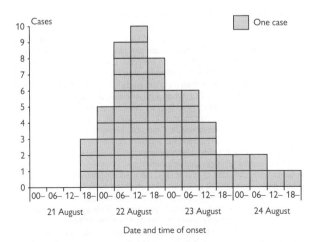

Figure 3.1.1 An example of a point source epidemic curve.

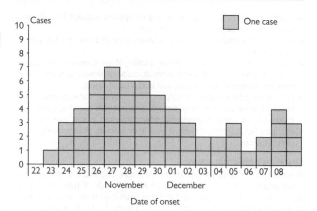

Figure 3.1.2 An example of a propagated source epidemic curve.

Determine who is at risk

Sometimes this is obvious—for example, a food poisoning outbreak at a wedding breakfast when those at risk are the guests. Also consider other people who might have dined at the same place but not been part of the wedding party.

Generate and test hypotheses for exposure

Collate information about symptoms, circumstances, and diagnosis to form hypotheses about the cause of the outbreak, which can be tested using analytical epidemiology. Do not re-use the cases who were interviewed as part of the hypothesis-generation exercise. Decide on the appropriate study design. If the event is so well delineated that all those at risk, both ill and well, can be identified, then a cohort study is appropriate. If all those at risk cannot be delineated (e.g. when a general excess of disease is apparent in the community but its origin is not) a case-control study is appropriate:

- *Data capture from the cohort, or cases and controls, is usually by a standard structured questionnaire:* if possible, develop questionnaires on the web to avoid the need for separate data entry, but ensure that data are secure. Emailing questionnaires and/or using web-enabled questionnaires achieve rapid responses.
- *Control selection (case-control study)* (Table 3.1.3): controls must have had the opportunity to be exposed to the hypothesized source and, in a community outbreak, select the controls from that community. Consider the need for matching (e.g. within 10% for age) but avoid overmatching. Controls can be nominated by cases or recruited at random (e.g. random digit dialling). Increasingly popular is the use of market research panels or so-called 'control banks' for recruiting controls. Speed of access to these sources of controls is an advantage but can be offset by low participations rates and poor representation among panel members of certain population groups.

Table 3.1.3 Pros and cons of control selection in epidemic/outbreak investigations

Control type	Advantages	Disadvantages
Hospital or laboratory	Easy to access. Cases and controls comparable in terms of medical care	Patients may have other conditions that are associated with the disease of interest
Case-nominated	Easy to access. Useful for rare conditions. Participation rate fairly good	Risk of overmatching—friends, relatives, or neighbours may share exposures with the cases
Community	Avoids bias inherent in using case-nominated controls	Method of recruitment may introduce new biases. Participation rate likely to be lower than with case-nominated controls
Control registers or market panels	Quick to implement facilitating timely investigation	Expensive to maintain control registers or to access market panels. Need to provide a very detailed specification to ensure that controls are appropriate. Low response rate. Demographic characteristics of panel members might be different from that of general population (e.g., fewer panel members from black and minority ethnic populations and fewer children).

- *Data analysis:* in a cohort study, where denominators are known, compare the attack rates in those who consumed a (Table 3.1.4), given food with the attack rate in those who did not. In a case-control study, calculate the odds of becoming ill (Table 3.1.5). In each instance, compute 95% confidence intervals (CIs) and use an appropriate statistical test (seek advice from a statistician). If more than one exposure is significantly associated with illness, look at strategies for dealing with confounding and potential interactions (e.g. stratified analysis or logistic regression modelling).

Alternative methods for analysis include case–case studies[3] and case cross-over studies[4].

Consider what additional evidence is needed

Do you need additional laboratory tests (e.g. food, water, or environmental samples)? What have investigations by your professional colleagues shown? For example, in a food poisoning outbreak, environmental health officers will collect important details, such as food preparation and storage practices, and carry out an inspection of the implicated premises. Whole-genome sequencing in microbiology is providing additional important insights into transmission of microorganisms at a forensic level, revealing just how complex it can be.[5] In an outbreak of Legionnaires' disease, a specialist inspection by an environmental engineer may be needed. Combining information from epidemiological, environmental, and microbiological investigations means that you can develop a picture of what went wrong and

Table 3.1.4 An example of how to present results from a single risk variable analysis in a retrospective cohort study

Variable	Category definitions	Ill	Not ill	Attack rate	Relative risk	95% CI for the relative risk	P value
Coleslaw	Yes	21	23	48	1.13	(0.62, 2.09)	0.89
	No	8	11	42			
	Missing	1	3				
Pasta salad	Yes	26	24	52	2.43	(0.86, 6.85)	0.08
	No	3	11	21			
	Missing	1	2				
Italian ciabatta and butter	Yes	16	14	53	1.39	(0.81, 2.40)	0.34
	No	13	21	38			
	Missing	1	2				
Lemon cheesecake	Yes	9	11	45	0.92	(0.52, 1.64)	1.00
	No	20	21	49			
	Missing	1					
Strawberry gateau	Yes	13	17	43	0.92	(0.54, 1.58)	0.96
	No	16	18	47			
	Missing	1	2				
Orange juice	Yes	28	22	56	3.92	(1.06, 14.48)	0.01
	No	2	12	14			
	Missing	0	3				

why, and this will help you formulate both immediate control measures and measures to prevent a recurrence in the longer term.

Implement control measures

These can be initiated at any stage of the investigation, as soon as there is sufficient evidence to act on. Seek specialist advice if necessary. The aims are to prevent new primary cases and secondary spread. Ongoing surveillance will tell you if the control measures have worked and, if not, you need to revisit your hypothesis and re-evaluate the situation.

Write up your findings

Keep contemporaneous (preferably handwritten) notes as you go along—this saves a lot of heartache in court later! At the end of the outbreak, write up your findings in an outbreak control team report. As well as being a record of what you did and what was found, lessons learned should be highlighted so that others may learn from what happened.

Table 3.1.5 An example of how to present results from a single risk variable analysis in a case-control study (in this instance, the analysis was matched)

Variable	Exposed (%)		MOR*	95% CI		P Value
	Cases	Controls		Lower	Upper	
Cold food from take-away cafes	46 (58)	34 (26)	3.46	1.84	6.50	<0.001
Eat any eggs	56 (71)	67 (51)	2.41	1.26	4.61	0.006
Egg prepared away from home	35 (60)	14 (18)	25.74	3.24	204.55	<0.001
Any cold cows' milk drunk	56 (71)	107 (81)	0.48	0.24	0.99	0.04
Sandwiches, rolls, etc., bought in plastic packs	47 (59)	26 (20)	4.34	2.33	8.07	<0.001
Ham sandwiches, etc.	10 (13)	5 (4)	3.68	1.12	12.07	0.02
Prawn/other seafood sandwiches, etc.	6 (8)	3 (2)	4.52	1.05	19.46	0.03
Egg mayonnaise sandwiches, etc.	13 (16)	1 (1)	18.11	2.33	140.51	0.0001

Note: the percentage of cases and controls exposed ignoring matching.
* Matched odds ratio.

What skills and competencies are needed?

Public health professionals investigating outbreaks need expertise in the following areas:
• Surveillance.
• Epidemiological study design.
• Statistics.
• Leadership.
• Management of programmes.
• Evaluation.
• Communication.
A sense of humour also helps! Remember that skills such as microbiology and environmental health are vested in other team members.

What is involved in getting something done?

Have an outbreak plan beforehand, exercise it regularly, and update it annually. It helps to know your colleagues before you come together in a crisis. Make sure that you can mobilize people 24 hours a day, set up an incident room, and access specialist advice.

Who else might need to be involved?

This depends to a certain extent on the nature of the outbreak/epidemic. For example, in an outbreak of food-borne disease, the core team often comprises a public health practitioner with specialized training, an environmental health officer or sanitarian, a microbiologist, and a statistician. It might be appropriate to include a specialist food microbiologist, a clinician, and a veterinarian, depending on the exact circumstances. Assistance from a press officer usually proves invaluable.

Potential pitfalls

Probably the biggest potential pitfall is trying to run an investigation single-handed. Outbreak/epidemic investigation is genuinely a team effort. Do not rely on being able to conduct an investigation solely during office hours. By the time an outbreak comes to light, many of the cases may have recovered. This means that they are back at work during the daytime, just like you are. The best times to conduct interviews in person tend to be during the evening, up to 9.00pm, and at weekends, although make sure that you are aware of the major sporting fixtures—ringing people during a major sporting fixture is unlikely to increase the response rate. Do not have more than one person speaking to the press. Agree at the outset who will do it, and stick to it. Finally, use your common sense—a good descriptive study can provide better evidence than a poor analytic one.

Dogma, myths, and fallacies

It is sometimes said that there is no point in investigating point-source outbreaks because they are, by definition, over. However, you cannot know that an outbreak is over unless you have at least conducted a preliminary investigation. Requests for standard questionnaires are often made. While it is true that certain elements (e.g., demographic and clinical details) rarely change—in reality there is no such thing as a standard outbreak. The danger is of being blinded by biological plausibility and, if taken to its logical conclusion, outbreaks of salmonellosis associated with contaminated lettuce or melons would never have been identified and controlled. Similarly, we would still be chasing contaminated hamburgers as the cause of outbreaks of *Escherichia coli* O157, ignoring transmission from the environment and animals. Standard questionnaires are not a substitute for thinking.

What are the key determinants of success?

These are skill, speed (including the ability to mobilize sufficient resources at very short notice), a pre-determined tested plan, flexibility, and political clout.

How will you gauge success?

Continue to monitor the epidemic curve and routine surveillance data, which should show no new cases or a reduction in incidence.

Further resources

Connolly MA. (ed.) (2005). *Communicable disease control in emergencies. A field manual*. World Health Organization, Geneva.

Giesecke J. (2017). *Modern infectious disease epidemiology*, 3rd edn. CRC Press, Boca Raton, FL.

Gregg MB. (ed.) (2008). *Field epidemiology*, 3rd edn. Oxford University Press, Oxford.

Heymann DL. (ed.) (2014). *Control of communicable diseases manual*, 20th edn. American Public Health Association, Washington DC.

Nelson KE, Williams CFM. (2014). *Infectious disease epidemiology: theory and practice*, 3rd edn. Jones and Bartlett Learning, Burlington, MA.

World Health Organization. Available at: ℜ http://www.who.int/immunization/policy/immuniza-tion_tables/en (accessed 4 October 2019).

References

1 Porta M. (ed.) (2014). *A dictionary of epidemiology*, 6th edn. Oxford University Press, Oxford.

2 Plummer M, de Martel C, Vignat J, et al. (2016). Global burden of cancers attributable to infections in 2012: a synthetic analysis. *Lancet Global Health*, **4(9)**, e609–16.

3 Fonteneau L, Jourdan Da Silva N, Fabre L, et al. (2017). Multinational outbreak of travel-related Salmonella Chester infections in Europe, summers 2014 and 2015. *Eurosurveillance*, **22(7)**. pii: 30463.

4 Zenner D, Zoellner J, Charlett A, et al. (2014). Till receipts—a new approach for investigating outbreaks? Evaluation during a large Salmonella Enteritidis phase type 14b outbreak in a North West London takeaway restaurant, September 2009. *Eurosurveillance*, **19(27)**, 21–8.

5 Kaiser T, Finstermeier K, Häntzsch M, et al. (2017) Stalking a lethal superbug by whole-genome sequencing and phylogenetics: influence on unraveling a major hospital outbreak of carbapenem-resistant Klebsiella pneumoniae. *American Journal of Infection Control*, pii: S0196–6553(17)30909-4.

Chapter 3.2

Environmental health risks and assessment

**Wendy Heiger-Bernays and
Kathryn Crawford**

Objectives

This chapter will help you appreciate:
- environmental health in the rapidly changing context of health protection
- the utility of having a framework for environmental health risk assessment
- the process for conducting an environmental health risk assessment
- the major strengths and limitations of risk assessment
- the process of identifying, evaluating, and planning a response to an environmental health threat.

Definitions

Environmental health is concerned with all aspects of the natural and built environment that may affect human health, including physical, chemical, biological, and psychosocial factors. It encompasses the assessment and control of those factors, and is focused on preventing disease and creating health-supportive and sustainable environments for current and future generations. The occupational environment is generally excluded from consideration, but practitioners in both domains often share similar approaches. Successful environmental health practice is usually invisible to the public, while failures often attract attention. Disasters such as hurricanes and earthquakes powerfully illustrate the essential nature of local environmental health measures in reducing morbidity and mortality during recovery phases. Likewise, during non-emergency situations, food-borne and water-borne illnesses highlight gaps in process or strategies for prevention:

- Environmental health practitioners may work in private, not-for-profit, government, or academic sectors and operate at local (municipal), regional, or national and international levels. These professionals may be involved in a wide range of issues across many sectors.
- Health protection is the avoidance or reduction of potential harm from exposures through organized efforts, including direct action with individuals or communities, regulation, legislation, or other measures. Health protection may include environmental health services, air, food and water safety, housing, toxic chemicals in consumer products, vector control, communicable disease control, tobacco control, injury prevention, emergency planning and response, and other activities that aim to minimize preventable health risks. Health departments often organize public health governance along the lines of health protection, health promotion, and (depending on the jurisdiction) quality of care assurance.
- *Hazard* is the intrinsic capacity of an agent or mixture of agents that make it capable of causing adverse effects or health outcomes to organisms or the environment following exposure to that agent.
- *Adverse effects* range from immediately observable effects (e.g. burns or skin irritation) to effects that take time to develop (e.g. cancer, heart disease, lowered IQ in offspring).

- *Hazard assessment* is the determination of the potential for a chemical, physical, biological, or social stressor to cause damage, resulting in immediate or delayed adverse health outcomes.
- *Exposure assessment* is the process of finding out how people come into contact with a hazard, how often and for how long, and the amount they are in contact with. Exposure pathways typically include inhalation, ingestion, or contact with the skin or eyes. Exposure assessments for many chemicals rely on the use of biomarkers.
- *Biomarkers* are measurable substances in the body that indicate exposures to hazards or disease. Chemicals or their metabolites, such as lead measured in children's blood, are examples of *biomarkers of exposure* because they indicate exposure, but not an adverse health effect. DNA adducts, a type of DNA damage, are an example of a *biomarker of effect* because they are directly associated with a human disease (cancer).
- *Dose* is the total amount of a substance or agent taken up, or absorbed, by an organism. Many processes including absorption, metabolism, storage, and excretion may affect the dose that ultimately reaches a target organ.
- *Dose–response* is the relationship between the dose of a substance and the resulting changes in body function or health (response).
- *Risk assessment* is the process of estimating the risk to individuals or populations resulting from a specific occurrence or use of a hazard, including the identification of uncertainties, and taking into account possible routes and duration of exposure. When good information is available, risks may be quantifiable, but risk assessment is not an exact science. To be effective, qualitative information influencing the nature of health effects and concerns in the context of particular communities must also be taken into account.
- *Health impact assessment* utilizes risk assessment techniques in relation to development or policy proposals that may have consequences for environmental health. Increasingly, consideration of equity is being introduced into health impact assessment (see ➲ Chapter 1.5).

Why is this an important public health issue?

Risks to public health from environmental hazards emerge and re-emerge with impacts ranging from small-scale or local to widespread exposures affecting whole populations. Childhood morbidities, including learning disabilities and mental health disorders, asthma, obesity, and low-birth weight have raised attention to exposures to environmental conditions.[1] Exposures early in life can negatively affect health across the life course. Many parts of the body are rapidly developing, including the human brain, which is not fully developed until the early 20s, making the fetus and young children more susceptible to environmental toxicants (e.g. lead, endocrine-disrupting chemicals, Zika virus).

Public health has its developmental roots in the identification and control of environmental health risks. 'Old' health protection issues, such as failures in sanitation, contamination of food or water supplies, and air pollution episodes continue to re-emerge, and new threats are evolving from our changing environments and patterns of human use.

Environmental health practitioners must identify environmental hazards and understand how to predict, prevent, monitor, and respond to the threats that they present. The tools from environmental epidemiology, toxicology, exposure science, environmental engineering, and environmental law are used to describe problems and solutions in environmental health. Enforcement of statutory provisions (often through environment agencies) remains an important tool, but the emphasis now on prevention requires a broad range of strategies, including advocacy, intersectoral collaboration, and community engagement and development models in addition to expansion of policy and incentives, standards, and guidelines.

Environmental health practice at the grassroots level—such as the work carried out by local governments to ensure the safety of food, water, and housing conditions—forms part of the bedrock of public health protection.

Public health practitioners understand that healthy environments, including healthy social and economic conditions, are needed to improve the health of the population. Effectively implementing systemic changes to reduce hazards at a broader population level usually requires a strong understanding of environmental health research, knowledge, and skills as well as policy making, community action, and regulation (see ➲ Chapters 3.4, 4.1, and 4.8).

It is also abundantly clear that climate changes' environmental and ecosystem degradation threaten health at the global level, on a massive scale, in ways that are likely to affect disadvantaged people and developing nations most severely[7], and which will require environmental health practitioners to work collaboratively across a wide range of sectors and disciplines (see ➲ Chapter 7.6).

Dividing this work into defined tasks

In order to assess and then protect against a potential environmental health threat, it is useful to adopt a consistent framework for assessing and managing a health risk. The steps involved are:[2]

- issues identification
- hazard identification
- dose–response assessment
- exposure assessment
- risk characterization
- risk management.

In practice, this is often an iterative, rather than a linear framework. Risk management strategies must typically be developed before all the information about risk is available.

Issues identification

Before embarking on a formal risk assessment, the specific issues should be identified with key stakeholders. Explore the underlying concerns and their context—including any existing health concerns or complaints that may be related to current exposures. Find out what interventions have been used and what alternative strategies may be available. Discuss whether the issue is amenable to risk assessment. Successful management of the issues (as distinct from producing a technically competent risk assessment) requires transparency and strong involvement of affected communities as far as possible in the process.

Hazard identification

Hazard identification generally relies on prior knowledge and published scientific evidence of adverse effects associated with exposure to a substance or agent.

Dose–response assessment

Dose–response information involves detailed study of available in-vitro toxicology, animal toxicology, and epidemiology data to understand what is known about how much of a chemical is required to cause adverse health effects. It is also important to thoroughly understand the gaps that exist in such data. These data gaps can be due to difficulties in measuring exposure and dose in human studies (which tend to be opportunistic and retrospective) or methodological weaknesses. It can also be difficult to draw inferences about human health effects from animal studies, and challenges exist when extrapolating dose–response relationships from high-exposure studies to situations involving low exposures, even when human data are available.

Exposure assessment

Commonly, in developed nations, environmental exposures (e.g. via food, soil, water, or ambient air) present lower exposures and total doses than those experienced through personal behaviours or occupational sources. Such exposures may incur relatively small increases in risk. However, because they are perceived as being outside the control of individuals, there is often a large outrage factor. It is important to understand and accept that such issues may require attention that seems out of proportion to their health impact if the exposure is involuntary (see ➲ Chapter 6.5). Knowing the source of emissions and environmental concentrations of contaminants is essential to environmental health protection, but does not indicate how much hazard is actually absorbed by an individual. The use of biomarkers of exposure can provide a more complete picture of the absorbed dose, but they cannot easily be used to attribute the source of the chemical (e.g. blood lead levels). An agent may be hazardous but not result in a risk until exposure occurs and a sufficient dose is delivered to target organs.

Risk characterization

Environmental factors with only a small, perhaps unmeasurable, additional risk at the individual level can still have a major impact on populations if many people are exposed—for example, low-level childhood lead exposure and cognition, or particulate pollution and cardiovascular disease.

Rose's 'prevention paradox' is very relevant to environmental health and can be used to illustrate how small reductions of exposure across a population may reap significant health benefits overall, while offering little benefit to the individual.[3] Likewise, by focusing on reducing the highest exposures of single hazards, the cumulative impact of environmental toxicants on health has been underestimated.

Risk management

The above steps provide a sound basis for effective risk management, which is the process of evaluating alternative actions, selecting options, and implementing them. The goal is defensible, cost-effective, integrated actions that reduce or prevent risks while taking into account social, cultural, ethical, political, and legal considerations. The decision-making process requires value judgements, and the more transparent these are the better it is for communication of health risk (see ➔ Chapters 3.8 and 6.5). Recognition that some communities are burdened with more environmental health risks than others is important in the consideration of equity. The influences of risk perception and community outrage must also be addressed.

Competencies needed to achieve risk assessment tasks

Teamwork is necessary because risk assessment requires technical and non-technical competencies, including communication, interpersonal skills, media relations, interdisciplinary teamwork, advocacy, policy, and planning together with a technical understanding of epidemiology, toxicology, microbiology, exposure assessment, and a range of other biological, physical, and social sciences. A low threshold for recognizing when additional specialist input is needed is desirable.

Systematic performance to make action more effective

Maintenance of a healthy environment requires a systematic approach that may include a range of strategies such as:
- healthy public policy
- legislation and other regulation, with enforcement
- appropriate guidelines and standards
- economic incentives
- demonstration projects
- interventions to bring about attitudinal change
- community involvement
- accurate information communicated effectively
- cross-sectoral action.

Although legislative controls and regulatory mechanisms may be available to deal with an environmental health threat (and are sometimes essential as a back-up measure), this is not usually the first course of action. It is prefer-able to establish collaborative approaches and to work with stakeholders, including affected communities, from an early stage in developing risk man-agement strategies.

Monitoring and surveillance systems are necessary for verifying that con-trol measures are working (e.g. monitoring water quality in drinking water supplies).

Some environmental hazards are amenable to control more readily than lifestyle exposure factors and therefore present opportunities for efficient and effective public health interventions. This is analogous to 'engineered' injury prevention measures that separate the person from the hazard.

In establishing priorities when there are multiple environmental health problems to contend with, consider:
- the urgency of the threat (see ⮞ Chapter 3.5)
- the number of people affected, and their experience of the impacts
- whether the exposure is increasing
- the consequences of 'doing nothing'
- the vulnerability and identifiability of population subgroups
- the amenability of issues to investigation
- the availability of interventions or remedies.

Periodic, systematic review is important to ensure that priorities are not only reactive. For example, there remains an urgent need to consider the long-term health perspective and address global environmental issues (such as the abatement of greenhouse gas emissions), as well as to respond to the immediate impacts of problems related to the environment (e.g. repeated flooding due to increased storm severity and rise in sea level).

Effective action for systemic changes to reduce a hazard (e.g. environ-mental tobacco smoke, including e-cigarettes) can require careful building of a mandate, and political engagement via multiple pathways, to ultimately succeed.

Risk management options can be systematically considered as follows.

Reducing the hazard at its source
- Alteration of systems and human behaviours that underlie the production of a hazard (e.g. transport systems, housing and overcrowding, land use practices, food production methods, water catchment management).
- Alternative source materials (e.g. unleaded paint and petrol, less toxic pesticides)
- Cleaner processing systems and improved emission controls.
- Enforced shutdown of activity.

Protection at the community level
- Removal of contaminant from a medium (e.g. drinking water treatment).
- Physical separation from the source (e.g. relocation of activity, buffer zones, barriers such as highway noise barriers, creation of shade.
- Altering behaviours to reduce exposure (e.g. education to reduce intake of mercury-contaminated fish in pregnancy, boil water alerts, signage and access controls to prevent recreational water contact during blue-green algal blooms, regulation of environmental tobacco smoke).

Protection at the individual level

- Lead abatement of a household to protect a toddler.
- Wearing personal protective equipment.
- Biological measures (e.g. vaccination against hepatitis A to reduce the risk of the disease from unsafe food or water).

Options that reduce hazards at their source are generally preferable because they address root causes and tend to be more equitable and sustainable.

Who else should be involved?

Given the breadth of inputs and strategies mentioned earlier, efforts to protect public health from environmental threats typically require more engagement with stakeholders outside the healthcare system than within it (and this may in part explain why environmental health has been described as the 'Cinderella' of the health system, in terms of resourcing).

In controversial environmental health issues, it can help to involve independent third parties who can objectively question an investigative or risk assessment process, or comment on the evidence available. This is often the case for locating larger infrastructure projects (e.g. power lines or waste facilities) or existing sources of air pollution. Because a disproportionate burden of disease often coincides with low socio-economic status, the location of facilities that emit regulated or unregulated substances requires engagement with representatives from the affected community and limitations on increasing health burdens disproportionately.[4]

Potential pitfalls

Epidemiological approaches

Community members often call for a study of the health status of a local area when concerned about impacts from an existing or perceived exposure. However, epidemiological investigations in relation to environmental exposures should not be undertaken lightly and many factors need to be considered in examining their feasibility. Such studies can be resource-intensive, inconclusive (particularly in small populations) and may actually cause delay in implementation of reasonable precautionary measures to reduce exposure. Cancer cluster investigations often suffer from these pitfalls and various agencies are refining their approach to deal with increases in demand (see ➲ Chapter 2.9).

It is often more appropriate and efficient to evaluate community concerns through exposure assessment, which may include environmental sampling and sometimes biomonitoring, and rely on pre-existing information (e.g. dose–response data of a known toxicant, or application of environmental standards or guidelines) to help interpret the exposure data.

Well-conducted epidemiological studies of adverse health outcomes from environmental exposures provide critical evidence. However, health studies also have limitations and can be a weak link in health risk assessments that often result in dismissal of a problem.

Inadequate measurement of exposure is a particularly common short-coming when attempting to assess whether current health outcomes are attributable to past environmental exposures. Other problems may include lag times between exposures and potential health effects, health effects may be poorly defined, and low-level effects may be very difficult to distinguish from 'background' incidences of common health problems.

There may be groups within a population who are more susceptible to certain hazards, or more highly exposed, or both (e.g. children), and to whom standard risk assessment assumptions do not apply. Compounding of risk by other exposures or possible interactions between co-pollutants may also lead to underestimates of risk. Alternatively, the significance of such risks may be overplayed.

Uncertainty and the precautionary principle

While an evidence-based approach should underpin environmental health action, there are many instances when adequate information is lacking. In such circumstances, a precautionary approach should apply, recognizing the existence of uncertainty and ignorance, and accepting that lack of full sci-entific certainty should not be used as a reason to postpone preventative measures (see Box 3.2.1).

Box 3.2.1 The precautionary principle

One of the outcomes of the United Nations Conference on Environment and Development (also known as the 'Earth Summit') held in Rio de Janeiro, Brazil, in June 1992, was the adoption of the Rio Declaration on Environment and Development, which contains 27 principles to underpin sustainable development.

One of these principles is Principle 15, which states: 'In order to pro-tect the environment, the precautionary approach shall be widely applied by States according to their capabilities. Where there are threats of ser-ious or irreversible damage, lack of full scientific certainty shall not be used as a reason for postponing cost-effective measures to prevent envir-onmental degradation.'

The 'cost-effective' component of this principle can be overlooked by pro-tagonists, leading to conflict between stakeholders about the appropriate response to an issue. Nevertheless, proponents of environmental modifi-cation need to be able to demonstrate that, to a very high degree of prob-ability, a project will not cause significant harm, either to the environment or to health.

In the development of standards and guidelines, it is common for govern-ment policy to be defined not in terms of the precautionary principle but on a science and economics-based approach, which underpins risk assessment and risk management regimes.

Health risk assessments need to be explicit about uncertainties. Looking for bias and identifying what further information could reduce the uncer-tainty also assists in setting priorities in research and monitoring.

Key determinants of success

In situations when environmental exposures clearly threaten health, adequate legislation and emergency powers to support public health interventions may be essential to ensure that exposures are abated as soon as possible.

Risk assessment and management practices need to be sound and accountable. Knowing where and when to seek advice on technically complex matters is vital. Cultivate contacts who can rapidly steer you in the right direction if they do not know themselves.

Empowerment and support of local authorities and communities to integrate environment, health, and sustainable development in local strategies is fundamental to the creation of healthy environments.[5]

Developing a shared understanding with all partners is a key strategy—for example, in promoting transportation systems with co-benefits to reduce air pollution and carbon emissions, and to increase human activity through local and regional planning, with public health at the table. There are many local examples of success from environmental health activities, with the Belfast Healthy Cities partnership being one such case from the World Health Organization's European Healthy Cities Network.[5]

Being proactive (e.g. being prepared for and offering briefings to senior managers, politicians, and community meetings) is often a more productive way to secure understanding and engagement, than being reactive through the media dialogue (see ➜ Chapter 4.5)

How will you know if you have been successful?

Positive indicators include:
- reduced population exposures to a hazard (usually easier and quicker to measure than health outcomes, although there are exceptions—for example, food safety improvements)
- 'process' measures such as improvements in policy or community satisfaction with the process of risk assessment and management
- other sectors own and maintain the environmental control measures that you initiated
- reduced morbidity or mortality associated with the exposure, when health surveillance/epidemiological methods and time frames allow.

Emerging issues

Environmental health inequities are widening, with major risks persisting or emerging in developing countries, as well as in developed nations, typically where income disparities are greatest [6]. The impacts of climate change have necessitated local adaptation strategies[7], requiring decisions regarding housing, food supplies, and livelihood. Fine particles in air pollution are associated with morbidities beyond asthma, such as low birthweight (a predictor for health later in life), and endocrine-disrupting chemicals found in tap water and in consumer products may interfere with the body's endocrine system and produce adverse developmental, reproductive, neurological, and immune effects.[8]

The proliferation of chemical synthesis and the advent of new technologies (e.g. pesticides dispersed in nanoparticles) coupled with the ability to measure previously unmeasurable hazards (e.g. perfluorinated chemicals) present challenges for established methods of toxicological assessment. In the twenty-first century, there is a need for better and more rapid toxicological assessment tools in order to increase the rate at which hazard assessments are conducted.

Improved epidemiological evidence is providing dose–response data that commonly shows there is no threshold or 'safe' level of exposure to a widely distributed hazard (e.g. air pollution from fine particulate matter and lead from multiple sources). In such cases, the policy and regulatory response is shifting from a standards compliance basis towards ongoing measures to further reduce population exposure.

The interrelationship between environment and chronic disease has long been recognized, but the momentum to achieve real change remains limited outside the public and environmental health sectors. However, the profoundly urgent and complex issue of climate change is driving strategic recognition of the co-benefits of environmental action for sustainability with simultaneous improvements in more immediate population health problems such as obesity.[5, 6]

Further resources

Agency for Toxic Substances and Disease Registry (2005). Public health assessment guidance manual. US Department of Health and Human Services. Available at: ℗ https://www.atsdr.cdc.gov/hac/phamanual/pdfs/phagm_final1-27-05.pdf (accessed 16 August 2019).

Public Health England. Available at: ℗ https://www.gov.uk/government/organisations/public-health-england (accessed 30 July 2019).

U.S. National Library of Medicine, Environmental health and technology. Available at: ℗ https://sis.nlm.nih.gov/enviro.html (accessed 30 July 2019).

U.S. National Library of Medicine, ToxTutor: risk assessment. Available at: ℗ https://toxtutor.nlm.nih.gov/06-000.html (accessed 30 July 2019).

World Health Organization (2011). *Guidelines for drinking water quality*, 4th edn. Available at: ℗ http://www.who.int/water_sanitation_health/publications/dwq-guidelines-4/en (accessed 22 December 2017).

World Health Organization (2018). Public health, environmental and social determinants of health. Available at: ℗ http://www.who.int/phe/en (accessed 30 July 2019).

References

1 Lanphear BP. (2015) The impact of toxins on the developing brain. *Annual review of public health*, **36**, 211–30 (Volume publication date March 2015. First published online as a Review in Advance on 12 January 2015). Available at: ℗ https://doi.org/10.1146/annurev-publhealth-031912-114413 (accessed 30 July 2019).

2 United States Environmental Protection Agency (USEPA). Human health risk assessment. Available at: ℗ https://www.epa.gov/risk/human-health-risk-assessment (accessed 22 December 2017).

3 Rose G. (1992). *The strategy of preventive medicine*. Oxford University Press, Oxford.

4 Martuzzi M, Mitis F, Forastiere, F. (2010). Inequalities, inequities, environmental justice in waste management and health. *European Journal of Public Health*, **20**(1), 1 February, 21–6, Available at: ℗ https://doi.org/10.1093/eurpub/ckp216 (accessed 30 July 2019).

5 Belfast Healthy Cities. Available at: ℗ http://www.belfasthealthycities.com (accessed 22 December 2017).

6 *The Lancet* (2017). Commission on pollution and health, **391(10119)**. Available at: ℛ doi: https://doi.org/10.1016/S0140-6736(17)32345-0 (accessed 30 July 2019).

7 *The Lancet* (2015). Health and climate change. Available at: ℛ http://www.thelancet.com/climate-and-health/2015 (accessed 30 July 2019).

8 Gore AC. (2016) Endocrine-disrupting chemicals. *JAMA Internal Medicine*, **176(11)**, 1705–6. Available at: ℛ doi:10.1001/jamainternmed.2016.5766 (accessed 30 July 2019).

Chapter 3.3

Safeguarding and promoting health in the workplace

Stefanos N. Kales and Michael S. Chin

Objectives

After reading this chapter you will be able to understand:
- the nature and scope of occupational health practice
- how illness and injury prevention in the workplace contribute to general public health.

Definition of occupational health

Occupational health deals with the two-way interactions between the health of the worker and the work environment. It encompasses:
- preventing and managing occupationally related illness or injury resulting from workplace hazards
- ensuring that, whenever possible, workers with pre-existing illnesses or disability are able to work safely without undue risk to their own health or those of third parties
- promoting good health, quality of life, and safe working practices in the workplace.

Why is this an important public health issue?

The average worker spends one-third of their life at work. Hence, work accounts for a considerable amount of time for exposures that may result in injury or illness, as well as ample opportunities for improving wellness.

Work environment hazards can be physical, chemical, biological, ergonomic, or psycho-social. In addition, the occupation, type of work performed, environments in which people work, timing of work shifts, and how people are treated in those workplaces can all contribute to workers' overall physical, psychological, and social well-being.

Approaches to occupational health

Preventing occupational illness or injury
- Identifying hazards in the work setting.
- Determining the population exposed to such hazards.
- Assessing the risks from exposure to the hazards (risk assessment).
- Taking appropriate preventive action by one or more of the following actions: elimination, substitution, or containment/mitigation of the hazards (engineering controls) and limiting the numbers of workers exposed.
- Providing personal protective equipment, when other options are not feasible or sufficient.
- Periodically auditing and reassessing the efficacy of the preventive measures.
- Considering the need for a suitable health surveillance programme or periodic monitoring system for the workforce.
- Educating the work population on the relevant safety and health hazards in the workplace.

Accommodating workers with pre-existing illnesses or disability

- Identifying relevant risk factors (e.g. atopy, previous asthma, or previous history of a musculoskeletal disorder,) so that suitable advice, job placement, and work modification can be considered if indicated.
- Assessment of job duties and providing advice on reasonable accommodations that would allow the worker to be employed safely.
- Evaluating the worker's ability to safely perform these job duties with or without modifications.
- Pre-placement assessment and advice.
- Health surveillance, including periodic review of health status and sickness absences.
- For some occupational groups (e.g. healthcare workers), verifying and enforcing the worker's immunizations status is required. An example is determination of measles/mumps/rubella immune status for healthcare workers.

Treating new occupational illness or injury

- Diagnosing new workplace-related illness or injuries.
- Efficient management of illness or injury with emphasis on functional recovery and return to work.
- Assessing the scope of the injury or illness as it may reveal risks to other employees in similar positions.

Promoting general health in the workplace

- Address non-occupational, lifestyle factors that affect health and quality of life, such as information on alcohol intake, smoking, diet, exercise, sleep, safe driving, safe sex, and precautions in the course of travelling or working abroad.
- Promote initiatives in the workplace that can include measures, such as improving the quality of food provided in workplace canteens, establishing no-smoking/tobacco-free policies, encouraging exercise at and away from the workplace, and/or providing subsidized membership to sports and exercise facilities.

What are the tasks needed to achieve effective change?

- Proper identification and assessment of risks.
- Clear strategy for implementing preventive measures.
- Good communication among preventive medicine professionals, management, and the workforce. Publicity through in-house newsletters, seminars, and effective use of the media are crucial elements for creating effective change.
- Timely implementation of measures and ongoing programme review.
- Appropriate engagement of the workforce.

Competencies required

- Occupational health training to assess hazards and risks at the workplace.
- Clinical skills to diagnose and treat injury and illnesses in the workforce.
- Technical expertise to modify workplaces and recommend safer work practices.
- Communication skills to persuade workers to participate in behavioural change to improve health.
- Advocacy acumen to effectively promote the health and safety of the workforce to the organization's management and stakeholders.

Who else might need to be involved?

- Management at all levels, because they ultimately have the responsibility for managing occupational health issues and controlling the access to resources.
- Workers and their representatives, because workers' cooperation and participation are essential for the measures to succeed.
- Occupational health and safety and public health professionals:
  - occupational physicians and nurses
  - public health practitioners
  - safety practitioners
  - occupational hygienists
  - occupational psychologists
  - ergonomists
  - health promotion personnel
  - toxicologists
  - epidemiologists
  - other health practitioners and specialists.
- General practitioners (primary care), because they can help provide advice to their patients on the importance of work to health and well-being, and support a timely return to work after a period of absence.

Ethical dilemmas

Consider these dilemmas, and see what advice is given by the professional bodies (e.g. The London and Irish Faculties of Occupational Medicine's publications on guidance on ethics,[1, 2] and other publications on ethics (e.g. the International Commission on Occupational Health (ICOH) code of ethics for occupational health professionals).

A worker with occupational asthma wants to continue in his job where workplace exposure to an asthmagen cannot be eliminated. The medical advice is to avoid exposure. The worker has no other available job alternatives:

- Should the worker be given all the necessary medical information, and then they choose whether to continue being employed or to leave the job?
- Is the physician avoiding responsibility by asking the patient to make a decision?
- Might the worker's specific occupation and training affect the decision— for example, a veterinarian with an animal allergy?

A safety practitioner is informed by a worker about poor control of exposures at their workplace and poor compliance with safe systems of work. However, they are asked to keep this information confidential and that no representations on this are made to management, because they might be identified as the source of this information with implications for their job security:

- Should the safety practitioner approach management and ignore the request of the worker?
- Or should the wishes of the worker be respected, and the unsafe work practices be allowed to continue?
- Should the practitioner encourage the worker to report anonymously to a watchdog agency or their labour union?

Common myths in occupational health

Myth 1: There is always abundant evidence

For many occupational hazards, there is often insufficient data regarding the effects of exposure on human health. This is either because a good system for gathering information on health effects is non-existent, that compliance with current reporting requirements for occupational ill health is poor, or that animal data and human epidemiological data is limited. The explanation that is sometimes offered that 'we have never had a case of ill health in our workplace resulting from the use of our chemicals or due to our work processes' may reflect an absence of a system for collecting data on occupational ill health, instead of an absence of ill health.

Myth 2: Most clinicians are well trained in occupational health

Training in occupational medicine and occupational health in medical and nursing schools is limited. Consequently, medical and nursing professionals often have only a very general understanding of what can be done to prevent ill health and injury at the workplace.

Myth 3: If we examine every potential worker, and exclude those who are not 100% fit, that will help reduce future ill health and sickness absence

Pre-employment examinations are used in many parts of the world to exclude individuals who have a health problem, even if there is no obvious mismatch between the ill health or disability detected and the job tasks involved. Most pre-employment assessments do not detect clinical abnormalities relevant to safe job performance. Such examinations may be restricted to specific jobs where there is residual exposure to significant risk despite the best measures to reduce the risk. The focus on prevention in the workplace should be on improving the workplace instead of excluding the worker. The new Equality Act in the UK will outlaw many processes used for pre-employment screening. Clinical assessments, if indicated, will need to be performed at a pre-placement stage (as under current United States law), and not as a condition for employment.

Case studies in occupational health

Bhopal disaster

An explosion in the workplace led to acute and chronic health effects among the workforce and surrounding community. The chemical agent involved was methyl isocyanate.[3]

Chernobyl incident

Effects from an out-of-control 'industrial process', partly related to operator fatigue, became a major public health problem (occupational and environmental). The agents involved were radioactive materials.[4]

Dibromochloropropane

Questions on male infertility and the inability to start a family among a US workforce led to factory- and industry-wide epidemiological investigations that then identified dibromochloropropane (DBCP) as the cause. This resulted in cessation of manufacture of DBCP for use as a pesticide.[5]

Sudden cardiac death in firefighters

The leading cause of on-duty mortality in US firefighters is sudden cardiac death, accounting for 45% of all duty-related fatalities. It has been shown that the physical and psychological stressors of firefighting can precipitate acute cardiovascular disease events in firefighters with underlying susceptibilities such as cardiac enlargement, reduced physical fitness, and subclinical atherosclerosis.[6]

Asbestos exposure

Pulmonary fibrosis, bronchogenic carcinoma, and pleural and peritoneal mesothelioma occurred in workers exposed to asbestos fibres. The risk of lung cancer for asbestos exposure was noted to be multiplied where there was concomitant cigarette smoking. Similar health effects occurred from secondary exposure of wives who had to clean the asbestos-contaminated overalls of these workers. Mesotheliomas have also been associated with non-occupational environmental exposure to asbestiform fibres.[7]

Vinyl chloride monomer

A cluster of four cases of a very rare malignancy—angiosarcoma of the liver—occurred among workers responsible for cleaning polymerization chambers for manufacture of polyvinyl chloride (PVC). Prompt preventive action led to rapid reduction in worker exposure to the chemical agent—vinyl chloride monomer.[8] This is a gas that is polymerized to form the relatively inert and non-toxic PVC. Corroborative animal evidence of similar tumours in rodents came to light at about the same time.

Obstructive sleep apnoea

First described in the 1970s, untreated obstructive sleep apnoea (OSA) is the major medical cause of excessive daytime sleepiness. Good evidence demonstrates that untreated OSA results in a several-fold increase in the risk of motor vehicle accidents in the general population and preventable accidents among commercial drivers.[9] In response to mounting evidence, starting in 2016, OSA now has legal reporting and treatment requirements for commercial drivers in the UK.

Take-away lessons

- Prompt public health action may be needed even if not all the desired information is available. Do not let the desire for perfection hinder the need for prudent pragmatism.
- Clusters of a rare disease (e.g. mesothelioma, angiosarcoma) are often easier to identify as resulting from occupational exposure than more common pathology such as lung cancer or spontaneous abortions.
- Effects on the workforce, the wider community, and the environment can result from workplace hazards.
- Public health vigilance and clinical case reports can both lead to identification of health hazards in the workplace.

How is success measured?

- Reduction in the incidence and prevalence of occupational ill health and injury.
- Improvement in morale and productivity of the workforce.
- Reduction of risk or frequency of hazardous exposures.
- Improvement in knowledge of risks and awareness by the working population.
- Positive changes in behaviour and attitudes towards occupational risks by the working population.
- Increased worker productivity and overall health.
- Absence of negative or adverse media publicity.
- Commitment and participation by managers and workers in initiatives to improve health at the workplace.

Predictors of success and failure

Success

- Appropriately trained occupational health professionals may identify problems earlier in order to initiate effective interventions.
- Sympathetic and supportive management and workforce aid this process. Successful implementation of an occupational health programme necessitates that workers' health and safety be at the core of the employment organization's values.
- Team approach involving primary and secondary care providers can facilitate in protecting and promoting workers' health.

Failure

- An over-reliance on the medical treatment model may prove to be ineffective in addressing the problems encountered in the workplace. Prevention is crucial. Workplace health hazards should be communicated effectively to the public, politicians, decision makers, employers, and employees.
- Health promotion in the workplace should not be done at the expense of control of workplace hazards.

- A multidisciplinary approach will not work if coordination and communication are poor. Understanding the roles of each team member is essential.

Emerging issues

- *The aging worker:* greater longevity of the population and fewer offspring per family have contributed to a higher proportion of older workers in the workforce. Many countries have also proposed increasing the retirement age (mainly for fiscal reasons). Workplaces have to adapt to accommodate the physical capabilities of older workers. Chronic and degenerative disorders will be expected to increase among the causes of ill health in the aging workforce of the future.
- *Stress and mental health:* the main cause of sickness absence in many countries has shifted from infections and respiratory, gastrointestinal, and skin problems to musculo-skeletal and mental health issues. The trend towards an increase in stress, anxiety, and depression is seen in developed and rapidly developing countries, and especially when physical and chemical risks start to decrease with good control of exposures. A UK government report on building mental capital and well-being has identified workplace factors that may help or hinder the promotion of mental health.[10]
- *The 'fit note':* Dame Carol Black reviewed the health of workers in the UK and made a number of recommendations.[10] The most progressive reform proposed was a replacement of the traditional 'sick note' signed by general practitioners by an electronic 'fit note'. Implemented since 2010, the aim has been to encourage individuals back to work instead of indicating just the number of days the person should take as certified sickness absence.
- *New technology/emerging materials:* concerns have been raised about the possible impact of new technology and emerging materials on health. One example is nanotechnology and nanomaterials. Nano particles have considerable potential for use in a wide range of applications including clothing, computing, industrial coatings, and medicines, Studies on laboratory animals have demonstrated a potential for toxic effects, and there is a concern that nanoparticles may produce adverse human health effects.[11]

Further resources

Books

Baxter PA, Aw TC, Cockcroft A, et al. (eds) (2010). *Hunter's diseases of occupations*, 10th edn. Hachette, London.

Koh D, Aw TC. (2017). Textbook of occupational medicine practice, 4th edn. World Scientific Publishing Company, Singapore.

Ladou J, Harrison R. (2014). CURRENT Occupational and Environmental Medicine, 5th edn. McGraw-Hill Education, New York.

Palmer K, Brown I, Hobson J. (eds) (2013). *Fitness for work: the medical aspects*, 5th edn. Oxford University Press, Oxford.

Occupational health journals

Occupational and Environmental Medicine

Scandinavian Journal of Work, Environment and Health
American Journal of Industrial Medicine
Journal of Occupational & Environmental Medicine
Occupational Medicine

Acknowledgements

This chapter was adapted from the *Handbook*'s previous edition, authored by Tar-Ching Aw, Stuart Whitaker, and Malcolm Harrington.

References

1 Faculty of Occupational Medicine (2006). *Guidance on ethics for occupational physicians*. Faculty of Occupational Medicine, Royal College of Physicians, London.
2 Faculty of Occupational Medicine, Ireland (2007). *Guidance on ethical practice for occupational physicians*. Faculty of Occupational Medicine, Dublin.
3 Dhara VR, Dhara R. (2002). The Union Carbide disaster in Bhopal: a review of health effects. *Archives of Environmental Health*, **57**, 391–404.
4 Tuttle RM, Becker DV. (2006). The Chernobyl accident and its consequences: update at the millennium. *Seminars in Nuclear Medicine*, **30**, 133–40.
5 Whorton D, Krauss RM, Marshall S, et al. (1977). Infertility in male pesticide workers. *Lancet*, **2**, 1259–61.
6 Smith DL, Barr DA, Kales SN. (2013). Extreme sacrifice: sudden cardiac death in the US Fire Service. *Extreme Physiology and Medicine*, **2**, 6.
7 Pasetto R, Comba P, Marconi A. (2005). Mesothelioma associated with environmental exposures. *La Medicina del Lavoro*, **96**, 330–7.
8 Makk L, Delmore F, Creech Jr JL, et al. (2006). Clinical and morphologic features of hepatic angiosarcoma in vinyl chloride workers. *Cancer*, **37**, 148–63.
9 Kales SN, Czeisler CA. (2016). Obstructive sleep apnea and work accidents: time for action. *SLEEP*, **39**(6), 1171–3.
10 Black C. (2008). *Working for a healthier tomorrow*. TSO, London.
11 Gulumian M, Verbeek J, Andraos C, et al. (2016). Systematic review of screening and surveillance programs to protect workers from nanomaterials. *PLoS One*. Nov 9, **11**(11).

Chapter 3.4

Engaging communities in participatory research and action

Meredith Minkler and Charlotte Chang

Objectives

After reading this chapter you will be able to:
- define participatory research and its core principles
- describe how engaging communities in participatory research and action can add value to research, while building community capacity and helping achieve action to promote community health
- identify some of the challenges that arise in such work and how they may be addressed
- describe a case study that started with an important issue in the community and demonstrates core principles of community-based participatory research (CBPR), challenges faced in such work, and subsequent community action for change.

Definition and core principles

Participatory research is a generic term for a wide range of approaches that go by many names (e.g. CBPR, mutual inquiry, participatory action research and community-partnered research), but have as their centrepiece three interrelated elements: participation and education, research, and action.[1, 2] Building on earlier work,[3] the Kellogg Community Health Scholars Program[4] defined CBPR in the health field as:

> a collaborative approach to research that equitably involves all partners in the research process and recognizes the unique strengths that each brings. CBPR begins with a research topic of importance to the community with the aim of combining knowledge and action for social change to improve community health and eliminate health disparities.

The core principles of CBPR are listed in Box 3.4.1.

Why is this an important issue?

Recent decades have seen growing appreciation of the importance of working 'with', rather than 'on', communities to understand and address complex health problems. Participatory, community-partnered and action-oriented approaches, including CBPR, to problems ranging from asthma and HIV/AIDS to obesity, depression, and violence are important parts of a health professional's toolkit.

Many of today's complex health problems have proven poorly suited to 'outside expert'-driven research and the often disappointing interventions to which it has given rise.[2] Too often, communities feel 'studied to death' by researchers, while seeing no real local benefit. With its accent on engaging community members throughout the research process, and using study findings to help promote new or improved programmes, practices, and policies, community engagement both strengthens the research itself and builds local capacity or problem-solving ability, while addressing concerns of genuine interest to the community and other stakeholders.

Box 3.4.1 Core principles of participatory research

- Recognizes community as a unit of identity.[a]
- Builds on strengths and resources within the community.
- Facilitates a collaborative, equitable partnership in all phases of research, involving an empowering and power-sharing process that attends to social inequalities.
- Fosters co-learning and capacity building among all partners.
- Integrates and achieves a balance between knowledge generation and intervention for the mutual benefit of all partners.
- Focuses on the local relevance of public health problems and on ecological perspectives that attend to the multiple determinants of health.
- Involves systems development using a cyclical and iterative process.
- Disseminates results to all partners and involves them in the wider dissemination of results.
- Involves a long-term process and commitment to sustainability.
- Openly addresses issues of race, ethnicity, racism and social class, and embodies 'cultural humility',[b] (acknowledging personal biases and the limitations of one's own knowledge about others' cultures, being open to learning, and committing to genuine and respectful partnership)[c]
- Works to assure research rigour and validity, but also 'broadens the bandwidth of validity'[d] by making sure that the issue comes from, or has real relevance, to the community, and that different ways of knowing, including the community's lay knowledge, are called upon and respected.

a) Israel BA, Eng E, Schulz AJ, et al. (eds). (2012). Methods in community-based participatory research for health, 2nd edn). Jossey-Bass, San Francisco.

b) Murray-Garcia J. (1998). Cultural humility versus cultural competence: a critical distinction in defining physician training outcomes in multicultural education. Journal of Health Care for the Poor and Underserved, 9, 117–25.

c) Wallerstein N, Duran B, Oetzel J, et al. (2018). On community-based participatory research. In: Wallerstein N, Duran B, Oetzel J, et al., eds, Community-based participatory research for health: advancing social and health equity, 3rd edn, pp. 3–16). Jossey-Bass, San Francisco.

d) Reason P, Bradbury H. (2006). Handbook of action research: participatory inquiry and practice, concise edn. Sage Publications, London.

Approaches to participatory action and research

Following the principles of engagement of communities in participatory research and action requires:

- ensuring that the problem under study comes from, or is of genuine interest to, the community
- identifying and building on community strengths and assets
- building genuine collegial relationships characterized by mutual respect and co-learning between the partners
- engaging communities throughout the research process, including on:
  - the research question
  - the study design and methods, including the design of culturally appropriate instruments

- data collection and interpretation
- dissemination and use of findings to help bring about change
- the ongoing evaluation of the project's processes and outcomes.[2, 3, 5, 6–11]

Who is the community and how do we begin?

- *Identification of the community is a critical starting point for participatory research and action:* although commonly identified in geographic terms, communities can also be based on identity, and a 'shared sense of personhood' resulting from common cultural beliefs, values, and traditions. A local neighbourhood, a community of people with disabilities, or people who identify as gay or lesbian or gender non-conforming, also may be an important starting point for participatory and action-orientated research.
- *Find out who the key opinion leaders are in that community:* who do people go to for advice or help? Who are the 'movers and shakers' who have helped in the past when the community has come together around a problem? Is there a strong, autonomous organization (e.g. a faith- or community-based organization, or community centre) that is widely respected and that might serve as a partner on an action-oriented participatory research effort?
- If an outside researcher or health department is interested in mobilizing the community to study and address a particular health issue, it is also important to find out whether that issue is, in fact, of genuine concern to the community. Key opinion leaders and respected local organizations can help us do this, or we may hold focus groups or interviews with community members to assess their views. Asking communities what their greatest concerns are can also open possibilities for bridging issues or laying the foundation for future collaboration.

The spectrum of community engagement

Participatory research and action can be seen as taking place along a spectrum, depending on the level of community engagement involved:[12]

- *Informing communities about a project or study and inviting members to take part as subjects or participants:* although commonly listed as a form of participatory research, such an approach tends to be *community placed*, but not genuinely *community based*. While important for achieving informed consent, it is not truly participatory in nature and typically does not promote improved community health.
- *Inviting community members to have input on some aspects of the study:* for example, the design of survey questions or dissemination of findings. This approach is important, and helpful in increasing response rate. However, it does not take full advantage of what communities bring or give back optimally to the community.
- *Engaging community members as collaborators on a research project or intervention that is designed by outside researchers:* even when outside researchers have already designed a study or intervention, significant mutual value can be added when community partners are then invited to participate collegially in providing input at each stage of the study project.
- *Collegial research for action, in which community members are involved as equal partners throughout the process:* here, the research comes from, or is of real importance to, the community partners who participate

as colleagues from the study's inception through the dissemination and action phases of the work. Community partners control or share control of the entire project and have explicit decision-making power.

Competencies required

- Ability to identify appropriate community members and other collaborators, and respectfully engage with them as equal partners.
- Familiarity with or commitment to the principles of participatory research.
- Technical expertise in research methods, along with an openness to alternative ways of knowing (e.g. community's lay knowledge) and an ability to engage in research that draws upon both.
- Communication skills, including skills in communicating cross-culturally and/or with low-literacy populations.
- Comfort and willingness in sharing power and engaging in respectful conflict resolution as challenging issues arise.
- Ability to commit to a participatory research project 'over the long haul' to ensure reaching the action phases of the work, which may extend well after formal funding for the project has ended.

Who needs to be involved?

- Community-based organizations and groups, including neighbourhood agencies and faith-based organizations, their staff, and affiliated and non-affiliated members.
- Community organizers and other staff, or 'bridge people' who have strong relationships with, and cultural knowledge of, both community members and academic researchers, and can facilitate the development of trust and relationships between diverse partners.
- Policy makers, funders, or other decision makers with the power to help the partnership use its findings to foster health-promoting change.
- Local health departments, hospitals, or academics knowledgeable about the topic and interested in engagement as equal partners.

What's the value added in using a participatory approach?

- Helping to ensure that the topic under investigation comes from, or is of genuine interest to, the community.
- increasing community buy-in and trust, which in turn can increase response rate.
- Enhancing people's ability to develop meaningful informed consent procedures and materials, and to consider potential community as well as individual risks and benefits.[8]
- Improving cultural sensitivity and acceptability of surveys, and other research instruments, which may improve their validity.

- Enabling the design of more locally appropriate interventions, increasing in the process the likelihood of success.
- Improving interpretation of research findings.
- Identifying new dissemination channels and approaches that can increase the value of study findings and recommendations for end users.
- Helping ensure that study findings are translated into action that can in turn result in programmes, policies, or practices that can benefit the community and other stakeholders.
- Empowering and increasing capacity of communities to understand and take action on local health issues.[2, 3, 5–10]

Challenges in participatory research and action

Time and labour-intensive nature of the work

Community-engaged participatory research requires more 'front-end time' than traditional research for building relationships, co-learning processes, and engaging community partners in each step of the process. This can include holding meetings outside business hours, providing language access services, or travelling long distances to locations convenient to communities to make possible meaningful participation by community members. As noted earlier, the action phase of the process, and the commitment of researchers to the community over the long term, also means that this work may continue well beyond a funded project period.

Conflict and power dynamics are part of the process

Health professionals who take part in a CBPR or related project should be comfortable dealing with conflict and should recognize that power sharing—and therefore likely struggles over power, resource allocation, etc.—are part of the process. Practitioners should be honest and upfront with community partners about institutional challenges to sharing power—for example, parameters required by human subjects review processes.[8] Developing 'ground rules' and memorandums of understanding (MOUs), using guidelines for assessing partnership processes[9, 10, 11] and building in ongoing participatory evaluation can help address some of these concerns, but cannot be expected to fully prevent them.

Community engagement may involve trade-offs between scientific rigour and community-responsive interventions and measurement tools

One of the greatest strengths of participatory research and action—its ability to contribute to culturally sensitive and acceptable research instruments and interventions—may also be problematic when community concerns challenge study designs, or preclude the use of validated instruments in data collection. For example, community members facing urgent health problems may not believe that randomized studies with control groups are fair to those who do not receive the intervention, and may argue strongly for a less rigorous study design (e.g. a staggered design in which all participants eventually receive the intervention). Genuine dialogue about the meanings attached to terms like 'rigour' and 'validity', the advantages of having stronger 'scientific' findings, and the equally important need for community trust and acceptance, as well as openness to compromise and different ways of knowing, will help address these knotty issues.

Conflicts over the dissemination and use of findings to promote change

Price and Behrens[13] write about the mismatch that frequently occurs between the 'necessary skepticism of science' and the 'action imperative of the community'. Community partners thus may wish to move quickly from preliminary findings to advocating for a change in practice or policy, while health professionals feel a responsibility to ensure that the findings are accurate—and sometimes, that they have first gone through peer review! Sometimes, too, findings may emerge that could cast the community in a bad light if made public.[8] In these cases, ongoing dialogue and MOUs may be helpful, but cannot fully prevent tough issues from emerging that need to be addressed in ways that satisfy all concerned partners.

Case study

A participatory approach to studying and addressing occupational health and safety among immigrant workers in San Francisco's Chinatown restaurants

One-third of all residents in San Francisco's Chinatown district are employed in the restaurant industry. Health and safety problems abound in these workplaces, and include traditional occupational health and safety concerns, such as cuts, burns, falls, and on-the-job stress. Health problems also encompass serious economic and other social vulnerabilities when employers do not pay the legal minimum wage and delay or evade payment of wages earned, sometimes for periods as long as several months.

The Chinese Progressive Association (CPA) had been organizing campaigns around such worker issues in Chinatown restaurants for over 30 years when, in 2007, it formed a partnership with the University of California Berkeley School of Public Health and its Labor Occupational Health Program, the San Francisco Department of Public Health, and the University of California San Francisco Division of Occupational and Environmental Medicine in 2007. The partnership used a participatory research approach to document working conditions and the health status of Chinatown restaurant workers, evaluate their process throughout, and use the study findings to take action. Research activities included initial focus groups, a community survey of 433 Chinatown restaurant workers, development and use of an observational checklist on the physical working environments of 106 of the 108 restaurants in Chinatown, and interviews and surveys of participating partners.[14]

The structure and dynamics of the partnership evolved over time and were adapted to changing circumstances. Many layers of complexity were involved in obtaining equitable participation on the project across the different partners who included Chinese immigrant restaurant workers, community organizers, university-based researchers, and health department professionals. These factors included the use of three languages, different educational and professional backgrounds, and differences in organizational as well as ethnic cultures. Mutual trust and respect, including 'leaps of faith' in other partners, the use of translation services, explicit attention to partnership evaluation, and much 'bridging' by key facilitating partners were keys to success in working across diversity and within the constraints of a tight budget and timeline. In the end, partners successfully collaborated to develop research instruments and questions, recruit participants, collect, analyse, and interpret data, and lay the foundation for policy action.[15]

Findings from the research showed that of all Chinatown restaurant workers surveyed:

- 50% did not receive the city's minimum wage
- 48% had been burned, 40% had been cut, and 17% had slipped or fallen at work in the past 12 months
- 40% did not receive any breaks during the day
- 64% did not receive any training on how to perform their jobs
- 54% paid for healthcare out of own pocket; just 3% had employer-covered insurance.[16]

From the observational checklist component of the study, it was learned that:

- 65% of the 106 restaurants did not have any of the required labour law postings displayed
- 62% had wet and greasy floors
- under half (48%) had non-slip mats
- 82% did not have fully stocked first aid kits.[17]

Outcomes from the project included:

- major contributions to the development by worker partners and allies of a low-wage worker bill of rights policy advocacy tool and its use in subsequent organizing to enact groundbreaking anti-wage theft enforcement legislation at the city level[17]
- development of leadership potential and 'courage to confront problems in their community' among worker partners[15]
- posting of the observational checklist on the websites of the health department and labour occupational health programmes that conducted continued research on its use in county health departments, and coordinated enforcement efforts between other agencies and health department food inspectors to address worker health and safety and related labour issues
- the formal 'launch' of the study's report and recommendations for action at a community event attended by over 170 community members, media representatives, and agencies as a prelude to subsequent community action
- development by the community partner and a design cooperative of a glossy, professional quality report on key findings and action steps for use in subsequent education of employers, employees, and community members, and with the lay and ethnic media.
- development of strong relationships among partners and their continued collaboration on the action phase of the work over a year past the end of funding

- community capacity building through the development of a worker leadership core and support for future worker organizing campaigns, including a major victory and $4.2 million settlement with a large Chinese restaurant in 2014.

Some important lessons

- Community participation in research, and inclusion of an action component, will likely slow down the process. However, the extra time and effort may be well counter-balanced by the added richness of the study; its capacity for investigating a problem of genuine local concern, doing so in ways that respect and honour local community beliefs and wisdom; and increase of the likelihood of intervention success and follow-up action to promote improved community health
- Although there is no one set of principles for engaging communities in research and action, attending to the basic principles described,[2,3,5] and tailoring them to meet the specific needs of your own partnership, can be an important way to monitor and assess your progress and facilitate the discussion of difficult issues before, or as, they occur
- Balancing research with action in participatory work with communities is a must, and all partners should commit 'to the long haul', including staying engaged in the action phase of the work even if the money has run out.

Predictors of success and failure

Success

- A strong partnership, with plenty of front-end and ongoing attention to building trusting and collaborative relationships.
- Shared goals, including assurance that the research topic matters to the local community, and that the methods selected and interventions developed similarly reflect local knowledge and priorities.
- Respect among all partners for the importance of community needs and priorities, as well as 'good science' as a prerequisite to effective action, particularly when the desired change requires action on the part of policy makers or other key decision makers.
- Engagement of multiple key stakeholders in the process, and the building of alliances well beyond the original partnership to instigate action.
- Mutual respect, trust, and flexibility in working with partners from different perspectives and backgrounds.[1–10]

Failure

- 'Name only' participatory research and action, in which community members are rarely consulted and simply used to help bring in a grant or help increase response rates, often incur resentment and do not lead to authentic and effective partnerships.
- Lack of community commitment to the research question under consideration misses both the spirit and the process of participatory research and action—often with disappointing results.

- Particularly when there are multiple partners or major differences in culture and educational level among partners, lack of sufficient attention to process and communication, and failure to use mechanisms that help ensure equal participation can doom an otherwise promising partnership.
- Failure to plan ahead for the dissemination and action phases of the study—including deciding on a dissemination strategy and commitment by all partners to the action phase of the work—can be disillusioning for the community while precluding a central tenet of participatory research and action—namely, committing to translating findings in ways that benefit communities and promote health equity. [1–10]

How will you know if you have been successful?

Criteria for success
- Partners have shown mutual respect and engaged in co-learning throughout the process.
- Many clear examples exist of the ways in which community participation improved research quality, and built individual and community capacity in the process.
- The final study shows evidence of the partners' commitment to academically strong research enriched by community members' deep knowledge of their community. Different ways of knowing have been valued and incorporated.
- Study findings have been used by the partners to work for changes in programmes, practices, and policies promoting improved community health and well-being.
- There is clear evidence of both community and individual capacity building as a result of community participation throughout the process.
- The partners respond in the affirmative to the question, 'Would you engage together again if you had the chance?'
- Partners agree that the group has successfully reached mutually determined goals for research and action. [2–11]

Emerging issues

- Participatory research has become a 'buzz word' in the USA, the UK, and elsewhere. With funders now mandating CBPR and related approaches in calls for proposals, it is essential that new mechanisms be developed to help foster authentic community engagement in the work. [2] From ethics review procedures that respect the different processes involved in CBPR[8] to easily accessible sample MOUs and other tools for monitoring process,[9–10] institutional help for partnerships interested in exploring this approach is needed.
- The substantially longer timetable involved in participatory research and action suggests the need for realistic, multi-year funding that includes

ample support for partnership building processes and subsequent action aspects of the work, as well as the more traditional research components.

- Appropriate institutional support for health practitioner and academic partners, and recognition and adequate compensation of community partners, should be provided in recognition of the time and labour-intensive nature of this work.
- The Institute of Medicine[18] has named CBPR as one important content area in which schools of public health should be offering training. How can such training be developed that builds in on-the-ground experience with participatory research and action processes, while also respecting the limitations of the typical academic timetable, the limited time and resources of community partners, and the long-term commitment required in improving community health?
- There is increasing interest in using a CBPR orientation with such traditional approaches as randomized controlled trials (RCTs). How can these diverse approaches be brought together effectively?[19]
- Due to the increasingly popular use of community-engaged and participatory research approaches to public health issues, there is a need to develop clearer ways to evaluate such efforts, and strong criteria for what qualifies as an 'authentic' or 'effective' effort. The application of mixed methods and the development of clear metrics and measures of CBPR processes and mechanisms continue to evolve.[11]

Further resources

Books and monographs

Corburn J. (2005). *Street science: community knowledge and environmental health justice.* MIT Press, Cambridge.

Israel BA, Eng E, Schulz AJ, et al. (eds). (2012). *Methods in community-based participatory research for health,* 2nd edn. Jossey-Bass, San Francisco.

Wallerstein N, Duran B, Oetzel J, et al. (eds). (2018). *Community-based participatory research for health: advances in social and health equity,* (3rd edn). Jossey-Bass, San Francisco.

Journals featuring articles on participatory research and action (selected)

Health Education and Behavior
American Journal of Public Health
Action Research Journal of the American Medical Association
Cancer Care
Health Affairs
Progress in Community Health Partnerships
Journal of Health Promotion Practice
Ethnicity and Disease
Journal of General Internal Medicine
Journal of Urban Health
Health Promotion International
International Journal of Preventive Medicine
American Journal of Community Psychology

Journal papers

Cacari-Stone L, Wallerstein N, Garcia AP, Minkler M. (2014). The Promise of Community-Based Participatory Research for Health Equity: A Conceptual Model for Bridging Evidence With Policy. *American Journal of Public Health,* **104**(9), 1615–23.

Cargo M, Mercer SL. (2008). The value and challenges of participatory research: strengthening its practice. *Annual Review of Public Health,* **29**(1), 325–50.

Cyril S, Smith BJ, Possamai-Inesedy A, et al. (2015). Exploring the role of community engagement in improving the health of disadvantaged populations: a systematic review. *Global Health Action*, **8**, 1–12.

Green LW. (2006). Public health asks of systems science: to advance our evidence-based practice, can you help us get more practice-based evidence? *American Journal of Public Health*, **96**(3), 406–9.

Minkler, M. (2010). Linking science and policy through community-based participatory research to eliminate health disparities. *American Journal of Public Health*, **100**(Supplement 1), S81–7.

O'Fallon LR, Dearry A. (2002). Community-based participatory research as a tool to advance environmental health sciences. *Environmental Health Perspectives*, **110**(Supplement 2), 155–9.

Salimi Y, Shahandeh K, Malekafzali H, et al. (2012). Is community-based participatory research (CBPR) useful? A systematic review on papers in a decade. *International Journal of Preventive Medicine*, **3**(6), 386–93.

Seifer SD. (2006). Building and sustaining community-institutional partnerships for prevention research: findings from a national collaborative. *Journal of Urban Health*, **83**, 989–1003.

Websites

Community campus partnerships for health. Available at: ℅ http://www.ccph.info (accessed 10 August 2019).

Developing and sustaining CBPR partnerships. CBPR resources for community partners. Available at: ℅   http://depts.washington.edu/ccph/cbpr/u1/u11.php (accessed 10 August 2019).

PolicyLink Inc. Available at: ℅ www.policylink.org (accessed 10 August 2019).

The Community Tool Kit. Available at: ℅ http://ctb.ku.edu (accessed 10 August 2019).

UNM Center for Participatory Research. Available at: ℅ https://cpr.unm.edu (accessed 10 August 2019).

References

1 Hall BL. (1992). From margins to center: the development and purpose of participatory action research. *American Sociologist*, **23**, 15–28.

2 Wallerstein N, Duran B, Oetzel J, et al. (2018). On community-based participatory research. In: Wallerstein N, Duran B, Oetzel J, et al., eds, *Community-based participatory research for health: advancing social and health equity*, 3rd edn, pp. 3–16). Jossey-Bass, San Francisco.

3 Israel BA, Schulz AJ, Parker EA, et al. (1998). Review of community-based research: assessing partnership approaches to improve public health. *Annual Review of Public Health*, **19**, 173–202.

4 W.K. Kellogg Community Health Scholars Program (2001). *Stories of impact.* University of Michigan, School of Public Health, CHSP, National Program Office, Ann Arbor.

5 Israel BA, Eng E, Schulz AJ, et al. (eds). (2012). *Methods in community-based participatory research for health*, 2nd edn). Jossey-Bass, San Francisco.

6 Cargo M, Mercer SL. (2008). The value and challenges of participatory research: strengthening its practice. *Annual Review of Public Health*, **29**(1), 325–50.

7 O'Fallon LR, Dearry A. (1992). Community-based participatory research as a tool to advance environmental health sciences. *Environmental Health Perspectives*, **110**(Supplement 2), 155–9.

8 Flicker S, Travers R, Guta A, et al. (2007). Ethical dilemmas in community-based participatory research: recommendations for institutional review boards. *Journal of Urban Health*, **84**, 478–93.

9 Mercer SL, Green LW, Cargo M, et al. (2008). Reliability-tested guidelines for assessing participatory research projects. In: Minkler M, Wallerstein N, eds, *Community-based participatory research for health: from process and outcomes*, 2nd edn. Jossey-Bass, San Francisco.

10 Israel BA, Lantz PM, McGranaghan RJ, et al. (2012). In-depth semistructured interview protocol: Detroit community-academic Urban Research Center, Detroit URC board evaluation, 1996–2002. In: Israel BA, Eng E, Schulz AJ, et al., eds, *Methods in community-based participatory research for health*, 2nd edn, pp. 623–7. Jossey-Bass, San Francisco.

11 Wallerstein, N. (2018). Instruments and measures for evaluating community engagement and partnerships (Appendix 10). In: Wallerstein N, Duran B, Oetzel J, et al., eds, *Community-based participatory research for health advancing social and health equity*, 3rd edn, pp. 393–8. Jossey-Bass, San Francisco.

12 Biggs SD. (1989). *Resource-poor farmer participation in research: a synthesis of experiences from nine national agricultural research systems.* VTechWorks, the Hague, Netherlands.

13 Price RH, Behrens T. (2003). Working Pasteur's quadrant: harnessing science and action for community change. *American Journal of Community Psychology*, **31**, 219–23.

14 Minkler M, Lee PT, Tom A, et al. (2010). Using community-based participatory research to design and initiate a study on immigrant worker health and safety in San Francisco's Chinatown restaurants. *American Journal of Industrial Medicine*, **53**, 361–71.

15 Chang C, Salvatore A, Lee PT, et al. (2012). Popular education, participatory research, and community organizing with immigrant restaurant workers in San Francisco's Chinatown: a case study. In: Minkler M, ed., *Community organizing and community building for health and welfare*, 3rd edn, pp. 246–64. Rutgers University Press, Piscataway, NJ.

16 Minkler M, Salvatore AL, Chang C, et al. (2014). Wage theft as a neglected public health problem: an overview and case study from San Francisco's Chinatown district. *American Journal of Public Health*, **104**(6), 1010–20.

17 Gaydos M, Bhatia R, Morales A, et al. (2011). Promoting health and safety in San Francisco's Chinatown restaurants: findings and lessons learned from a pilot observational checklist. *Public Health Reports*, **126**(Supplement 3), 62–9.

18 Gebbie K, Rosenstock L, Hernandez LM. (eds). (2003). *Who will keep the public healthy? Educating public health professionals for the 21st century*. National Academies Press, Washington DC.

19 Buchanan DR, Miller FG, Wallerstein N. (2007). Ethical issues in community-based participatory research: balancing rigorous research with community participation in community intervention studies. *Progress in Community Health Partnerships*, **1**, 153–60.

Disasters

Paul Bolton and Frederick M. Burkle, Jr

Objective

After reading this chapter you will be familiar with a basic public health approach to disasters and other crises.

Classification and definition

The term 'disaster' is used in many different ways. A brief overview is provided in Box 3.5.1.

Box 3.5.1 Natural and human disasters

Disasters of natural origin
- Sudden onset (earthquakes, landslides, floods, etc.).
- Slower onset (drought, famine, etc.).

Disasters of human origin
- Industrial (e.g. Chernobyl).
- Transportation (e.g. train crash).
- Complex emergencies (e.g. wars, civil strife, and other disasters causing displaced persons and refugees).

Adapted from Noji E (ed.) (1997). *The public health consequences of disasters.* Oxford University Press, New York with permission from Oxford University Press.

It could be argued that even 'disasters of natural origin' are man-made because most recur and failure to prepare for them could be considered a human failure. However, preparation is beyond the scope of this chapter.

Disasters are a sub-category of crises. A public health crisis is an event(s) that overwhelms the capacity of local systems to maintain a community's health. Therefore, outside resources are temporarily required. Crises can range from specific health issues, such as a disease outbreak in an otherwise unaffected community, to a full-scale disaster with property destruction and/or population displacement and multiple public health issues. This chapter focuses on the more complex disasters and crises (with the understanding that any of the issues and approaches described applies equally to other types of disasters and lesser crises). During disasters, mortality and morbidity are widely understood to result either from the loss of public health social and physical protections (i.e. water, sanitation, health, food, shelter, and fuel) or from the overwhelming of these protections by increased demand. However, the loss or overwhelming of other resources— for example, transportation, communications, and public safety— can limit or prevent access to, and availability of, public health services resulting in indirect, preventable, or excess mortality and morbidity in a public health crisis. The tsunami in December 2004 that had an impact on the public health protections in 20 countries, or the Haiti earthquake of 2010, exemplify how big the challenge can be, but smaller disasters can also pose severe threats to public health.

After years of decline, the global number of displaced persons has once again peaked.[1] Increasing numbers of refugees and internally displaced populations live in tenuous post-conflict environments suffering various low levels of intensity of violence, poor governance, limited public health protections, and wide proliferation of weaponry. The numbers of refugees and internally displaced populations fleeing post-conflict despair or climate change consequences have risen dramatically. Many now live in cities rather than camps where dense urban populations have marginal shelter and other essentials resulting in some of the highest infant mortality and under age five mortality rates.

Principles of response

The immediate public health response to any disaster or crisis is based on these principles:

1 Secure the basics that all humans require to maintain health.
2 Determine the current and likely health threats to the affected community, given the local environment and the community's resources, knowledge, and behaviour.
3 Find and provide the resources required to address points 1 and 2.

The first action is a rapid assessment of points 1 and 2 in order to initiate step 3 as soon as possible. Too often, assessment is delayed due to a misguided fear of delaying assistance. Instead, organizations may rush to supply materials and personnel without checking what is really needed. After a major disaster, these supplies can choke the transport system with unneeded goods while goods that are needed cannot get through. Even in a limited crisis, time and money may be wasted sorting through, storing, and/ or destroying useless donated supplies. The World Health Organization (WHO) has issued guidelines on drug donations during disasters that have helped improve this situation.[2] However, compliance with these regulations are frequently ignored, resulting in a burden on recipient countries to sort and destroy unwanted or expired medicines.[3]

Remember to quickly assess first, by the aphorism 'don't just do something, stand there (and assess)'. Any assessment should include coordination with local government, community leaders, and other assisting and coordinating organizations such as the United Nations (UN) or 'non-governmental organizations' (NGOs). This is necessary to determine their capacities and intentions to avoid misunderstandings, conflicting activities, duplication of efforts, and to gain their cooperation in future programmes to address the issues that emerge.

This chapter concentrates on the initial rapid assessment as the basis for response. More detailed assessments and response should be done after the practitioner has been joined by persons skilled in the necessary techniques.

The initial rapid assessment

Assessment involves determining what and how much is needed, based on the principles mentioned earlier. This has been standardized into an initial rapid assessment (IRA) format, which explores both the direct and indirect (public health preventable) consequences of a disaster. This section provides a brief summary of the needs of populations that can be compared with the findings of an IRA. A detailed version of the IRA is available.[4]

Consider the basics required for health

Clean water and sanitation

Each person requires a minimum of 14 litres a day—3 litres for drinking (more in hot weather or with exertion), 2 litres for food preparation, 5 litres for personal hygiene, and 4 litres for cleaning clothes and food utensils. Drinking water need not be pure, as long as it is reasonably clear, free of toxic substances and faecal contamination, and has acceptable taste. Simple kits for testing water quality are widely available. Where water is compromised, you should consult with a water and sanitation engineer as soon as possible to reconstruct damaged systems or set up temporary new ones.

Food

Food aid is most often required after disasters of human origin and when people have been displaced from their usual food sources. After natural disasters (except flooding), crops usually remain intact and people usually do not leave the area, so that large supplies of food are not required.

When outside supplies of food are required, the major considerations are adequate calories, adequate micronutrients, acceptability to the local population, and ease of preparation. To survive, a population requires an average of at least 2,100 kcal/person/day. If a population is already malnourished, or the emergency lasts months, they will require more. Acceptability to the population refers to supplying foods that people are familiar with and will therefore eat. Ease of preparation is an important factor: if foods require cooking, then supplies of fuel (such as piped gas or firewood) must be available. Alternatively, cooked meals may be provided directly in the short term.

When food must be supplied, a nutritional survey conducted by nutritional experts should be done as soon as possible to determine the correct food needs. Securing and transporting adequate supplies of food will require the expertise of a food logistician.

Shelter and clothing

People are best housed in their own homes, except if a disaster has rendered those structures unsafe. They should never be moved from their homes just to ease provision of assistance. If shelter must be provided, people should be housed in small groups (i.e. families or groups of families) to reduce general crowding and exposure to disease and crime, both of which tend to worsen with time. In cold weather, attention to insulation and heating is necessary.

Additional clothing is rarely required because people already have clothes appropriate to their environment and usually manage to retain sufficient supplies (an exception is when a population is displaced from a hot to a cold area). Displacement does require facilities for washing clothes. Estimating (and supplying) shelter and clothing material needs falls under general logistics.

Health services

Adequate healthcare provides treatment for illness and reassurance to the population who will feel unsafe without it. It is important that the whole population has access to the drugs, equipment, trained staff, and infrastructure necessary to treat likely problems. Good 'access' means that people know about the services, know that they are eligible to use them, and do not have to travel so far, wait so long, or pay so much as to discourage their usage. Since healthcare services form the basis of the health information system, good access to accurate data on current and incipient health problems is also important (see Information).

It is also important to consider which, if any, outside medical staff are required. For example, an internist accustomed to Western illnesses and advanced diagnostic facilities is not appropriate for a crisis in a tropical area with limited resources: a skilled local nurse will usually be more useful. Outside staff are most useful when they are clinical, pharmaceutical, and medical supply personnel with emergency experience.

Medical personnel need to assess the potential for epidemics and assess the need for vaccination. Keep in mind that epidemics cannot occur unless the causative organism is present. For example, cholera cannot occur in a community, no matter how crowded or how poor the sanitation, without the presence of *Vibrio cholerae*. Therefore, epidemic risk assessment includes finding out about the previous disease patterns of both the area of the disaster and the affected population. A notable codicil to this rule recently occurred in Haiti, where Nepali UN troops responding to the earthquake introduced cholera that became epidemic: in the future, the epidemiology of relief troops and workers may also become a consideration.

Among disaster-affected populations exposed to exhaustion, malnutrition, and crowding, vaccination for preventable diseases, such as measles, assumes prime importance because of increased susceptibility, morbidity, and mortality under these conditions. Measles vaccination is recommended for children aged from 6 months to 12 years. This is particularly important among populations for which measles vaccine coverage prior to the disaster was low. Coverage of other routine child vaccinations should be maintained.

For large-scale emergencies, WHO provides a recommended list of drugs and materials, including quantities, to serve 10,000 people for 3 months. These materials are available in kit forms.[5]

Information

This is often neglected but is a fundamental requirement of the disaster response. In unaccustomed circumstances, people require new information on how to maintain their health. They also require information on what is happening and what is likely to happen. In the absence of information, rumour will fill the gap, causing insecurity, anxiety, and mistrust of those handling the emergency. Rumours may even force inappropriate diversion of resources to minor or non-existent problems to appease the population. Therefore, a system of good communication is vital between those assessing the situation and in charge, and the affected population. Any accessible means of transmitting information is appropriate as long as it communicates directly with the population and not through a third party, to avoid distortion. Collaboration with local persons in designing the messages is important to ensure a style and approach that is understandable to the population. Methods can include radio and TV, pamphlets, posters, advice by health workers in the clinics, even megaphones. As smartphones have become more available in both high- and low-income countries, texting and websites have become increasingly important methods of spreading and updating information.

Consider the current and likely health threats, given local conditions

Current health problems

Description of a population's health should include measurement of crude mortality rates, causes of mortality, and the nature of health problems—their current incidence and severity (including case fatality rates). Rates are important for determining disease trends in the face of varying population size. Measuring rates requires both numerators (the frequency of events, such as illness or death) and denominators (an estimate of population size).

For the initial assessment, numerator information can be gathered by visiting the available treatment centres, talking with staff, and reviewing daily records of diagnoses and treatment. These records form the basis of the Health Information System (HIS), which should be established as part of the initial assessment. In most cases, setting up the HIS requires developing case definitions for the important health problems and establishing treatment protocols to ensure appropriate medical supplies for treatment and prevention. Case definitions are required because laboratory facilities are often not adequate to test all suspected cases of illness. Rather, the (usually limited) testing facilities are primarily used to confirm the presence of specific illnesses among the population (particularly those with epidemic potential, such as meningitis) by testing the first suspect cases, and to develop case definitions for these diseases once confirmed. These case definitions are then used to diagnose subsequent suspected cases.

If the affected population is spread over a wide area and transport is poor, it is important to regularly visit areas far from the treatment centres to ask people about the problems affecting them and examine suspect cases. In these situations, or any situation where access is limited for at least some people, rates calculated using a clinic-based HIS are likely to be underestimates because many people will not attend the health centres. Supplementing HIS data with visits to outlying areas will provide a more accurate picture of the main problems and trends and any incipient problems.

Denominators can be difficult to calculate or even estimate, and made more difficult when people are on the move. Increasing availability of drone technology will enable more accurate population estimates as well as assessing needs, to the point where drones will likely become an essential tool in disaster management.[6] Although much less useful, proportional mortality ratios (the number of deaths in a population from a specific cause divided by the total number of deaths in the population) can be used if the denominator cannot be determined with any confidence. Data on mortality and morbidity needs to include age in order to disaggregate crude rates into infant, under aged five, maternal, and elderly mortality and morbidity rates. Disaggregating crude mortality rates defines which are the vulnerable populations and the nature of their health problems.

All efforts should be made to identify the leaders among the population, meet them early on, get their impressions of the main problems, and enlist their support for your efforts.

Another important aspect of current health and disease threat is the health knowledge and behaviour of the population. Failure to take precautions, such as washing hands, can render populations more susceptible to illness. Such behaviours are relatively more important where there is overcrowding, or in a specific health crisis like a single transmissible disease. Local knowledge and behaviour can be assessed by direct observation, and by interviews in which local people are asked how they prevent particular illnesses of concern, such as diarrhoea. Addressing gaps in knowledge and behaviour form part of the information needs discussed earlier.

General condition of the population

Talk with health workers and walk through the community. Observe and talk with people. The aim is to form an overall impression of the state of nutrition and available supplies, including clean water and food, cooking supplies and fuel, shelter and clothing, particularly in a cold environment:

- Assess whether people appear to be getting enough supplies.
- Observe how people get water, to estimate the risk and potential for contamination.
- Ask how people are disposing of their faeces.
- Estimate the adequacy of access to medical treatment, given the distance, available transport, cost, and degree of crowding of the clinics.

Condition of the environment

Assess the need for shelter in terms of the weather. Research the climate. Observe the water sources and whether the water from those sources looks clean or turbid. Observe where people are defecating, the adequacy of available latrines, water drainage, and the likelihood that the water supply and faeces will come in contact. If there is a sewerage system, investigate whether the system has been damaged, whether it is being attended to, and whether water treatment supplies are adequate.

Just as you would investigate the climate, research the epidemiology of transmissible diseases. Information on disease endemicity is usually available from local authorities, and from regional health organizations like the Pan-American Health Organization (PAHO). If the area is known to harbour transmissible diseases, then monitor those diseases as part of the disease surveillance system. Supplies needed to address these illnesses must be investigated, and prepared by the health team and logisticians. Injuries and diseases augmented by crowding—such as any respiratory or gastrointestinal infections—will be more likely where populations have left their homes and are crowded into an unfamiliar environment.

Security issues

These may be both health problems in their own right, such as violence, or threats that preclude access to resources and affect behaviour and daily function. For example, people may be unable to go to a clinic or collect supplies if this exposes them to danger. Similarly, health personnel may be unwilling to work or unable to do their jobs. Even limited health emergencies may engender violence, often through ill-feeling and rumour due to lack of information or criminal opportunism where police presence is reduced. Security can be assessed by talking with local people, particularly women who face greater threats than men. Addressing these issues requires close cooperation with the police and/or the military. Having assessed what is needed, consult with these groups about how it can best be provided.

Size of the affected or vulnerable population

This is one of the most important pieces of information about the population. Without this 'denominator', the amounts of resources required cannot be assessed. Moreover, rates cannot be calculated, making it impossible, in public health terms, to determine the size of a problem or trends in prevalence or incidence.

Early in an emergency, rough estimates are acceptable, and can be based on pre-existing information, estimates of knowledgeable persons, or even, in the case of a mass displacement of people to an open area, 'eyeballing' from a high piece of ground. Later, more sophisticated sampling and survey methods should be used by a demographer or epidemiologist, or even a count if possible. As noted previously, portable aerial observation through drones will become an increasingly standard tool in population size assessment.

Demography of the affected population

Normally, some groups will be more vulnerable to problems than others. In a limited crisis, such as a disease outbreak, this may be because of variations in disease susceptibility. For example, children are more susceptible to vaccine-preventable diseases (e.g. measles and influenza) and the undernourished to other transmissible diseases. In a full-scale disaster with crowding and limited resources, some groups are at a disadvantage in securing their needs. This is particularly true in low-income countries and can include women (particularly if pregnant or lactating), children (especially those without adult protectors), elderly people, and those with disabilities. The size and location of these groups should be determined and particular attention given to meeting their needs and monitoring whether they are met.

Assessing capacity

In meeting needs, the emphasis is on reconstructing or supporting the system that met those needs before the emergency rather than on creating a parallel system. Determine what that system was or is and who is in charge. Work with that person(s) to identify what they need to meet the current crisis, and try to provide it. This is particularly true after a disaster yet this simple principle is often ignored. Where a system has been damaged rather than simply overwhelmed, this does not mean reconstituting it the way it was, at least not in the short term, but rather rapidly providing those elements required to meet demand. For example, in an emergency, it is usually not possible to rebuild a damaged hospital quickly, but tents, supplies, etc. can be provided to temporarily restore lost functions.

Compared with the creation of a new system, reconstruction:
* requires fewer outside resources
* uses locally appropriate resources and so will be sustainable
* builds local capacity to address this emergency, other problems, and future emergencies
* provides employment
* uses people who know the local population best
* restores a sense of self-reliance.

Assessing local systems in detail requires persons skilled in that field—for example, a sanitation engineer to assess sewerage, a health information specialist or epidemiologist to assess a health information system. Suitable local people with these skills are preferable to outsiders because they are the ones who will maintain the systems in the long term.

Surveillance

After the initial assessment, a surveillance system must be created to monitor health trends and detect incipient epidemics and other public health problems. In any displaced and crowded population, surveillance should include measles and the common serious diseases known to occur among the population and in the geographic area. These should include important epidemic diseases known to be present in the population or the geographic areas, such as cholera and other diarrhoeal diseases, dysentery, malaria, dengue fever, meningitis, hepatitis, typhoid and paratyphoid, typhus, and viral encephalitis. Of particular concern are disasters involving displacement of populations into regions with endemic transmissible diseases for which they are immunologically naïve. The reverse situation is also a concern for the local population where conditions for transmission are favourable. Although measles and other vaccine-preventable diseases are on the wane in many parts of the developing world, most countries, especially the least developed, remain at risk of reversals when politico-military situations worsen.

Surveillance information must be provided to all stakeholders, including the affected population and those in charge politically. It will provide the most important information to determine whether the response to the crisis is effective. The surveillance system must be capable of rapidly detecting, investigating, and either confirming or debunking rumours.

Setting up surveillance will require consultation with the other organizations providing health assistance so that they become part of the monitoring and reporting system, and to agree on standard case definitions and reporting formats. Access to a laboratory will be required to confirm diagnoses, particularly in the early phases of an epidemic. The system should be under the direction of an epidemiologist.

The International Health Regulations (IHR) treaty covering 196 countries was put into effect in 2007 following the SARS pandemic, and provides for improved surveillance capacity and response assistance from neighbouring countries to those nations with limited resources. Although much needs to be accomplished to improve surveillance in many regions of the world, clearly the IHR has improved capacity to monitor and manage outbreaks.

Logistics

For all external supplies, consider:
• where to get them in sufficient quality and quantity
• how to pay for them
• how quickly they are needed
• available transportation methods for these requirements
• how the situation is likely to change.

All these considerations will require cooperation between an experienced logistician and local people familiar with local suppliers and markets. Setting up a system for moving and monitoring supplies, and keeping the system from being choked by low-priority items will require considerable human and financial resources.

Skills and knowledge

After a disaster, the following are required:
• Rapid assessment and survey skills.
• Clinical skills.
• Water and sanitation.
• Food and nutrition.
• Logistics knowledge.
• Familiarity with the local language, culture, environment, and affected population.
• Relationships with important local persons whose assistance and support will be needed.
• Sensitivity in dealing with the affected population.
• Ability to communicate ideas and problems well, and to write coherent and clear reports.
• Ability to deal with the media.

Personnel

The following personnel are required:
• Project director.
• Epidemiologist.
• Logistician.
• Local people familiar with local culture and language.
• Water and sanitation expert.
• Nutritionist.
• Clinical staff familiar with likely problems and resources.

Fallacies

In his book, *The public health consequences of disasters*, Eric Noji describes some of the important myths and realities about disasters collected by the PAHO. Awareness of these myths is useful in approaching emergency response:
  1 Foreign medical volunteers are always needed.
  2 Any kind of international assistance is urgently required.
  3 Epidemics are inevitable after disasters.
  4 Disasters bring out the worst in people.
  5 Affected populations are too shocked and helpless to help themselves.
  6 Disasters kill randomly.
  7 Locating disaster victims in temporary settlements is the best shelter solution.
  8 Food aid is always required after natural disasters.
  9 Clothing is always needed.
  10 Conditions return to normal after a few weeks.

All these myths, except 4 and 10, have been dealt with previously in this chapter. Most workers would agree that disasters overwhelmingly bring out the positive side of human nature, and that community spirit is usually enhanced. Far from resolving quickly, the effects of most disasters are long-term, lasting for years, or even decades. This is true even in developed countries, where increased debt and interruption in economic activity can create long-term financial burdens.

Future humanitarian crises

Large-scale war is now uncommon but persists in Syria, Yemen, South Sudan, and Afghanistan, and in a more long-lasting form than in the past. The risk of asymmetrical or unconventional wars and conflicts remains high. 2016 has been reported as the fifth most violent year since the end of the Cold War. Continuing the trend since at least World War II, the proportion of battlefield deaths has greatly declined.[7] However, indirect civilian deaths from destruction of infrastructure, including public health infrastructure, have increased. This destruction is frequently deliberate, reflecting increased acceptance of civilian infrastructure as a military target. The result is that conflicts continue to result in pervasive insecurity, especially for civilians and aid workers, and in prolonged and catastrophic loss of public health protections, infrastructure, and services.

More people now live in urban than in rural settings. Rapid urbanization in many African and Asian countries has proved unsustainable. Sanitation is often poor and the prevalence of infectious diseases is increased, contributing to severe health indices and large gaps between the 'have' and 'have-not' populations. Many urbanites are relegated to living in slums that are densely populated disaster-prone areas devoid of public health protections. With more people living in cities, the increasingly urban nature of conflicts has made them correspondingly more deadly.

Climate change migration from rising oceans has already taken place in Kiribati and other Polynesian islands where public health emphasis is on educating populations in adaptation, resilience, and the inevitable migration planning. It has been estimated that up to 75 million island refugees will require placement and aid by 2050.[8] For the rest of the world, rising sea levels will be overshadowed by drought and flooding. Between 1995 and 2015, 90% of major disasters were caused by weather events— notably, floods, storms, heatwaves, and droughts—and this trend is likely to increase.[9] These events are closely linked to 'emergencies of scarcity', the term used to describe increasing areas of the world suffering from scarcity of water, food, and energy. Drought in Africa in 2016–17 has been linked to climate change in Angola, Namibia, Botswana, Zimbabwe, Lesotho, and South Africa. In Mozambique, half the population experienced severe drought and all maize was destroyed.

These and other public health crises will become more severe and common. They will dominate humanitarian requirements in the coming decades.[10] The aforementioned principles of assessment and response will remain critical, ensuring that population-based public health protections will become more challenging to humanitarian practice.

Conclusion

As a public health professional or team, there is much you can do to help in a disaster. Effective disaster and crisis response is predicated on rapid assessment of the situation prior to initiating a response and on focusing on the public health principles outlined in this chapter.

Further resources

Further reading

Hanquet G. (ed.) (1997). *Refugee health: an approach to emergency situations*. Macmillan/Médecins Sans Frontières, London.

Heymann DL. (ed.) (2014). *Control of communicable diseases manual*. American Public Health Association, Washington, DC.

Inter-Agency Standing Committee (2012). Multi-cluster/sector initial rapid assessment. Available at: ℘ https://interagencystandingcommittee.org/needs-assessment/documents-public/iasc-multi-clustersector-initial-rapid-assessment-mira-manual-2015 (accessed 16 August 2019).

U.S. Agency for International Development Office for Foreign Disaster Assistance (2014). *Field operations guide for disaster assessment and risk*. Available at: ℘ https://www.usaid.gov/sites/default/files/documents/1866/fog_v4_0.pdf (accessed 16 August 2019).

References

1 United Nations High Commissioner for Refugees. Global trends: forced displacement in 2015. Available at: ℘ http://www.unhcr.org/en-us/statistics/unhcrstats/576408cd7/unhcr-global-trends-2016.html (accessed 1 October, 2017).

2 World Health Organization. Guidelines for medicine donations. WHO, Geneva. Available at: ℘ http://www.who.int/selection_medicines/emergencies/guidelines_medicine_donations/en, (accessed 1 October 2017).

3 Bero L, Carson B, Moller H, et al. (2010) To give is better than to receive: compliance with WHO guidelines for drug donations during 2000–2008. *Bulletin of the World Health Organization*, **88**(12), 922–9. doi:10.2471/BLT.10.079764.

4 IASC (2012) Multi-cluster/sector initial rapid assessment. March. Available at: ℛ https://interagencystandingcommittee.org/needs-assessment/documents-public/iasc-multi-clustersector-initial-rapid-assessment-mira-manual-2015 (accessed 16 August 2019).

5 World Health Organization. Interagency Emergency Health Kit 2017. WHO, Geneva. Available at: ℛ http://www.who.int/emergencies/kits/iehk/en (accessed 1 October 2017).

6 United Nations High Commissioner for Refugees. (2016). UNHCR uses drones to help displaced populations in Africa. 21 November. Available at: ℛ http://www.unhcr.org/afr/news/latest/2016/11/582dc6d24/unhcr-uses-drones-help-displaced-populations-africa.html (accessed 1 October 2017).

7 Norway Peace Research Institute Oslo (PRIO) (2017). Trends in armed conflict, 1946–2016. February. Available at: ℛ https://www.prio.org/utility/DownloadFile.ashx?id=1373&type=publicationfile (accessed 1 October 2017).

8 Oxfam (2009). The future is here: climate change in the Pacific. Briefing paper. Available at: ℛ https://www.oxfam.org.nz/sites/default/files/reports/The%20future%20is%20here-Oxfam%20report-July09.pdf (accessed 1 October 2017).

9 UN Office for Disaster Risk Reduction (UNISDR) and the Belgian-based Centre for Research on the Epidemiology of Disasters (CRED). The human cost of weather related disasters. Available at: ℛ https://www.unisdr.org/archive/46793 (accessed 1 October 2017).

10 Burkle FM. (2010). Future humanitarian crises: challenges to practice, policy, and public health. *Prehospital and Disaster Medicine*, **25**, 194–9.

Assuring screening programmes

**Angela Raffle, Alex Barratt, and
J.A. Muir Gray**

All screening programmes do harm, some do good as well.

UK National Screening Committee

Objectives

After reading this chapter, you will:
- understand why screening needs a programme, not just a test
- recognize the biases that limit the validity of observational evidence
- be clearer about the public health tasks in screening
- understand that values and beliefs shape screening policy as much as evidence.

What screening is and is not: definitions

Screening is testing people who do not suspect they have a problem. It is done:
- to reduce risk of future ill health (e.g. screen for raised blood pressure, intervene with drugs, reduce risk of stroke)
- to give information (e.g. screen pregnant woman, identify unborn baby has Down's syndrome, couple keeps baby and is forewarned).

Tests or inquiries once disease is symptomatic are not screening. They are for prompt recognition or for clinical management.

Screening involves a system not just a test

There are two ways of looking at a screening system:
- Consider everything that must be in place to deliver a service. This helps you ensure that high-quality programmes are delivered to your population. The elements include:
  - a register for issuing invitations and reminders
  - a system for checking that follow-up steps happen
  - screening tests
  - investigations
  - interventions
  - information and support for participants
  - staff training
  - policy making
  - coordination locally and nationally
  - setting standards and ensuring they are met
  - commissioning research to improve screening.
- Consider the basic steps that a participant goes through. This looks like a flow diagram (see Figure 3.6.1) and it helps with understanding what screening does.

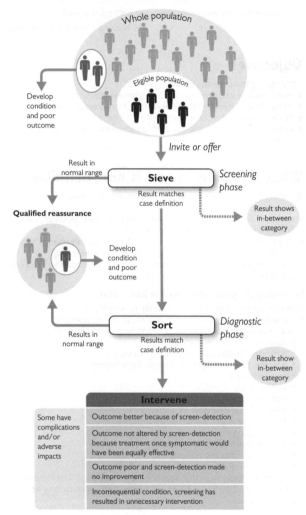

Figure 3.6.1 The screening process.

What screening does

You need to know the range, and likelihood, of different consequences in order to make decisions about policy. Individuals need this information so they can decide whether to participate. Whether a consequence is judged 'good' or 'bad' varies from person to person. Figure 3.6.1 can help you map the consequences.

The screening test is not a diagnostic test. It is only like a sieve. It sorts large numbers of low-risk people into a group at higher risk, who then go on to a diagnostic phase, and those at lower risk (but not no risk).

The main consequences, using breast screening as an example, are listed below. The individual may:

- be reassured at the time of screening and not get the disease (i.e. have a negative result and not develop breast cancer)
- be reassured but get the disease (i.e. have a negative result but subsequently be diagnosed with breast cancer)
- have a life-impacting disease averted (i.e. screen-detected breast cancer whose **timely** treatment prevents breast cancer death)
- have an intervention but develop life-impacting disease (i.e. screen-detected breast cancer but still die of breast cancer despite intervention)
- have a potentially harmful intervention for a symptomless phenomenon (i.e. screen-detected ductal carcinoma *in situ* (DCIS) that would have caused no problem)
- have an intervention but with no extra benefit, with an equally good prognosis if diagnosed symptomatically (i.e. screen-detected low-grade breast cancer, or DCIS, that would have been curable on symptomatic presentation)
- have an abnormality of uncertain significance detected, leading to follow-up, surveillance, possible intervention, and uncertain benefit (i.e. mammographic changes leading to annual repeat mammography).

Who is helped and who is harmed?

As a public health practitioner, you will see that the people genuinely helped are those who, as a direct result of screen detection, avoid death or serious disease. The perception of most participants and clinicians can be very different. Almost everyone with a screen-detected abnormality feels thankful, and some clinicians believe they have cured all the people detected. This is the *popularity paradox*. *Over-detection* is a major screening-related harm, yet it contributes to the popularity of screening through the illusion that large numbers of people are helped. A nurse in the UK cervical screening programme will see over 150 women with screen-detected abnormality for each one who has serious disease prevented.[1] For 10,000 men age 50, the number who would die of prostate cancer is 30, yet 4,200 of them will have histologically confirmed prostate cancer if screened,[2] which leads to substantial harm from treatment-related deaths and side-effects, such as incontinence and impotence.

Balancing harm, benefit, and affordability

There is always a trade-off between benefit, harm, and affordability. The numbers flowing into different parts of the system are influenced by:

- the acceptability and accessibility of screening (e.g. convenience, publicity, information, frequency of testing)
- the definition of the eligible group (e.g. age range)
- changing the numbers of people with positive screening results (e.g. by more tests, by double or treble reading, or by changing the cut-off between positive and negative)
- changing the number of people defined as screen-detected 'cases' (e.g. multiple investigations or changing the cut-off used to define those with the condition).

Measuring the impact of screening

Observational evidence can be highly misleading because of biases that make outcome in screened people look good even if screening makes no difference.

Three key biases in screening

- *The healthy screenee effect:* people who come for screening tend to be healthier than those who do not.
- *Length-time bias:* screening is best at picking up long-lasting, slow-growing conditions. This pulls good-prognosis cases into the observed group, whereas rapidly progressive, and therefore poor-prognosis, cases are less likely to be picked up.
- *Lead-time bias:* the apparent survival time for people with screen-detected disease is longer simply because they are detected at an earlier point in the course of the disease.

Three sources of evidence for evaluating screening in the population

Measures of test performance tell you little about the whole programme's impact on health so do not count as evidence.

- *Randomized control trials (RCTs):* people are recruited, then randomly assigned to receive screening or usual care. RCTs need to be large and last a long time, but are less expensive than allowing unevaluated screening to develop haphazardly. They are the most reliable source of evidence of benefit and harm.
- *Time-trend studies:* these involve observation of trends in incidence and deaths once screening is in place. They are useful if properly conducted, and comparison with countries or regions without screening can help.
- *Case-control studies:* these compare past screening in people with the disease, or who have died from the disease, and controls. Even with matching and validation of screening history, they still consistently overestimate the effect of screening[3] because of confounding.

If there is more than one study using a particular method, then a systematic review of all the evidence should be prepared.

Two additional sources of information about screening in the population
- *Modelling studies*: These make theoretical predictions about screening outcomes and examine the effect of varying frequency, age range, intervention threshold, etc. They are strongest if based on RCT evidence.
- *Pilot or demonstration projects*: These can solve practical issues. They are not reliable for assessing benefit and harm.

Presenting information about benefits and harms

Concern about uptake rates has meant that benefits of screening have been emphasized more than harms. This slanted approach disregards the rights of autonomous adults to reach informed decisions and is no longer considered appropriate or ethical. Policy in the UK and elsewhere now requires that balanced information be available to people considering screening. Decision aids can be valuable in helping people to feel informed and to reach decisions that fit with what matters most to them.[4]

Practical tasks: implementing screening programmes

Starting a programme from scratch

It helps if you have:
- an agreed evidence-based national or regional policy and roll-out plan
- ring-fenced resources that can be spent only on screening
- training centres and demonstration sites
- citizen involvement
- reliable information technology.

Some of your challenges locally are:
- *agreeing the boundary of the local programme*: administrative and provider catchments seldom match
- getting cooperation from all organizations with a part to play
- *communicating understanding of the programme*: to staff, participants and public.

Sorting out a mess

Haphazard testing often starts ahead of evidence-based policy. Converting this to a quality-assured equitable screening programme is difficult, but can be done. Major problems are that:
- there is inconsistent training and practice but everyone thinks their way is right
- commercial, private practice, and research vested interests abound
- you meet resistance when changing from intense screening for a few to less intense for all.

Carrying on screening

Once a programme is up and running, things will go wrong unless you keep an eye on them. Make sure there is:
- a nominated public health lead who knows the key players and understands the performance data

- a coordinating group meeting 1–3 times a year
- an annual report including a forward plan
- regular training and updating for all staff.

Quality assurance
Achieving quality and best value depends on:
- system design and resources (e.g. staff training)
- monitoring and readjustment (e.g. region-wide collation of annual performance data).

Box 3.6.1 illustrates an example of a quality assurance standard, taken from the programme to reduce risk of sight-threatening retinopathy in people with insulin-dependent diabetes.[5]

Box 3.6.1 Example of a quality standard

Objective: to ensure digital images of the retina are of adequate quality
  Criteria: proportion of known eligible people with diabetes where a digital image has been obtained but the image is ungradable
  Acceptable standard: less than or equal to 4%
  Achievable standard: less than or equal to 2%

Quality is not solely about effectiveness. The seven components in Donabedian's definition of quality[6] include optimality and equity. Exclusive pursuit of effectiveness increases resource use irrespective of opportunity cost.

Practical tasks: controlling harmful screening

You need to be able to stop unwanted screening in order to protect your public from diversion of resources and direct harm.

Harmful screening arises because of the following:
- *New screening self-starts irrespective of evidence:* drivers include market forces, consumer pressure, clinician enthusiasm, and media pressure, including celebrity endorsement, with usually a complex and manipulative interrelationship between them.
- Within existing programmes, there is pressure to intensify irrespective of marginal cost–benefit. This is a response to inherent limitations (undetectable cases, cases outside the eligible group).

Key steps in controlling harmful screening:
- *Understand why people want the screening:* go and meet with and listen to clinicians, pressure groups, campaigning journalists.
- *Explicitly acknowledge the reasons why people want it:* don't dismiss concerns or belittle their interpretation of evidence.
- *Assemble and communicate evidence and information:* about the consequences the screening would really have, and about alternative ways of addressing the problem.

- *Carefully introduce specific enforcement measures:* for publicly funded programmes, this could include declining requests for unscheduled tests.
- *Regulate the advertising of tests:* so that citizens are guaranteed to receive balanced, accurate, and evidence-based information about benefits, harms, quality, and price for the tests they are being offered.[7]

Screening and the law

Out-of-court settlements are commonplace. In rare cases that have been defended, some judgements have related to standards you would expect from diagnosis, not screening. Judges are influenced by the fact that an expert witness finds abnormality in the test the screener judged normal. This ignores:

- *outcome bias:* the witness knows the outcome for the subject—the screener does not
- *context bias:* the witness is an experienced doctor and has days to look at the sample—the screener is competent only at screening and has a few minutes.

Equipped with careful preparation and an expert lawyer who understands screening, it is possible to successfully defend a service that meets recognized standards. We think it vital that health departments enable this to happen more often.

Making screening policy

Who makes policy decisions about screening?

Generally, decisions are regional or national. They may relate to:

- state-funded provision of quality-assured national programmes (as in the UK)
- state reimbursement for approved screening, with provision by both public and private providers (as in Australia)
- recommendations to consumers, who decide if they can afford a health policy that includes the screening (as in the USA).

What factors influence screening policy

In theory, you base your policy on evidence and resources. In practice, values and beliefs have a profound influence. Box 3.6.2 illustrates the case of mammography recommendations in the USA.

The public health role is to present information for decision making as clearly as we can, but the politician, who needs to survive the next election, may take a decision that matches public values and beliefs. In the UK, for example, we have an evidence-based national decision against introducing a prostate cancer screening programme, but the NHS provides prostate-specific antigen (PSA) testing for individual men. The strong belief in PSA testing among public and politicians made it politically unacceptable to have an outright embargo.

Box 3.6.2 Case study: mammography recommendations in USA

When the USA National Institutes of Health (NIH) recommended in January 1997 that evidence was insufficient to recommend screening mammography for all women in their 40s, the response was dramatic:

• At the news conference, the panel was accused of condemning American women to death.
• The panel's chairman was summoned to a Senate sub-committee.
• The Senate voted 98 to 0 in favour of supporting mammography for this age group.
• The head of the NIH said he was shocked by the report and asked the NIH advisory board to look at the evidence.

In March 1997, the advisory board overruled the consensus panel's recommendation and stated instead that women in their 40s should get a screening mammogram every 1–2 years.

The *New England Journal of Medicine* published a review article[8] lamenting the lack of logic. However, what the Senate was articulating were the values of American society. If mammography offers any potential for health gain, how dare anyone recommend that the individual should not have it?

Many other societies take a collectivist approach and 'take it as read' that the rights of an individual to have any intervention that could be beneficial has to be balanced with the needs of others who require a share of the healthcare resource.

8 Fletcher SW. (1997). Whither scientific deliberation in health policy recommendation? Alice in the Wonderland of breast-cancer screening. New England Journal of Medicine, 336, 1180–3.

The last word

Screening, like most other public health services, is at best a zero gratitude business.

Further resources

Barratt A, Irwig I, Glasziou P, et al. (1999). Users' guides to the medical literature. XVII: How to use guidelines and recommendations about screening. *Journal of the American Medical Association*, 281, 2029–34.

Bryder L. (2009). *A history of the 'unfortunate experiment' at the National Women's Hospital*. Auckland University Press.

Raffle A. (2009). Screening. Interactive learning. Health knowledge. Available at: ✍ https://www.healthknowledge.org.uk/interactive-learning/screening/introduction (accessed 10 August 2019).

Raffle A, Mackie A, Gray JAM. (2019). *Screening; evidence and practice*. Oxford University Press, Oxford.

UK National Screening Committee. Available at: ✍https://www.gov.uk/government/groups/uk-national-screening-committee-uk-nsc (accessed 10 August 2019).

Welch HG. (2015). *Less medicine, more health: 7 assumptions that drive too much medical care*. Beacon Press, Boston, MA.

References

1 Raffle AE, Alden B, Quinn M, et al. (2003). Outcomes of screening to prevent cancer: analysis of cumulative incidence of cervical abnormality and modelling of cases and deaths prevented. *British Medical Journal*, **326**, 901–4.

2 Frankel S, Davey Smith G, Donovan J, et al. (2003). Screening for prostate cancer. *Lancet*, **361**, 1122–8.

3 Moss SM. (1991). Case-control studies of screening. *International Journal of Epidemiology*, **20**, 1–6.

4 Stacey D, Légaré F, Lewis K, et al. (2017). Decision aids to help people who are facing health treatment or screening decisions. *Cochrane Database of Systematic Reviews*. Issue 4. Art. No.: CD001431. DOI: 10.1002/14651858.CD001431.pub5

5 Public Health England (2017). Diabetic eye screening programme: pathway standards. Available at: ✒ https://www.gov.uk/government/publications/diabetic-eye-screening-standards-and-performance-objectives (accessed 10 August 2019).

6 Donabedian A. (2003). *An introduction to quality assurance in health care*. Oxford University Press, Oxford.

7 Raffle, A. (2010). Guest editorial: advertising private tests for well people. *Clinical Evidence*, **2**.

8 Fletcher SW. (1997). Whither scientific deliberation in health policy recommendation? Alice in the Wonderland of breast-cancer screening. *New England Journal of Medicine*, **336**, 1180–3.

Genomics

Hilary Burton and Mark Kroese

Objective

Genomic technologies are having a major impact on our understanding of health and disease. Genomic sequencing is much cheaper and quicker, while our ability to sort and interpret the data using huge computer power and very big databases means that genomic testing influences clinical decisions in many areas of medicine. Similarly, in public health, it is beginning to provide information about disease risk that could be valuable in preventive programmes including large population screening programmes. In the area of infectious disease, sequencing of pathogen genomes is rapidly becoming an indispensable tool in detecting and managing outbreaks, disease surveillance, and managing antimicrobial resistance.

The field of genomics is moving quickly and involves many players from basic researchers to clinicians, ethicists, regulators, the commercial sector, and the public. The multidisciplinary nature of public health means that specialists are ideally placed to ensure that genomics becomes centre stage for health. This is the only specialism whose core is the well-being (in the most holistic sense) of the entire population. In this chapter, we will try to give you the basics about genomics, to whet your appetite about the future, and introduce you to some of the key debates and stakeholders.

After reading this chapter, you will have a better understanding of:

- the absolute basics of genomics (and how it relates to genetics) from DNA to sequence to healthcare decision
- genomics in healthcare: how understanding the molecular basis of disease forms the basis of personalized medicine
- genomics and disease prevention
- genomics and reproductive choice
- genomics and formal population health screening programmes
- genomics and common non-communicable disease prevention
- genomics and infectious disease
- genomics and society: ethical issues in the use of genomics
- the roles that public health specialists might play
- where to get further information.

Genomics and genetics

The genome is often thought of as the blueprint for an individual, specifying overall development and the structure of the different cells and tissues, as well as controlling activity by switching on and off millions of processes involved in homeostasis. The precise sequence of the genome varies between individuals, usually without any effect on function. Some sequence differences (or variants) have a small influence on disease susceptibility. More rarely, where a change in sequence catastrophically disrupts protein production or cellular processes, the result may be a severe, 'single gene' disorder (see Box 3.7.1 for examples). Such changes and the ensuing diseases are characteristically inherited—the conditions, such as cystic fibrosis or hypertrophic cardiomyopathy may occur in several family members. The management of these patients and families with genetic disease forms an important aspect of care in most clinical specialties.

> **Box 3.7.1 Examples of single-gene disorders**
>
> **Single-gene disorders**
> Duchenne muscular dystrophy
> Cystic fibrosis
> Adult polycystic kidney disease
> Phenylketonuria
> Sickle cell disease
> Neurofibromatosis
>
> **Single-gene subsets of common chronic disease**
> Familial hypercholesterolaemia (atherosclerosis)
> BRCA1 and BRCA2 (breast cancer)
> Hereditary non-polyposis colorectal cancer
> Maturity onset diabetes of the young

Genome sequencing and interpretation

Understanding how changes in genome sequence may affect an individual's health is becoming an important aspect of healthcare and disease prevention. Our current knowledge is far from complete. The foundations were built from decades of analysis of how particular changes are associated with disease in families. Such research elucidated many of the changes that are responsible for severe disease running through generations within families. These may also appear as single gene 'subsets' of more common chronic disease (see Box 3.7.1 for examples). More recently, research has shown that even comparatively straightforward genetic disease can be extraordinarily complicated, with multiple genes and many different variations within genes being responsible for apparently the same clinical disease. For example, more than a dozen causal genes have been implicated in an inherited disease of cardiac muscle known as hypertrophic cardiomyopathy (HCM).[1]

Identifying the type and nature of variation between individuals and determining whether a particular variation is responsible for clinical symptoms in an individual has been further advanced by the availability of technologies for sequencing the whole genome at relatively low cost and high speed. However, the complexity of analysis of such whole genome sequencing (WGS) remains a critical factor. Clinical interpretation of genome sequences is dependent on the accuracy with which the patient's sequence is determined (this often depends on a process of sequencing small fragments of DNA and then piecing them back together), the ways in which putative variants are identified, filtered, and then evaluated to determine those that may be disease causing, and the ways in which the remaining variants are subsequently interpreted. For example, interpretation will require comparison with large databases to see if the same variant has been previously associated with similar clinical findings, or may require modelling of the potential functional implications of the protein produced by the changed sequence. Genome sequencing and interpretation in the clinical setting are thus entirely dependent on the ability and capacity to manage, process, store, and share vast quantities of genomic and clinical data.[2, 3]

With increased breadth of testing comes more difficulty in interpretation—and the greater likelihood of identifying variants that, although unusual, cannot be classified with certainty as disease causing or benign. Such 'variants of uncertain significance' pose challenges for health professionals in the short term, in knowing how to characterize such variants and what to report back to patients and, in the longer term, in developing robust and consistent systems to keep them under review so that they can be acted upon and the patient potentially re-contacted in the light of new knowledge. Sequencing of the whole genome rather than restricting testing to genes that are known to harbour changes relevant to the clinical question also raises significant risks of identifying a different and unconnected genetic condition. This may be useful for the patient depending on whether there is an effective preventive intervention but it also has the potential to cause unnecessary anxiety or, even worse, lead to invasive diagnosis, treatment, or lifelong restriction for a condition that may never have become clinically manifest.

Using the genome in healthcare

Genomic-based testing is now relevant throughout healthcare and is becoming routine in many areas of mainstream medicine. It underpins many of the developments widely considered as 'personalized' or 'precision' medicine, by assisting in the characterization of disease at a molecular level and by providing information about the patient's likely response to treatment. In many clinical areas, rare forms of inherited disease exist as subsets of common disease. For example, in diabetes, a rare inherited form called 'maturity onset diabetes of the young' affects 1–2% of people with diabetes, particularly those under the age of 25. Recognising this form by undertaking genetic testing is important because patients will respond to treatment with sulfonylureas rather than requiring insulin.[4]

Whereas in rare disease the patient's own inherited (germline) genome is interrogated, in cancer the testing of tumour DNA (somatic testing) can give information about the characteristics and likely response to treatment of the tumour and, in infectious disease, the genomes of pathogens may be sequenced to give information about the likely organism causing disease as well as its potential source or resistance to antimicrobials.

Genomic testing is set to become part of the diagnostic portfolio for the entirety of clinical medicine. The key challenge for its effective implementation will be in establishing the clinical care pathways to deliver the clinical utility, and ensuring effectiveness and equity across the health system as a whole. Health professionals will need to be properly competent to embed genomics in their everyday practice. At a health system level, this will require concerted development of training curricula, good practice guidelines, clinical pathways, and near patient prompts coupled with timely information to support day-to-day interactions with patients.[5]

Pharmacogenomics

Genomic testing is increasingly used to guide drug treatment. This may be choosing the right drug based on understanding the molecular pathology of disease (e.g. some personalized cancer treatments); using genetic testing to predict the likelihood of adverse drug reactions; or using testing to decide on drug dosage (which may relate to the way in which an individual's genetic background influences how drugs are taken up, metabolized, or excreted in the body). As whole genome sequencing (WGS) becomes more common, it is anticipated that in the future relevant genetic information will be available at the time of prescribing.

The laboratory testing services

Genome based testing is an important aspect of healthcare provision in the UK health system. Historically in the NHS, molecular testing for inherited diseases developed as part of the regional clinical genetics services, where genetic tests were offered originally for single gene disorders. As technologies developed, these single gene tests were expanded into 'panel' tests of multiple genes, followed by the development of tests for clinical exomes (all the expressed genes in the genome) and even WGS to investigate a particular condition or presentation. These technological developments have resulted in the expansion of clinical applications of genetic testing and reduction in diagnostic delays as a consequence of not having to undertake sequential testing. The development of tumour (somatic) genetic testing, pathogen genomic testing and WGS technologies, alongside their specialist interpretation and more complex data-handling requirements, is now necessitating the development of new, more centralized genomic laboratory services in the NHS.

As genetic testing applications increase in the various medical disciplines, there is an associated requirement for clinicians in these disciplines to understand how to use these new diagnostics. In the NHS upto 2018, the UK Genetic Testing Network undertook evaluations of new genetic tests for inherited diseases and provided information on these on its website, where the NHS directory of tests could also be accessed.[6,7] This service has now been replaced with the NHS Genomic Medicine Service in England and alternative arrangements in the other devolved countries.

Genomics and disease prevention

Testing a person's genome can provide opportunities for disease prevention at an individual level. For certain inherited diseases, this relies on identifying those individuals with the relevant genetic changes that may only become manifest clinically later in life. The timescales and certainty for this vary—but the opportunity for prevention rests in the fact that, once identified, an intervention may be offered that reduces the likelihood or severity of the disease in question. Preventive interventions might be drugs (e.g. the use of statins to reduce high blood cholesterol levels in individuals with familial hypercholesterolaemia [FH] and thus prevent early cardiovascular disease);[8] enhanced surveillance (e.g. regular colonoscopy to detect and remove polyps that may progress to colon cancer in hereditary non-polyposis colorectal cancer [HNPCC]); or surgery (e.g. prophylactic mastectomy in women who have BRCA1 or BRCA2 mutations indicating high risk of hereditary breast cancer).

As well as providing a more detailed diagnosis for the individual (and sometimes influencing treatment), the importance of molecular testing in inherited conditions is that it enables the disease to be linked with a specific (causal) variant in the DNA that can then be sought in first-degree relatives who may have inherited the same variant. This is known as 'cascade testing' and is an important aspect of managing inherited disease. For more common genetic conditions such as FH, where there are thought to be more than 260,000 affected individuals in the UK, putting cascade testing in place in a systematic way, through provision of dedicated services led by nurse specialists, has been shown to be crucial in identifying previously unknown individuals with disease. This has been shown to be highly cost-effective.[8, 9]

Genomic testing for inherited diseases for prevention purposes is thus usually restricted to people who already have disease or to their family members rather than to individuals who are fit and healthy with no family history of disease. For the latter, the potential of genomic testing has focused on risk for common disease and large genome-wide association studies have established a wide range of variants associated with common chronic disease such as cancer or diabetes.[10] However, it has been found that the contribution of each variant to disease is quite small. In the longer term, it is expected that the results of susceptibility testing may be incorporated into risk calculators alongside well-established risk factors such as age, body mass index, and smoking status.

Genomics and reproductive risk

Over the years, one of the most important ways in which genetic testing has been used is in assessing reproductive risk and providing advice. Couples may already know that they are at risk of having an affected child, possibly because of a family history, because one of them is affected, or because they already have an affected child. In these cases, they are usually advised by specialist feto-maternal or clinical genetic services that will wish to establish the precise molecular diagnosis in the affected individual so that a specific mutation test can be undertaken prenatally.

Prenatal genetic testing may be undertaken using various forms of fetal sampling during pregnancy: chorionic villus sampling can be performed in the first trimester and amniocentesis in the second. Both these forms of testing carry a small risk of miscarriage. The development of non-invasive methods of obtaining fetal DNA has thus been widely welcomed. Non-invasive testing involves the extraction of small quantities of fetal DNA from the maternal serum and can be undertaken in the first trimester (see Box 3.7.2).

A further option for couples who are at risk of having a child with an inherited disease is pre-implantation genetic diagnosis (PGD). This involves in vitro fertilisation to create embryos that can be tested by removal of cells at a very early stage of development prior to implementation, with only an unaffected embryo being re-introduced to establish pregnancy. In the UK, NHS provision of PGD services is limited to genetic conditions that have been licensed by the UK Human Fertilisation and Embryology Authority (HFEA).

Box 3.7.2 Non-invasive testing

'Free fetal DNA' technology is technically demanding because the fetal DNA is in small fragments and in minute quantities relative to the maternal DNA from which it has to be differentiated. This innovative form of prenatal testing, which avoids unnecessary invasive prenatal testing and the risk of miscarriage, has now been validated for use by NHS services in the UK.[a] Non-invasive prenatal diagnosis (NIPD) is provided for certain inherited diseases and there are plans to introduce non-invasive prenatal testing (NIPT) as part of the NHS Down's screening programme in the near future. The important distinction between NIPD and NIPT is that in the case of NIPT an abnormal result requires confirmation by an invasive test such as amniocentesis.

a) Chitty LS, Wright D, Hill M, et al. (2016). Uptake, outcomes, and costs of implementing non-invasive prenatal testing for Down's syndrome into NHS maternity care: prospective cohort study in eight diverse maternity units. *British Medical Journal*, **354**, i3426.

Genomics and population screening programmes

Inherited disease or other forms of disease based on genomic structure is also the subject of a number of population-level screening programmes aimed at the preconception, antenatal, or neonatal period. These have different underlying rationales and use a number of different technologies, incorporating other biomarkers as well as genomic testing. Examples are given in Table 3.7.1.

The use of genomic testing in population screening programmes in the UK requires data and evidence to fulfil the rigorous criteria of the UK National Screening Committee. In other countries with different approaches to the evaluation and provision of antenatal screening programmes, there has been greater expansion of screening options for genetic conditions. It is inevitable that, with the further development of genomic medicine, there will be opportunities for new screening options for specific high-risk populations that do not warrant a national delivery programme because of the smaller size of these populations. These will need to be evaluated and considered for NHS service provision.

Table 3.7.1 Examples of population screening for inherited diseases

Condition	Stage	Rationale	Technology
Tay Sachs disease	Preconception carrier screening	To identify couples at risk of Tay-Sachs disease—a progressive nervous system disease; individuals with Ashkenazi Jewish origin are at increased risk	Enzyme test (biochemical) or DNA test
Sickle cell and thalassaemia	Linked antenatal and newborn	To identify couples at risk of having an affected child and to identify an affected newborn early	Testing for different haemoglobin variants
Phenylketonuria and other inherited metabolic disorders	Newborn	Early identification of affected infants so that specialised diet can be provided to prevent brain damage	Tandem mass spectrometry (enzyme test); biochemical testing
Cystic fibrosis	Newborn	Early diagnosis so that treatment can be started to prevent lung damage	Immunoreactive trypsinogen test; test for gene mutations

Genomics and common non-communicable disease prevention

Genomic research in common chronic disease has taken the form of very large genome-wide association studies. These usually involve cohorts of many thousands of individuals to look at the associations of possible susceptibility variants in the genome, personal, lifestyle, and other biomarkers with common chronic disease. The complexity of interactions between all these variables is high. Although there are a large number of genetic variables involved, each has only a small effect. Such studies have so far not led to evidence-based preventive applications. While it is certainly true that individuals vary in their risk of common complex disease and that this risk is, at least in part, genetically determined, it is not yet clear that an understanding of personal susceptibility enhances prevention. It does not lead to a differentiation of the preventive interventions that may be offered (the general advice around healthy diet, no smoking, advice on alcohol, exercise, limited exposure to environmental toxins etc. does not change). Although the existing evidence is poor, a recent systematic review has shown no evidence that communicating DNA-based risk estimates changes behaviour.[11]

One area that has been investigated and may lead to useful population stratification for prevention is that of breast cancer, where there is a potential to offer different mammographic screening at different ages or at different intervals according to risk of disease. Modelling has shown that so-called 'risk-stratified screening' could help to optimise the ratio of benefit to harm for mammography, recognising the potential harm arising from unnecessary testing, associated anxiety, and, occasionally, biopsies or even unnecessary treatment arising from false positives and overdiagnosis (disease that would not have led to clinical consequences). Although theoretically effective, the same research programme showed that some of the organisational, ethical, legal, and social issues for stratified screening might be quite complex to deal with (see Box 3.7.3).[12]

Box 3.7.3 Examples of ethical, legal, and social issues in stratified cancer screening[a]

- The consent process should address the benefits, harms, and uncertainties of genotyping.
- How best to communicate the risks and benefits of stratified screening to patients.
- Obtaining informed consent for the necessary genetic testing.
- Protecting children's autonomous choices by restricting personalized screening to adults.
- Potential for discrimination in insurance or employment for higher-risk individuals.
- Concerns for equitable access and need for fairness.
- Regulatory issues around storing, linking, and sharing genetic data.

a) See also the collaborative oncological gene-environment study (COGS) project. Available at: ✍ http://www.phgfoundation.org/project/cogs (accessed 24 August 2019).

Genomics and infectious diseases

A significant part of public health involves detecting, managing, and treating the effects of pathogens in populations: genomics is beginning to play a number of important roles with respect to management of the individual and to the control of infectious disease.

Pathogen genomes are much smaller than human genomes and so can be sequenced relatively easily, quickly, and cheaply. In some conditions, particularly where the bacterium takes a long time to culture (e.g. *M. Tuberculosis*), rapid sequencing of the genome of individual pathogens can lead to a much quicker diagnosis and even provide information on key virulence factors or the likely response to different antimicrobials so that the patient can be started on the right treatment much more quickly.[13]

But it is perhaps in the area of surveillance and control that pathogen sequencing has the most to offer public health. The pathogen genome is evolving rapidly, enabling it to evade treatments and the immune system. The small changes that take place as the pathogen evolves can be used to plot a phylogenetic tree that provides information on the likely route or mechanism of transmission—for example, by showing that cases that may previously have been thought to be sporadic are linked and that all may be due to infection from a single source (See Box 3.7.4).

Sequencing can also be useful in detection of emerging threats—for example, how human infection may arise from an animal source or the emergence of antimicrobial-resistant strains of pathogens.

> **Box 3.7.4 Use of whole genome sequencing in outbreak control**
>
> Pathogen whole genome sequencing (WGS) was used during a suspected outbreak of methicillin-resistant *Staphylococcus aureus* (MRSA) infections on a special care baby unit first to confirm that an outbreak was underway and then, in combination with epidemiological information, to identify a probable source of the infections enabling the infection control team to end the outbreak.[a]
>
> a) Koser CU, Holden MTG, Ellington MJ, et al. (2012). Rapid whole-genome sequencing for investigation of a neonatal MRSA outbreak. *New England Journal of Medicine*, **366(24)**, 2267–75.

Genomics and society: ethical issues in the use of genomics

The Human Genome Project recognised the potential for genomics to raise ethical, legal, or social issues, which, although not necessarily unique to this area, may sometimes be more serious or more personal than other types of medical information. There has therefore been a tradition of research into ethical, legal, and social issues in parallel with emerging scientific, technological, and clinical work.

Genetic information, like other personal identifiable medical information, should generally be kept confidential. In reality, the main reason this information is regarded as sensitive is due to its predictive value. Some genetic information may confer a high risk of future disease in an individual who is otherwise healthy, something that may cause anxiety, lead to people seeking preventive interventions that could be harmful, or be used by outside agencies such as employers or insurance companies to discriminate against individuals. Importantly, this information is also relevant to family members—requiring that those responsible for the care of the initially diagnosed patient (the proband) also take the proband's family into account. The responsible healthcare professional will need to consider their obligations of confidentiality to the proband against the potential benefits of disclosing to relatives that they might share a disease causing genetic variants, taking account of the worry and potential harm associated with that knowledge. Finally, there is the question of whether the 'at-risk' individual 'wants' the information.

These ethical questions come into even greater focus with new sequencing technologies.[14] It is now possible to identify the risks of developing hundreds of diseases through analysing the entire genome sequence. In a clinical setting, this information may be secondary to the original reason for testing, which formed part of a diagnostic pathway in response to the presentation of symptoms and signs. Policy makers address this by determining that the individual should give informed consent, but there are considerable challenges in ensuring that patients and families fully understand the potential implications of receiving a large number of possible results that are not likely to materialise into disease.

A further challenge to clinical care is that our knowledge about the disease-causing nature of variants and their interactions with each other is constantly evolving. Some services maintain a database of patients and test results, keeping them under review so that referring clinicians can be alerted if the status of a result changes and then take appropriate action. This is less problematic in clinical areas such as diabetes where the advice may be to change medication, but it may be significant where invasive action such as surgery may be undertaken. It highlights the importance of developing systematic and robust infrastructures and processes across genomic services in the UK to help ensure that information is as up to date as possible, and that new knowledge is acted upon promptly rather than later when it has been 'cascaded' beyond the individual patient.

Modern genomics relies on the creation, storage, sharing, and use of large quantities of clinical and laboratory data relevant to each patient in routine clinical care. Interpretation of test results involves comparison with reference databases holding relevant clinical and genomic information. In England and Wales, hierarchies of different regulations on data protection, consent, and confidentiality create a complex landscape that makes it challenging for healthcare providers to share and utilise data in an optimal fashion.

Genomics—what does it mean for public health specialists?

Although public health specialists have traditionally focused on populations rather than individuals, new understanding of genomics will have an impact on many areas of practice.

Genomics is an important determinant of disease, particularly rare disease

Rare disease, as a group of conditions, is estimated to affect 1 in 17 of the UK population at some point in their lives. This is a significant burden of morbidity and ill health. Public health specialists need to understand the important opportunities for prevention, through healthcare services, screening programmes, and identifying and targeting high-risk forms of common chronic disease.

Genomics and healthcare

The further development of personalised medicine will need to be integrated in healthcare services and will require general public health skills. Public health specialists will need to show leadership in the expected transformation of healthcare to more personalised care, particularly when this involves changes in health service infrastructure including data sharing.

Genomics and reproductive decision making

Preconception and antenatal genetic testing is increasingly being sought by couples to understand their risk of having children with serious genetic disease and to inform their choices. The development of appropriate services for the population will require careful evaluation and public engagement.

Genomics and screening

Public health specialists can expect to become involved in debates about the incorporation of genomic testing into screening programmes for both rare and common complex disease. This will require a good understanding of the genetic tests, the diseases or conditions under consideration, the target populations, and surrounding societal values and practices.

Genomics and disease prevention

Wider prevention of disease through genomic testing is usually under-taken by cascade testing from known cases within families. This needs to be undertaken by health services in a systematic way and requires genetic data to be shared across health systems.

Genomics and health protection

Pathogen sequencing is increasingly used for identification and investigation of outbreaks of infectious disease, detecting new and emerging pathogens, and monitoring antimicrobial resistance. Public health specialists working in the field of health protection will need to develop such applications and support their implementation.

Further resources

Burton H, Jackson C, Abubakar I. (2014). The impact of genomics on public health practice. *British Medical Bulletin*, **112**(1), 37–46.

References

1 Sabater-Molina M, Pérez-Sánchez I, Hernández Del Rincón JP, et al. (2018). Genetics of hyper-trophic cardiomyopathy: a review of current state. *Clinical Genetics*, January, **93**(1), 3–14.

2 Luheshi L, (2014). Clinical whole genome analysis: delivering the right diagnosis. PHG Foundation.

3 Johansen Taber KA, Dickinson BD, Wilson M. (2014). The promise and challenges of next-generation genome sequencing for clinical care. *JAMA Internal Medicine*, **174**(2), 275–80.

4 Thanabalasingham G, Owen KR, (2011). Diagnosis and management of maturity onset diabetes of the young (MODY). *British Medical Journal*, **343**, d6044.

5 Slade I, Burton H. (2016). Preparing clinicians for genomic medicine. *Postgraduate Medical Journal*, **92**(1089), 369–71. (accessed 24 August 2019).

6 UKGTN, https://ukgtn.nhs.uk/. [cited 2017].

7 Kroese M, Zimmern RL, Farndon P, et al. (2007). How can genetic tests be evaluated for clinical use? Experience of the UK Genetic Testing Network. *European Journal of Human Genetics*, **15**(9), 917–21.

8 Brice P, Burton H, Edwards CW, et al. (2013). Familial hypercholesterolaemia: a pressing issue for European health care. *Atherosclerosis*, **231**(2), 223–6.

9 Kerr M, Pears R, Miedzybrodzka Z, et al. (2017). Cost effectiveness of cascade testing for familial hypercholesterolaemia, based on data from familial hypercholesterolaemia services in the UK. *European Heart Journal*, **38**(23), 1832–9.

10 Langenberg C, Sharp SJ, Franks PW, et al. (2014). Gene-lifestyle interaction and type 2 diabetes: the EPIC interact case-cohort study. *PLOS Medicine*, **11**(5), e1001647.

11 Hollands GJ, French DP, Griffin SJ, et al. (2016). The impact of communicating genetic risks of disease on risk-reducing health behaviour: systematic review with meta-analysis. British Medical Journal, 352, i1102.

12 Burton H, Chowdhury S, Dent T, et al. (2013). Public health implications from COGS and potential for risk stratification and screening. *Nature Genetics*, **45**(4), 349–51.

13 Walker TM, Merker M, Kohl TA, et al. (2017). Whole genome sequencing for M/XDR tuberculosis surveillance and for resistance testing. *Clinical Microbiology and Infection*, **23**(3), 161–6.

14 Hallowell N, Hall A, Alberg C, et al. (2015). Revealing the results of whole-genome sequencing and whole-exome sequencing in research and clinical investigations: some ethical issues. *Journal of Medical Ethics*, **41**(4), 317–21.

Health communication

**Rachel McCloud, Mesfin Bekalu, and
Kasisomayajula Viswanath**

Objectives

After reading this chapter, you will be able to:
- understand why health communication is important in health promotion and disease prevention
- explain how communication messages are produced by different organizations
- identify different types of communication content and genres, such as entertainment, news and advertising
- understand the effects of exposure to communication messages on health outcomes.

Introduction

The twin revolutions in communication and biomedical sciences have made the role of communication critical for mitigating or exacerbating health problems.[1] The dizzying array of delivery platforms, from conventional channels, such as interpersonal networks and radio, to more recent developments, such as the rapid rise in prominence of smartphones and the proliferation of social media channels, has magnified the interest in health communication among researchers, funders, and practitioners.

The primary focus of this chapter will be on 'mediated communications', rather than communication between patients and physicians.

Why is health communication important?

The interest in health communication stems partly from the sheer amount of time one spends interacting with mass media or information and communication technologies (ICTs) of one kind or other. For example, in the USA, 89% of adults use the internet.[2] The vast majority of Americans (95%) now own some sort of cell phone, with smartphone ownership now reaching 77%—a dramatic 42% increase since 2011.[3] Although 65% have access to broadband internet at home, many smartphone users access the internet from their device, and 20% use the internet solely from their smartphones.[2] Time spent with media even among children is yet another indicator of media dominance in our contemporary lives. According to one study:[4]
- 74% of all infants and toddlers have watched television before age 2.
- 99% of all children aged 0–6 years live in a home with a television set.
- 97% have products, like clothes and toys, based on characters from television shows or movies.
- Children under 6 spend about 2 hours a day with screen media, about the same amount of time that they spend playing outside, and three times as much time as they spend reading or being read to.
- Total time spent with all media by those aged 8–18 years has increased from 6.19 to 7.38 hours on a 'typical day'.

Thus, the sheer breadth and depth of penetration of various ICTs have public health practitioners wonder about the value and efficacy of the platforms to communicate health information to diverse audiences. The value of health communications to promote health stems from several reasons:

- Recognition of importance of health communication by such organizations as the World Health Organization (WHO) to the United States' National Academy of Medicine.
- Research suggesting that communication is a significant factor in major public health problems, such as obesity, tobacco use, unsafe sex, and violence.

Given these diverse opinions, and fast-evolving technologies and platforms, characterizing the role of communication for public health practice is important although challenging.

Dimensions of communication and health

Given its vast scope, interdisciplinary roots, cross-cutting appeal, and the fast-evolving technologies, from a public health point of view, it is critical to get a clear understanding of the scope of health communication and how it can be used in health promotion and disease prevention.

At the outset, health communication is pursued and understood at multiple levels: individual, organizational, and societal.[5, 6] Literature at these different levels offers useful insights into how communication messages are produced, processed, and disseminated within organizational contexts, and how they are consumed with different effects at individual, group, and social levels. Within this framework, studies have focused on two broad areas as they affect health:

- Research has offered insights on how use of media and exposure to messages during *routine* use of media may have an impact on health.
- Another line of work has looked at how communications may be used strategically to promote health.

One way to map health communication is to look at it along three dimensions:

- *Production of communication messages:* a process of generating information as a result of interaction between those who generate information, or act as sources of information, and media personnel who gather, process, and disseminate information across different platforms.
- *Communication content:* that includes genres of advertising, news, and entertainment that could promote health, such as latest scientific developments or content that could detract from health.
- *Communication effects* of messages on individual and population health.

This section will summarize what we know about health communication along these three dimensions to map the field and understand health communication from a population perspective. Such an understanding will help practitioners to more skilfully use media for public promotion.

How are communication messages produced?

Much of what we see in the health information environment is a product of interaction between the 'suppliers' or generators of health information and producers representing media organizations that amass, process the content per imperatives of organizations they are working in, and disseminate the information. We will briefly elaborate on these points.

In general, there are three types of information that pertain to health directly or indirectly—news, entertainment, and advertising. Each of these types is a product of organizational cultures, structures, and process that are somewhat unique to each with varying impact on health. It must be noted that, while most advertising is not focused on promoting health per se, it nonetheless affects health, often adversely.

Despite the creative nature of media products, such creativity generally occurs within the constraints of organizations with defined hierarchies, cultures, norms, rules, and operating procedures. These bureaucratic structures drive how information is gathered, processed, and distributed.

News coverage of health is a good example. Coverage of topics increases the salience for those issues in the minds of the audience, 'frame' the topic, and influence audiences' beliefs, attitudes, and behaviours. News media are also critical channels that translate scientific developments in health and medicine for different audiences including consumers, but also often to healthcare providers and policy makers. Journalists who report on health rely on 'sources' such as media or public relations personnel, 'spokespersons', or news or video releases from scientific organizations or from medical journals for their initial ideas on what issues to report on. Health journalists use certain 'newsworthiness criteria' or rules of thumb to develop their stories, including 'potential for public impact', 'new information or development', and whether the story allows them 'to provide a human angle', among others.[7]

Journalists also work under constraints of shaping the story to the imperatives of their medium. These include:

* potential length of the story
* deadline pressures
* the literacy levels of their audience, and
* the need for visuals in case of television.

These imperatives and priorities often clash with the practices of scientists who emphasize specialized use of language, long lead times to conduct and report research, stringent requirements for the rigour of studies and quality of data that is referenced, and careful and qualified expression of their results. This 'clash of cultures' could lead to potential misunderstandings and frustrations, and mutual stereotyping. If one were to understand and work within the journalistic constraints, news media would be a helpful ally in shaping public beliefs and behaviours on health.

While the genres may differ, entertainment and advertising are also influenced by their respective organizational cultures though the degree of control exercised by producers, and sponsors may vary with some exercising a great deal of control in advertising and entertainment. Understanding and using these organizational rules and cultures could be particularly helpful for public health practitioners.

Communication content: genres and public health

Three broad genres of messages are worth paying attention to in understanding health communication: advertising, news, and entertainment.

Advertising

Advertising has drawn considerable attention in health, primarily for promoting beliefs and behaviours that are generally considered harmful to health, and in contributing to an increase in disease burden. The sources of material and funding for generating the information are manufacturers, such as the tobacco industry or the food industry who have worked closely with the advertising and marketing agencies to promote certain values, beliefs, and lifestyles. The increasing prominence of social media has also driven such 'risk-promoting' industries to reach their target audiences through platforms such as Facebook, YouTube, or Instagram, which provide a way to gain access to niche markets.[8] The social media environment is fertile ground for companies to evade advertising restrictions and reach their target audience, particularly through loopholes such as Facebook fan pages, coupons accompanying YouTube videos, and embedded links in other websites.[9]

The influence of advertising on certain lifestyle factors has garnered quite a bit of attention among researchers and policy makers. For example, an exhaustive review by the United States' National Cancer Institute (NCI) concluded that advertising and promotion are 'causally' related to the promotion and increased use of tobacco.[5] Similarly, food marketing has been implicated as one of the principal contributors to the growing problem of obesity worldwide.

Entertainment

Entertainment media expose people to content that could be harmful as well as conducive to health. The reason entertainment media are particularly effective is because the exposure to health messages is 'incidental' or unintentional. Audiences who are watching stories in entertainment media such as movies or television shows are 'transported' to the fictionalized world and often let their guard down.[10] The consequence is that they are less likely to engage in critical viewing and thus more susceptible to media messages. Exposure to tobacco use in movies leading to greater initiation among youth is one of the most well-documented effects of entertainment on health in the literature. However, entertainment content has also been purposefully harnessed by public health researchers and practitioners to increase health knowledge on a certain topic or influence health behaviours. Some interventions have used entertainment or narratives to promote family planning, cancer screening, life skills, and maternal and child health among others, often using radio or embedding storylines within popular television shows.

News

News is a major source of information on health to general as well as specialized audiences, such as physicians and policy makers. Exposure to news is generally intentional and, hence, the audience is more engaged. Considerable work shows that people's exposure to health news, such as coverage of harmful effects of tobacco, are likely to lead to anti-tobacco beliefs and even change behaviour.[5] More effective is news in 'setting' the agenda, shaping the social norms about health, and creating public opinion that is conducive to change or deters change. Social norms around smoking, including second-hand smoking, has led to the enactment of stricter laws restricting smoking in public places. Cultivating and working with reporters to improve health news coverage is one effective way to promote health.

Social media

While not a traditional, one-way channel of information, it is also important to note the role of social media in leading to the advent of more user-generated health content. Through health or fitness blogs, social media communities for patient audiences (such as the platform PatientsLikeMe), and photo-sharing sites such as Instagram, end users are increasingly able to generate their own content, make recommendations, and share health-related information widely among followers or community members. Although this is not bound by the rules and institutional norms of the channels above, it is important to consider this flow of information, because content generated and shared in this manner may not always be accurate, safe, or in line with physicians' recommendations.

What are the 'effects' of communication?

Given the immense exposure to mediated information, it is reasonable to assume that such exposure may potentially lead to 'effects' shaping audiences' knowledge, attitudes, and normative beliefs, and their behaviours. Communication effects could result not only through direct exposure to media, but also indirectly through 'interpersonal' channels, such as family members, peers, and co-workers. In fact, reactions to exposure to communication content may be 'mediated' or, in other words, influenced by others in one's social networks. The body of research documenting communication effects on various health outcomes is extensive and, in some cases, incontrovertible. Despite the well-documented observations, the difficulty in drawing causal connections between exposure and outcomes has resulted in controversial interpretations of media effects. Given the large body of work, it may be more useful to discuss 'effects' of communication on some major public health problems.

Tobacco use

Tobacco use is the most preventable public health threat and is implicated in almost 7 million deaths a year according to WHO, with the heavier burden being faced by low- and middle-income countries.[11] In many ways, media had a significant role in normalizing and glamorizing cigarette use starting with advertising and then Hollywood movies. Prominent Hollywood actors and actresses, such as former president Ronald Reagan, served as spokespersons promoting cigarettes.

Content analytic studies show that tobacco use is portrayed in prime time television, music videos, and movies, even in those rated for children over 13 years. While the recent trends show some decline in smoking incidence in the movies, almost half of those for youth over 17 years still show tobacco use.

With a global focus, span, and reach, the tobacco industry has effectively used advertising and marketing to both initiate and sustain tobacco use, although several countries have begun to place restrictions on tobacco advertising. One of the most, if not *the* most, extensively documented bodies of work in public health communication on health is in the areas of tobacco, summarized in 'The role of the media in promoting and reducing tobacco use'[5] published by the NCI in the USA. This review of hundreds of studies and evidence reviews came to some far-reaching conclusions about the influence of media in tobacco use:

- Movies glamorized tobacco use, particularly cigarette use, and smoking is quite prevalent in them.
- The total weight of evidence from multiple studies, using a variety of research designs and from different countries, shows a causal relationship between tobacco advertising and promotion, and increased tobacco use.
- In a similar vein, the total weight of evidence from cross-sectional, longitudinal, and experimental studies indicates a causal relationship between exposure to depictions of smoking in movies and youth smoking initiation.
- On the other hand, both controlled field experiments and population studies demonstrate that mass media tobacco control campaigns could change beliefs, curb initiation, and encourage cessation. Mass media campaigns are particularly effective when combined with other tobacco control programmes.

Obesity

That there is a growing 'epidemic' of obesity in industrialized countries is widely accepted. It is a major risk factor for a variety of chronic diseases including cardiovascular disease, diabetes, and cancer, among others. The WHO estimated that, in 2016, there were approximately 1.9 billion adults (age 18+) who were overweight and more than 650 million adults who were obese.[12] More critically, an estimated 41 million children under age 5 were considered overweight or obese, foreshadowing a looming public health crisis.[12]

Communications media, particularly television and screen media, were implicated as contributing to the growing obesity crisis. To be more specific, communications may contribute to the overweight and obesity problem through two mechanisms:

- by reducing time spent on physical activity
- in encouraging consumption of unhealthy foods, primarily through advertising.

Advertising and promotion as aspects of food marketing have been a focus of attention by those concerned with the growing obesity problem.

Children and young adults are a particular target with more than $10 billion per year being spent on marketing food and beverages to them. For example, over 6 billion fast food ads appeared on Facebook in 2012, often targeting teens, young adults, and certain racial and ethnic groups.[13]

These intense marketing and advertising efforts have likely led children and adults to become consumers in the marketplace. In fact, children as young as 2 and 3 years, according to the National Academy of Medicine (formerly Institute of Medicine), recognize packages and spokespersons and, by pre-school, recall brand names from exposure to televised advertising.[14] The effect is that children are likely to ask for branded products when making requests, and are often loyal to brands among beverages and the fast food industry. According to one study, in 2009, children aged 2–11 saw on average more than 10 television food ads per day.[15] Children are exposed to advertising and marketing messages for food through various channels, including radio, movies, billboards, and print media. Many new digital media venues and platforms for food marketing have emerged in recent years, including internet-based advergames, couponing on cell phones, and marketing on social networks, and much of this advertising is invisible to parents.[16] Consumption of sugar-sweetened beverages is one of the largest contributors to the problem of obesity.

Some have argued that time spent using media such as television and computers—'screen time'—may eat into time spent being physically active, contributing to a sedentary lifestyle. Although there are a large number of studies documenting the relationship between screen time and lower PA, with some exceptions, most are cross-sectional studies and seldom control for all other variables, such as social context, which influence PA. On the other hand, reducing screen time among children has been found to have had positive outcome on body mass index, thus making this relationship plausible.

It is little wonder that this double dose of lowering physical activity and increasing food consumption that is unhealthy has led many to zero in on the role of communications media in obesity and how to address this relationship.

Alcohol

According to the Centers for Disease Control and Prevention, excessive alcohol consumption is responsible for more than 88,000 deaths and 2.5 million years of potential lives lost each year,[17] and leads to 4,300 deaths of underage youth per year.[18] Alcohol and cigarettes serve as gateway drugs to other more serious drug abuse, such as of marijuana. Alcohol consumption is related to a variety of other social ills and problems, including risky sex and abuse. As is the case with other risk factors, communications media are important environmental contributors to alcohol use through advertising and entertainment.

Opportunities for exposure to pro-alcohol content are widely prevalent in the media. The American Academy of Pediatrics' position statement (2010) reported that about $6 billion are spent annually on alcohol advertising and promotion, and that youth are exposed to 1,000–2,000 alcohol commercials a year.[19] Most of the advertising is in sports programmes that attract young viewers. Facebook users who list 'alcohol' or 'bars' as an interest receive an alcohol-related ad as frequently as one in every eight ads.[20]. In entertainment programmes, on American television for example, alcohol use is widely prevalent including during prime time. The portrayal of alcohol use is usually positive and seldom shows the negative consequences. Music videos and movies also contain high depictions of alcohol use.

The consequence of such broad and extensive portrayal of alcohol use and its promotion in the media is that the audiences', especially young viewers', knowledge, and beliefs are influenced by it. For example, exposure to heavy alcohol advertising has major consequences such as:

- brand recognition ('Budweiser frogs') among children as shown in one study
- more favourable beliefs towards drinking
- potentially 'normalizing' alcohol use among the viewers, especially teenagers
- *drinking itself*—watching alcohol use in music videos and television is associated with the beginning of alcohol use and even higher consumption.

Media violence

The impact of exposure to violent programmes on television and movies, and, more recently, in computer games, has drawn attention from researchers, policy makers, and activists. As George Gerbner and colleagues have argued, television is the 'storyteller' of our times, providing a 'common symbolic environment' for all people irrespective of their personal and social backgrounds.[21] With more than 98% of US households owning at least one television set, and most households an average of almost three sets, television so far is the primary socialization agent. Because of massive exposure and broad reach, and arguably high levels of violent content, considerable research has been done to assess the impact of exposure to violent programmes and games, particularly on children, considered a 'vulnerable audience'. Several congressional committees have held hearings and the Office of Surgeon General has released reports.

The evidence for the impact of violent programmes comes from studies using a variety of research designs, including longitudinal studies, cross-sectional studies, and field and laboratory experiments. The research conclusions are as follows:

- There is a 'causal connection between media violence and aggressive behaviour in some children'.[22]
- Exposure to violence in childhood could lead to aggression among adults, thus suggesting a longitudinal impact. Several explanations have been offered for documented effects of violent programming, including how the programmes can 'model' actions to children leading to social learning, provide 'cognitive shortcuts' for quick and unthinking action to resolve social problems, and priming.
- Heavy exposure to television, especially violent programmes, could lead to a heightened sense of vulnerability and susceptibility to violence among viewers.[21]
- Television and games can also promote pro-social behaviour, such as sharing, co-learning, fair exchange, building relationships, and engagement among children.

Similar effects of violent computer and video games are now being documented with studies showing that playing games is associated with a temporary decrease in pro-social behaviour, and engendering aggressive thoughts and feelings, and arousal.

With a capacity for mass production and distribution, the influence of American entertainment programmes spans across the globe, thus enhancing the importance of studying the impact of such entertainment on violence and taking steps to mitigating this impact.

Media campaigns and health

Mass media campaigns have been used strategically in health promotion and disease prevention.[23–27] They have been shown to be a cost-effective strategy in, for example, tobacco control[25] and HIV/AIDS prevention[26] efforts. Research suggests that mass media campaigns are successful when done right and when they achieve sufficient exposure in:

- changing social norms
- promoting pro-healthy behaviours
- preventing unhealthy behaviours
- changing people's knowledge and attitudes towards health risks.

Communication campaigns are particularly effective when they are accompanied by environmental supports, such as creating structural opportunities in the community and appropriate policy changes.

Communication technologies and health

The explosion in new information delivery platforms such as the internet and mobile communications, such as smartphones and other such telecommunication developments, offer tremendous challenges and opportunities in public health communications. As of 2018, 77% of US adults go online every day, including 26% who report being on the internet 'almost constantly'.[28] Feature phones and smartphones have increased the ability for individuals to go online more often. Because of their ability to connect individuals to the internet at lower cost and with less hardware than a desktop, these devices offer new opportunities for low-cost, flexible online access in rural and underserved areas across the globe.[29] The widespread adoption of the internet in a number of countries is changing the way we conduct commerce, communicate, seek information, and entertain ourselves. The added potential to reach individuals at the point of behaviour through tailored texts or health-related applications through smartphones has also shown great promise to aid in both health communication and survey research.

Some broad figures of 'new media' reach demonstrate why this matters. A recent government report in the USA[30] showed that about 81% of American households have a broadband internet subscription at home, which allows faster downloads and uploads. Similar such numbers are reported by the International Telecommunication Union[31] with particularly impressive penetration of 103.5 mobile-cellular phone subscribers and 48 internet users for every 100 inhabitants worldwide as of 2017.

Equally compelling are the uses of new communication technologies for health. As smartphone use has increased, more users are also using these devices to search for health information and 62% of smartphone users have used their phone to look up health information within the past year.[29] Pew data also shows the continued emphasis on social media as a part of everyday life, with many accessing these sites from their smartphone.[32] Facebook remains a top platform, with 68% of US adults visiting the site,[32] and with 1.45 billion daily and 2.20 billion monthly active users worldwide as of March 2018. Users have the option of following health-related Facebook pages, with the page 'Health Digest' having 11.1 million page likes and 'Women's Health' having 8.2 million pages likes, as of 2017.[33]

The opportunities to use these technologies to widen and deepen reach and overcome barriers of geography are tremendous. Nonetheless, they also pose some compelling challenges:

- One major challenge is that people are getting their information from a variety of sources and often from multiple sources, leading to increasing fragmentation of audience. One advantage of such fragmentation and specialization is that health information can often be customized more narrowly to the interests and needs of the audience, allowing for better reception, attention, and communication effects. However, this fragmentation also makes it more difficult to track exposure to both health information and risk-promoting messages.

- More interesting is the fact that people are forming online communities and relying on experiences of others similar to them when engaging in online health information. This has the potential to increase engagement of the audience. For example, Pew data[34] shows that four out of ten 'e-patients' have followed someone else's experience on a blog or another site, and two out of ten have consulted rankings of reviews of providers or hospitals.

- On the other hand, the diversity of sources, 'gatekeepers', makes it challenging to provide accurate information that has been vetted for accuracy and relevance. The millions of websites on health mean that there are multiple interpreters of health information that may or may not be accurate.

- It also could potentially confuse some people and overwhelm them with choices. For example, Pew reports that there are almost 300,000 apps for mobile phone users on a variety of health topics including nutrition, physical activity, counting calories, estimating risk, assisting in smoking cessation, and keeping personal health records. The value, utility, accuracy, and reliability of such applications and websites. and the consequences for population health, remain to be investigated.

Communication inequalities and health disparities

One of the most significant, if not transformative, movements in public health is the insight from research in social epidemiology on identifying social factors or 'social determinants' that affect population health[35, 36] leading to disparities in mortality and morbidity among social classes, races, geographies, and countries. A number of social determinants, such as social class, race, ethnicity, urbanicity, access to medical care, neighbourhood, social capital, social and economic policies, among others, have been examined by researchers. The significance of this research has been a shift in focus from more medical and biological lens for disease causation to a focus on social, economic, and cultural factors.

In parallel, in public health communication, researchers are beginning to document 'communication inequalities' as one type of social determinant that could potentially explain disparities in health outcomes. Communication inequality may be defined as differences among social classes in the generation, manipulation, and distribution of information at the group level, and differences in access to and ability to take advantage of information at the individual level.[37] Several studies have documented significant differences among social classes, and racial and ethnic groups, in preferences for accessing, using, and understanding health information from a variety of media including newspapers, television, radio, and the internet.

For example, the American government report on broadband internet use cited earlier[2] suggests that those with higher education and income, Whites, and those living in urban areas are likely to access the internet through broadband technology. The reasons for not accessing through broadband include lack of affordability, perceived need, and availability. While smartphones have lessened the gaps in the digital divide, low-income individuals often have more issues maintaining connectivity with their devices compared with their higher-income counterparts, and also experience greater issues with device quality and upkeep.[29] Similarly, at global level, the International Telecommunication Union reports that, in developed countries, the proportion of households with internet access at home is twice as high as in developing countries. There are more than 80 internet users per 100 people in the 'developed world' compared with about 41 users per 100 people in the developing world.[31] For example, Europe is estimated to have more than 80 users per 100 people compared with a little fewer than 22 per 100 people in Africa.[31]

The consequences of communication inequalities are growing 'knowledge gaps' in health between the haves and have-nots, and the ensuing gaps in health behaviours and health outcomes. The inequities become even more pernicious at a time when more information on health is being made available for public consumption, and greater responsibility in the guise of 'informed' and 'shared' decision making is expected of patients and their families.

At the same time, communication inequalities are much more addressable than other social determinants through the development of appropriate interventions at group and policy levels. Also, under certain conditions, technological developments have the potential to narrow the gap.

Conclusions

This brief chapter cannot do justice to the rapidly changing field of health communications and the opportunities and challenges it offers to public health. In parallel to biomedical revolution at the molecular and clinical levels, revolutionary changes in communication technologies may radically transform how scientific developments in health and medicine are translated to influence public health. These radical developments are upending the conventional approach of controlled dissemination of health information to public and patients. While the advantage is that this democratizes health information to spread beyond specialists and those with advantages, the speed with which it is spread, as well as multiple players, institutions, and interpretations, also overwhelm people, leading to confusion and frustration. The greatest challenge of public health in the twenty-first century, one may contend, is the explosion in health information, and taming the tide of this explosion is one of the most significant roles that public health practitioners may be able to play.

References

1 Viswanath K. (2005). Science and society: the communications revolution and cancer control. *Nature Reviews Cancer*, 5, 828–35.

2 Pew Research Center (2018). Internet/broadband fact sheet. Pew Research Center, Washington, DC. Available at: ℘ http://www.pewinternet.org/fact-sheet/internet-broadband (accessed 3 June 2018).

3 Pew Research Center (2018). Mobile fact sheet. Pew Research Center, Washington, DC. Available at: ℘ http://www.pewinternet.org/fact-sheet/mobile (accessed 3 June 2018).

4 Rideout V, Foehr UG, Roberts DF. (2010). Generation M2: media in the lives of 8- to 18-year-olds. Henry J. Kaiser Family Foundation, Menlo Park. Available at: ℘ http://www.kff.org/entmedia/upload/8010.pdf (accessed 11 August 2019).

5 National Cancer Institute (2008). *The role of the media in promoting and reducing tobacco use*, Tobacco Monograph Series 19. Department of Health and Human Services, NCI, Washington, DC.

6 Finnegan JR, Viswanath K. (2008). Communication theory and health behavior change: the media studies framework. In: Glanz K, Rimer B, Viswanath K, eds, *Health behavior and health education: theory, research, and practice*, 4th edn, pp. 363–87. Jossey-Bass, San Francisco.

7 Viswanath K, Blake KD, Meissner HI, et al. (2008). Occupational practices and the making of health news: a national survey of US health and medical science journalists. *Journal of Health Communication*, 13, 759–77.

8 McCloud R, Kohler K, Viswanath K. (2017). Cancer risk-promoting information: the communication environment of young adults. *American Journal of Preventive Medicine*, 53(3) (Supplement 1), S63–S72.

9 Liang Y, Zheng X, Zeng DD, et al. (2015). Exploring how the tobacco industry presents and promotes itself in social media. *Journal of Medical Internet Research*, 17(1), e24.

10 Green MC. (2006). Narratives and cancer communication. *Journal of Communication*, 56, S163–83.

11 World Health Organization (2018). Tobacco. WHO, Geneva. Available at: ℘ http://www.who.int/news-room/fact-sheets/detail/tobacco (accessed 4 June, 2018).

12 World Health Organization (2017). Obesity and overweight. WHO, Geneva. Available at: ℘ http://www.who.int/en/news-room/fact-sheets/detail/obesity-and-overweight (accessed 28 May, 2018).

13 Richardson J. (2011). Food marketing and social media: findings from fast food FACTS and sugary drink FACTS. American University Digital Food Marketing Conference.

14 Institute of Medicine (2006). *Food marketing to children and youth: threat or opportunity?* Institute of Medicine, Washington, DC.

15 Powell LM, Schermbeck RM, Szczypka G, et al. (2011). Trends in the nutritional content of television food advertisements seen by children in the United States: analyses by age, food categories, and companies. *Archives of Pediatrics and Adolescent Medicine*, 165(12), 1078–86. doi: 10.1001/archpediatrics.2011.131. Epub 2011 Aug 1.

16 Institute of Medicine (2013). Challenges and opportunities for change in food marketing to children and youth: workshop summary. The National Academies Press, Washington, DC. Available at: ℘ https://doi.org/10.17226/18274. (accessed 11 August 2019).

17 Centers for Disease Control and Prevention (2018). Fact sheets – alcohol use and your health. Available at: https://www.cdc.gov/alcohol/fact-sheets/alcohol-use.htm (accessed 5 June 2018).

18 Centers for Disease Control and Prevention (2018). Fact sheets – underage drinking. Available at: https://www.cdc.gov/alcohol/fact-sheets/underage-drinking.htm (accessed 5 June 2018).

19 Strasburger VC. (2010). The Council on Communications and Media, American Association of Pediatrics. Children, adolescents, substance abuse, and the media. *Pediatrics*, **126**, 791–9.

20 Hoffman EW, Pinkleton BE, Weintraub Austin E, et al. (2014) Exploring college students' use of general and alcohol-related social media and their associations with alcohol-related behaviors. *Journal of American College Health*, **62(5)**, 328–35.

21 Gerbner G, Gross L, Morgan M, et al. (2002). Growing up with television: cultivation process. In: Bryant J, Zillmann D, eds, *Media effects: advances in theory and research*, pp. 43–67. Lawrence Erlbaum, Mahwah.

22 Anderson CA, Bushman BJ. (2001). Effects of violent video games on aggressive behavior, aggressive cognition, aggressive affect, physiological arousal, and pro-social behavior. A metanalytic review of the scientific literature. *Psychological Science*, **12**, 353–83.

23 Hornik RC. (2002). Public health communication: making sense of contradictory evidence. In: Hornik RC, ed., *Public health communication: evidence for behavior change*, pp. 1–19. Lawrence Erlbaum, New York.

24 Randolph W, Viswanath K. (2004). Lessons learned from public health mass media campaigns: marketing health in a crowded media world. *Annual Review of Public Health*, **25**, 419–37.

25 Atusingwize E, Lewis S, Langley T. (2015). Economic evaluations of tobacco control mass media campaigns: a systematic review. *Tobacco Control*, **24**, 320–7.

26 Hogan DR, Baltussen R, Hayashi C, et al. (2005) Achieving the millennium development goals for health: cost effectiveness analysis of strategies to combat HIV/AIDS in developing countries. *British Medical Journal*, doi:10.1136/bmj.38643.368692.68

27 Wakefield MA, Loken B, Hornik RC. (2010). Use of mass media campaigns to change health behaviour. *Lancet*, **376**, 1261–71.

28 Perrin P, Jiang J. (2018). About three-in-ten U.S. adults say they are 'almost constantly' online. Pew Research Center. Available at: http://www.pewresearch.org/fact-tank/2018/03/14/about-a-quarter-of-americans-report-going-online-almost-constantly (accessed 4 June 2018).

29 Pew Research Center (2015). U.S. smartphone use in 2015. Available at: http://www.pewinternet.org/2015/04/01/us-smartphone-use-in-2015 (accessed 3 June 2018).

30 National Telecommunications and Information Administration (United States Department of Commerce) (2016). Mapping computer and internet use by state. Available at: https://www.ntia.doc.gov/blog/2016/mapping-computer-and-internet-use-state-introducing-data-explorer-20 (accessed 16 August 2019).

31 International Telecommunication Union (2018). Statistics. Available at: https://www.itu.int/en/ITU-D/Statistics/Pages/stat/default.aspx (accessed 4 June 2018).

32 Smith A, Anderson M. (2018). Social media use in 2018. Pew Research Center. Available at: http://www.pewinternet.org/2018/03/01/social-media-use-in-2018 (accessed 4 June 2018).

33 Hitlin P, Olmstead K. (2018). The science people see on social media. Pew Research Center. Available at: https://www.pewresearch.org/science/2018/03/21/the-science-people-see-on-social-media (accessed 16 August 2019).

34 Fox S, Jones S. (2009). The social life of health information. Pew Research Center's Internet and American Life Project, Washington, DC. Available at: https://www.pewresearch.org/fact-tank/2014/01/15/the-social-life-of-health-information (accessed 19 August 2019).

35 Berkman LF, Kawachi I. (2000). A historical framework for social epidemiology. In: Berkman LF, Kawachi I, eds, *Social epidemiology*, pp. 3–12. Oxford University Press, New York.

36 CSDH (2008). *Closing the gap in a generation: health equity through action on the social determinants of health*, Final report of the Commission on Social Determinants of Health. WHO, Geneva.

37 Viswanath K. (2006). Public communications and its role in reducing and eliminating health disparities. In: Thomson GE, Mitchell F, Williams MB, eds, *Examining the health disparities research plan of the National Institutes of Health: unfinished business*, pp. 215–53. Institute of Medicine, Washington, DC.

Chapter 3.9

Public health practice in primary care

Steve Gillam

Objectives

Having read this chapter, you should:
- understand why effective systems of primary care—entailing universal health coverage—are integral to delivering public health objectives
- know those public health interventions that primary care professionals provide
- be able to define those elements of primary care that need strengthening in order to deliver public health objectives
- appreciate how the skills of public health and primary care practitioners complement and contrast with one another.

Definitions

The central importance of primary care for public health has long been acknowledged. In 1978 at Alma Ata, primary health care was declared to be the key to delivering 'health for all'. Primary healthcare 'based on practical, scientifically sound and socially acceptable methods and technology made universally accessible through people's full participation and at a cost that the community and country can afford' was carefully distinguished from primary medical care.[1] The social and political goals of those epochal declarations—acknowledging as they did the social and economic determinants of health—were subsequently diluted. So-called 'selective primary health care' and packages of low-cost interventions, such as GOBI-FFF (growth monitoring, oral rehydration, breast feeding, immunization; female education, family spacing, and food supplements), in some respects distorted the spirit of Alma Ata.[2] Nevertheless, a central justification for universal primary care is ethical: the public health preoccupation with equity.

Primary care is often defined in terms of 'four Cs': it is continuous, comprehensive, the point of first contact, and coordinates other care. This coordinating function underlines a second set of arguments in support of primary care concerning efficiency and cost-effectiveness. International comparisons of the extent to which health systems are primary care-oriented suggest that those countries with more generalist family doctors with registered lists acting as gatekeepers are more likely to deliver better health outcomes, lower costs, and greater public satisfaction.[3] Universally accessible primary care is central to delivering the Sustainable Development Goals.[4]

Bridging the divide

General practitioners and public health specialists improve health by different means. General practitioners concentrate on personal, continuing healthcare while public health physicians focus on the population through changes in the environment, society, and health service provision. At the heart of the relationship between general practice and public health is an ethical conflict between individual and collective freedom.[5] The utilitarian values underpinning population-orientated care are at odds with the individualistic nature of the traditional doctor—patient relationship.[6] The roles of carer, advocate, and enabler may overlap and conflict with one another.

The clinical generalist develops a unique understanding of the personal and social determinants of their patients' health.[7] However, traditional primary care based on the perspective of the clinician exposed exclusively to individual patients presenting for care has evident limitations. Knowledge about the distribution of health problems in the community cannot be derived from experience in the practice alone because most episodes of ill health do not lead to a medical consultation. An understanding of how disease presents cannot be obtained without a population focus. Doctors overestimate their role in the provision of care. Primary health care is not, of course, synonymous with general practice and is provided by a range of other health personnel. Finally, professional knowledge about disease does not necessarily reflect people's illness experiences and needs to be supplemented with the insights of the community.

Several international trends in the delivery of health services are facilitating community-oriented approaches to primary care. Public health competencies, especially as they relate to the management of chronic disease, are of increasing importance to the twenty-first century primary care workforce.[8] More training is now taking place in community settings. An emphasis on more effective and more efficient healthcare will entrench community-oriented approaches if they prevent disease and encourage more discriminating use of medical technologies. In high-income countries, a 'secondary to primary shift' is relocating specialist care closer to patients. Primary healthcare teams have always been pivotally placed to combine high-risk and population approaches to disease prevention.[9] Meeting the challenge of non-communicable disease in low- and middle-income countries will require universal coverage of horizontally integrated programmes accessible through primary care.[10]

How does primary care deliver public health?

With the decline in infectious diseases and the ageing of the population, an increasing proportion of the workload in general practice deals with the consequences of chronic disease. This has required the development of new services and changing systems of care. Many diseases, such as diabetes, which were once the exclusive preserve of hospital specialists, are now managed by teams in the community. If the 1970s saw the birth of a 'New Public Health', the first decade of the millennium saw the emergence of a 'New Primary Care', at least in the UK (Box 3.9.1). How each of these five elements contributes to public health is considered below.

Self-care

Less than one in ten ailments experienced is brought into contact with the formal system of healthcare. Most are self-managed using whatever knowledge and support are available to the sufferer. Increasingly, many patients are more knowledgeable than their doctors about the management of their chronic disease. Nevertheless, they sometimes need help in making sense of the surfeit of information available. The computer screen threatens the

Box 3.9.1 Elements of today's primary care
- Self-care
- First contact care
- Chronic disease management
- Health promotion in primary care
- Primary care management.

personal nature of the consultation, but new tools are changing clinicians from being repositories of facts to being managers of knowledge.[11] Some clinicians are nervous about giving patients better information and not all patients want it. However, most people want to be in charge of decisions about their health—for the default approach to be empowerment, rather than paternalism.[12] Giving patients more knowledge or a consultation style that facilitates shared decision making improves not only patient satisfaction but also clinical outcomes. Indeed, as people gain access to information about risk, a higher proportion may choose not to accept the offer of screening or treatment.[13]

First contact care

If the bulk of first contact care is provided by friends and relatives, the next port of call has traditionally been general practice. However, there is an increasing plurality of routes through which primary care can be obtained (Figure 3.9.1). These include the NHS telephone helpline 111, walk-in centres, and community pharmacies. Multiple access points with poorly

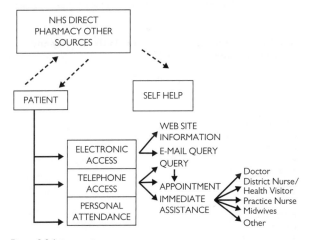

Figure 3.9.1 Routes of access into primary care.

coordinated record-keeping may result in fragmented care, and questions over the cost-efficiency of these services remain. Nevertheless, they have exposed the limitations of conventional general practice in providing basic care for populations who have not, for reasons of culture or convenience, gained satisfactory access to primary care in the past.

Chronic disease management

Numerous studies attest to the variable quality of care provided for people with chronic diseases. The GP contract in the UK introduced financial incentives for practices to enhance the quality of their care in specific areas through the Quality and Outcomes Framework (QOF, see Box 3.9.2). Much infrastructural investment was required to develop registers and call–recall systems, but the benefits in terms of public health were potentially significant. There is evidence that the QOF has led to better-recorded care, improved intermediate outcomes, and reductions in health inequalities (although pay-for-performance schemes can yield perverse consequences for continuity, patient-centredness and professionalism).[14] However, evidence for real mortality gains remains elusive.[15] Routine disease monitoring is increasingly undertaken by practice nurses with extended training. Disease management is becoming more complicated as pharmaceutical advances allow more care to be shifted from secondary to primary care. There is growing interest once more in North American techniques of managed care: risk stratification, targeting the heaviest consumers of care, and utilization review—but little clear-cut evidence to guide policy makers.[16]

Health promotion in primary care

General practitioners have always understood the importance of social factors such as housing, employment, and education as influences on their patients' health. The registered list, which defines the practice population,

---

Box 3.9.2 Chronic diseases targeted in the Quality and Outcomes Framework (QOF)

- Coronary heart disease.
- Stroke and transient ischaemic attack (TIA).
- Hypertension.
- Hypothyroidism.
- Diabetes.
- Mental health.
- Chronic obstructive pulmonary disease.
- Asthma.
- Epilepsy.
- Cancer.
- Palliative care.
- Dementia.
- Chronic kidney disease.
- Atrial fibrillation.
- Obesity.
- Learning disabilities.

provides the basis for effective health promotion programmes in primary care. Preventive activities within primary care can be divided into individual, organizational, and community interventions.[17] *Individual* interventions take place between health professionals and patients, often classified into primary, secondary, and tertiary prevention (see Box 3.9.3). The public health approach to screening focuses on maximizing participation in screening, rather than on informed participation. For example, current recommendations for the primary prevention of coronary heart disease in groups at high risk depend on screening through primary care and provision of risk-related advice or treatment. However, we lack evidence for the cost-effectiveness of multiple risk factor interventions delivered through primary care.[18]

Organizational interventions are concerned with improving the management of care and access to services for disadvantaged groups. Such interventions may take place at the level of the practice or the whole health system. An example of the former might be changes to make cervical screening more accessible to certain ethnic groups by providing information in different languages and increasing the availability of female health professionals. New organizational models are being developed—for example, to address previously unmet needs in deprived, under-doctored locations.[19]

The third category of interventions is *community*-wide. For example, in their roles as employers, users of resources, procurers, producers of waste, deployers, and vendors of land, primary care organizations have opportunities to enhance community health that have as yet been neglected by practitioners in the UK. They are just beginning to understand their role in promoting sustainable healthcare in a future low-carbon health system.[20]

Community development has a stronger pedigree in developing countries. Every year, over 500,000 women die from maternal causes, four million infants die in the neonatal period, and a similar number are stillborn. If the millennium development goals to reduce maternal and child mortality are to be achieved, public health programmes need to reach the poorest households. Most maternal and neonatal deaths take place at home, beyond

---

Box 3.9.3 Individual interventions between health professionals and patients

Primary prevention
- *Health education and behavioural change*: e.g. dietary, smoking cessation, exercise.
- *Immunization*: for an ever-increasing range of infections.
- Welfare benefits advice.
- Community development.

Secondary prevention
- Detection and management of ischaemic heart disease.
- *Screening*: e.g. for cervical, breast, and colon cancer.

Tertiary prevention
- *Chronic disease management*: e.g. diabetes mellitus.

the reach of health facilities. Evidence is growing that primary care strategies centred on community-based interventions are effective in reducing maternal and neonatal deaths in countries with high mortality rates, even if institutional approaches are necessary to reduce them further.[21]

Primary care management

New public management with its emphasis on targets and objective setting has permeated all parts of the health service. One important consequence of the growth of large practice-based teams has been the differentiation of administrative functions. Increasingly, primary care teams need to accept responsibility for auditing the health status of their patients, publicizing the results, monitoring and controlling environmentally determined disease, auditing the effectiveness of preventative programmes, and evaluating the effect of medical interventions. Their newly devolved role in commissioning health services gives general practitioners particular responsibilities for local strategy development and budgetary management.[22] Public health specialists remain crucial in supporting these functions.

Key challenges for public health practitioners

- *What kind of primary care?* The difficulty of transposing health systems across international boundaries is universally acknowledged. Care at the level of the community within any system reflects different histories and cultural contexts. No single model of primary healthcare will be universally applicable. For example, community-orientated primary care (COPC) seeks to integrate public health practice by delivering primary care to defined communities on the basis of its assessed health needs.[23] COPC remains a powerful, enduring concept, but its protagonists have made little mark beyond developing countries. In part, this reflects the lack of financial incentives within hospital-orientated health systems.
- *The politics of public and patient involvement:* there is a fundamental difference between healthcare that is multi-sectoral, preventive, participatory, and decentralized, and low-cost (low-quality) curative treatment aimed at the poorest and most marginalized segments of the population, particularly if that care is provided through programmes that are parallel to the rest of the healthcare system and without the active participation of the full population. Many authors have argued for the need to look in a new way at the relationship between doctors and patients as 'co-producers of health' and develop alliances between health workers and the public in defence of health.[24]
- *Information systems:* the creation of a single, longitudinal electronic patient record could create powerful new means of monitoring and improving care. An easily accessible, portable record ought to increase the involvement of users in their own management.
- *Evaluation:* assessing the health impact at the level of the organization or individual health worker is challenging. Even large UK general practices serve populations that are usually too small to allow the comparison

Box 3.9.4 Factors complicating the assessment of primary care

- Small denominators and the play of chance.
- 'Street lamp effect': focusing on what is measured (paid for), ignoring the penumbra.
- Measuring the easily measurable, but unimportant...
- ...while ignoring the difficult to measure (e.g. communication skills, continuity of care).

of health outcomes such as all-cause or disease-specific mortality rates. The focus is on intermediate outcomes—changes in established markers of quality care. The QOF provides an example of an evidence-based approach to measuring (and rewarding) improvements in the management of common chronic diseases. Public health practitioners will be familiar with the measurement challenges listed in Box 3.9.4.

- *Ensuring equity at practice level:* one well-attested form of differential access to care is the so-called 'inverse prevention' effect whereby communities most at risk of ill health tend to experience the least satisfactory access to the full range of preventive services.[25] Access may be affected in more material ways (e.g. through the provision of aids for wheelchair users or translated materials for people for whom English is not their first language). User charges for primary care have been repeatedly shown to deter those most likely to benefit from preventive activities.[26]
- *Continuing professional development and the workforce:* primary care like public health is a multidisciplinary endeavour. In the UK, labour is being divided in new ways between many different health workers. Primary care nurses are taking responsibility for minor illness management, triage, and routine care of common chronic diseases. The particular skills of others, such as community pharmacists, are being recognized. Beyond strengthening appraisal and revalidation mechanisms within different disciplines, there lies the challenge of ensuring that professional development activities are congruent and coordinated across teams.
- *Maximizing effectiveness:* the dearth of evidence in support of many preventive interventions highlights the need for further research.[27] Reasons for the failure to implement best practice go beyond the quality of the research, and accumulating further technical evidence may not be the most useful response. Barriers to implementation include a consistent failure to address the opportunity costs of new or different activities in primary care. For example, increasing primary care's public health role may mean doing less of something else. Related to this is a failure to address adequately, and with all relevant stakeholders, the question of the role of primary care. This is not a technical agenda but one of achieving shared values as a starting point for any changes in professional roles.

Conclusions

Health systems are in constant flux. Everywhere, the generalist seems to be under threat. What were once seen as strengths of general practice within the NHS are now regarded as liabilities—the registered list (restricting choice), personal (paternalistic) care, gate-keeping (rationing). Public health practitioners should be mindful of the law of unintended consequences. For example, one result of increasing access points may be discontinuous, poorly coordinated services for those most in need. Paying practitioners by results may create disincentives to practise exactly where care is already weakest. Fragmented primary care will yield poorer public health. Public health practitioners who understand the complementary nature of these disciplines (see Table 3.9.1) will mobilize the resources of primary care more effectively.

Table 3.9.1 Public health and primary care practitioners—core competencies contrasted

Public health practitioners	Primary care practitioners
Care for populations	Care for individuals on practice lists.
Use of environmental, social, organizational, legislative interventions.	Use of predominantly medical technical interventions.
Prevention through the organized efforts of society.	Care of the sick as their prime function with the consultation as central.
Application of public health sciences (e.g. epidemiology/medical statistics).	Application of broad clinical training and knowledge about local patterns of disease.
Skills in health services research, report and policy writing.	Skills in clinical management and communicating with individuals.
Analysis of information on populations and their health in large areas.	Analysis of detailed practice and disease registers and information on individuals.
Use of networks that are administrative: health and social care authorities, voluntary organizations.	Use of networks that are less bureaucratic: frontline health and social care providers, other primary care teams.

References

1 World Health Organization (1978). *Primary health care*. Report of the International Conference on Primary Health Care, Alma-Ata, USSR, 6–12 September. WHO, Geneva.
2 Gillam S. (2008). Is the declaration of Alma Ata still relevant to primary health care? *British Medical Journal*, **336**, 536–8.
3 Starfield B. (1994). Is primary care essential? *Lancet*, **344**, 1129–33.
4 World Health Organization (2015). *Health in 2015: from MDGs to SDGs*. WHO, Geneva.
5 Pratt J. (1995). *Practitioners and practices. A conflict of values?* Radcliffe Medical Press, Oxford.
6 Fitzpatrick M. (2001). *The tyranny of health—doctors and the regulation of lifestyle*. Routledge, London.
7 Heath I. (1995). *The mystery of general practice*. Nuffield Provincial Hospitals Trust, London.

8 World Health Organization (2006). *Preparing a workforce for the 21st century: the challenge of chronic conditions*. WHO, Geneva.

9 Rose G. (1992). *The strategy of preventive medicine*. Oxford University Press, Oxford.

10 World Health Organization (2013). *Global NCD action plan 2013–2020*. WHO, Geneva.

11 Muir Gray JA. (1999). Post-modern medicine. *Lancet*, **354**, 1550–2.

12 Joseph-Williams N, Lloyd A, Edwards A et al. The challenges of shared decision-making in the NHS. *British Medical Journal*, **357**, 132–4.

13 Coulter A, Ellins J. (2007). Effectiveness of strategies for informing, educating, and involving patients. *British Medical Journal*, **335**, 24–7.

14 Gillam S, Siriwardena N, Steel N. (2012) Pay for performance in the UK: the impact of the Quality and Outcomes framework. Ann Fam Med; 10: 461–8.

15 Roland M. (2016) Does pay-for-performance in primary care save lives? Lancet; 388: 217–8. doi:10.1016/S0140-6736(16)00550-X pmid:27207745.

16 Gillam S. (2004). What can we learn about quality of care from US health maintenance organisations? *Quality in Primary Care* **12**, 3–4.

17 Hulscher MEJL, Wensing M, van der Weijden T, et al. (2001). *Interventions to implement prevention in primary care*. Cochrane Review. The Cochrane Library, Issue 1, Update Software, Oxford.

18 Capewell S, McCartney M, Holland W. (2015) Invited debate: NHS Health Checks—a naked emperor? *Journal of Public Health*, 37(2), 187–92.

19 Royal College of General Practitioners (2017). *GP Forward View interim assessment*. RCGP, London.

20 Gillam S, Barna S. (2011). Sustainable general practice: another challenge for trainers. *Primary Care Education*, **22**, 7–10.

21 Costello A, Osrin D, Manandhar D. (2004). Reducing maternal and neonatal mortality in the poorest communities. *British Medical Journal*, **329**, 1166–8.

22 Rosen R (2015). *Transforming general practice: what are the levers for change?* Nuffield Trust, London.

23 Mullan F, Epstein L. (2002). Community-oriented primary care: new relevance in a changing world. *American Journal of Public Health*, **92**, 1748–55.

24 Tudor Hart J. (1988). *A new kind of doctor*. Merlin Press, London.

25 Marmot M. (2011). *Fair society, healthy lives—the Marmot Review*. Available at: ℜ http://www.instituteofhealthequity.org/resources-reports/fair-society-healthy-lives-the-marmot-review/fair-society-healthy-lives-full-report-pdf.pdf (accessed 16 August 2019).

26 NHS Centre for Reviews and Dissemination (2000). *Evidence from systematic reviews of the research relevant to implementing the 'wider public health' agenda*. University of York, NHS Centre for Reviews and Dissemination, York.

27 Peckham S, Hann A, Kendall S, et al. (2017). Health promotion and disease prevention in general practice and primary care: a scoping study. *Primary Health Care Research & Development*, **18**(6), 529–40.

Chapter 3.10

Translating research into practice— implementation science

Shoba Ramanadhan

Objectives

After reading this chapter, you should be able to:
- define the terms 'dissemination', 'implementation', 'evidence-based intervention', and 'implementation science'
- describe the utility of implementation science for improving public health outcomes
- recognize key implementation science frameworks and models
- identify opportunities to incorporate implementation science into public health practice activities.

Definitions

There are several terms utilized to describe efforts to study the path evidence takes from research to practice environments, including dissemination and implementation, knowledge translation, knowledge integration, and knowledge exchange.

The first step is to define terms related to the evidence that is expected to be spread and utilized in practice settings. An *evidence-based intervention* (EBI) is a programme, practice, or policy that has been found effective through rigorous research.[1] For example, in the area of tobacco cessation, there are EBIs for individual-level counselling, community education, and smoke-free environment policies.

Dissemination refers to an active approach to spread EBIs to a defined target audience.[1] Target audiences might include potential adopters and implementers, decision makers, and other stakeholders. As an example, a dissemination research study might assess the impact of using practice facilitators to engage primary care practices and raise awareness/demand for a given EBI.

Implementation refers to integrating EBIs into practice settings.[1] Research in this area focuses on the range of factors that have an impact on the use of a given EBI in a practice setting.

Evidence-based public health is another relevant term and refers to efforts to integrate the scientific evidence base with community needs and preferences, with the goal of improving population health.[2] This approach prompts practitioners to engage with public health data to increase the efficiency and impact of public health programmes.

This chapter focuses on *implementation science*, or efforts to understand and influence the path between research and practice.

Why is this an important public health issue?

A common call to action around implementation science starts with a study that found it took an average of 17 years to move medical research findings into practice settings and that, even with that lag, uptake was partial.[3] In the area of cancer prevention and control, a similar call to action comes from the finding that about half of the cancers occurring today could be prevented through the application of knowledge that is already available.[4] By improving the flow of high-quality, current research evidence into practice settings, public health practitioners can increase access to needed services, improve the likelihood of intervention success, and increase the efficiency of investment of limited public health resources.

Clearly, an effective intervention cannot produce public health impact simply because results are published in a scientific journal. The field of implementation science puts structure around the process of moving evidence from the literature into practice settings by providing frameworks and theories to identify a range of important factors, assess strategies with which to influence practice change, and then evaluate success. Public health practitioners can benefit from understanding the scope and key questions of implementation science so that they can apply the literature to create change in practice settings.

Considering the evidence base

It can be helpful to think about implementation science in relation to other pieces of the evidence-generation process:[1]

- Efficacy research focuses on demonstrating a causal link between an intervention and outcomes of interest in a highly controlled environment.
- Effectiveness research is usually the next step. It focuses more on generalizability and addresses the question of whether an intervention can produce important incomes in practice settings.
- Implementation science addresses the uptake and use of tested, proven interventions in practice settings and systems. This research may focus on a single EBI (e.g. a programme that uses text messaging between providers and patients to improve asthma management), or it may draw on an evidence-based strategy for creating change (e.g. a systematic review highlighting the impact of text messaging within a healthcare system to improve short-term medication adherence). Outcomes of implementation science move beyond clinical and behavioural outcomes to include behaviours and outcomes among providers, organizations, and systems.

Traditionally, these steps were taken in a linear fashion but, increasingly, researchers are encouraged to address multiple aspects simultaneously (e.g. through hybrid designs to collect effectiveness and implementation data simultaneously).[5] The attention to the path that evidence takes is also a useful prompt when practitioners are creating or investing in a new programme. By considering the resources, requirements, and necessary supports for scale-up within the organization and long-term integration, practitioners can make decisions about interventions that will maximize their return in the long run.

Approaches to implementation science

The field of implementation science is growing rapidly, with a range of available theoretical approaches. A review from 2012 found 61 models, theories, and frameworks addressing dissemination, implementation, or both[6], and the number is increasing steadily. One useful taxonomy splits them into 1) process frameworks, which guide the process of implementation; 2) determinant frameworks, which support understanding of the key influences on implementation; and 3) evaluation frameworks, which assess how well implementation efforts have worked. Practitioners may wish to draw on a combination of framework types to ensure that they are asking the right questions to set up, conduct, and evaluate a given implementation effort.

The models and frameworks that dominate implementation science typically take an ecological perspective, which focuses on the system in which behaviours take place, emphasizing the mutual influence between individuals and their environment, and accounting for the fact that individuals impact—and are impacted by—multiple levels of influence, from personal attributes to their personal networks, organizations, communities, and broader policy and cultural environments.[7] In relation to implementation of EBIs in practice, this perspective prompts attention to attributes of the EBI, the background and circumstances of participants who will receive the EBI, characteristics of individuals and organizations involved in adopting and delivering the EBI, and the broader institutional, social, and political contexts in which an EBI will be implemented. A useful starting point is the Consolidated Framework for Implementation Research,[8] which integrates a number of the leading theories on dissemination and implementation science, including aspects of Rogers' Diffusion of Innovations theory.[9]

Using frameworks for planning

Another popular framework is the Exploration, Preparation, Implementation, and Sustainment (EPIS) Framework, which supports preparation, delivery, and maintenance of an EBI. As an example, a practitioner interested in implementing an EBI for obesity prevention among youth in schools could draw on the EPIS framework to prepare for and assess implementation efforts. Table 3.10.1 highlights exemplar questions that might arise.

The assessments needed for planning the implementation of an EBI are detailed and multi-level given that the EBI must be integrated into a complex, dynamic, adaptive system.[10]

Considering implementation strategies

The notion of incorporating an EBI into an ever-changing system prompts attention to how best to support a transition into using the new programme, practice, or policy. Implementation strategies are methods that can improve the adoption, implementation, or maintenance of an EBI. These strategies may be specified in an intervention package, or practitioners may need to identify the most useful set for a given implementation effort. A recent typology[11] highlights the following categories of strategies:

- Evaluation strategies, many of which are iterative, such as creating cycles of experimenting, assessing impact, and planning new tests.
- Interactive support for implementers, such as provision of technical assistance.
- Adaptation assistance, such as supporting tailoring of EBI elements.

Table 3.10.1 Examples of assessments during the planning and implementation of an evidence-based intervention (EBI) to prevent child obesity delivered in schools

Domain	Exemplar questions
Outer context	
Socio-political context	How will current laws or policies affect implementation of this EBI? What measures of success must be met?
Funding	What funds are available through state agencies, school districts, etc. to support the intervention?
Inter-organizational networks	Which institutional partners, such as local after-school childcare providers, are important sources of influence or present referral or collaboration opportunities?
Inner context	
Organizational characteristics	What are the size, structure, and leadership characteristics for target schools? Do they have the necessary capacity, readiness, and supportive context to deliver the EBI?
Adopter characteristics	Who are the key decisionmakers (e.g. district superintendent or school principal?) How does the EBI fit with the decisionmakers' needs, goals, and constraints?
Implementer characteristics	What are the characteristics of staff who will lead implementation of the EBI? What is their level of readiness for this innovation?
Student characteristics	What is the socio-demographic profile of the student body? What are the major barriers they face to healthy eating and physical activity?

- Partnership promotion, such as creating or supporting relationships among stakeholders to share local knowledge or partner in implementation efforts.
- Training supports for diverse stakeholders (ranging from participants and implementers to organizations and the broader community), including capacity-building or train-the-trainer models.
- Provider supports, such as clinical reminders or shifting of roles to support clinicians to use an EBI.
- Participant engagement, such as involvement of community members in implementation processes.
- Financial tactics, such as offering incentives or changing payment structures.
- Infrastructure change, such as changing the location of service delivery or changing the physical structure or equipment used for an EBI.

Evaluation frameworks and implementation outcomes

Lastly, practitioners may wish to use a framework designed to evaluate results of an implementation effort. For example, the PRECEDE-PROCEED model can be used to plan delivery of a public health intervention, with the second portion (PROCEED) focusing on the implementation (delivering the EBI), process evaluation (assessing which components were delivered and how they were delivered), impact evaluation (success in reaching the target audience), and outcome evaluation (the impact on programme goals). Alternatively, for efforts reaching across multiple sites or institutions, it may be useful to use the RE-AIM framework. This framework assesses Reach (the number, proportion, and representativeness of participants in the EBI), Effectiveness (impact on intervention outcomes of interest), Adoption (the number, proportion, and representativeness of sites or implementers who have adopted the EBI), Implementation (the delivery of the EBI, in terms of fidelity and adaptation, as well as costs), and Maintenance (the extent to which the EBI has been integrated into a given site's activities and policies).[12]

Practitioners may wish to evaluate a select set of implementation outcomes as complements to traditional programme outcomes. This allows for a distinction between challenges related to the intervention versus challenges related to the implementation effort.[13] Common implementation outcomes[14, 15] and their definitions are highlighted in Table 3.10.2.

Table 3.10.2 Key categories of implementation outcomes and definitions

Outcome	Definition
Acceptability	Perceptions among participants, implementers, and stakeholders that the EBI is agreeable or satisfactory.
Adaptation	Intentional changes made to the EBI (details in next section).
Adoption	Uptake or use of the EBI.
Appropriateness	Perceived fit of the EBI with the participant, implementer, and/or system.
Costs	Costs of implementation (which vary by the EBI), implementation strategies used, and site of delivery
Feasibility	Extent to which the EBI can be used in the target setting
Fidelity	Degree to which the EBI is delivered according to the original protocol/intervention developer's plan, with expected dose and quality.
Penetration	Extent to which eligible target sites or participants use an EBI.
Sustainability	Extent to which the EBI is maintained by the organization over the long term.

Considering adaptations

While the process for using EBIs seems straightforward on paper, it is not always simple to translate an intervention into a new context. After all, an intervention may have initially been tested within a narrowly defined population subgroup, setting, and/or system that is quite different from the implementation target. The challenge, then, is in applying the evidence to a broader set of populations and contexts, often with fewer resources than were available for the initial study. It may be necessary to make *adaptations*, or strategic changes made to an intervention to increase utility, relevance, and impact, while preserving the core elements of the intervention. The goal is to find a balance between maintaining sufficient fidelity such that the 'active ingredients' are preserved, while allowing for the fact that interventions are implemented in dynamic systems and thus both change and are changed by the larger system. The goal is to conduct strategic adaptations and evaluate the altered intervention.

Given the goal of making necessary adaptations, but preserving the original intervention where possible, practitioners may wish to use an existing framework to guide their adaptation work, such as the ADAPT-ITT model[16] or Dynamic Adaptation Process[17]. Adaptations may be prompted by differences between research and target settings in terms of:

• system-level factors, such as funding or policies
• organization-level attributes, such as resources or training opportunities, leadership buy-in and characteristics, and organizational culture or climate
• provider-level characteristics, such as the educational background of available staff and their experience with and attitudes towards EBIs
• participant characteristics, including their unique socio-cultural context and according risks and resources. This may include behaviour patterns, socio-demographics, cultural background, other health concerns, and competing demands.

Based on these assessments, which can draw on qualitative and quantitative data, practitioners may wish to make adaptations to the programme. Changes may be made to the content of the programme, such as tailoring elements, integrating elements of another EBI, and changing the timing or length of intervention components. Changes may also be made to the context, with modifications to the format, setting, staff selected to implement the programme, or participants targeted. Other changes may affect the way in which implementers are trained or the way the programme is evaluated. Adaptations may be made at any of the multiple levels involved in the EBI.[15]

Leveraging implementation science research for public health practice

There is tremendous potential to harness the research evidence base and implementation science to improve public health practice. The steps below support taking an evidence-based approach to public health and utilizing implementation science to increase impact.

• Gather the necessary data to examine the public health issue of interest and identify potential leverage points. Drawing on the multi-level approaches of health promotion and implementation science, the data-gathering effort should include information about the target population, organizations that may be able to support delivery of EBIs, and the broader context in which the health issue will be addressed.

- Begin to engage stakeholders so that the decision-making process is informed by realities of participant, setting, and system resources and constraints.
- Access the literature to find available evidence-based programmes, practices, policies, or approaches, and assess the strength of the evidence. There are a number of publicly available databases for EBIs, such as the Research-Tested Intervention Programs section of Cancer Control PLANET, offered by the US National Cancer Institute. Evidence syntheses, such as the Community Guide from the US Community Preventive Services Task Force, may also provide useful information about potential options for achieving key public health goals (see Further resources).
- Weigh candidate interventions and approaches, considering the relative impact of available evidence, the types of adaptations that will need to be made to ensure that the offering is relevant and useful for the target population, and the match between required and available resources. Data collected earlier regarding implementation about the settings and context will be useful here and may need to be augmented.
- Access the implementation science literature to find useful theories or frameworks for planning, implementation, and sustainment periods. At the outset, engage in planning processes to account for multiple levels of influences on implementation success. Adapt the selected EBI as needed, or—if the adaptation requirements are too great—reconsider other options.
- Identify potential implementation strategies that can support the uptake and use of the selected EBI approach. Create the package of materials, trainings, and other supports.
- Implement the EBI.
- Evaluate the success of the effort, collecting implementation and outcomes data in an ongoing manner. Use a multi-level approach to capture impact for the participant and relevant social networks, organizations, community influences, and broader system factors.
- Feed findings from the effort into future work. Share initial findings with relevant stakeholders.

Competencies required

- Ability to gather and synthesize data describing the target population.
- Familiarity with the range of potential partners and stakeholders that may be involved or affected by the implementation effort.
- Expertise with the health issue, target population, implementation settings, and broader context.
- Capacity to learn about the EBI and make strategic adaptations, while preserving core components.
- Ability to plan and conduct iterative evaluations.

Who are the people who might need to be involved?

As seen above, translating evidence into practice requires a diverse set of competencies, often achieved through coordinated action by a team with diverse skills sets. Practitioners who are finding, adapting, implementing, and evaluating EBIs may find it helpful to partner with:

- individuals expected to benefit from EBIs and their relevant social networks
- potential implementers
- practitioners and providers at other organizations (e.g. from community-based organizations or healthcare delivery sites)
- researchers, who can point practitioners to relevant literature, while simultaneously benefiting from exposure to real-world use of implementation science findings
- funder organizations, which may see the use of EBIs as a distinguishing feature and may be interested in supporting such programming or offering technical assistance to encourage use of EBIs
- policymakers, who are trying to assess the best available evidence and determine how best to allocate limited resources.

Taking a partnered approach

A partnership model is a natural fit for bringing the benefits of implementation science to bear in public health practice. Taking the EPIS model as an example, it quickly becomes clear that a team is needed to be able to effectively and efficiently characterize the recipients, implementers, and adopters of an EBI as well as the organizations, communities, and socio-political context surrounding the implementation effort. Practitioners can engage with stakeholders, researchers, policy makers, and others in a range of ways, from providing expert advice for specific needs, all the way to giving more high-level advice throughout the project. Or practitioners may wish to utilize the team's expertise in a more collaborative or collegial way, with increased power sharing and joint decision making. Increased engagement on behalf of partners can increase the likelihood of implementation success, but such efforts can be more costly and time-consuming, as highlighted by the literature on participatory implementation science.[18] Regardless of the model of engagement, partnered approaches to leveraging implementation science fit naturally with the collaborative, interdisciplinary nature of public health practice.

Emerging issues

The field of implementation science is growing rapidly and practitioners may find a few emerging areas of particular interest. First, it is increasingly clear that practitioners require dedicated training and supports to be able to effectively engage with and benefit from the research evidence base. Skills development and technical assistance for practitioners to find, adapt, implement, and evaluate EBIs not only support improved outcomes for a given implementation effort but also build infrastructure for more effective use of the research evidence base overall.[19] This reflects the move in the field towards models in which practitioners integrate practice-based knowledge actively and strategically into existing interventions and approaches supported by research.

Second, there is an increased focus on mis-implementation, the continuing use of ineffective interventions, or the premature ending of effective interventions. There are a range of historical, economic, professional, and social forces that determine which interventions are utilized. This emerging area of research focuses on how to identify instances of mis-implementation and then create change strategies to address them. Practitioners can benefit from this area of work as they move resources away from unnecessary or harmful interventions towards those supported by the evidence.

Finally, implementation science is increasingly focused on opportunities to use EBIs to improve health equity. Although the potential of EBIs to improve population health and increase health equity has been highlighted by the National Academies of Medicine and others, there is still a great deal of work to be done to ensure that implementation science is utilized to improve health equity. Explicit attention to avoid creating or exacerbating disparities through implementation efforts is critical.

Further resources

Websites

Community Guide from the US Community Preventive Services Task Force. Provides evidence syntheses for a wide range of health topics. (https://www.thecommunityguide.org/) OK

Substance Abuse and Mental Health Services Administration (SAMHSA). *Evidence-based Practices Resource Center.* Available at: (https://www.samhsa.gov/ebp-resource-center) (accessed 24 August 2019)

Cancer Control PLANET - Research-Tested Intervention Programs. A database of EBIs from the US National Cancer Institute and partners. (https://rtips.cancer.gov/rtips/index.do) OK

Health Evidence for Public Health – McMaster University. Source for systematic reviews and evidence syntheses across a wide range of health topics. Available at: (https://www.healthevidence.org) (accessed 24 August 2019)

Consolidated Framework for Implementation Research. Cancer Prevention and Control Research Network (CPCRN). Detailed description of framework, with related tools. (http://cfirguide.org)

US National Cancer Institute. Available at https://rtips.cancer.gov/rtips/index.do (accessed 24 August 2019)

US Community Preventive Services Task Force. Available at: https://www.thecommunityguide.org (accessed 24 August 2019)

Cancer Prevention and Control Research Network (CPCRN). Putting public health evidence in action training workshop. Available at: ⅋ https://cpcrn.org/training (accessed 24 August 2019).

Books

Brownson RC, Colditz GA, Proctor EK, eds. Dissemination and implementation research in health: Translating science to practice. 2nd ed. New York: Oxford University Press; 2018.

Journals

Implementation Science (open-access)
Translational Behavioral Medicine
Preventing Chronic Disease (Implementation Evaluation section)

References

1 Rabin BA, Brownson RC. (2018). Terminology for dissemination and implementation research. In: Brownson RC, Colditz GA, Proctor EK, eds, *Dissemination and implementation research in health: translating science to practice*, 2nd edn, pp. 19–46. Oxford University Press, New York.

2 Kohatsu ND, Robinson JG, Torner JC. (2004). Evidence-based public health: an evolving concept. *American Journal of Preventive Medicine*, **27**(5), 417–21.

3 Balas EA, Boren SA. (2000). Managing clinical knowledge for health care improvement. In: Bemmel J, McCray A, eds, *Yearbook of medical informatics 2000: patient-centered systems*, pp. 65–70. Schattauer, Stuttgart, Germany.

4 Emmons KM, Colditz GA. (2017). Realizing the potential of cancer prevention-the role of implementation science. *New England Journal of Medicine*, **376**(10), 986–90.

5 Curran GM, Bauer M, Mittman B, et al. (2012). Effectiveness-implementation hybrid designs: combining elements of clinical effectiveness and implementation research to enhance public health impact. *Medical Care*, **50**(3), 217.

6 Tabak RG, Khoong EC, Chambers DA, et al. (2012). Bridging research and practice: models for dissemination and implementation research. *American Journal of Preventive Medicine*, **43**(3), 337–50.

7 Stokols D. (1996). Translating social ecological theory into guidelines for community health promotion. *American Journal of Health Promotion*, **10**(4), 282–98.

8 Damschroder LJ, Aron DC, Keith RE, et al. (2009). Fostering implementation of health services research findings into practice: a consolidated framework for advancing implementation science. *Implementation Science*, **4**(1), 50.

9 Rogers E. (2003). *Diffusion of innovations*, 5th edn. The Free Press, New York.

10 Best A. (2011). Systems thinking and health promotion. *American Journal of Health Promotion*, **25**(4), eix–ex.

11 Kirchner JE, Waltz TJ, Powell BJ, et al. (2018). Implementation strategies. In: Brownson R, Proctor E, Colditz G, eds, *Dissemination and Implementation Research in Health: Translating Science to Practice*, 2nd edn, pp. 245–66. Oxford University Press, New York.

12 Gaglio B, Glasgow RE. (2018). Evaluation approaches for dissemination and implementation research. In: Brownson R, Proctor E, Colditz G, eds, *Dissemination and Implementation Research in Health: Translating Science to Practice*, 2nd edn, pp. 317–34. Oxford University Press, New York.

13 Fixsen DL, Naoom SF, Blase KA, et al. (2005). *Implementation research: a synthesis of the literature*. University of South Florida, Louis de la Parte Florida Mental Health Institute, National Implementation Research Network, Tampa, FL.

14 Lewis CC, Proctor EK, Brownson RC. (2018). Measurement issues in dissemination and implementation research. In: Brownson RC, Colditz GA, Proctor EK, eds, *Dissemination and implementation research in health: translating science to practice*, 2nd edn, pp. 229–44. Oxford University Press, New York.

15 Baumann AA, Cabassa LJ, Stirman SW. (2018). Adaptation in dissemination and implementation science. In: Brownson RC, Colditz GA, Proctor EK, eds, *Dissemination and implementation research in health: translating science to practice*, 2nd edn, pp. 285–300. Oxford University Press, New York.

16 Wingood GM, DiClemente RJ. (2008). The ADAPT-ITT model: a novel method of adapting evidence-based HIV interventions. *Journal of Acquired Immune Deficiency Syndrome*, **47** (Supplement 1), S40–46.

17 Aarons GA, Green AE, Palinkas LA, et al. (2012). Dynamic adaptation process to implement an evidence-based child maltreatment intervention. *Implementation Science*, **7**(1), 32.

18 Ramanadhan S, Kohler RK, Viswanath K. Partnerships to support implementation science. In: Chambers D, Vinson C, Norton WE, eds, *Optimizing the cancer control continuum: advancing implementation research*. Oxford University Press, New York, in press.

19 Ramanadhan S, Viswanath K. Engaging communities to improve health: models, evidence, and the participatory knowledge translation (PaKT) framework. In: Fisher EB, Cameron L, Christensen AJ, et al., eds, *Principles and concepts of behavioral medicine: a global handbook*. Springer Science & Business Media, in press.

Part 4

Policy arenas

Developing healthy public policy

Don Nutbeam

Objectives

Reading this chapter should help you better understand:
- the process of policy making and the role of public health information and evidence in shaping policy
- the role of public health practitioners in influencing the policy process through the provision of evidence and advocacy.

Definition of key terms

- Public policy: public issues identified for attention by the government and the courses of action taken to address them.
- Public policy making: the processes through which decisions are made by governments about policy, often enacted through legislation or other forms of rule making that define regulations and incentives and enable the provision of resources, programmes, and services to address public issues.
- Healthy public policy: healthy public policy is a concept promoted by the World Health Organization (WHO) to highlight the potential impact that all government policies have on health. Healthy public policy is policy that optimizes the positive impact it may have on health. The WHO's *Ottawa Charter* emphasizes that health should be a consideration in policy making in all sectors at all levels of government, and that governments should be held to account for the health consequences of their policies.[1]
- Health impact assessment: a methodology for prospectively assessing the potential impact of policy proposals in order to improve their positive impact on the health of a population and to minimize inequalities in health (see ➔ Chapter 1.5).[2]
- Health in all Policies (HiaP): HiaP is an approach advocated by WHO to develop public policies across sectors that systematically take into account the health implications of decisions, seek synergies (co-benefits), and avoid harmful health impacts in order to improve population health and health equity.[3] HiaP promotes accountability of policy makers for health impacts at all levels of policy making.
- Evidence: in public policy making, 'evidence' is derived from information from a variety of sources including, though not limited to, peer-reviewed research. In practice, a great deal of policy-relevant evidence can be gathered from programmes already in existence by observing the way they operate, identifying what has worked in the past and what has not, and learning from the experience of practitioners in delivering programmes. Evidence from more conventional research is often blended with this contextual, 'real world' knowledge.[4] (For more on evidence, see ➔ Chapter 2.7.)

Why is it important to be able to use evidence to inform or influence policy?

Public health practitioners are often frustrated that public health evidence and a population-based perspective on health do not adequately influence the development of public policy, particularly in sectors other than health. An improved understanding of the policy-making process and how to influence it will enable you to engage more effectively in the development of healthy public policy and advocate for health in all policies.

How is healthy public policy made?

Policy develops and changes on the basis of underlying beliefs about both the cause of a problem and the feasibility and potential effect of proposed interventions. These beliefs contribute to the policy-making process and final policy direction along with the social and political context in which the decision is made. The ability to interpret the causes of a problem and identify effective solutions are skills that will enable you to influence policy decisions. These basic skills will be enhanced by an understanding of the social and political context of a problem and the processes through which decisions are made.[5]

Policy making is rarely an 'event' or even an explicit set of decisions derived from an appraisal of evidence and following a pre-planned course. Policy tends to evolve through an iterative process and to be subject to continuous review and incremental change. Policy making is an inherently political process and the timing of decisions is usually dictated as much by political considerations as the state of the evidence.

As such, policy making requires a point-in-time appraisal of the following:
• What is scientifically plausible, based on an appraisal of the best available evidence at the time it is needed?
• What is politically acceptable, based on an appraisal of the political context in which policies are being made?
• What is practical for implementation, based on an appraisal of the experience of practitioners in delivering programmes?

Models to help explain the relationship between public health evidence and the policy-making process

Evidence can be used in a variety of ways to lead, justify, or support policy development. A range of models explain the different ways in which evidence has been used to guide the policy-making process[6] including the following:
• *The knowledge-driven model:* the emergence of new knowledge from research will create pressure for its application in policy. In public health,

developments such as the development of new vaccines or screening tools may lead to public pressure for their immediate adoption, often regardless of their cost relative to benefit.

- *The problem-solving model:* evidence derived from a variety of sources is gathered and forms a starting point for the development of policy as part of a rational process with a clear beginning and end. For example, the government of the Netherlands introduced interventions to tackle health inequalities for which there was good evidence and an established system for monitoring progress.[7]
- *The interactive model:* the decision-making process is informed not only by research knowledge but by experience, social pressures, and political considerations. Approaches to tackling health inequalities in the UK reflect this complex process and mix of influences.[8]
- *The political model:* evidence is selectively used to justify a pre-determined position. Reliance on mass-media campaigns and/or school-based interventions to address complex problems such as drug misuse and anti-social behaviour reflect this model. An example is evaluation of the US drug-use-prevention programme, DARE.[9]
- *The tactical model:* the normal uncertainty of research findings is exploited to delay a decision or where weak evidence is used to justify an unpopular decision. The responses of some governments to the difficult policy decisions needed to address the challenge of childhood obesity exemplify this model.[10]

In reality, policy decisions emerge from complex and sometimes unpredictable interactions between political imperatives and from public debate alongside analysis of more conventional evidence from a range of sources. You need to be aware of rare 'windows of opportunity' for the uptake of evidence into policy, when policy makers' interests and the social climate coincide to support the use of public health evidence in policy making. Timing is everything.

Who is involved in developing healthy public policy, and what role can I play?

There are four main players in the development of healthy public policy:[5]

- *Policy makers:* people, usually politicians and bureaucracies, who have initiated or hold a mandate for a specific policy and move the policy at a pace that meets their interests. As a public health practitioner, you can get to know this group and, where feasible, develop a relationship with individual policy makers not only in health but also in sectors such as housing, education, and transport.
- *Policy influencers:* groups such as industry lobby groups or public advocacy groups (mostly outside government) with an interest in a specific issue and which try to influence the content of policy and its implementation. As a public health practitioner, you can engage with them to support or resist the development of policy content and the process of implementation.

- *The public*: audiences, consumers, taxpayers, and voters whose opinion will ultimately affect the adoption of the policy. As a public health practitioner, you can play an important role as a community leader and public-opinion maker, especially through effective use of the media.
- *The media*: (print and electronic) media influence both policy makers' and the public's understanding of, and attitude towards, an issue. The growth of digital media has made this a more complex and contested environment. As a public health practitioner, you can engage with the media to provide credible information and expert advice, as well as more active media advocacy (see b Chapter 4.5 for more on media advocacy).

Given such complexity, it would be foolish to imagine that there will ever be a simple and smooth transfer of evidence into the policy-making process. The types of evidence used, and the way evidence is applied in policy processes, vary according to the beliefs of those who create and influence policy.[8] Information can be used internally to monitor, analyse, and critique policy options, or externally to persuade or mobilise others into action. The media has an important role in creating public opinion not only in relation to what they report but also by choosing who is allowed to speak, how much prominence an issue is given, and how an issue is framed.[5]

What determines success in developing healthy public policy?

Public health practitioners and academics often complain that their evidence is ignored by policy makers. However, our choice of research, methods of communication, and general dislocation from the policy-making process all exacerbate this situation.[10]

A 'hierarchy of evidence' is well established in the public health and broader scientific community. Systematic reviews and meta-analyses of randomized trials have become far more accessible and policy-makers have become more adept at using this type of evidence. There is little doubt that this high-quality evidence has been influential in policy-making and countries like the UK (through its National Institute for Health and Care Excellence) have established formal structures to systematize the use of evidence in health policy making. (For more on the transfer of evidence into policy, see ➲ Chapter 4.2).

However, not all randomized trials produce evidence that is policy relevant and not all policy-relevant evidence comes from randomized trials. Evaluations based on prospective experimental designs are simply not possible in many areas of public health policy. From a policy-making perspective, a large amount of public health research appears to offer no practical way forward and to provide no solutions to the problems examined.

In contrast, a great deal of policy-relevant evidence is gathered from case studies of practice, reflecting expert opinion or even anecdotal evidence. Such 'evidence' generally ranks at the bottom in established hierarchies of evidence but it is frequently highly valued by policy makers, particularly as it is often available when needed, addresses issues of current concern, and offers solutions that are practical for implementation.

Policy is most likely to reflect public health priorities and the evidence that informs them if:

- evidence is available and accessible when needed
- the evidence is presented in a way that fits with the political vision of the government (or can be made to fit)
- the evidence points to actions for which powers and resources are (or could be) available, and the systems, structures, and capacity for action exist
- there is successful public health advocacy within and outside the political system, and
- policy makers have basic critical appraisal skills and are supported in using evidence in policy development.

While there are many obstacles to using public health evidence in developing healthy public policy, there are real signs of progress in many countries, including:

- explicit commitments by governments to use evidence in policy making
- the growth of active public health communities and a strengthened voice in public debate
- changes to research funding to better align research with policy needs, and
- investments in institutions to build the public health evidence base.

What competencies are required for public policy making?

Public health practitioners need to develop skills in public communication and political advocacy. This does not mean that you have to become 'politicians', but it may involve building relationships with civil servants and policy makers within government departments, establishing partnerships and alliances with organizations and individuals with similar objectives, and effectively engaging with the media (see ➔ Chapter 4.5). Importantly, researchers need to develop closer working relationships with policy makers, from the earliest stages of research design through to programme implementation and beyond (see the case study ↑↔ Box 4.1.1).

Our collective challenge is to find ways of ensuring that evidence forms part of an inherently fluid political decision-making process. This is the responsibility of both those who generate evidence and those who use it. We need to provide timely access to information and to use effective techniques for communicating and managing the inevitable uncertainties that arise through scientific research. For the public servants who use evidence in policy making, there is the challenge to develop skills in the critical appraisal of evidence, and to judge how to achieve the best 'fit' between available evidence, current political priorities, and practical actions to achieve the desired outcomes in the real world. Public health practitioners who can make evidence accessible and comprehensible to policy makers will have an advantage when it comes to advocating and influencing.

Box 4.1.1 (case study) Successful healthy public policy and lessons learned: physical activity in schools

Research and the policy process

The New South Wales (NSW) schools fitness and physical activity survey was undertaken to provide reliable scientific evidence in response to growing professional and community concern about reduced physical activity and rising levels of obesity in Australian children.[a]

The study measured the body composition, health-related fitness, physical activity habits, and fundamental motor skills of primary and high school students in NSW. It also investigated the school facilities, policies, and practices relevant to students' participation in physical activity.

Fundamental movement skills include running, jumping, catching, throwing, kicking, and forehand strike, and are essential prerequisites for participation and enjoyment of sports and other forms of physical activity. The results from the study showed only that about 30% of students had completely mastered running and jumping, with another 30% close to mastery. Girls in particular scored poorly on some skills, with fewer than 20% showing mastery or near mastery of kicking and forehand strike. Most of these skills should be mastered by the age of ten and the results showed that NSW school children had surprisingly poor physical skills.

Two relatively small and achievable recommendations were made to policy makers:
• Two hours per week were to be allocated to physical education in primary schools.
• One hour of this was to be used for developing fundamental movement skills.

These recommendations were taken by contacts within the department to higher levels in the organization until they reached the Minister and were accepted. The resulting skills development programme in primary schools was well supported. Resources developed to support the teachers in implementing the programme included videos, workbooks, phone support, and face-to-face training.

Subsequent research showed improvements in the fundamental movement skills of NSW primary school children and an association between skill proficiency and higher levels of physical activity. Long-term effects on obesity were mixed.

Lessons learned

Several conditions assisted this transfer of evidence into education policy:
• Public health researchers engaged in a sustained media advocacy campaign, using their evidence to portray the lack of physical skills in Australian children as an important problem for society. This created the social and political climate needed for the adoption of healthy policy change.
• Public health researchers worked collaboratively with contacts in the Department of School Education throughout the process, from the design and implementation of the study through to the evaluation of the subsequent skills development programme.

Box 4.1.1 *(Contd.)*

- The involvement of policy makers in the design phase of the survey meant that factors amenable to policy change and implementation were measured. For example, school facilities, sports equipment, and time allocated to physical education were assessed.
- Lastly, the policy changes were consistent with the Australian Department of School Education's broader goals and within their capability to implement.

a) Hardy LL, Okely AD, Dobbins TA, et al. (2008). Physical activity among adolescents in New South Wales (Australia): 1997–2004. Journal of Science and Medicine and Science in Sports and Exercise, 40, 835–41.

Myths and misconceptions

The emergence of evidence-based medicine in the early 1990s put pressure on policy makers to become more evidence-based in their decision making. In the scientific and medical communities, where evidence-based practice is highly regarded, there is a common misconception that policy making is and should be a purely evidence-based and rational process.

Policy makers often have many valid and competing concerns when formulating policy. Political survival, financial constraints, and public opinion are strong motivators in policy decisions and tapping into these motivators will greatly increase the chances of influencing policy. If you take an honest look at most published 'evidence', you will see that it too often describes the problem well but offers few, if any, of the practical solutions, options, and alternatives needed for policy making.

References

1 World Health Organization (1986). *Ottawa Charter for Health Promotion*. WHO, Geneva.
2 Mindell JS, Boltong A, Forde I. (2008). A review of health impact assessment frameworks. *Public Health*, **122**, 1177–87.
3 World Health Organization (2014). Health in all policies: Helsinki statement. Framework for country action.WHO, Geneva. Available at: http://apps.who.int/iris/bitstream/10665/112636/1/9789241506908_eng.pdf?ua=1 (accessed 21 August 2019).
4 Brownson RC, Fielding JE, Maylahn CM. (2009). Evidence-based public health: a fundamental concept for public health practice. *Annual Review of Public Health*, **30**, 175–201.
5 Milio N. (1987). Making healthy public policy: developing the science by learning the art. *Health Promotion International*, **2**, 263–74.
6 Weiss CH. (1979). The many meanings of research utilization. *Public Administration Review*, **39**, 426–31.
7 Mackenbach J, Stronks K. (2002). A strategy for tackling health inequalities in the Netherlands. *British Medical Journal*, **325**, 1029–32.
8 Nutbeam D, Boxhall AM. (2008). What influences the transfer of research into health policy? Observations from England and Australia. *Public Health*, **122**(8), 747–53.
9 West SL, O'Neal KK. (2004). Project DARE outcome effectiveness revisited. *American Journal of Public Health*, **94**, 1027–9.
10 Brownell KD. Farley T, Willett WC, et al. (2009). The public health and economic benefits of taxing sugar sweetened beverages. *New England Journal of Medicine*, **361**(16), 1599–605.

Chapter 4.2

Translating evidence to policy

Lauren Smith and Ichiro Kawachi

Objectives

As a result of reading this chapter, you will:
- identify the challenges that arise in translating research findings to public policy
- understand the frequently cited barriers to evidence-based public health policy making from the perspective of legislators
- take steps to bridge the gap between evidence and policy formation.

Introduction

The three critical ingredients to public health policy formation are 1) the establishment of an evidence base to support action, 2) the existence of political will to act, and 3) the identification of sustainable strategies.[1] Yet evidence-based public health policy remains limited because of the challenges that arise in bridging research and policy.

Considering the 'supply side' of evidence production, some researchers hesitate to become involved in the policy process because a) they do not want short-term political interests to direct their research agendas, or b) they feel that becoming 'mired' in policy considerations will compromise the integrity of their research, or c) few institutional incentives exist for them to address the policy relevance of their work.[2] From the perspective of the potential users of evidence (i.e. the 'demand side' of the equation), legislators and regulators are often forced to make policy under budgetary and time constraints. For instance, if there is a pressing political agenda to tackle childhood obesity, laws will be formulated with or without scientific input. At the same time, supplying the most rigorous evidence does not guarantee that policy actions will follow. The goal of this chapter is to start you thinking about overcoming the barriers to translating evidence into policy.

Barriers to translating evidence into policy

What are the barriers that impede an effective incorporation of public health knowledge into policy?
- The rapid pace of decision making, which can be uncomfortable for academics.
- The unavoidable tension between the sufficiency of information available for decision making versus the need to act now.
- Researchers and policy makers placing different weights on evidence versus experience.
- The unquestionable appeal of policy making based on anecdotes.

What do researchers need to understand about the policy-making process?

Evidence for action is produced by several sets of people—not just academic researchers but also practitioners. From the perspective of decision makers, the following is a list of things you need to understand about translating evidence into action.

Public health researchers are not well prepared to convey the impact of 'intersectoral effects'

As a public health researcher, you need to explicitly 'connect the dots' to inform policy makers of the 'upstream' social determinants that influence population health. Often, decision makers in the sectors controlling these determinants (e.g. community development, education, employment, zoning) do not view population health as belonging to their domain. The strategic use of health impact assessments can be a useful tool to educate key stakeholders and policy makers on the health impacts of these social determinants (see also ➲ Chapter 1.5).

Public health researchers often do not recognize the 'supply versus demand' dynamic of data

Public health researchers (including practitioners engaged in the production of evidence) are usually more accustomed to the passive diffusion of data through peer-reviewed journals or presentations at professional conferences. A more effective strategy is to position your work so that the decision makers (policy makers and legislators) can reach out to you for information and advice at the specific time they need it. This requires the cultivation of relationships ahead of time, before the decision maker needs information immediately and wants to turn to a credible, experienced, and known source.

Public health researchers devote inadequate attention to the 'framing' of their arguments

You need to understand that the language you use to present your data matters and must be chosen carefully. You may need training and experience in how to frame your ideas and evidence effectively, particularly when presenting evidence that may be inconsistent with the cognitive frames of the audience. As a result, you need to learn and consistently apply the lessons supplied by the field of cognitive linguistics and strategic frame analysis.[3] If you do not, your hard-earned knowledge may be dismissed.

Existing public health research training does not adequately prepare or support public health professionals who seek to work at the intersection of evidence production and public health policy

From the perspective of professional training in public health, you need to be aware of the following gaps between evidence production and policy translation that you will need to bridge during your training:
- An unclear pathway of career advancement for those interested in this kind of work.

- The inconsistent emphasis within public health training curricula on the requisite skills required to operate at this intersection.
- Public health training curricular requirements that do not consistently emphasize the specific skills necessary to bridge the gap between evidence and policy (see Box 4.2.1 and Table 4.2.1).

Box 4.2.1 Public health professional competencies in US Schools of Public Health

In the USA, schools of public health fully accredited by the Council on Education of Public Health (CEPH) must identify required competencies that define the knowledge, skills, and abilities that a successful graduate should be able to demonstrate at the conclusion of their programme.[a] The 2016 CEPH criteria emphasize 'foundational competencies' that all professional public health trainees are required to be taught. Several of these core competency domains touch on the skills necessary to bridge the gap between public health and policy.

a) Council on Education for Public Health (2016). Accreditation criteria: schools of public health and public health programs. CEPH, Washington, DC. Available at: ℅ https://ceph.org/assets/2016.Criteria.pdf (accessed 21 August 2019).

Table 4.2.1 Foundational competencies for professional public health training (Master of Public Health degree)

Competency domain	Competencies addressing the intersection between research and policy
Evidence-based approaches to public health	• Interpret results of data analysis for public health research, policy or practice.
Policy in public health	• Discuss multiple dimensions of the policy-making process, including the roles of ethics and evidence.
	• Propose strategies to identify stakeholders and build coalitions and partnerships for influencing public health outcomes.
	• Advocate for political, social or economic policies and programmes that will improve health in diverse populations. Discuss the policy process for improving the health status of populations.
Communication	• Communicate audience-appropriate public health content, both in writing and through oral presentation

Source: data from Council on Education for Public Health (2016). *Accreditation criteria: schools of public health and public health programs*. CEPH, Washington, DC. Available at: ℅ https://ceph.org/assets/2016.Criteria.pdf (accessed 21 August 2019).

Unclear pathway of career advancement for those interested in working at the intersection of public health and public policy

Even if you successfully bridge the gap between the worlds of evidence production and policy translation, you need to be aware of the barriers to career advancement as a result of working at the intersection between the two worlds. Different things are valued in the worlds of evidence production and policy translation. In the research world, what counts for career advancement are publications, publications, and publications. However, in a world where policy translation is valued, you should get credit for doing things such as:

• providing testimony at legislative hearings
• providing expert guidance, in the form of policy briefs or reports to decision makers
• participating in developing legislation or regulations
• providing policy briefings based on sound interpretation of available evidence to legislators, agency staff, and elected officials.

The disconnect between emphasis on social determinants of health and insufficient support for assessing and communicating public health effects of policies originating outside the public health domain

There is increasing consensus on the need to focus on the fundamental drivers of population health, which often lie outside the domains of public health and healthcare. As a public health professional, you need to develop a deeper understanding of how these sectors are organized and how to develop effective collaborations with colleagues in those sectors who may be better positioned to identify potential policy issues to be addressed, and the kinds of questions that would be most useful to answer (see Box 4.2.2).

Box 4.2.2 Case study: a child health impact assessment of energy costs and the Low Income Energy Assistance Programme

The Department of Pediatrics at Boston Medical Center (Massachusetts, USA) convened an interdisciplinary, inter-institutional working group to develop a child health impact assessment strategy to make the relationship of public policy to child health more comprehensible to policy makers and the public in Massachusetts. Below is a case study of one of the health impact assessments they conducted in 2007.[a]

• Purpose:
  • To conduct a timely health impact assessment to determine the influence of home energy costs on children's health and well-being, particularly among children from low-income families,
  • to identify and inform key stakeholders of the findings and recommendations.

- Participants:
  - representatives from Boston University School of Medicine, Boston University School of Public Health, Brandeis University, Boston Children's Hospital, Harvard Medical School, Harvard School of Public Health, and University of Massachusetts
  - state and federal programme officers from the Low Income Home Energy Assistance Program (LIHEAP);
  - energy assistance programme directors at Massachusetts community action agencies
  - energy advocates and researchers at the local, state and federal levels.
- Findings:
  - Low-income families facing disproportionately high energy costs are forced to make household budget trade-offs that jeopardize child health.
  - Families facing high heating costs resort to alternative heat sources that jeopardize child health and safety.
  - High energy costs combined with unaffordable housing creates important budget constraints that force low-income families to endure unhealthy housing conditions that threaten child health.
  - The growing gap between rising energy prices and LIHEAP benefits means more Massachusetts families accumulate substantial unpaid utility bills, leading to arrearages and disconnections that adversely affect child and family well-being.
- Resulting policy actions:
  - Members of the Child Health Impact Assessment Working Group presented their findings to the state legislature in testimony before the Joint Committee on Housing. State expenditures for LIHEAP were subsequently increased.
  - Members of the Child Health Impact Assessment Working Group presented the findings to the National Energy Assistance Directors Association, stimulating what has become an ongoing interest in the connection between health and energy costs. Some energy assistance programmes developed outreach programmes located in community health centres.

a) Child Health Impact Working Group (2007). Unhealthy consequences: energy costs and child health impact assessment of energy costs and the low income home energy assistance program. CHIWG, Boston.

Bridging the gap between evidence and policy

Evidence producers and policy makers differ in their priorities, their time horizons, and their information communication and presentation styles.[4, 5] If your work involves evidence production, you can increase the impact of your findings by taking the following steps:

- Getting more involved in the policy process to gain an understanding of political decision making.[6]
- Translating and communicating findings so they are accessible and understandable by policy makers.[7]
- Building formal partnerships and informal relationships with policy makers.[8]
- Preparing for windows of opportunity when evidence can have maximal impact.[9]
- Conducting systematic reviews and meta-analyses to synthesize findings from large bodies of research.[10]
- Conducting health impact assessments that can increase recognition of social determinants of health and of inter-sectoral responsibility for health (see also ➲ Chapter 1.5).[11]
- Employing cost-effectiveness studies to compare costs of a programme or policy with some measure of health impact or outcome (see also ➲ Chapter 1.6).[12]

Further resources

Further reading

Braveman PA, Egerter SA, Woolf SH, et al. (2011). When do we know enough to recommend action on the social determinants of health? *American Journal of Preventive Medicine*, **40**(Supplement 1), S58–66.

Brownson Royer C, Ewing R, McBride TD. (2006). Researchers and policymakers: travelers in parallel universes. *American Journal of Preventive Medicine*, **30**, 164–72.

Choi BC, Pang T, Lin V, et al. (2005). Can scientists and policy makers work together? *Journal of Epidemiology and Community Health*, **59**, 632–7.

Dannenberg AL, Bhatia R, Cole BL, et al. (2008). Use of health impact assessment in the U.S.: 27 case studies, 1999–2007. *American Journal of Preventive Medicine*, **34**, 241–56.

Frenk J. (1992). Balancing relevance and excellence: organizational responses to link research with decision making. *Social Science & Medicine*, **35**, 1397–404.

Innvaer S, Vist G, Trommald M, et al. (2002). Health policy-makers' perceptions of their use of evidence: a systematic review. *Journal of Health Services Research & Policy*, **7**, 239–44.

Kelly MP, Morgan A, Bonnefoy J, et al. (2007). *The social determinants of health: developing an evidence base for political action: final report to World Health Organization Commission on the Social Determinants of Health*. WHO, Geneva.

Nelson DE, Brownson RC, Remington PL, et al. (eds) (2002). *Communicating public health information effectively: a guide for practitioners*. American Public Health Association. Washington, DC.

References

1 Atwood K, Colditz GA, Kawachi I. (1997). From public health science to preventive policy. Placing science in its social and political contexts. *American Journal of Public Health*, **87**, 1603–6.

2 Rychetnik L, Wise M. (2004). Advocating evidence-based health promotion: reflections and a way forward. *Health Promotion International*, **19**, 247–57.

3 Dorfman L, Wallack L, Woodruff K. (2005). More than a message: framing public health advocacy to change corporate practices. *Health Education & Behavior*, **32**, 320–36.

4 Brownson RC, Royer C, Ewing R, et al. (2006). Researchers and policymakers: travelers in parallel universes. *American Journal of Preventive Medicine*, **30**, 164–72.

5 Whitehead M, Petticrew M, Graham H, et al. (2004). Evidence for public health policy on inequalities: 2: assembling the evidence jigsaw. *Journal of Epidemiology and Community Health*, **58**(10), 817–21.

6 Black N. (2001). Evidence based policy: proceed with care. *British Medical Journal*, **323**, 275–9.

7 Sorian R, Baugh T. (2002). Power of information: closing the gap between research and policy. *Health Affairs*, **21**, 264–73.

8 Martens PJ, Roos NP. (2005). When health services researchers and policy makers interact: tales from the tectonic plates. *Healthcare Policy*, **1**, 72–84.

9 Brownson RC, Chriqui JF, Stamatakis KA. (2009). Understanding evidence-based public health policy. *American Journal of Public Health*, **99**, 1576–83.

10 Anderson LM, Brownson RC, Fullilove MT, et al. (2005). Evidence-based public health policy and practice: promises and limits. *American Journal of Preventive Medicine*, **28**(Supplement 5), 226–30.

11 Cole BL, Fielding JE. (2007). Health impact assessment: a tool to help policy makers understand health beyond health care. *Annual Review of Public Health*, **28**, 393–412.

12 Brownson RC, Gurney JG, Land GH. (1999). Evidence-based decision making in public health. *Journal of Public Health Management and Practice*, **5**, 86–97.

Translating policy into indicators and targets

John Battersby

Objectives

Indicators and targets have been used in industry for many years and they are widely used to measure and manage health systems. Reports to hospital boards, for example, routinely include performance indicators and many organizations use sets of indicators or dashboards.

An understanding of what indicators are and how indicators and targets are constructed is essential for public health practitioners. You will be called on to interpret indicators, the performance of your department or team may be monitored using indicators, and you will be expected to meet targets. You may also have to construct indicators and set targets for others.

Reading this chapter should improve your understanding of:

• what targets and indicators are
• what they can be used for
• how to go about constructing a good indicator
• how to go about setting a target
• when to avoid using indicators and targets.

The focus of this chapter is on constructing indicators and setting targets. To learn about using existing goals, targets, and indicators to best advantage, see ⮕ Chapter 4.4.

Definitions

There are a number of definitions of the terms 'indicator' and 'target'. For the purposes of this chapter, the following definitions have been used:

• *Indicator*: a summary measure that describes the condition or performance of a system, implying a direction.
• *Target*: a specific, time-bound, destination.

In other words, a target suggests what you are trying to achieve and an indicator shows you how close you are to achieving it.

Why should you use indicators and targets?

Turkey farmers in Norfolk, UK, know the old saying, 'You can't fatten a turkey by weighing it.' What applies to turkeys also applies to health systems: measuring performance does not necessarily improve it. There are two reasons for measuring performance:

• So you know when things are going wrong. For example, if you do not regularly measure infection rates following surgery, you will not know if and when they are getting worse.
• So you know when things are going right. If you redesign a care pathway, you need to measure its outcomes to know whether you have improved care or not.

Indicators can be used to measure various elements of health and health-care. What a particular indicator measures will be determined by how that indicator is constructed, but it will measure either health status (inequality), the provision of health services (equity), or the performance of the system itself.

Performance can be measured:
- at different places, either geographic or organizational
- at different stages in a pathway (e.g. in relation to structures, processes, outputs, or outcomes)
- at different times (e.g. the same measure repeated annually).

Understanding variation

Have you ever considered why you measure things? If nothing ever varied, we would not need to measure but, just as physiological parameters like blood pressure or weight vary, so do aspects of health and health systems.

Indicators are typically used to make a comparison with an average or benchmark so the key to making effective use of indicators is understanding variation. There are three causes of variation:
- chance
- artefact
- real differences.

Variation due to chance, sometimes called 'common cause variation', occurs with all measurement. There are a variety of statistical techniques for distinguishing whether variation is due to chance or whether it reflects a real difference between measurements (sometimes called 'special cause variation'). These include tools such as funnel plots[1], process control charts[2], and, particularly for measuring individual performance, cumulative sum monitoring[3]. Figure 4.3.1 shows an example of a funnel plot.

These techniques, which are all forms of *statistical process control* (SPC), separate out common cause variation from special cause variation.[4] Such techniques originated in the commercial sector and are now often used to understand indicators and targets in healthcare. Common cause variation is normal and inevitable. In contrast, special cause variation requires further investigation to understand what is causing it and what action to take.

Variation due to artefact may often show itself as special cause variation and investigation of special cause variation needs to exclude artefacts as a possible cause. Common types of artefact are changes in the definition of an indicator, changes in the method of data collection, and errors in the coding or classification of data.

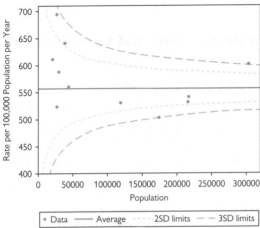

Local Authority rate of hip fracture in persons ages 65 and over in East of England (2014–15)

• Data —— Average ---- 2SD limits — — 3SD limits

Source: Public Health Outcomes Framework
Note: Population is adjusted due to Standardisation Calculations

Figure 4.3.1 A funnel plot (generated using the APHO tool[5,6]) showing the rate of hip fractures in persons aged 65 and over in local authorities in the East of England during 2014 and 2015. Each dot on the funnel plot equates to one local authority.

How is an indicator constructed?

An indicator is constructed from a numerator and a denominator. The resulting proportion or ratio can then be compared with a standard (e.g. a regional average or benchmark). Table 4.3.1 gives an example of how data on the number of obese children in a school can be used to construct an indicator suitable for comparison. Statistical tests, such as the SPC techniques

Table 4.3.1 Using data on the number of obese children in a school to construct an indicator suitable for comparison

Measurement	Comparator
a (numerator), e.g. number of obese children aged 6 at a school	C (average or benchmark), e.g. mean proportion of obese children aged 6 at schools in the region
b (denominator), e.g. all children aged 6 at the school	

used for understanding variation, can be applied to assess whether the difference between the measurement and the comparator is due to common cause or special cause variation.

How do you select and use indicators?

Selecting indicators is not always straightforward. Issues to consider when choosing an indicator include the following:
* Is the issue you want to measure important?
* Does the indicator you want to use measure a relevant aspect of the issue?
* Is the indicator you plan to use valid (i.e. does it measure what it is supposed to measure?)?
* Can you obtain the data you need for the indicator and will it be timely?
* Is the indicator you plan to use sufficiently sensitive (i.e. will it detect changes in the system?)?
* Is the indicator meaningful? A useful test is whether you can explain it to somebody else.
* Do you know how to respond if the indicator is high or low? If not, do not use it!

Sometimes managers ask for an indicator that sums up a whole system but it is rarely possible to achieve this through a single indicator and you might instead consider using a selection of indicators that measure different but important parts of the system. Such selections are known by a variety of names including *baskets of indicators, dashboards, balanced* scorecards, or *performance frameworks*.

You will often find someone else has already done the work for you. There are many examples of *baskets of indicators* that allow you to choose from a selection of validated indicators. In some countries, there may be nationally developed sets of validated indicators that can be used. For example, in England, the Public Health Outcomes Framework is a national-level set of validated public health indicators.[7]

The secret to using indicators successfully lies in communication. Indicators on their own are rarely sufficient to persuade people or organizations to change but, if communicated effectively, they can help to drive change. A useful tip when using indicators to change behaviour is to involve stakeholders in the choice or development of the indicators that you will be using to monitor them.

Understanding targets

Targets are widely used in the management of healthcare systems and can be useful for clarifying priorities and setting expectations. Targets may also be linked to sanctions and this is often the case for performance management targets, or rewards, such as the use of stretch targets where success is linked to additional financial reward. Whatever their purpose, targets should be SMART: Specific, Measurable, Achievable, Relevant/Realistic, and Time bound.

Some measures can act as both targets and indicators depending on how they are used. For example, life expectancy is commonly used as an indicator of the health of a population and to compare the health of different populations. Life expectancy has many of the properties of an indicator, is objectively quantifiable, and is a proxy measure, because health itself cannot readily be measured. Life expectancy can also be used as a target.

How do you set and use targets?

The process of setting a target can be split into three stages:

- scoping
- gathering baseline data
- pitching.

Scoping

This involves deciding what the target should cover and what indicator (or indicators) you are going to use to monitor it. You need to be very clear about what you are trying to achieve. For example, are you trying to motivate an effective team to deliver even better results or do you want to set a clear standard against which to judge performance? Because targets are increasingly used to hold people or organizations to account, it is important to include stakeholders in the scoping process.

Gathering baseline data

You will need to understand both current and historical patterns in the indicators you have chosen. For example, mortality rates from cardiovascular disease in most developed countries are falling. If the historical trend in mortality is not considered when setting a target, it is easy to choose a target that can be reached without additional action.

Availability of data over the full time period can be a problem. It may be impossible to establish a trend accurately if methods of data collection have changed. Similarly, the quality of data coding needs to be considered because poor-quality coding may prevent certain data from being used to measure progress towards a target.

Pitching

Pitching is the process of deciding how much change you are aiming for. This requires an understanding of how much change is possible and, given the likely effort and resources required to achieve change, how much change is realistic. Too often you see targets that have been chosen seemingly at random (e.g. a 10% reduction in emergency admissions over the next year) when proper pitching of the target would have shown clearly that it was either impossible to achieve or could only have been achieved by investing more resources than available.

Deciding the way in which a target is expressed is also part of the pitching process—for example, as:

- *absolute*: reducing waiting times for potential cancer patients to two weeks
- *proportional*: reducing teenage pregnancy by 25%
- *relative to a benchmark or expected level*: reducing cardiovascular disease mortality to the level of the lowest in Europe.

When using targets you should:
- have a clear monitoring process
- provide regular feedback to those involved in delivery
- avoid blame—try to understand why a target is not being met
- periodically review the target
- do not expect all targets to be met—if targets are always met, they are probably not sufficiently challenging!

What are the potential pitfalls of using indicators and targets?

Several problems are associated with the use of indicators and targets:
- Their appeal: indicators and targets appeal to people in authority (e.g. managers and politicians) but this may not be matched by an understanding of how the indicator or target has been arrived at.
- They can make people feel threatened and a missed target or judgement of poor performance can be demoralizing.
- Resources are required to construct, and particularly to collect, the necessary data to populate indicators or to assess the achievement of a target—those resources could be used elsewhere.
- They may encourage people to focus on the wrong issue. For example, in England, targets associated with smoking cessation services have at times diverted attention away from the broader work of reducing smoking prevalence.
- They can create unintended outcomes. For example, a focus on shortening emergency waits may result in unnecessary hospital admissions.
- Targets may work against each other. For example, a target to increase the numbers of laboratory samples requested by clinicians may result in 'apparent' increases in certain infections because the laboratory is detecting infections that are not clinically important.
- The final pitfall is associated with not using them. Failure to use indicators and targets correctly can result in wasted resources and potential harm to patients.

The key to avoiding most of these pitfalls is for those who are measuring (often managers) and those who are being measured (often clinicians or other practitioners) to have a shared understanding of how the indicator or target has been developed and how it is going to be used.

Some myths about indicators and targets

- *You can develop a single indicator to measure a whole system:* unfortunately you cannot—no one measure can reflect the complexity of health systems.

- *You always need to develop an indicator from scratch:* much work has been done on developing validated indicators for use across health and social care, and you will often find one that exists already.
- *Indicators tell you what to do:* in fact, indicators generally raise questions. Their usefulness is in pinpointing what questions to ask.
- *Targets are bad:* targets can be used badly or be poorly constructed, but they are not in themselves bad.
- *Data needs to be perfect:* data is never perfect but is often good enough. Part of the skill in constructing an indicator is in ensuring that the data source is good enough, and recognizing that it is acceptable to improve the indicator rather than the system.

How will you know when you have identified a good indicator?

You will know you have got it about right when:
- those affected by the indicator feel motivated and encouraged
- nobody complains about it
- managers can use it to demonstrate service improvement
- politicians ask you to develop some more!

Emerging issues

Indicators have been used for many years to measure processes, outputs, and outcomes. There is an increasing focus on using indicators to measure quality of care (see also ➲ Chapter 5.10)—in England, this is reflected in the way in which organizations such as NHS Improvement and the Care Quality Commission approach their work.

Quality has often been defined in terms of clinical outcomes but there are now also requirements to include measures based on data from users of services. A good example of this is the NHS Friends and Family Test.[8] Collecting user data is usually done using a survey approach and it is both time-consuming and expensive.

Another emerging issue is the increasing public availability of data. Both raw data and indicators are becoming more available online. There is a risk that this availability of data will not be matched by the increasing level of skill required to interpret and understand it.

Further resources

Further reading

Battersby J, Williams C. (2003). *Quantifying performance: using performance indicators*. Briefing papers on topical public health issues, 4. Eastern Region Public Health Observatory, INpho, Cambridge.

Dancox M. (2008). *Technical briefing 4: target setting in a multi-agency environment*. APHO, York. Available at: ℜ www.apho.org.uk/resource/item.aspx?RID=54328 (accessed 21 August 2019).

ECHI—European Core Health Indicators. Available at: ℜ https://ec.europa.eu/health/indicators/echi/list_en (accessed 21 August 2019).

NHS Institute for Innovation and Improvement (2008). The Good Indicators Guide: understanding how to use and choose indicators. Association of Public Health Observatories and the NHS Institute for Innovation and Improvement, Coventry. Available at: ℜ http://webarchive. nationalarchives.gov.uk/20170106081109/http://www.apho.org.uk/resource/view. aspx?RID=44584 (accessed 21 August 2019).

Public Health England (2017). Technical guide: RAG rating indicator values. Available at: ℜ https:// fingertips.phe.org.uk/documents/PHDS%20Guidance%20-%20RAG%20Ratings.pdf (accessed 21 August 2019).

References

1 Spiegelhalter D. (2002). Funnel plots for institutional comparison [comment]. *Quality and Safety in Health Care*, **11**, 390–1.

2 Mohammed MA, Cheng KK, Rouse A, et al. (2001). Use of Shewhart's technique. *Lancet*, **358**, 512.

3 Bolsin S, Colson M. (2000). The use of the Cusum technique in the assessment of trainee competence in new procedures. *International Journal of Quality Health Care*, **12**, 433–8.

4 Flowers J. (2007). *Technical briefing 2: Statistical process control methods in public health intelligence*. APHO, York. Available at: ℜ www.apho.org.uk/resource/item.aspx?RID=39445 (accessed 21 August 2019).

5 Public Health England. *Public Health Outcomes Framework 2016 to 2019*. Available at: ℜ https:// www.gov.uk/government/uploads/system/uploads/attachment_data/file/545605/PHOF_ Part_2.pdf (accessed 21 August 2019).

6 APHO Funnel Plot tool for rates. Available at: ℜ www.apho.org.uk/resource/item. aspx?RID=47240 (accessed 21 August 2019).

7 Public Health Outcomes Framework. Available at: ℜ www.phoutcomes.info (accessed 21 August 2019).

8 NHS Friends and Family Test. Available at: ℜ www.england.nhs.uk/ourwork/pe/fft (accessed 21 August 2019).

Chapter 4.4

Translating goals, indicators, and targets into public health action

Rebekah A. Jenkin, Christine M. Jorm, and Michael S. Frommer

Objective

The objective of this chapter is to help you improve your use of goals, targets, and indicators in guiding and informing the choice, implementation, and evaluation of public health action.

Why is this an important public health skill?

In public health practice, the effort to base policy on evidence is crucial. Goals, indicators, and targets enable governments and health agencies to specify responsibilities for the health of populations and communities. They can also help galvanize public health action, and the compilation of indicator data provides metrics for gauging progress. The depth of organizational and community commitment to the policies and programmes that goals promote and represent is important. Specific, challenging, well-defined, time-limited goals lead to higher levels of task performance than vague and easily realized goals or a lack of goals.[1] Goals are only motivational if individuals and organizations are committed to them. Commitment is determined by such factors as the perceived value of specific goals, the perceived potential for goal attainment, the source and legitimacy of goals, and the use of sanctions and incentives.

Uses of goals, targets, and indicators

We can use goals, targets, and indicators to:
- guide the design and selection of interventions
- help focus implementation efforts
- provide a means of evaluating programmes and policies.

Using goals, targets, and indicators at different levels of public health practice

The international level

The eight ambitious United Nations' Millennium Development Goals (MDGs)[2] were adopted in 2000 to halve abject poverty by 2015 and address problems such as infectious disease, education, and gender equality. The MDGs were widely publicized and promoted, and many international luminaries and bodies publicly committed to pursuing them. Ultimately, some of those goals were met and others were not, but the designers of the subsequent Sustainable Development Goals (see ➍ Further resources) were able to build on and learn from what had worked and what had not in relation to the MDGs. For some regions (particularly sub-Saharan Africa and South Asia), the lack of prioritization of development needs coupled with a lack of ownership and complexity stymied progress.[3] Self-evidently, goals with such breadth may have limited utility at the local or even national level. Moreover, high-level global goals may overlook questions of local sustainability, local priorities, and capacity for implementation.[4] For instance, while maternal mortality remains an important problem internationally, the numbers of maternal deaths amenable to prevention in developed countries is very small. Programmes to prevent maternal deaths may therefore not constitute a public health priority in developed countries but in all settings there are shifting needs and priorities and goals need to reflect these.[5]

The real value of international goals and targets in public health may be in setting a worldwide policy agenda to which individual nations can subscribe, enabling them to use relevant goals to energize national agendas.

The national level

In most countries, mechanisms exist to ensure that the priorities of regional or local health authorities reflect national priorities. In Australia, for example, regional health authorities are accountable to state and territory governments that, in turn, have performance-based funding agreements with the Australian government. These agreements require reporting on the implementation of specified health programmes and, when possible, health outcomes.[6, 7] Analogous arrangements exist in other countries where funds flow from a central health policy agency to local health service agencies.

An example of national health goals promoted with the aim of directing regional and local public health activities in Australia is the country's National Preventative Health Strategy (2009). The strategy recommended a range of interventions aimed at reducing the chronic disease burden associated with three lifestyle risk factors—obesity, tobacco, and alcohol—(see Box 4.4.1).

> **Box 4.4.1 Examples of targets and associated projected national outcomes from the Australian National Preventative Health Strategy**
>
> *Aim:* halt and reverse the rise in overweight and obesity
>
> *Target:* prevention of half a million premature deaths if obesity is maintained at current levels between now and 2050
>
> *Aim:* reduce the prevalence of daily smoking to 10% or less
>
> *Target:* 1 million fewer people smoking in Australia by 2020, resulting in prevention of 300,000 premature deaths from four of the most common smoking-related diseases alone
>
> *Aim:* reduce the proportion of Australians who drink at short-term risky or high-risk levels from 20% to 14%, and the proportion of Australians drinking at high-risk levels from 10% to 7%
>
> *Target:* prevention of (a) more than 7,200 premature deaths; (b) the loss of 94,000 person-years of life; (c) 330,000 hospital admissions; (d) 1.5 million bed days. Savings of nearly $2 billion to the national health sector by 2020.[a]
>
> a) National Preventative Health Taskforce (2009). The healthiest country by 2020—national preventative health strategy—the roadmap for action. Australian Government, Canberra.

National-level activity can be particularly effective in situations where a policy or legislative change is required to achieve a public health goal. For example, legislation is an effective tool in regulating the sale of cigarettes or alcohol by banning smoking from public places or the serving of alcohol to intoxicated persons. Enforcement of legislation such as the wearing of seat belts, or correct labelling of foods so consumers can monitor their fat or salt intake, can also be effective.

The key in each case is to link the goal or target with an effective mechanism. At a national level, such mechanisms tend to focus on the population rather than the individual, although the message and effect may have individual-level outcomes—for example, children cannot purchase cigarettes or alcohol under laws setting minimum consumer ages for sale of these products. Often, though, local mechanisms must be identified to translate higher-level goals into action.

The local level

Any large-scale effort to hit a target in public health typically relies heavily on local actions and success. While national- and regional-level activities are important in establishing and maintaining policy and funding environments that enable change to occur, most of the activity occurs at a local level.

Local and regional health services have limited financial and human resources. Specialist expertise may be in short supply and community services often rely on a core of dedicated but overworked staff. Teams may be reluctant to take on new responsibilities and engage with new policies and programmes. Nationally proscribed activities, such as action plans and related goals and targets, may seem irrelevant to those who face the day-to-day reality of dealing with disadvantaged communities that have heavy burdens of morbidity and complex social problems.

Conversely, once convinced of the value of a programme or the urgent need for a solution, local health services are often opportunistic and creative in identifying and using resources to support global, national, and regional political commitment to goals and targets. These resources (funds or intellectual capacity) can be used for local priorities that mirror high-level priorities and may often provide incidental support for other (regional) priorities.

Ideally, a regional or local action plan will identify regional or local goals and targets. These set appropriate local expectations, taking account of baseline rates. Local targets may differ substantially from national or regional targets because of characteristics unique to the locality, and translation of interventions and problems into a local context.

Even in taking local action, it is important to recognize the heterogeneity of the population within defined geographic areas, not only because of variations in baseline occurrence of diseases or risk factors but also because of the varying responsiveness of particular groups to specific interventions. For some conditions, variations in baseline rates are enormous. For example, the prevalence of type 2 diabetes in many Australian indigenous communities is up to seven times that of the rest of the population.[8] The setting of targets for diabetes control in these communities requires both knowledge of the medical interventions and an understanding of indigenous social values, attitudes to illness, and community processes.[9–11]

Using targets to select interventions

There are likely to be a range of actions that could be taken to address a particular public health problem. Using established goals and targets, and being aware of the agreed indicators of performance, can help you select or set priorities among intervention options. Guidelines can assist in this process (e.g. *Deciding and specifying an intervention portfolio*[12]) as can schemes for evaluating evidence to assess possible public health interventions.[13]

Criteria for selecting interventions include the following:

- *Assessment of feasibility*: of the interventions if they were applied locally, including estimates of necessary resources: financial, infrastructural, and human.
- *Assessment of the effectiveness of the interventions*: whether they will provide short-, medium-, or longer-term solutions to the health problem; the likely magnitude of their effect in a given time period; their sustainability; and other effects on current services, positive or negative.
- *The ethics, acceptability, and distribution of the interventions*: are the expected benefits likely to reach all groups? Are they evenly distributed? Do they particularly affect some groups to the detriment of others? Are the proposed interventions appropriate and acceptable, politically, socially, and culturally, to the target communities? Are the resources required to implement the interventions equitable given the burden of the problem for different population groups or subgroups? (For more on priorities and ethics, see ➦ Chapter 1.2.)
- *Assessment of the costs associated with the potential interventions*: has an economic evaluation of the potential interventions been conducted?
- *Timing*: how soon can the potential interventions be introduced? How soon will the benefits be realized?
- *Risks*: relating to successful implementation of the interventions, which may include changes in the political and policy environment, shifts in priorities, escalation of costs, and unanticipated effects.
- *Availability of mechanisms to promote implementation*: which may include regulations, funding incentives, a requirement for public reporting, and individual performance agreements.[12-14]
- *Capacity to evaluate the intervention*: are the necessary data and expertise available to allow assessment of both baseline levels and the effects of the intervention?[13, 14]

Taking into account these criteria, and the goals, targets, and indications, local action plans will include the following:

- New interventions (i.e. those to be initiated).
- Maintenance of existing interventions, either at their current level or with some enhancement or diminution.
- Cessation of existing interventions because they are inappropriate, ineffective, or too costly. (Cessation of interventions and disinvestment in them can be difficult and is often avoided, but continuing ineffective interventions risks diluting the impact of new interventions and sending mixed and confusing messages to all stakeholders. Staged removal may be an acceptable compromise rather than immediate shutdown.)

Implementation

Implementation requires the translation of knowledge on interventions into specific local contexts, taking into account:
- local resources
- specific characteristics of the population
- incidence or prevalence of the health problem of interest
- the latency period before an effect of the intervention is observable
- local variations in the likely effectiveness of interventions.[15, 16]

Once appropriate interventions have been identified, you may find it useful to check that these interventions and the local goals and targets they are aimed at achieving:
- are consistent with higher-level (regional and national) goals and targets, if these are explicit
- reflect policies and principles such as equity of access and outcome, service quality, cost-effectiveness, and efficiency
- take account of particular areas of need, such as those of disadvantaged groups.

Implementation is likely to require the following steps:
- *Definition of terms* using existing datasets and dictionaries where available. It is essential that the same definitions and measures of terms are used throughout the periods of implementation and evaluation. For example, terms such as 'disadvantage', 'independence', and 'need' may be interpreted in a range of ways and even contested, so ensuring that they are clearly defined for the purposes of your programme—even if these definitions are not universally agreed upon—is important.
- *Analysis of regional expectations* and assessment of any significant differences between local intentions and the intentions expressed in higher-level (regional or national) goals and targets. This may include analysis of particular local problems or populations (and sub-populations at very high risk) not specifically addressed in the higher-level goals and targets.
- *Understanding context and local circumstances* that may influence the problem, and understanding the acceptability of a programme at a local level. This will include setting priorities to mitigate the effects of the determinants, taking account of the risks and benefits.
- *Reviewing the existence, effectiveness, and cost* of current local objectives and programmes relevant to the new action plan.
- *Consulting* on the validity of the goals and targets and the action plan, their acceptability to local communities (both from a consumer and professional practice perspective), and their priorities for implementation. Consultation can inform the action plan (content) *and* is a central part of the action itself (agreement and implementation).[17]
- *Utilizing* existing partnerships and recruitment of community organizations to support the action plan (see ➲ Chapter 7.4)
- *Quantifying* resources needed and resources available. The latter include existing programmes that might be relevant and amenable to leverage, resources that could be shared or shifted, and coincidental availability of appropriate funding opportunities.

Evaluating public health action

Examining progress relative to goals and targets and the monitoring of process indicators will enable you to assess the success of an action plan. Time pressures and political imperatives will make rigorous evaluation difficult[18, 19] but there are many published examples for reference and guidance when developing an evaluation framework in such circumstances.[13, 14]

There is also an ethical imperative to design action plans so that they can be the object of valid, unbiased evaluation. Although pragmatism may dictate the conduct of retrospective evaluations, these are often limited in scope and restricted in validity. In planning evaluations, it is important that you allow sufficient time for changes in health outcomes to be observed, especially if interventions are very complex.[20, 21]

Successful evaluation requires upfront planning and budgeting. The evaluation plan should be formulated *before* putting the interventions in place, allowing for the compilation of baseline data and detailed documentation of the implementation process. The concept of realist review[21] is especially helpful and aims to identify what works, for whom and in what circumstances, and why (on realist approaches, see also ➔ Chapter 2.6).

Case study: implementing a national strategy

In the course of public affairs, health interventions are sometimes carried out as components of broader political initiatives. A recent Australian example was the Northern Territory Intervention, described in Box 4.4.2. Although unsuccessful in various ways, this case offers useful learning points in relation to what can go wrong on the journey from goals, indicators, and targets to public health action.

Box 4.4.2 The Northern Territory Intervention

Background

The indigenous people of Australia are highly disadvantaged compared with other Australians. They have poorer health outcomes, lower life expectancy, higher levels of socio-economic disadvantage, and lower school completion rates. Alcohol abuse and violence, including self-harm, are particularly common in the more isolated communities.[a, b] A cycle of increasing indigenous disadvantage—so-called 'cumulative causation'—has occurred over many generations. In response to discoveries about child abuse,[d, e] the Australian government announced a reform strategy recognizing that the abuse of children in remote communities was an issue of national importance.

The resulting intervention had national and local aspects. It aimed to provide urgently needed protection for children and simultaneously announced a much wider reform agenda. The Northern Territory Intervention was implemented via legislation that also suspended existing anti-discrimination laws and blocked the right of appeal to the social security appeals tribunal. The new legislation applied to 87 prescribed Aboriginal communities within the Northern Territories. In addition, substantial government funding was provided for health and new housing.

Specific actions implemented at a local level included alcohol restrictions, pornography bans, quarantining of welfare payments (so that they could only be spent on ways deemed socially responsible and were tied to child school attendance), compulsory child health checks (including for signs of abuse), appointment of government business managers, and support to enable community stores to deliver healthier and cheaper food.

The intervention split communities nationally and locally. There was widespread criticism of its paternalistic orientation and the overriding of individual and community preferences. Equally vocal were those who hailed the intervention as a long overdue step to protect those at greatest risk of harm. International agencies, including the United Nations Committee on the Elimination of Racial Discrimination were highly critical.[f]

Results to date

It would be fair to say that the intervention has not resulted in a dramatic improvement in the living circumstances, health, and well-being of the indigenous communities it was designed to benefit. Data on the health outcomes is patchy and difficult to interpret. Preliminary data analysis suggested that income management had no beneficial effect on tobacco and cigarette sales nor on soft drink or fruit and vegetable sales—purchases have not become healthier.[g] Other data suggests that health outcomes such as childhood hospitalizations and ear and eye infections may have improved.[h]

The NTI highlights some of the difficulties in implementing complex programmes with multiple interlinked goals. Problems arise with data quality and interpretation—in particular, when increased reporting might indicate increased care and awareness rather than changes in the phenomena being measured. In the NTI, the programmes were implemented without time to prepare an evaluation framework or define appropriate indicators. Debate on the outcomes of the intervention is therefore beset with intractable differences of interpretation. The NTI experience also emphasizes the risks associated with designing and implementing an intervention without appropriate and adequate local consultation and ownership.

a) Have, M. (2010). An overview of ethical frameworks in public health: can they be supportive in the evaluation of programs to prevent overweight? BMC Public Health, 10, 638.

b) Hunter B. (2007). Cumulative causation and the productivity commission's framework for overcoming indigenous disadvantage. Australian Journal of Labour Economics, 10.

c) Hunter B. (2007). Conspicuous compassion and wicked problems. Agenda, 14, 35–51.

d) Report of the Northern Territory Board of Inquiry into the Protection of Aboriginal Children from Sexual Abuse (2007). Available at: ⅋ http://www.nt.gov.au/dcm/inquirysaac/pdf/bipacsa_final_report.pdf (accessed 21 August 2019).

e) Ampe A, Meke M (2010). Little children are sacred. Available at: ⅋ http://www.inquirysaac.nt.gov.au/pdf/bipacsa_final_report.pdf (accessed 21 August 2019).

f) Committee on the Elimination of Racial Discrimination (2010). Concluding observations of the Committee on the Elimination of Racial Discrimination. Australia, 2010, UN Doc CERD/C/AUS/CO/15-17. Available at: ⅋ https://dfat.gov.au/about-us/publications/Documents/final-cerd-report-appendix-5.pdf (accessed 21 August 2019).

g) Brimblecombe J, McDonnell J, Barnes A, et al. (2010). Impact of income management on store sales in the Northern Territory. Medical Journal of Australia, 192, 549–54.

h) Department of Families, Housing, Community Services and Indigenous Affairs. (2009). Closing the gap in the Northern Territory, whole of Government July-June 2009 monitoring report. Australian Government, Canberra.

Further resources

Further reading

Commission on Macroeconomics and Health (2001). *Macroeconomics and health: investing in health for economic development*. World Health Organization, Geneva.

Gostin LO, Powers M. (2006). What does social justice require for the public's health? Public health ethics and policy imperatives. *Health Affairs (Millwood)*, **25**, 1053–60.

New Zealand Ministry of Health Health Targets – updated annually. Available at: ⌕ https://www.health.govt.nz/new-zealand-health-system/health-targets (accessed 21 August 2019).

The Good Indicators Guide: understanding how to use and choose indicators (2017). Published by the NHS Institute for Innovation and Improvement and The Association of Public Health Observatories. Available at: ⌕ https://www.england.nhs.uk/improvement-hub/publication/the-good-indicators-guide-understanding-how-to-use-and-choose-indicators (accessed 21 August 2019).

Website

Sustainable Development Goals. Available at: ⌕ https://sustainabledevelopment.un.org/post2015/transformingourworld (accessed 21 August 2019).

References

1 Office of Disease Prevention and Health Promotion. (2018). Secretary's advisory committee report #4: Target-setting methodologies for objectives in healthy people 2030. Available at: ⌕ https://www.healthypeople.gov/sites/default/files/TargetSettingReport-8-6-18%20FINAL.pdf (accessed 21 August 2019).

2 United Nations (2000). *United Nations millennium declaration*. United Nations, New York.

3 *Lancet*/London International Development Commission (2010). The Millennium Development Goals: a cross-sectorial analysis and principles for goal setting after 2015. *Lancet*, **376**, 991–1023. Available at: ⌕ http://www.thelancet.com/mdgcommission (accessed 21 August 2019).

4 Oxman A, Lavis JAF. (2007). The use of evidence in WHO recommendations. *Lancet*, **369**, 1883–9.

5 Milne E, Schrecker T. (2017). Public health goals for a post-Brexit world. *Journal of Public Health*, **39**(2), 217–8.

6 Child and Youth Health Intergovernmental Partnership (2004). *Healthy children—strengthening promotion and prevention across Australia; developing a national public health action plan for children 2005–2008*. National Public Health Partnership, Melbourne.

7 Council of Australian Governments (2018). National Healthcare Agreement. Australian Government Printing, Canberra. Available at: ⌕ https://meteor.aihw.gov.au/content/download.phtml?customDownloadType=mrIndicatorSetAdvanced&itemIds=%5B%5D=658550&shortNames=long&includeRMA=0&userFriendly=userFriendly&form=long&media=pdf (accessed 31 May 2011).

8 Australian Institute of Health and Welfare (AIHW) (2008). *A set of Performance indicators across the health and aged care system*. Australian Government Printing, Canberra.

9 Commonwealth Department of Health and Aged Care and Australian Institute of Health and Welfare (1999). *National health priority areas report: diabetes mellitus 1998*. AIHW cat. No PHE 10. AusInfo, Canberra.

10 Hunter B. (2007). Cumulative causation and the productivity commission's framework for overcoming indigenous disadvantage. *Australian Journal of Labour Economics*, **10**.

11 Hunter B. (2007). Conspicuous compassion and wicked problems. *Agenda*, **14**, 35–51.

12 National Public Health Partnership (2000). *Deciding and specifying an intervention portfolio*. National Public Health Partnership, Melbourne.

13 Harris MJ. (2016). Evaluating Public and Community Health Programs, 2nd edn. Jossey-Bass, San Francisco.

14 Hasson H. (2010). Systematic evaluation of implementation fidelity of complex interventions in health and social care. *Implementation Science*, **5**, (67). Available at: ⌕ http://www.implementationscience.com/content/5/1/67.

15 Jorm C, Banks M, Twohill S. (2008). The dynamic of policy and practice. In: Sorenson R, Iedema R, eds, *Managing clinical processes in the health services*. Elsevier, Sydney.

16 McCaughey D, Bruning N. (2010). Rationality versus reality: the challenges of evidence-based decision making for health policy makers. *Implementation Science*, **5**, 39.

17 Evidence-Based Policymaking Collaborative (2016) Principles of evidence-based policymaking. Available at: ⅏ https://www.evidencecollaborative.org/file/191/download?token=DZtcuR7u (accessed 21 August 2019).

18 Shepperd S, Lewin S, Straus S, et al. (2009). can we systematically review studies that evaluate complex interventions? *PLoS Medicine*, **6**, e1000086.

19 Greenhalgh T, Russell J. (2005). Reframing evidence synthesis as rhetorical action in the policy making drama. *Healthcare Policy*, **11**, 31–5.

20 MacKenzie M, O'Donnell C, Halliday E, et al. (2010). Do health improvement programmes fit with MRC guidance on evaluating complex interventions? *British Medical Journal*, **340**, c185.

21 Pawson R, Greenhalgh T, Harvey G, et al. (2005). Realist review—new method of systematic review designed for complex policy interventions. *Journal of Health Services & Research Policy*, **10**(Supplement 1), 21–34.

Chapter 4.5

Media advocacy
for policy influence

Simon Chapman and Becky Freeman

Objectives

Many public health interventions are controversial or potentially controversial. The way the media handle such issues can strongly influence public and policy-maker attitudes towards them, and effective media advocacy can be a powerful way of taking forward public health initiatives.

After reading this chapter, you should have a better understanding of:

- how the media deal with public health issues
- how the framing of an issue influences whether and how it leads to changes in policy
- what you can do when a public health issue is framed in an adverse or harmful way.

Why is this an important public health skill?

A simple yet vital lesson about influencing politicians is to understand the centrality of news media in their lives. From the moment of waking, politicians are exposed more than most to how the news media are covering issues relevant to their portfolio. A clock radio may wake them; social media alerts are scanned on smartphones before getting out of bed; a newspaper is read at the breakfast table; news is consumed on the car radio on the way to work; on arrival, press secretaries brief them about opportunities and threats in the news media that day. Politicians also spend many hours in hotel rooms with their main companions being their smartphones and a television, and they will often focus on news content.

Many public health advocates put much energy into trying to secure face-to-face appointments with health ministers so they can put the case for a particular proposal. However, if a health minister has never encountered the issue previously, it is likely that a low priority will be given to meeting with people representing the issue. Politicians and their staff devote a great amount of effort to trying to get difficult issues out of news pages and to backing high-profile issues they believe will advantage them politically.

Public health advocates' tasks are therefore bound up with both keeping their issues in the news as unavoidable issues for politicians while doing all that can be done to avoid framing the politicians who need to take action as the problem. Like everyone else, politicians tend not to be attracted to people or movements that are constantly critical of them and prefer to deal with people who put them in a good light. Attacking a politician when they are the person who needs to take a political decision is generally a step of last resort and one that destines a proposal to be considered by a future (rather than current) government.[1]

The importance of understanding the media

Potent public health advocates need to make the business of news making part of their core business and, in doing so, acquire a thorough knowledge and understanding of the way news organizations operate and the nature of newsworthiness. Information about the size and demographics of the audience and readership of different media at different times of the day is basic, as is familiarity with news routines and deadlines. Advocates also need to know the predilections or interests of journalists in all news media. Some will have a particular interest in public health matters. Others will be hostile towards some of the regulatory strategies and will therefore require careful attention.

Perhaps the most basic lesson we have learned through our careers in public health advocacy is the importance of standing back from the 'text' of news and trying to understand the power of its subtexts. For example, a story about a research report on smoking in bars, and the concentration of particles inhaled by bar staff, is likely to be deemed newsworthy but this is not because of the scientific particulars of the story, the journal in which it was published, or anything to do with the quality of the research. Journalists are typically not trained in science or epidemiology and do not run critical appraisal 'quality meters' over potential research stories in deciding to run them. What they do react to is the subtext of research, which in this case is bound up with the injustice of bar staff having to endure working conditions that other workers have long been protected from when smoking has been banned from other workplaces. The force and news values of the story lie in its implied injustice and the implications for those responsible.[2] The details and science of the exposure are simply the hook to the 'real' story.

The media are peerless as sites for public health debates in which large and often influential numbers of people will engage. If a public health issue is ignored by the news media, or if the media choose to frame its meaning from the perspectives of those working against the interests of public health, it is highly unlikely that political, public, or funding support will follow. There are few, if any, examples of robust public health policy or well-funded programmes that have not been preceded and sustained by widespread and supportive news coverage. As a reporter who had 40 years' experience with *The Wall Street Journal* said: 'Well done investigative reporting produces public outrage (or policy maker outrage) that forces new regulations and laws or tougher enforcement of existing ones. Ten-thousand-watt klieg lights turned on a situation focuses the minds of policy makers very fast 38 wrds.'[3]

Framing

A core skill of effective public health media advocates is to appear to have an instinct for framing their concerns in ways that make their issues instantly comprehensible in terms of wider discourses that reach beyond the manifest or overt subject of their concerns. For example, while few people may comprehend the complexities of tobacco litigation rampant in the USA, people do understand from years of negative press reportage about the tobacco industry that the cases are being fought about allegations of negligence, cover-up, and deceit.[4] Such dimensions or subtexts allow audiences who may not have detailed knowledge or awareness about the particulars of a given issue to identify that here is something similar to an issue they *do* understand. Frames and their subtexts serve to link topics to familiar, wider socio-political discourses so that coverage of particular events are decoded by audiences as instances of more general themes or types of story.

Entman's classic description notes that framing allows us to 'select some aspects of a perceived reality and make them more salient...in such a way as to promote a particular problem definition, causal interpretation, moral evaluation and/or treatment recommendation'.[5] Dominant framings can come to define what an issue is 'about' and condition public perceptions of the appropriate political response to that issue. Work by cognitive psychologists such as Lakoff[6, 7] has underscored the importance of understanding the value dimensions to framing and newsworthiness for those wishing to become effective advocates. Such analysis represents the policy process as a semiotic battle in which conflicting parties attempt to have their conceptions of policy problems, acceptable solutions, evaluation criteria, and legitimate policy actors dominate those of their opponents.[8, 9] The policy process is portrayed as a social drama centred on conflict over the appropriate terms of the debate.[10]

Much news is not instructively seen as news but as 'olds'—essentially the retelling of age-old stories with new casts, circumstances, infectious agents, and so on. For example, the ongoing news saga about doping and anabolic steroid use in sport is essentially the retelling of the myth of Narcissus—a moral tale about the dangers of vanity, inflected to involve another widely understood subtext: that cheats should not prosper. Effective public health advocates must learn to think about their issues in such terms, rather than assume that news media have an intrinsic interest in specific issues like cancer, infection, injury, and so on.

There is no 'objective reality' that any platform of public health policy can be said to be *really* about. News discourse about public health issues is often heated and this testifies to the essentially contested nature of advocacy. To injury-prevention specialists, compulsory bicycle helmets might mean reduced brain injury and deaths; to indifferent parents, their meaning might be framed more in terms of additional expense; and to fashion-conscious young people, the intrusion of a paternalistic state on their ability to dress as they please and thumb their nose at danger. Reality is always a socially constructed notion.

The emphasis or framing that is placed around particular events or issues and that seeks to define *what this issue is really about* will represent only one of many competing meanings that jostle for public dominance. While health interests may frame the meaning of a bill to introduce proof of immunization in terms of the protection of children's health, anti-immunizationists may choose to describe the bill in terms of the encroachment of the 'nanny state', 'compulsory medication', and other negative metaphors.[11]

Examples of the use of media advocacy

Politics, and therefore the progression of public health policy, is largely about the problem of competing interest groups seeking to advance multiple definitions of the same events. In public health, policy advocacy is ultimately the process by which advocates for different positions and values seek to define what is at issue for the public, media gatekeepers, and policy makers and legislators.

Examples

Are taxes on sugar-sweetened beverages: [12]
- an economic disaster in the making that will cause the collapse in gross domestic product and employment?
- an inappropriate governmental intrusion that is another example of the 'nanny state' going too far in its attempts to control our lives?

Or
- an effective way to address rising obesity rates and generate funds for much-needed childhood-obesity prevention programmes?

Are policies to restrict alcohol advertising:[13]
- overkill and unwarranted for a responsible drinks industry that contributes to the community?
- non-urgent and not the government's preferred policy option?

Or
- the sensible public health response and a necessity for the protection of children?

In 2012, Australia was the first country in the world to implement tobacco product plain-packaging laws. This law requires that cigarette packs have a large pictorial health warning on both the front (75% of the surface) and the back (90% of the surface), and that the remaining pack surface be a drab dark brown colour. No company logos, trademarks, or brand colours are permitted. Unsurprisingly, the tobacco industry was vehemently opposed to the introduction of such a law and launched a full-scale mass media and lobbying effort to prevent such a policy from being enacted.[14] The tobacco industry employed a wide range of frames and arguments in an attempt to position plain packaging as an unviable policy measure. The tobacco control workforce and other supportive stakeholders were able to systematically and strategically counter these arguments through: 1) studying and proactively anticipating negative reaction to policy, and 2) leveraging the decimated reputation of the tobacco industry to continuously question the validity of their opposition.[15]

Effectively countering, or reframing, the arguments of those opposed to public health policies is essential in generating positive news coverage. Table 4.5.1 sets out how public health advocates countered opposition to plain packaging reforms and ensured supportive arguments.

Table 4.5.1 Public health advocacy reframing

Argument against plain packaging	Public heath reframing in support of plain packaging	Supportive resource or tool
Plain packaging won't work to reduce tobacco use.	Why is the tobacco industry spending so much time and resources opposing a policy it says will no impact? The more the tobacco industry opposes a policy, the more likely it is to work.	Evidence and detailed literature reviews. Plain language, bullet summaries of why plain packaging will work to reduce the appeal of smoking.
It's never been done before.	Opportunity for Australia to show leadership. Australia need not follow other nations but can be a trailblazer and innovator.	Compare with other successful Australian innovations
Slippery slope: other products will be subject to these same laws.	Emphasize the unique and heavy public health burden of tobacco products. Highlight that no other products are totally banned from promoting their products through mass media.	History of reforms showing the long timelines in gradually reducing where and how tobacco companies can promote their products.

References

1 Chapman S. (2007). *Public health advocacy and tobacco control: making smoking history.* Blackwell Publishing: Oxford.
2 Champion D, Chapman S. (2005). Framing pub smoking bans: an analysis of Australian print news media coverage, March 1996–March 2003. *Journal of Epidemiology and Community Health*, **59**, 679–84.
3 Otten AL. (1992). The influence of the mass media on health policy. *Health Affairs*, **11**(4), 111–8.
4 Carter SM, Chapman S. (2003). Smoking, health and obdurate denial: the Australian tobacco industry in the 1980s. *Tobacco Control*, **12**(Supplement 3), iii23–30.
5 Entman RM. (1993). Framing: toward clarification of a fractured paradigm. *Journal of Communication*, **43**, 51–8.
6 Lakoff G. (2004). *Don't think of an elephant. Know your values and frame the debate.* Chelsea Green Publishing, Vermont.
7 Lakoff G. (1996). *Moral politics: what Conservatives know that Liberals don't.* University of Chicago Press, Chicago.
8 Schon DA, Rein M. (1994). *Frame reflection: toward the resolution of intractable policy controversies.* Basic Books: New York.
9 Majone G. (1989). *Evidence, argument and persuasion in the policy process.* Yale University Press, New Haven.
10 Greenhalgh T. (2006). Reframing evidence synthesis as rhetorical action in the policy making drama. *Healthcare Policy*, **1**, 34–42.

11 Leask J, Chapman S, Cooper S. (2010). 'All manner of ills': attribution of serious disease to vaccination. *Vaccine*, **28**, 3066–70.

12 Niederdeppe J, Gollust SE, Jarlenski, MP et al. (2013). News coverage of sugar-sweetened beverage taxes: pro-and antitax arguments in public discourse. *American Journal of Public Health*, **103**(6), e92–8.

13 Fogarty AS, Chapman S. (2012). Advocates, interest groups and Australian news coverage of alcohol advertising restrictions: content and framing analysis. BMC Public Health, **12**(1), 727.

13 Chapman S, Alpers P, Agho K, et al. (2006). Australia's 1996 gun law reforms: faster falls in firearm deaths, firearm suicides, and a decade without mass shootings. *Injury Prevention*, **12**, 365–72.

14 Chapman S, Freeman B. (2014). Removing the emperor's clothes: Australia and tobacco plain packaging. Sydney University Press, Sydney. Available at: ℬ http://purl.library.usyd.edu.au/sup/9781743323977. (accessed 21 August 2019).

15 Freeman B. (2011). Tobacco plain packaging legislation: a content analysis of commentary posted on Australian online news. *Tobacco Control*, **20**(5), 361–6.

Influencing international policy

Tim Lang and Martin Caraher

Objectives

This chapter will help you understand:

• the relationships between international policy and policy action at multiple levels;
• why public health practitioners should build an international dimension into their work;
• how to influence and advance public health internationally, even through local action.

The chapter uses examples from the world of food and health policy (on which the authors work) to illustrate the structures and processes of engagement you may encounter. In the policy worlds of both global public health and food, there is a mix of improvement and threats, inequalities alongside progress, fragmentation, and coherence. Similar trends in the global South and developed countries may have underlying drivers at work, resulting in the double burden of disease.[1] It is preferable to ensure that international policies tackle rather than ignore those determinants.

Why does international policy matter for public health?

The international dimension of public health work is today essential, not least because the world is complex and connectivities are global. This requires support and coordination between actors from global to local. This coordination function can challenge your negotiation skills, because tensions between local, national, regional, and global levels of health governance may be exposed as well as challenges to the boundaries of how we define public health.

The drivers and shapers of ill health today may be physically far away but manifest locally. The food system, for example, has transcended older boundaries. New giant companies have emerged. Tastes and marketing alter what appears in shops. Media realities infuse local realities. Work has shifted from the land to the gig economy (but remains low waged).

The connection between ecosystems and public health is coming clear with data on climate change, biodiversity loss, and water stress. New 'ecological public health' thinking is required to help policy makers shift the food system, and wider economies, into new sustainable consumption (diet) and production (farm to shop) patterns.[2, 3, 4]

Over the past half-century, globalized food chains became more sophisticated and complex, driven by demands to cut costs, by new technologies, and by trade deals—a good example is the 2012–13 EU horsemeat scandal.[5] Food companies now exert health controls that used to be the preserve of health inspectorates. At the same time, disease patterns have shifted from acute to chronic, and from communicable to non-communicable. Food and dietary changes are integral to these health trends.

As with all public health, many policies influencing food and health are not directly health related: for example, trade regulations may influence food availability. The infrastructure of health—issues such as food, transport, housing, water, energy, air, and climate—can be shaped by the actions of giant companies, powerful countries, and seemingly distant institutions. It can sometimes feel as though public health services pick up the pieces scattered by others.[1, 2, 3, 6]

Why do we need to think and act internationally?

As a public health practitioner, you should think and act internationally because:

- we live in a globalised world and actions in one area of the globe affect others
- the international dimension adds to, and can alter analysis of the presenting problems
- drivers of communicable diseases and non-communicable diseases can be distant from where effects are manifest
- ill health crosses borders in new ways in the globalised world; 'vectors' are culture- and trade-related as well as biological
- the movement of people, goods, ideas, and services has implications for international public health institutions.

If goods, foods, ideas, and messages cross borders, so must public health thinking. That requires collaboration. When we promote fruit and vegetable consumption, for example, we implicitly support and affect long food-supply chains, livelihoods, and working conditions.[6] In Germany, for example, health advice to drink fruit juice led to an increase in the importation of oranges from Brazil. A study calculated that 80% of Brazilian orange production was consumed in Europe[7] and that German consumption occupied 370,000 acres of Brazilian productive land, three times the land given over to fruit production in Germany. Orange growers in Brazil typically have low incomes: most of the profits went to intermediaries such as producers and retailers, and the demand meant that local crops were replaced by crops for export.[7] This illustrates how an apparently simple health education message had complicated consequences internationally. In the case of food, a purely nutritional perspective no longer provides a full health analysis and ecological public health thinking now suggests new goals: sustainable diets from sustainable food systems.[3]

Disease knows no boundaries

Infectious diseases constantly migrate, borne by human exchange. Diet-related non-communicable diseases[8] cross borders in different ways and through different mechanisms, typically involving social and economic as well as physical pathways.

The immediate impact of HIV/AIDS, for example, led to millions of deaths. Prevention strategies followed, involving international data and knowledge sharing. However, although population weight gain is shaped by changes in the environment far beyond the immediate control of health actors,[4, 9] deaths from diet are often seen as normal or the result of individual choice. Non-communicable diseases used to be judged as rich-society diseases but today the incidence of coronary heart disease, strokes, diabetes, some cancers, and obesity have spread round the world, associated with changes in diet, physical activity, and lifestyle.[4] (See also ➔ Chapter 4.7) Obesity now coexists with malnutrition in low-income countries and, in high-income countries, high levels of obesity have produced a culture where historically high body mass indices are accepted as normal.

Questions for public health practitioners include the following:

- Do your local public health planning and surveillance systems have direct links to similar systems elsewhere in the world, enabling comparisons and shared learning?
- Do you have interdisciplinary networks that provide information at the international level? Conversely, is your information available beyond your area to add to international intelligence?

The scaling up and globalizing of economic activity require a health response

The acceleration of world trade and international economic activity has had big implications for health. Rising incomes are generally beneficial for health, although the effects appear to level off beyond a certain level of income and are affected by relative levels of equality within societies.

A particularly sensitive issue in diet and health is the influence of what some analysts now term 'Big Food' (echoing 'Big Pharma' influence in medicine). International health agencies can be nervous about challenging Big Food, fearing threats to their funding sources. There is often talk of 'partnerships' as the way to address this. Marketing is an issue on which the World Health Organization has been vocal with its government membership. The consequences of promoting unhealthy foods and the targeting of young people are adequately regulated and this is something that international public health collaboration can monitor.[9, 10, 11]

Goods cross borders too. The removal of barriers to trade at the 1994 General Agreement on Tariffs and Trade (GATT) talks accelerated emerging patterns of food trade by including food under world trade rules for the first time. The World Trade Organization (WTO) was created to facilitate the spread of goods and services. International food and health standards are now negotiated at the global level. This can act as a brake on efforts to raise standards.

People also cross boundaries. Migration of labour from the global south to the global north has many implications for healthcare, not least of which is the denuding of a country of its healthcare skills and expertise (see ➔ Chapter 7.7). Mass migrations are often undertaken in pursuit of a better life and to escape poverty and repression.[4, 10] Around one-seventh of humanity crosses borders annually, potentially spreading and catching diseases while being introduced to new lifestyles and foods.

Food trade, particularly food retailers, illustrate how globalized supply systems have relocated and altered work. Sophisticated 'just-in-time' managerial controls, developed in the car industry, are now routine in food trade. They control how food factories work, assembling ingredients and delivering products to supermarket shelves just when needed. There are potential public health risks from reliance on self-regulation here. Extended supply chains introduce many more points for possible contamination or fraud, and have led to the introduction of risk assessment and management systems such as Hazards Analysis Critical Control Point (HACCP) approaches. These have their limits, however, and twenty-first century public health protection probably needs to go further than HACCP and reconnect with lessons from the nineteenth-century health movements that asked about the social distribution of health benefits, not just economic ones.

With unequal distribution of wealth from economic activity in international supply chains, there is increasing interest among health bodies about how to ensure positive health impacts.[1, 3] Broader questions touch on the power and influence of public health professionals in fiercely competitive commercial environments:

- Can public health interests compete with powerful economic forces?
- How can we use crises (when they happen) to promote health protection measures?
- Are our professional bodies involved in international policy making to ensure that public health is part of policy frameworks?

Getting organized

In an ideal world, public health policy and practice would be evidence-based but the reality is that the relationship between evidence, policy, and practice can be tortuous.[4] Health considerations are often not represented at the policy table where critical decisions are taken.

We cannot assume that political and institutional frameworks for addressing the 'transnationalization' of health patterns are either adequately resourced or fit to keep abreast of economic, social, and cultural change. Public health work and institutions tend to be locally and nationally focused and based, partly due to funding and tax-collection systems, but economic and social changes are increasingly trans-national. There is much to learn from the long, frustrating process of trying to control the scourge of tobacco. While food is not toxic in the way that tobacco is, the ways of working by the two industries are similar: they both engage in self-regulation and challenge changes to food legislation under the banners of choice and free will.

One important lesson is that a local focus is necessary but on its own not sufficient to get change. Local initiatives need international links. Another lesson is to ensure consistent messaging. Being well organized internationally helps the process of incremental change, too. A gain in one country can be replicated and exceeded elsewhere: the small steps on soda taxes in Mexico and Berkeley offer hope to others.[12]

All this needs international liaison, trusted forums, and efficient use of new communication and monitoring technologies. 'Big Food' lobbies rarely use or challenge public health initiatives in the courts, although they may well lobby about them. This happened in the late 2000s when attempts to get optimum front-of-pack nutrition labelling failed in the EU. Heavy and sustained lobbying by some (but not all) giant food industry interests swayed the European Commission not to act for optimum health. Policy fights about labelling formats continue worldwide. They illustrate how there may be limits to the 'right to know'.

One area where public health has powerful leverage is to protect children. Children cannot be expected to make 'fully informed choices'. Not that long ago, children were seen as legitimate targets for food advertising but, after effective health campaigns using sound data, the cultural attitudes and political support have shifted. Even the advertising industry accepts the need for limits.[4, 11] There are no grounds to be relaxed, however. Stronger international codes are needed.

Refining arguments to win 'hearts and minds'

Public health professionals pride themselves on pursuing evidence-based action. But the world of policy sometimes works with weak evidence, no evidence, and biased evidence. Policy makers juggle competing demands and it is wrong to think that good and effective public health action internationally only needs facts, evidence, and risk assessments. These are essential but may be insufficient for success.[12]

You should also think about arguments that can:
• gain public support in the 'battle of ideas'
• win over key decision makers, building confidence in our data and values
• be effective in non-health arenas, such as trade and finance, and build inter-sectoral and inter-disciplinary Alliances.

Public health advocacy may range from public campaigns to behind-the-scenes influencing. It has to address global impact and agreement (see ➲ Chapter 4.5). The general public, and even public health practitioners, may be unaware of this global dimension, or be concerned about it, but it cannot be ignored. The Fairtrade movement is an example of a social movement that has linked consumer purchasing decisions in high-income countries with effects on health and incomes in low-income ones.

Global institutions: what levers do we have?

There are many institutions—governmental, non-governmental, and commercial—shaping or responding to health policy at the global level (see Table 4.6.1). Most were created in the twentieth century but others are more recent, such as the WTO. Private institutions have also emerged.[14]

Table 4.6.1 Some international institutions involved in health policy

Remit	Examples of organizations
Public health	World Health Organization (WHO), Food and Agriculture Organization (FAO), World Bank
Children and health	UNICEF, UNESCO
Global economic bodies with health impact	World Bank, International Monetary Fund, World Trade Organization (WTO), Organization for Economic Co-operation and Development (OECD), International Labour Organisation, UN Development Programme
Inter-governmental agreements with a health impact	Cartagena Bio-safety Convention 2016, Basel Convention on Hazardous Waste 1989, Convention on Biodiversity 1992, International Conference on Nutrition 2014, International Health Regulations 2005, UN Sustainable Development Goals 2015
Emergency aid	World Food Programme, International Committee of the Red Cross/Crescent
Environmental health	Global Panel on Climate Change, UN Conference on Environment & Development (UNCED), International Maritime Organization
Commercial interests	Transnational corporations, International Federation of Pharmaceutical Manufacturers Associations, World Economic Forum
Networks to promote public health	Healthy Cities Network [WHO][a], International Baby Food Action Network (IBFAN), Pesticides Action Network, Tobacco Free Initiative [WHO]

a. Abbreviations in square brackets '[]' indicates support from that organization'

Many international bodies have resolutions, reports, conventions, and agreements that have implications for public health at the local level. They provide a rationale for health monitoring and action, and knowing and being able to cite these can be very helpful in local and national policies. National governments and firms might not like to be measured against international statements, which can be sources of irritation to some interested parties.

Table 4.6.2 gives illustrations of some conventions and international agreements supporting or contextualizing public health action. There are many others. One should note that some are 'soft' commitments, lacking binding power at national or legal level (e.g. declarations). Some are criticized as being remote or undemocratic. Others have been made important by being used as yardsticks for health improvement (e.g. binding agreements that have to be ratified by national governments, before being turned into national laws). They can legitimate local or national actions, and people working inside bodies set up to service international commitments can be useful allies.

Public health depends on practitioners and researchers finding new ways to win arguments, build evidence, and improve policy and practice. International links can help generate new methods and approaches. An

Table 4.6.2 Examples of international commitments with public health relevance

Occasion	Date	Relevance
Universal Declaration of Human Rights	1948	Right to health
Stockholm Conference on the Human Environment	1972	Started environmental protection focus in public health
World Food Conference (Universal Declaration on the Eradication of Hunger and Malnutrition)	1974	Commitment to eradicate malnutrition
Ottawa Charter on Health Promotion 'Health for All'	1986	Far-reaching approach to health promotion
Innocenti Declaration on Breastfeeding	1990	WHO/Unicef commitment to support breastfeeding
Kyoto Protocol	1997	Climate change
WHO Framework Convention on Tobacco	2003	Set international benchmarks
UN Sustainable Development Goals	2015	**17** Goals and 169 targets, many of which relate to health
Paris Climate Change Accord	2015	Sets targets to reduce greenhouse gas emissions to protect human and planetary health

example of how methods can be refined and improved is the growth of impact assessments, including health impact assessments and environmental impact assessments (HIAs and EIAs; see ⟳ Chapter 1.5 and Chapter 3.2). If HIAs and EIAs were accompanied by social impact assessments, public health might have the information needed to tackle multi-level, multi-sectoral problems.

Conclusions

International aspects of public health continue to be addressed by existing organizations within the United Nations but there are now many inter-governmental bodies besides the UN. Who could argue that the World Bank or International Monetary Fund are unimportant for public health? They shape economies that determine health but also have influential positions on health action, such as healthcare costs. There are also strong international commercial bodies that take positions on health. These, and civil society organisations, compete for policy attention and influence on health.[12, 13] Sound public health protection can get lost as such bodies tussle. That is why public health practitioners need to be—and to remain—well organized, informed, and funded internationally. This must not be an after-thought. It is not a luxury. Alemanno argues that we need to exercise our voice 'to create a better society'.[13]

The causes of health problems are complex. Having an international perspective was always useful. Today it is essential. Alliances across sectors as well as regions are key ingredients for success.

Influencing health at the international level means:

- acting to promote and protect health at all levels, linking the local, national, regional, to the international
- making the links across sectors so that impacts in one area can be related to those in others
- using existing international health institutions while also strengthening, supporting, and sometimes cajoling them
- being prepared to enter sensitive policy terrain where there are existing powerful interests.

Further resources

Howard, PH. (2016). Concentration and power in the food system; who controls what we eat? Bloomsbury, London.

Labonte R, Laverack G. (2008). Health promotion in action: from local to global empowerment. Palgrave, Basingstoke.

Lang T, Barling D, Caraher M. (2009). Food policy: integrating health, environment and society. Oxford University Press, Oxford.

Unicef (2005). 1990–2005 Celebrating the Innocenti Declaration on the protection, promotion and support of breastfeeding: past achievements, present challenges and the way forward for infant and young child feeding. Unicef, Innocenti Research Centre, Florence.

References

1 Murray CLJ, Lopez AD. (2017). Measuring global health: motivation and evolution of the Global Burden of Disease Study. *Lancet*, 16 September 2017. Available at: ℞ doi: http://dx.doi.org/10.1016/S0140-6736(17)32367-X (accessed 21 August 2019).

2 Ingram J. (2017). Look beyond production. *Nature*, **544(S17)**, 27April.

3 Mason P, Lang T. (2017). *sustainable diets; how ecological nutrition can transform consumption and the food system*. Routledge, Abingdon.

4 Lang T, Barling D, Caraher M. (2009). *Food policy: integrating health, environment and society*. Oxford University Press: Oxford.

5 HM Government (2014). Elliott review into the integrity and assurance of food supply networks – final report. Available at: ℞ https://assets.publishing.service.gov.uk/government/uploads/system/uploads/attachment_data/file/350726/elliot-review-final-report-july2014.pdf (accessed 21 August 2019).

6 Ingram J. (2016). Sustainable food systems for a healthy world. *Sight and Life Magazine*, **30(1)**, 28–33.

7 Kranendonk S, Bringezau B. (1994). *Major material flows associated with orange juice consumption in Germany*. Wupperthal Institute, Wupperthal, Germany.

8 Melaku YA, Renzaho A, Gill TK, et al. (2018). Burden and trend of diet-related non-communicable diseases in Australia and comparison with 34 OECD countries, 1990–2015: findings from the Global Burden of Disease Study 2015. *European Journal of Nutrition*. doi:10.1007/s00394-018-1656-7

9 Egger G, Swinburn B. (2010). *Planet obesity: how we're eating ourselves and the planet to death*. Allen and Unwin, NSW.

10 Williams S, Nestle M. (2015). 'Big food': taking a critical perspective on a global public health problem. *Critical Public Health*, **25**, 245–7. doi:10.1080/09581596.2015.1021298

11 Cairns G, Angus K, Hastings G. et al. (2013). Systematic reviews of the evidence on the nature, extent and effects of food marketing to children. A retrospective summary. *Appetite*, **62**, 209–15. doi:10.1016/j.appet.2012.04.017

12 Caraher M, Perry I. (2017). Sugar, salt, and the limits of self-regulation in the food industry. *British Medical Journal*, **357**, doi:10.1136/bmj.j1709

13 Alemanno A. (2017). *Lobbying for change: find your voice to create a better society*. Omnibus Books, London.

14 Reiff D. (2016). *The reproach to hunger: food justice and money in the 21st century*. Verso, London.

Improving public health in low-and middle-income countries

Eric Heymann and Nicholas Banatvala

The United Nation Development Programme's (UNDP) Human Development Indices and Indicators 2018 Statistical Update (HDII 2018) reports that even as the global population increased from 5 billion to 7.5 billion between 1990 and 2017, the number of people in low human development fell from 3 billion to 926 million—or from 60% of the global population to 12%—and that the number of people in high and very high human development more than tripled, from 1.2 billion to 3.8 billion—or from 24% of the global population to 51%.[a] The 2019 global poverty update from the World Bank using the international poverty line, which was updated to $1.90 a day in 2015, to reflect new price levels in developing countries and a globalized inflation in common goods, estimates that 10.0% (735 million people, in 2015) of the world population lived under the poverty line.[2]

The data above demonstrates that significant development gains have been made across the world, with a reduction in poverty in recent decades. While these advances paint a positive picture of the global efforts to eradicate poverty in the world (and indeed human development has increased across all HDII 2018 country groups), progress within these groups has been uneven and large pockets of poverty and exclusion persist. While there has been notable progress in China, Indonesia, and India over many years, for example, progress in conflict-affected countries, such as Yemen, Libya, and Syrian Arab Republic, has fallen in recent years.

A significant challenge is reaching those that remain in extreme poverty. Many live in fragile states and remote areas where access to services is extremely limited. A further challenge is ensuring that those that have moved out of poverty remain so and that economic shocks, food insecurity, climate change, and lack of universal health coverage (UHC) do not push them back into poverty.

This chapter looks at the broader determinants of health and current approaches to tackling public health in poorer countries.

Objectives

Reading this chapter will help you understand:
- the major public health issues in low- and low middle-income countries;
- the approaches used to tackle them.

---

a The Human Development Index is a summary measure of average achievement in key dimensions of human development: a long and healthy life, being knowledgeable, and have a decent standard of living. http://hdr.undp.org/en/content/human-development-index-hdi

Why is this an important public health issue?

Health is a long-recognized human right.[3] Better health is associated with decreased poverty as it enables people to secure better livelihoods. This is true at both a micro (family) level (less time caring for the sick means more time to learn and earn) and at a macro level (less sickness leads to regional and national economic growth).

The Global Burden of Disease website and the WHO's Global Health Observatory webpages (including the World Health Statistics series) provide global, regional, and country estimates of deaths and public health challenges in the world today.[4, 5]

According to WHO, more than half of all deaths in low-income countries in 2016 were caused by the so-called Group I conditions, which include communicable diseases, maternal causes, conditions arising during pregnancy and childbirth, and nutritional deficiencies. By contrast, less than 7% of deaths in high-income countries were due to such causes. Lower respiratory infections were among the leading causes of death across all income groups.

Noncommunicable diseases (NCDs) caused 71% of deaths globally, ranging from 37% in low-income countries to 88% in high-income countries. All but one of the ten leading causes of death in high-income countries were NCDs. In terms of absolute number of deaths, however, 78% of global NCD deaths occurred in low- and middle-income countries.

Injuries claimed 4.9 million lives in 2016. More than a quarter (29%) of these deaths were due to road traffic injuries. Low-income countries had the highest mortality rate due to road traffic injuries with 29.4 deaths per 100,000 population—the global rate was 18.8. Road traffic injuries were also among the leading ten causes of death in low-, lower-middle-, and upper-middle-income countries (Table 4.7.1).[6]

Top ten causes of deaths

Table 4.7.1 Top 10 causes of death by country economic grouping

	Low-income countries	Lower-middle-income countries	Upper-middle-income countries	High-income countries
1	Lower respiratory infections	Ischaemic heart disease	Ischaemic heart disease	Ischaemic heart disease
2	Diarrhoeal diseases	Stroke	Stroke	Stroke
3	Ischaemic heart disease	Lower respiratory infections	Chronic obstructive pulmonary disease	Alzheimer disease and other dementias
4	HIV/AIDS	Chronic obstructive pulmonary disease	Trachea, bronchus, lung cancers	Trachea, bronchus, lung cancers
5	Stroke	Tuberculosis	Alzheimer disease and other dementias	Chronic obstructive pulmonary disease

	Low-income countries	Lower-middle-income countries	Upper-middle-income countries	High-income countries
6	Malaria	Diarrhoeal diseases	Lower respiratory infections	Lower respiratory infections
7	Tuberculosis	Diabetes mellitus	Diabetes mellitus	Colon and rectum cancers
8	Preterm birth complications	Preterm birth complications	Road injury	Diabetes mellitus
9	Birth asphyxia and birth trauma	Cirrhosis of the liver	Liver cancer	Kidney disease
10	Road injury	Road injury	Stomach cancer	Breast cancer

Cause Group	I. Communicable, maternal, neonatal, and nutritional conditions	II. Noncommunicable diseases	III. Injuries

In order to address these global health challenges, WHO promotes UHC. UHC means that all people and communities can use the promotive, preventive, curative, rehabilitative, and palliative health services they need, of sufficient quality to be effective, while also ensuring that the use of these services does not expose the user to financial hardship. Moving towards UHC is a political choice with important social and economic benefits. In 2019, world leaders adopted a high-level United Nations Political Declaration on UHC, the most comprehensive set of health commitments ever adopted at this level.[7] At least half of the world's population lacks access to essential health services, more than 800 million people bear the burden of catastrophic spending of at least 10% of their household income on health care, and out-of-pocket expenses drive almost 100 million people into poverty each year. Action to achieve UHC by 2030 is inadequate and that the level of progress and investment to date is insufficient to meet target 3.8 of the Sustainable Development Goals (SDGs). Currently, on average, one-third of national health expenditure is covered by out-of-pocket expenses, while less than 40% of funding on primary health care is from public sources in low- and middle-income countries.

In April 2001, the African Union countries pledged to set a target of allocating at least 15% of their annual budget to improve the health sector and urged donor countries to scale-up support. Fifteen years later, most African governments had increased the proportion of total public expenditure allocated to health. In addition, the average level of per capita public spending on health rose from about $70 in the early 2000s to more than $160 in 2014 (Parity Purchasing Power).[8] The adoption of the Addis Ababa Action Agenda on Financing for Development and of the SDGs, both in 2015,[9] has been accompanied by a growing recognition of the need to explore the nature of the resources available and the use to which they are put, rather than focusing solely on the volume of resources required to make progress towards UHC. How public monies are allocated, spent, and used has a direct impact on the level of coverage and financial protection as well as on equity.

How do we define important tasks?

UNDP highlights that just as health shapes development, development shapes health. The conditions in which people live and work, including factors such as poverty, exclusion, inequality, social status housing and environmental, and political conditions, have a major impact on health and well-being. Conversely, healthy people are better able to contribute to the social, political, and economic development of their communities and countries.

Experience with the Millennium Development Goals (MDGs), which concluded in 2015, shows progress in health is heavily dependent on progress in other areas of development and vice versa. The positive outcomes from theses MDGs (see 1st edition of the OHPH) paved the way for the 2030 Agenda for Sustainable Development and the SDGs.[10] Together they further reflect a response to the increasing complexity and interconnectedness of health and development, including widening economic and social inequalities, rapid urbanization, threats to climate and the environment, the continuing challenges of communicable and noncommunicable diseases, malaria, maternal and child health, and lack of access to UHC. Universality, sustainability, and ensuring that no one is left behind are hallmarks of the 2030 Agenda.

The 17 SDGs and 169 targets frame international development action between 2015 and 2030. The 2030 Agenda for Sustainable Development is integrated and indivisible and balance the three dimensions of sustainable development: the economic, social, and environmental. Goal 3 is to ensure healthy lives and promote well-being for all at all ages and has 17 targets around: (1) reproductive, maternal, newborn, and child health; (2) infectious diseases; (3) NCDs, mental health, and environmental risks; and (4) health systems and funding.[11]

The interconnectedness between health and the other 16 SDGs are shown in Figure 4.7.1.

The World Health Statistics 2017 highlight six lines of action to promote health in the 2030 Agenda and help monitor health for the SDGs.[12] They are as follows:

	Six main lines of action	Opportunities provided by the 2030 Agenda
Building better systems for health	Intersectoral action by multiple stakeholders	Placing health in all sectors of policy-making; combining the strengths of multiple stakeholders
	Health systems strengthening for UHC	Disease-control programmes embedded in a comprehensive health system that provides complete coverage through fully staffed and well-managed health services, with financial risk protection

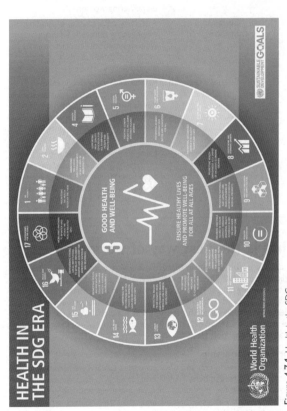

Figure 4.7.1 Health in the SDG era

Source: http://www.who.int/topics/sustainable-development-goals/test/sdg-banner.jpg?ua=1

	Six main lines of action	Opportunities provided by the 2030 Agenda
Enabling factors	Respect for equity and human rights	Improving health for whole populations by including all individuals ('leave no one behind') and empowering women
	Sustainable financing	Attracting new sources of funding; emphasizing domestic financing, with alignment of financial flows to avoid duplication of health system functions
	Scientific research and innovation	Reinforcing research and innovation as foundations for sustainable development, including a balance of research on medical, social, and environmental determinants and solutions
	Monitoring and evaluation	Exploiting new technologies to manage large volumes of data, disaggregated to ascertain the needs of all individuals; tracking progress towards SDG 3 and all other health-related targets

What is the best way of working?

No agency is able to put in place these key actions by itself. The Paris Declaration on Aid Effectiveness highlighted the importance of harmonizing and aligning aid efforts. Improving transparency in what is needed; who is willing to help, who can help, and in what way, may prevent overlap of projects and enable successful cooperation in a global effort to combat the issue at stake. Those developing strategies need to do four things to implement international policy.

Work in partnership

Partnerships between rich and poor countries can involve private and voluntary sectors, researchers, multilateral development organizations, and donors. To avoid the burden of multiple initiatives and projects, donors increasingly work with governments and other stakeholders in poor countries in a sector-wide approach, so efforts are focused on agreed priorities. Public-private partnerships include the Global Fund, Gavi—a global Vaccine Alliance, and the RBM Partnership to End Malaria. In 2019, 12 multilateral and United Nations system agencies launched Stronger collaboration, better health: global action plan for healthy lives and well-being for all.[13]

Non-state actors (non-governmental organizations, private sectors, foundations, and philanthropic) are all potential partners for health development. The tobacco industry should under no circumstances be a part of any development activity.

Use both multilateral and bilateral initiatives effectively

Bilateral aid describes support which is given directly by one government to another, whereas multilateral aid comes from numerous different governments and organizations and is usually arranged by an international organization such as the World Bank, regional development banks, the United Nations, or global health initiatives such as the Global Fund and Gavi.

Ensure local ownership of initiatives

Ensure local ownership of initiatives and local capacity development, and base activities on available evidence. This is critical for sustainable development. Sustainable Livelihoods approaches take a holistic view rather than just focusing on a few factors (e.g. economic issues, communicable disease, food security). The principles of sustainable livelihoods are that activities should be people-centred, responsive and participatory, multilevel, conducted in partnership, sustainable, holistic, and dynamic.

Match political commitment with funding and debt relief

Maintaining funding for international development and for global health is a significant challenge. These problems become harder to promote whenever there is pressure on international financial systems, such as in times of world economic crises. UN summits,10 as well as the G8 and other gatherings, provide opportunities to promote political and financial commitment for development, including debt relief, as well as using development assistance more effectively. UN high-levels meetings on NCDs (2011 and 2018), antimicrobial resistance (2016), and UHC (2019), as well as the 2030 Sustainable Agenda (2015) are important milestones in the global effort to tackle global health and development challenges but require commitment to funding and action to achieve their goals.

The SDG Health Price Tag released in 2017 estimates that achieving the SDG health targets (preventing 97 million premature deaths) would require new investments increasing over time from an initial $134 billion annually to $371 billion, or $58 per person, by 2030 (the so-called ambitious scenario). A 'progress' scenario in which countries get two-thirds or more of the way to the targets (preventing about 71 million premature deaths) would require new investments increasing from an initial $104 billion a year to $274 billion, or $41 per person, by 2030.[14]

Factors essential to success

The aforementioned agenda is more likely to succeed if a number of fundamental principles are adhered to. Success unlikely unless we can
* ensure government ownership. This requires development partners to align their activities with government policy and programming.

- address the causes rather than just the symptoms of ill-health. This requires working across the SDGs in their entirety.
- remove barriers that prevent the poor accessing services. This requires UHC.
- assure public standards, accountability, and responsiveness as well as strengthening state policy making, regulation, and service provision. This requires strong systems of governance and commitment to measuring progress.
- work in partnership with others. This requires harmonization of activities.
- encourage aid and development system to be ever more effective. This requires transparency, investment in research and development, and commitment to implementing evidence-based, cost-effective interventions.[15]

Nine fallacies

International public health policy is as prone to dogma as any area of domestic public health.

Fallacy 1: Models focused on a single discipline are most effective in tackling public health problems in developing countries

Approaches to international health have changed over time and biomedical, economic, and institutional/governance approaches have each been promoted. The present consensus is that poverty reduction should be at the core of international development policy and addressed through a range of different disciplines.

Fallacy 2: Either vertical or horizontal public health programmes are always better

Vertical programmes have been successful in areas such as immunization and communicable diseases (e.g. the cost-effective TB treatment strategy known as DOTS (directly observed treatment, short course) and insecticide-treated bed nets for malaria). In the longer term, however, sustainable services need health systems that integrate into national health systems rather than focus on a few specific interventions and services.

Fallacy 3: The cost of action and attaining the SDGs and universal health coverage cannot be met

The SDG targets and wider international health commitments will not be easy to achieve—and in some areas, especially in sub-Saharan Africa, are seriously off-track—but there remains the chance of meeting them if there is effective international cooperation, maintaining (and where necessary increasing) funding for programme activity, as well as R&D, and employing principles of sustainable livelihoods.

Fallacy 4: Models of health care delivery developed in Western settings can be effectively transferred to other situations

Enthusiasm for health sector reform based on management trends in Europe (decentralization, managerial autonomy, contracting, and internal market mechanisms) has been dampened by a realization that reforms must be tailored to local circumstances. Nevertheless, there are often examples where middle- and low-income countries can adapt the experience of OECD countries when it comes to contracting, providing incentives for effective healthcare delivery, and developing indicators that measure aspects of a successful healthcare. No single mix of policy options will work in every setting.

Fallacy 5: Cost-recovery systems are an effective approach to providing long-term delivery of health services

Cost-recovery systems (self-sustaining systems financed by the local community) have fallen out of favour because of concerns about equity, with poorer patients excluded and subsidies benefiting the non-poor. In any event, revenue yields have often been minimal.

Fallacy 6: In developing countries there is no place for anything other than publically funded and run services

The private sector can under government leadership provide services and stronger health systems. The private sector has an important role in research and development. This sector is also critical in implementing government policy (e.g. in efforts to reduce harmful use of alcohol and promote healthy diet).

Fallacy 7: There are too many players in international health with policies muddled through the competing agendas of UN agencies, NGOs, and others

Compared with the number of agencies in developed countries, the number of agencies in development projects in resource-poor countries is often small. All the same, the number of agencies responding to global health needs has grown and can lead to a challenge of co-ordination and competition for financial and media opportunities. Governments and other institutional donors have a responsibility to distribute funds to agencies with proven track records in the field of work and geographic region.

Fallacy 8: The real threat to development is globalization

Globalization and urbanization are far from detrimental. There are plenty of opportunities, if harnessed appropriately, that come from a global community: (1) economic; (2) trade agreements; (3) international response to debt relief; (4) communication and rapid transfer of information, maximizing flows of finance and capital; and (5) investment, competition. But for globalization and urbanization to work for all, it is crucial that public health is at the centre of government policy making.

Fallacy 9: Funding development activities is more effective than funding relief

Disaster preparedness and prevention are an essential component of development assistance. Disasters, natural and of human origin, including war, are more common in poor countries. The 'relief–development continuum' (cycles of relief and development) with agencies co-operating in different areas of expertise and 'developmental relief' (development models used in chronic relief efforts and often in complex emergencies) are both increasingly accepted approaches.

Examples of successes, failures, and lessons learnt

Readers interested in specific geographic or sector initiatives should search health databases or contact governments and development partners. Many publish annual reports and are widely available on the Internet. The US Centres for Disease Control and Prevention is now publishing a searchable library of global health success stories, which is available online.[16]

Which criteria are most useful for measuring success?

Most countries and development partners are using 26 different indicators chart progress on 13 SDG targets as a way of measuring success. The health targets under Good Health and Well-being (Goal 3) are as follows:

3.1 By 2030, reduce the global maternal mortality ratio to less than 70 per 100,000 live births

3.2 By 2030, end preventable deaths of newborns and children under 5 years of age, with all countries aiming to reduce neonatal mortality to at least as low as 12 per 1,000 live births and under-5 mortality to at least as low as 25 per 1,000 live births

3.3 By 2030, end the epidemics of AIDS, tuberculosis, malaria, and neglected tropical diseases and combat hepatitis, water-borne diseases, and other communicable diseases

3.4 By 2030, reduce by one-third premature mortality from NCDs through prevention and treatment and promote mental health and well-being

3.5 Strengthen the prevention and treatment of substance abuse, including narcotic drug abuse and harmful use of alcohol

3.6 By 2020, halve the number of global deaths and injuries from road traffic accidents

3.7 By 2030, ensure universal access to sexual and reproductive health-care services, including for family planning, information and education, and the integration of reproductive health into national strategies and programmes

3.8 Achieve UHC, including financial risk protection, access to quality essential health-care services and access to safe, effective, quality and affordable essential medicines and vaccines for all

3.9 By 2030, substantially reduce the number of deaths and illnesses from hazardous chemicals and air, water and soil pollution and contamination

3.A Strengthen the implementation of the World Health Organization Framework Convention on Tobacco Control in all countries, as appropriate

3.B Support the research and development of vaccines and medicines for the communicable and noncommunicable diseases that primarily affect developing countries, provide access to affordable essential medicines and vaccines, in accordance with the Doha Declaration on the TRIPS Agreement and Public Health, which affirms the right of developing countries to use to the full the provisions in the Agreement on Trade Related Aspects of Intellectual Property Rights regarding flexibilities to protect public health, and, in particular, provide access to medicines for all

3.C Substantially increase health financing and the recruitment, development, training, and retention of the health workforce in developing countries, especially in least developed countries and small island developing states

3.D Strengthen the capacity of all countries, in particular developing countries, for early warning, risk reduction, and management of national and global health risks

How will we know if we have been successful?

WHO's Global Health Observatory provides gateway to health-related statistics for more than 1,000 indicators for its 194 Member States. Theme pages provide information on global situations and trends, using core indicators, database views, major publications, and links to relevant web pages on the theme. The Observatory also includes a dashboard of the SDG health and health-related target indicators. Lessons learned from the MDGs were that the goals and their targets were too vague and there was often insufficient information as to what was being measured. The SDGs now include clear metrics, and data will be reviewed regularly by a number of independent agencies to chart progress.

Acknowledgement

The authors alone are responsible for the views expressed in this chapter and they do not necessarily represent the views, decisions, or policies of the institutions with which they are affiliated.

References

1 United Nations Development Program. (2018). Human Development Indices and Indicators 2018 Statistical Update. Available at: ℘ http://hdr.undp.org/sites/default/files/2018_human_development_statistical_update.pdf (accessed 28 November 2019).

2 The World Bank. Poverty and equity data portal. Available at: ℘ http://povertydata.worldbank.org/poverty/home/ (accessed 28 November 2019).

3 Article 25. United Nations' Universal Declaration of Human Rights. 1948. Available at: ℘ https://www.un.org/en/universal-declaration-human-rights/ (accessed 28 November 2019).

4 Global Burden of Disease. Available at: ℘ http://www.healthdata.org/ (accessed 28 November 2019).

5 World Health Organization. Global Health Observatory data. Available at: ℘ http://www.who.int/gho/en/ (accessed 28 November 2019).

6 World Health Organization. The top 10 causes of death. 24 May 2018. Available at: ℘ https://www.who.int/news-room/fact-sheets/detail/the-top-10-causes-of-death (accessed 28 November 2019).

7 United Nations General Assembly. A/RES/74/2. Resolution adopted by the General Assembly on 10 October 2019. Political declaration of the high-level meeting on universal health coverage. Available at: ℘ https://undocs.org/en/A/RES/74/2 (accessed 28 November 2019).

8 World Health Organization. *Public financing for health in Africa: from Abuja to the SDGs.* Available at: ℘ https://apps.who.int/iris/bitstream/handle/10665/249527/WHO-HIS-HGF-Tech.Report-16.2-eng.pdf (accessed 28 November 2019).

9 United Nations. Addis Ababa Action Agenda of the Third International Conference on Financing for Development. New York, 2015. Available at: ℘ https://sustainabledevelopment.un.org/index.php?page=view&type=400&nr=2051&menu=35 (accessed 28 November 2019).

10 Sustainable Development Goals Knowledge Platform. Transforming our world: the 2030 Agenda for Sustainable Development. Available at: ℘ https://sustainabledevelopment.un.org/post2015/transformingourworld (accessed 28 November 2019).

11 World Health Organization. SDG 3: Ensure healthy lives and promote wellbeing for all at all ages. Available at: ℘ https://www.who.int/sdg/targets/en/ (accessed 28 November 2019).

12 World Health Organization. World Health Statistics 2017. Available at: ℘ http://www.who.int/gho/publications/world_health_statistics/en/ (accessed 28 November 2019).

13 World Health Organization. Stronger collaboration, better health: global action plan for healthy lives and well-being for all. Available at: ℘ https://www.who.int/publications-detail/stronger-collaboration-better-health-global-action-plan-for-healthy-lives-and-well-being-for-all/ (accessed 28 November 2019).

14 Stenberg K, Hanssen O, Edejer T-T, et al. (2017). Financing transformative health systems towards achievement of the health Sustainable Development Goals: a model for projected resource needs in 67 low-income and middle-income countries. *Lancet Global Health,* 5, e875–87. Available at: ℘ https://doi.org/10.1016/S2214-109X(17)30263-2 (accessed 28 November 2019).

15 Disease Control Priorities Network. Disease control priorities. Available at: ℘ http://www.dcp-3.org/ (accessed 28 November 2019).

16 US Centres for Disease Control and Prevention. Global health success stories. Available at: ℘ https://www.cdc.gov/globalhealth/stories/topic-list.html (accessed 28 November 2019).

Regulation

Lawrence Gostin

Objectives

The objectives of this chapter are to help you understand:

- the impact of legislation, regulations, and litigation on the public's health
- the powers, duties, and restraints imposed by the law on public health officials
- the potential of legal change to improve the public's health
- the role of international law and institutions in securing public health in the face of increasing globalization.

Why is this an important public health issue?

Public health practitioners often regard law as arcane, indecipherable, and unhelpful in pursuing their objective of improving the public's health and safety. Certainly, law can obfuscate rather than clarify, impede rather than facilitate. However, even when the law stands as an obstacle, practitioners must understand it. They may even seek to circumvent legal barriers provided it is lawful and ethical to do so. More important, the law can be empowering, providing innovative solutions to the toughest health problems. For example, most of the ten great public health achievements in the United States in the twentieth century were realized, in part, through law reform or litigation:[1]

- vaccinations
- safer workplaces
- safer and healthier foods
- motor vehicle safety
- control of infectious diseases
- tobacco control
- fluoridation of drinking water.

The law—both legislation and regulation—is far more important in public health than usually acknowledged. Law creates a mission for public health authorities, assigns their functions, and specifies the manner in which they may exercise their power (see Box 4.8.1). The law is a tool to influence norms for healthy behaviour, identify and respond to health threats, and set and enforce health and safety standards. Some of the most important social debates about public health take place in legal forums—legislatures, courts, and administrative agencies—and in the law's language of rights, duties, and justice. It is no exaggeration to say that 'the field of public health...could no longer exist in the manner in which we know it today except for its sound legal basis'.[2]

Box 4.8.1 Powers, duties, limitations

'Health officers must be familiar not only with the extent of their powers and duties, but also with the limitations imposed upon them by law. With such knowledge available and widely applied by health authorities, public health will not remain static, but will progress.'

Source: Tobey JA. (1947). *Public health law*, 3rd edn. Commonwealth Fund, New York.

Definitions

There is a subtle difference between 'public health law' and 'law and the public's health'. The former is the body of legislation that creates governmental public health agencies and enables them to carry out their activities. The latter is the wider body of law that can be used in a variety of ways to safeguard and promote the public's health.

Public health law can be defined as the legislation and administrative rules that delineate a public health agency's mission, duties, and powers to assure the conditions for people to be healthy and the limits on an agency's power to constrain the autonomy, privacy, liberty, or proprietary interests of individuals.

Law and the public's health can be defined as the legislation, regulations, and case law that can be used as a tool to safeguard and promote the public's health including altering the socio-economic, informational, natural, and built environments.

The law for public health practitioners

As a public health practitioner, you should understand and obey the law. This means you must act within the scope of your legal authority, never abuse your power, treat persons with respect, and consult with community leaders. If the law is unclear, you should seek the guidance of public health lawyers. Because few lawyers have a specialized knowledge of population health, education and training programmes in public health law are needed.

Public health law: deficiencies and opportunities

Inadequacy of existing legislation

In many countries, public health legislation is so old it tells the story of health threats through time, with new layers of regulation for each page in history—from plague and smallpox to tuberculosis and polio, and now HIV/AIDS, SARS, Ebola, Zika, and novel influenzas. Legislation often pre-dates modern public health science and practice, and does not conform to modern ideas relating to the mission, functions, and services of agencies. Existing laws also often pre-date advances in human rights and may fail to safeguard civil liberties. These deficiencies become particularly apparent in the face of emergent crises such as those related to terrorism or emerging infectious diseases.

The purposes of sound public health legislation

Sound public health legislation should provide agencies with a clear and modern mission to create the conditions in which people can be healthy. The statute should enable agencies to exercise a full range of necessary functions, services, and powers. It should similarly provide funding and other structures necessary to carry out the agency's mission. At the same time, public health legislation should protect individual rights to privacy, autonomy, liberty, and non-discrimination. In particular, it should enunciate clear standards for the exercise of powers, due process, and fair treatment—see Box 4.8.2.

Box 4.8.2 Model public health legislation

In response to the attacks on the World Trade Center and subsequent dispersal of anthrax in the US, the Centre for Law and the Public's Health at Georgetown and Johns Hopkins Universities drafted the Model State Emergency Health Powers Act (MSEHPA). The MSEHPA was structured to reflect five basic public health functions to be facilitated by law:[a]

- preparedness
- surveillance
- management of property
- protection of persons
- public information and communication.

a) Gostin LO, Sapsin JW, Teret SP, et al. (2002). The Model State Emergency Health Powers Act: planning and response to bioterrorism and naturally occurring infectious diseases. Journal of American Medicine Association, 288, 622–8.

In the US in 2003, the 'Turning Point' Public Health Statute Modernization Collaborative drafted a comprehensive public health act focusing on the organization, delivery, and funding of essential public health services, together with a full set of powers and safeguards.[3] In 2017, the World Health Organization (WHO) published a report showing the value of law to advance the right to health. The report provides illustrations of evidence-based laws to safeguard the public's health, such as salt reductions, trans-fat bans, and package labelling to prevent non-communicable diseases.[4] WHO demonstrated the power of these tools in reducing non-communicable diseases in the Eastern Mediterranean region, shifting behaviour toward healthier diets.[5]

Public health law: power, duty, and restraint

Public health law creates public health agencies and grants them specific powers relating to issues such as:

- surveillance and monitoring
- testing and screening
- vaccination and treatment
- partner notification and contact tracing
- isolation and quarantine
- reducing injuries
- controlling non-communicable diseases.

The effective and careful use of these powers allows public health officials to protect and improve the public's health. The law also constrains the exercise of these powers. Public health officials should be conscious of how the exercise of these powers has an impact on the enjoyment of liberties (e.g. the right to privacy and freedom of movement), and should implement appropriate limits and procedural safeguards to ensure that a proper balance between individual liberties and the public's health is reached.

Law and the public's health: regulation and litigation as a tool

If government has an obligation to promote the conditions for people to be healthy, what tools are at its disposal? There are at least seven models for legal intervention designed to prevent injury and disease, encourage healthful behaviours, and generally promote the public's health. Although legal interventions can be effective, they often raise critical social, ethical, or constitutional concerns that warrant careful consideration.

Model 1: the power to tax and spend

The power to tax and spend is ubiquitous in national constitutions and provides governments with an important regulatory technique. The power to spend supports the public health infrastructure: a well-trained workforce, electronic information and communications systems, rapid disease surveillance, laboratory capacity, and response capability. The state can also set health-related conditions for the receipt of public funds. The power to tax provides inducements to engage in beneficial behaviour and disincentives to engage in risk activities. Tax relief can be offered for health-producing activities such as medical services, childcare, and charitable contributions. At the same time, tax burdens can be placed on the sale of hazardous products such as cigarettes, alcoholic beverages, unhealthy foods, and firearms.

Model 2: the power to alter the informational environment

The public is bombarded with information that influences their life choices and this undoubtedly affects health and behaviour. The government has several tools at its disposal to alter the informational environment, encouraging people to make more healthful choices about diet, exercise, cigarette smoking, and other behaviours. It can:

- use communication campaigns as a major public health strategy (e.g. educate the public about safe driving, safe sex, physical activity, and nutritious diets)
- require businesses to label their products to include instructions for safe use, disclosure of contents or ingredients, and health warnings
- limit harmful or misleading information in private advertising (e.g. ban or regulate advertising of potentially harmful products, including cigarettes, firearms, and even high-fat or other unhealthy foods, including trans fatty acids).

Model 3: the power to alter the built environment

Public health has a long history in designing the built environment to reduce injury (e.g. workplace safety, traffic calming, and fire codes), infectious diseases (e.g. sanitation, zoning, and housing codes), and harms from the environment (e.g. lead paint and toxic emissions). As countries face an epidemiological transition from infectious to non-communicable diseases, environments can be designed to promote liveable cities and facilitate health-affirming behaviour by, for example:

- encouraging more active lifestyles (walking, cycling, and playing)
- improving nutrition (fruits, vegetables, and avoidance of high-fat, high-sodium, high-caloric foods)
- decreasing use of harmful products (cigarettes and alcoholic beverages)
- reducing violence (domestic abuse, street crime, and firearm use), and
- increasing social interactions (helping neighbours and building social capital).

Model 4: the power to alter the socio-economic environment

A strong and consistent finding of epidemiological research is that socio-economic status (SES) is correlated with morbidity, mortality, and functioning. SES is a complex phenomenon related to, among other things, income, education, and occupation. Some scholars have even suggested that 'justice is good for our health'.[6] By narrowing socio-economic disparities, the state seeks to reduce inequities and improve the population's health.

Model 5: direct regulation of persons, professionals, and businesses

Government has the power to directly regulate individuals, professionals, and businesses. It can:

- regulate individual behaviour (e.g. use of seatbelts and motorcycle helmets) to reduce injuries and deaths
- use licences and permits to enable government to monitor and control the standards and practices of professionals and institutions (e.g. doctors, hospitals, and nursing homes)
- inspect and regulate businesses to assure humane conditions of work, reduce toxic emissions, and ensure the safety of consumer products.

Model 6: indirect regulation through the tort system

Attorneys general, public health authorities, and private citizens possess a powerful means of indirect regulation through the tort system. Civil litigation can redress many different kinds of public health harms—for instance:

- environmental damage (e.g. air pollution or groundwater contamination)
- exposure to toxic substances (e.g. pesticides, radiation, or chemicals)
- hazardous products (e.g. tobacco or firearms), and
- defective consumer products (e.g. children's toys, recreational equipment, or household goods).

For example, in 1998, tobacco companies negotiated a master settlement agreement with American states that required compensation in perpetuity, with payments totalling $206 billion through to the year 2025.[7]

Model 7: deregulation—law as a barrier to health

Sometimes laws are harmful to the public's health and stand as an obstacle to effective action. In such cases, the best remedy is deregulation. Examples include laws that penalize exchanges or pharmacy sales of syringes and needles, that restrict access to sterile drug injection equipment and fuel the transmission of HIV infection, or that close bathhouses to prevent the spread of sexually transmitted infections but end up driving the epidemic underground, making it more difficult to get condoms and save-sex literature to sexually active men who have sex with men. Finally, the criminal prohibition of narcotics can often create impediments to healthcare professionals in offering pain relief to suffering patients.

Global health law: comparative and international perspectives

The use of the law to improve the public's health is also important at the international level. Some health hazards—biological, chemical, and radionuclear—have profound global implications. Whether the origin of such threats is natural, accidental, or intentional, potential harms may transcend national frontiers and warrant a transnational response. The potential scope of international public health law is vast, ranging from communicable (e.g. global surveillance and border control) and non-communicable diseases (e.g. occupational health and narcotics) and injuries to trade, environmental, and human rights concerns. This section briefly discusses three important international legal instruments.

The International Health Regulations

The World Health Assembly adopted the revised International Health Regulations (IHR) in 2005.[8] The IHR had been critiqued because of their narrow scope (applying only to cholera, plague, and yellow fever), lack of enforcement, failure to set minimum national public health capacities, and failure to provide sufficient financial and technical assistance to poor countries. The main improvements in the new IHR are:
- expanded jurisdiction: covering 'all events which may constitute a public health emergency of international concern'.
- national focal points: for official WHO communications in each country
- core capacities: for public health preparedness in order to detect, report, and respond to public health risks
- global surveillance: by using official and unofficial sources of information and modern data systems.
- recommended measures: to reduce health risks on a standing or temporary basis.

The Framework Convention on Tobacco Control

The WHO has turned to international law solutions in the area of chronic diseases as well as infectious diseases. Particularly remarkable is the Framework Convention on Tobacco Control (FCTC), adopted by the World Health Assembly in 2003.[9] The FCTC is one of the most widely accepted treaties in the world. It establishes a 'framework' for ongoing diplomacy to reduce the global health threat posed by tobacco, and supports governments and civil society in pushing for strong tobacco laws; examples include Australia's 'plain packaging' law and Uruguay's comprehensive tobacco control laws. The tobacco industry sued Australia and Uruguay in international tribunals but lost those cases in large part because of the FCTC.[10]

Human Rights Law

The effective protection of public health also rests on laws underpinned by, and consistent with, human rights. Human rights are legal guarantees protecting universal values of human dignity and freedom, and they define the entitlements of all human beings and the corresponding obligations of the state as the primary duty-bearer. An important human rights standard for the purposes of this handbook is the right to the enjoyment of the highest attainable standard of health, often referred to as the 'right to health'. First recognized in the WHO Constitution, it is enshrined in six core international human rights treaties, including the International Covenant on Economic, Social and Cultural Rights (ICESCR).[11]

In order to clarify the content and meaning of the right to health, the UN Committee on Economic, Social and Cultural Rights (CESCR)'s General Comment 14 explains that the right to health is an inclusive right, extending beyond healthcare to the underlying determinants of health such as access to safe and potable water; adequate sanitation; adequate supply of safe food; nutrition; housing; healthy occupational and environmental conditions; access to health-related education and information, including on sexual and reproductive health; and freedom from discrimination.[11] States have an obligation to take immediate steps to progressively ensure that services, goods, and facilities are *available*, *accessible*, *acceptable*, and of *good quality*.

There are a variety of other health-related rights in international law that support actions by government to improve the health of their populations. These rights include the right to adequate food, clothing, and housing, and the right to 'environmental and industrial hygiene' in the ICESCR. Other rights include the right to liberty and security of the person, freedom from coerced labour, liberty of movement, and freedom from discrimination on groups including race, colour, sex, language, religion, and political opinion, as recognized in the International Covenant on Civil and Political Rights (ICCPR). Public health laws framed in ways that respect human rights are likely to be most effective in achieving the goals of disease prevention and health promotion.

Conclusion

The law is an under-appreciated tool for health improvement. Many public health practitioners distrust or are ignorant of the law and the law-making process. They are often not skilled in using, or reforming, the law to improve the public's health. Yet law at the national and international level can have profound effects in changing attitudes and behaviours of individuals and businesses with remarkable benefits for the health of populations. In 2017, the *Lancet*/O'Neill Institute of National and Global Health Law/Georgetown University Commission reported, urging policy makers to adopt evidence-based legal tools and public health practitioners to vigorously apply those legal tools:[12] a call to action for the public's health and wellbeing that should not be ignored.

Further resources

Books and articles

Bailey TM, Caulfield T, Ries N. (2009). Public Health Law and Policy in Canada. Butterworths, Markham.

Burci G, Vignes CH. (2004). World Health Organization. Kluwer Law International, The Hague.

Gostin LO Wiley L. (2016). Public health law: power, duty, restraint, 3rd edn. University of California Press, Berkeley.

Gostin LO Wiley L. (2017). Public health law and ethics: a reader, 3rd edn. University of California Press, Berkeley.

Reynolds C. (2004). Public health law and regulation. Federation Press, Sydney.

World Health Organization (2017). Advancing the Right to Health: The Vital Role of Law. Available at: 🖰 https://www.who.int/healthsystems/topics/health-law/health_law-report/en/ (accessed 21 August 2019).

Websites on public health law

Centre for Law and the Public's Health (Georgetown and Johns Hopkins universities). Available at: 🖰 https://www.jhsph.edu/research/centers-and-institutes/center-for-law-and-the-publics-health/index.html (accessed 21 August 2019).

O'Neill Institute for National and Global Health Law at Georgetown University. Available at: 🖰 https://oneill.law.georgetown.edu/ (accessed 21 August 2019).

US Department of Health and Human Services Centers for Disease Control and Prevention. Public health law program. Available at: 🖰 https://www.cdc.gov/phlp/index.html (accessed 21 August 2019).

World Health Organization. Available at: 🖰 http://www.who.int/en (accessed 21 August 2019).

World Health Organization (2008). Commission on Social Determinants of Health Closing the gap in a generation: health equity through action on the social determinants of health, final report. WHO, Geneva. Available at: 🖰 http://www.who.int/social_determinants/thecommission/finalreport/en/index.html (accessed 21 August 2019).

References

1 Centers for Disease Control and Prevention (1999). Ten great public health achievements—United States, 1900–1999. *Morbidity and Mortality Weekly Reports*, **48**, 241–8.

2 Grad FP. (2004). *Public health law manual*. American Public Health Association, Washington, DC.

3 Turning Point Model State Public Health Act. Available at: 🖰 https://journals.sagepub.com/doi/10.1111/j.1748-720X.2006.00010.x (accessed 21 August 2019).

4 *Advancing the Right to Health: The vital role of law*. (2017). Available at: 🖰 https://www.who.int/healthsystems/topics/health-law/health_law-report/en/ (accessed 21 August 2019).

5 Gostin LO, Abou-Taleb H, Roache SA, et al. (2017). Legal priorities for prevention of noncommunicable diseases: innovations from WHO's eastern Mediterranean region. *Public Health*, **144**, 4–12. Available at: 🖰 http://dx.doi.org/10.1016/j.puhe.2016.11.001 (accessed 21 August 2019).

6 Daniels N, Kennedy B, Kawachi I. (2000). Justice is good for our health. *Boston Review*, **25**(1), 6–15.

7 Gostin LO. (2007). The 'tobacco wars'—global litigation strategies. *Journal of the American Medicine Association*, **298**, 2537–9.

8 World Health Assembly (2005). Strengthening health security by implementing the International Health Regulations. Available at: 🖰 who.int/ihr/en/ (accessed 21 August 2019).

9 World Health Organization (2005). *Framework convention on tobacco control*, WHO doc. A56/VR/4 (2003). Available at: 🖰 https://www.who.int/fctc/en/ (accessed 21 August 2019).

10 Roach SA, Gostin LO, Bianco-Fonsalia E. (2016). Trade, investment, and tobacco: Philip Morris v Uruguay, *JAMA*, **316**(20), 2085–6.

11 Committee on Economic, Social, and Cultural Rights (2000). *General Comment No. 14, The right to the highest attainable standard of health,* UN doc. E/C.12/2000/4. Available at: ℘ https://digitallibrary.un.org/record/425041/files/E_C.12_2000_4-EN.pdf (accessed 21 August 2019).

12 Gostin LO, Monahan JT, DeBartolo Mary C, et al. (2015). Law's power to safeguard global health: A *Lancet*–O'Neill Institute, Georgetown University Commission on Global Health and the Law. *Lancet,* 385(9978). Published online, 22 April. Available at: ℘ http://dx.doi.org/10.1016/S0140-6736(15)60756-5 and https://scholarship.law.georgetown.edu/facpub/1479 (accessed 21 August 2019).

Chapter 4.9

Health, sustainability, and climate change

David Pencheon, Sonia Roschnik, and Paul Cosford

If not us, who? If not now, when?

(Attr. various)

Objectives

This chapter will help you understand the importance of, and the relationships between, health, health and care systems, sustainable development, and climate change, and to do so locally and globally.

The specific objectives of the chapter are to help you:

- *make the case for action* by understanding how science, law, policies, and values can be framed and translated into specific and system wide actions
- *translate what is known and what protects and creates health into policy and practice*, and help address barriers to implementation and quality improvement in health and care systems
- *engage a wide range of stakeholders* to ensure appropriate cross-system action involving a diverse group of people, skills, and influences across the health and care system.

We all have a duty of care to people locally and globally, now and in the future, to ensure that health and care organizations and the people who work within them create a worthwhile healthy future. This chapter aims to help you fulfil that duty at a personal, organizational, professional, and civic level, linking your values and your commitment with your competencies and your capacity, so that you are able to influence change positively.

Definition of key terms

Sustainable development

This is 'development that meets the needs of the present without compromising the ability of future generations to meet their own needs'.[1] definition should be extended to refer not just to time (the future) but also to place (people [and other systems on which all life depends] elsewhere in the world now).

Climate change

Climate change, *carbon reduction*, and *sustainable development* are related but not synonymous. Much of the failure of progress to date can be attributed to the inconsistent and unengaging use of language, including a poor appreciation of the power of framing and reframing. The science is clear that we are now risking dangerous and unhealthy disruption to all that makes life feasible and liveable as a result of the human use of limited natural resources. This is happening despite the tremendous progress that has been made in human health over the past century around the world. Too little attention is being paid to the consequences of the unbridled development that has accompanied these gains, especially in terms of the greenhouse gases (predominantly carbon dioxide) and other natural systems (soil, biodiversity, clean air, and water). However, science alone does not engage most people, be they politicians, policy makers, professionals, or public.

Most of us live in unsustainable ways, creatively rationalize it, and collectively increase the threat of irreversible and chaotic climate change. We need to be realistic, honest, engaging and collaborative if we are going to address the 21C's biggest health threat[2] *and* biggest health opportunity.[3] Preaching doom and gloom without rescue and guidance on positive actions can only fuel our collective sense of hopelessness, denial, disavowal,[4] and inaction. It is important to be realistic and positive about the future, and ensure that serious and coordinated action can be taken now. Health professionals are not only well placed to do this but might consider it a duty of care, both as respected professionals and as active citizens.

Why is this an important public health issue?

Climate change and lack of sustainability are already having adverse health impacts and, like many threats to public health, are having a particular impact on the most vulnerable communities.[5] These communities are already living on the edge and one year's bad weather or crops can be life threatening. Even in the wealthiest countries, older, younger, and less healthy people are vulnerable to sudden climate-related events, particularly when physical frailty is combined with poor social connections and care systems.[6, 7, 8]

Sustainability is now increasingly included as one of the dimensions of quality, alongside and related to other dimensions such as compassion, effectiveness, and safety.[9, 10] The public health role is to quantify the multiple benefits of taking action aligning environmental sustainability with financial and social sustainability: the 'triple bottom line',[11] also termed 'the health dividend',[12] 'virtuous circle', 'win-wins' and 'health co-benefits'. Sustainable development is, first, a way of understanding health and care strategically, and only then as a more operational part of an integrated, system-wide approach to protecting and improving health and organizing care. How this can be achieved can only be touched on here but there is already substantial evidence and best practice collated by many national and global health and sustainability organizations. An essay by Eric Chivian summarizes the approaches and framing that health professionals can consider.[13] Box 4.9.1 summarizes the key issues you should understand in relation to health, sustainability, and climate change.

Box 4.9.1 Key issues for public health practitioners to understand

- Embracing new definitions of health and wellbeing and its causes[a]
- The environmental unsustainability of human behaviours in general and health and care systems in particular.[b]
- Mechanisms of anthropogenic climate change and how they cause problems for (and are caused BY) health and care systems
- New models of health improvement and health/social care
  - The anchor institution role of health systems
  - The contribution to economic, social value, and natural assets by health systems
- Current effects of climate change on human health:
  - direct local extreme events and effects (heat wave, drought, flood)
  - global effects (migration, biodiversity)
- Relationship between adaptation and mitigation and resilience
- Practical steps that can be taken at an:
  - individual level
  - organizational level
  - system level ('accountable care system')
  - national/international level
- What health professionals[c] and health systems[d] can do.

a) Crisp N. (2010). Turning the world upside down: the search for global health in the 21st century, Hodder Education, London.

b) Hannah M. (2014). Humanising healthcare, Triarchy Press, Bridport.

c) Chivian E. (2014). Why doctors and their organisations must help tackle climate change: an essay by Eric Chivian. British Medical Journal, 348, g2407.

d) Pencheon D. (2015), Making healthcare more sustainable: the case of the English NHS. Public Health, 129, 1335–43. doi:10.1016/j.puhe.2015.08.010 2015

Public health competencies needed

There are two important public health skills you will need to make the case for rapid and meaningful progress towards a sustainable world:
- Engaging people positively, practically, and collaboratively in addressing the consequences and opportunities.
- Generating, analysing, and presenting data and research in ways that make sense to a wide range of stakeholders.

In practice, this means being able to frame and reframe the facts, challenges, opportunities and uncertainties, and what success looks like.

Measuring and monitoring progress consistently is a crucial part of the process. We risk valuing only what we can measure, rather than measuring what we should value. We are often drawn to familiar metrics such as life expectancy, QALYs, and DALYs (see ➜ Chapter 1.6), rather than creating or embracing other more meaningful indicators of progress. Success criteria of health and care systems should include compassion, patient- and public-defined outcomes, dignity, community engagement, empowerment, and the natural, social, and economic value added. Measures that already exist (such as the Happy Planet Index, which 'reveals the ecological efficiency with which human well-being is delivered'[14]) and approaches that consider planetary health more ambitiously[15] need to be more seriously considered.

To be successful in all this, you will need to use techniques to frame the issues in ways that make sense to a broad range of people (see ➔ Chapter 4.5). This requires you to understand issues of concern to stakeholders and that there are many perspectives from which issues can be seen: personal, cultural, governance, resources (especially money), professional, and organisational. Examples of how these perspectives can be used to engage different people include:

- governance ('don't break the rules or the agreement')
- resources ('don't break the bank')
- personal and ethical ('don't break your word or your principles').

Remember you may be engaging an individual, community, business, government, funder, regulator, commissioner, provider, professional, patient, member of the public... Everyone you aim to help is first a citizen and second a representative of many different groups, and engagement emotionally via the former nearly always trumps rational engagement via the latter.

You also need to appreciate the complexity of how change happens, behaviourally and culturally. Being clear about your assumptions in your models of change and how appropriate they are for the context in which you are working is an important part of the process.[16, 17]

You will find it easier to help people and organizations change if you can present them with a compelling story of how much better things can be based on real data and real examples. This emphasizes the importance of a vision, strategies based on good consultation,[18, 19] and the practical narratives and route maps[20] of how we can get there. Such scenarios are not predictions but descriptions of trends that help people ask good questions, engage the right people, address the most important uncertainties (e.g. via convening, via research ...), and frame realistic plans that can be prioritized and monitored.

People do not take the threat of climate change and the opportunities for sustainable development seriously if respected people like health professionals do not visibly do so themselves and speak up about it. Health professionals need to show they consider this to be one of the most significant health risks and opportunities of the twenty-first century in visible ways. Healthcare may be getting less carbon intensive but there is much more of it happening as the world grows and industrializes, so the absolute impact can still increase. Moreover, many of the significant innovations (e.g. more energy-efficient combined heat and power plants in large hospitals) are hidden from view, missing the opportunity to multiply the absolute effect through public example. Just as in the changing role of tobacco in the more industrialized world, health professionals and health systems can make a significant contribution to social change.[21]

Our experience of engaging healthcare organizations in England suggests the approaches that appeal to leaders in large healthcare organizations need to be feasible and practical, deliver short-term as well as long-term benefits, and be aligned with organizational objectives. This can be done through:

- saving resources (reducing waste, harm, emissions and pollution, and saving money[22])
- improving governance (complying with regulation and legislation) (see ➲ Chapter 7.1)
- protecting and enhancing reputation (developing people better)
- embedding the values of staff and organization into every contract and contact
- ensuring the health and care system adds value to the community beyond simply healthcare: being a good employer, buyer, partner, and joint investor[23]
- delivering resilient services (the capacity of a system to absorb sudden shocks and still function and learn)
- protecting and improving health and reducing health inequalities (especially exploiting the opportunities of health co-benefits)
- setting a visible example of what the future can be.

Three key areas on which to focus in sustainable approaches to public health

1. Focus on aligning multiple actions by many groups

Sustainable development is related to other major public health issues such as inequalities and social justice. The issue of sustainability and health resembles emergent public health challenges of the past in that:

- it is relatively new
- it is not a single issue (more a [super-]wicked issue)
- it challenges conventional thinking, norms, and interests
- it has a rapidly changing and often contested evidence base
- it involves closely interrelated technical, legal, policy, and behavioural issues
- action is needed before the whole picture is clear
- there is no obvious end point of success
- there is no magic bullet.

There are multiple opportunities to be exploited and risks to be avoided through early action by professionals, by governments, by individuals, and by health and care systems. In addressing these, you should remember two important principles:

- Those embarking on programmes of large-scale change must recognize that large organizations or sectors (e.g. the health sector) are complex, adaptive systems that behave in unpredictable ways[24] despite our enduring belief that they can be micromanaged in traditional ways.
- Do not focus on efficiency gains alone. Although this is a good place to start, it is a bad place to finish. Efficiency is essential but should be approached as the springboard to transformation (occasionally via creative disruption). At best, there is a limit to what is achievable by efficiency gains. At worst, you are deluding yourself by making a broken system into a marginally better broken system. Improving efficiency is necessary but insufficient and it is important to have a broad approach

to both efficiency (doing the same things with fewer resources) and transformational change (revisiting the fundamental objectives and considering meeting them in quite different ways).[25]

2. Focus on co-benefits and common interests

Public health action is rarely successful if its practitioners tell others what to do (and what *not* to do). Fortunately, in the area of health and sustainability, there are often multiple benefits from clear policies.[26] Focus on these. These approaches should be made a priority instead of focusing entirely on trade-offs and compromises. Co-benefits for health from work on sustainability and climate change exist at three levels: improving public health, improving health and care organizations and systems, and improving global health and injustice (see Box 4.9.2).

> **Box 4.9.2 Three levels of health co-benefits from addressing sustainability and climate change**
>
> - *For better health:* e.g. more physical activity, better diet, improved mental health, less road trauma, less air pollution, less obesity/heart disease/cancer, greater social inclusion.
> - *For better health and care organizations/systems:* e.g. more prevention, care closer to home, more empowerment/self-care, reducing over-diagnosis and over-treatment, better use of drugs, better use of information and IT, better skill mix, better models of care.
> - *For more global fairness:* the adoption of economic systems (such as 'Contraction and Convergence') that distribute resources (such as carbon credits) equitably amongst the world's populations whilst redistributing wealth and opportunity more fairly.

At each level, there are both immediate and longer-term benefits. Obvious examples include the ways we eat (a low-carbon diet, low in intensively raised processed animal products and high in fruit and vegetables, is good for human and environmental health, now and in the future) and the ways we move (a more active lifestyle improves physical and mental health now, reduces air pollution and transport trauma, improves social cohesion, and reduces reliance on high-carbon transport systems).

> Never in human history have we moved our bodies around the world so much without moving our bodies.

3. Focus on a whole-systems approach to adaptation, mitigation, and resilience

> Adaptation is managing the unavoidable; mitigation is avoiding the unmanageable.

Mitigation means reducing the causes of dangerous climate disruption. In public health terms, this equates to addressing the causes—focusing on prevention. Adaptation is akin to addressing the consequences, the inevitable impact of the climate change already locked in to the system. They are equally important but should be seen as complementary approaches that need to be integrated. It is wrong to view the approaches as separate and dangerous or to see them as competing: they are both important parts of the same strategy. Above all, don't focus on adaptation *at the expense of* mitigation: for example, cooling buildings by increasing the use of air conditioning is a dangerously short-term approach. Designing naturally and passively cooled structures using knowledge that has been around for 2,000 years both adapts and mitigates.

Extreme events: evidence of a slow-burn emergency

While individual disasters or incidents can never be specifically attributed to climate change alone, there is good evidence that climate change increases the risk and severity of flooding, heatwaves, and changing in patterns of infection.

Flooding incidents create significant harm economically, physically, and especially psychologically for those affected. Heatwaves, such as the one in central Europe in 2003 in which at least 30,000 excess deaths occurred,[27] disproportionately harm elderly and the most vulnerable people who are least able to adapt physiologically, and who rely on resilient social networks. Similarly, the potential for increases in infectious diseases such as malaria and dengue fever all require a public health response that predicts the likely impact and future pattern of diseases and identifies those most likely to be affected. Emergency preparedness must include planning to mitigate the impact of severe weather events such as flooding and heatwaves and their consequences.[28]

> Nature has enough for our need but not for our greed.
>
>   Mahatma Gandhi (attrib.)

Health systems and health professionals should be clear about their responsibility to maintain population size and behaviour within the limits that available resources can support. Average family size should mean that the total population does not exceed available resources. Although health professionals and systems should not prescribe family size, they should make clear, through their policies and actions, that population size is a crucial determinant of our ability to maintain health for all, now and in the future. The total impact of human activity is the product of population and individual intensity and footprint. An increase in global population from 7 billion to 10 billion will not make things easier but increasing per capita impact from less than 2 tonnes CO_2e (CO_2 equivalent) (much of the world's population) to nearly 20 tonnes CO_2e (some of the world's population) is disastrous.

Sustainability and quality

Rather than seeing sustainability as an issue to be balanced and traded off against other issues such as affordability or urgency, it should be treated as any other mutually reinforcing dimension of quality:[29]

> Any quality aims that cannot be maintained with the resources available to us are set up to fail. It is important to realize that working

to improve sustainability will seldom be in conflict with the other dimensions of quality; in particular, low carbon health care is likely to improve cost efficiency and patient empowerment.

From O'Donoghue D. (2010).[10]

Improving quality requires an investment of attitude and effort (and sometimes other resources such as money, at least initially). However, as with most public health activities, this should be treated as an investment rather than a cost. Getting things right first time in ways that make the future possible ultimately makes the best use of all resources and capitals. The initial investment will nonetheless involve shifting framing, cultures, and attitudes more than shifting budgets.

Summary

As a public health practitioner, you will want and need to develop the skills, use your values, and identify the opportunities to engage others positively in a system-wide transformation of the health and care system—for direct benefit and as an example to others. This means that using and framing the evidence of health co-benefits to ensure sustainable development, as summarized by the UN Sustainable Development Goals[30], is a crucial principle of public health research and action in the twenty-first century.

Further resources

Further reading

Birnbaum LS, Balbus JM, Tart KT (eds). (2017). Marking a new understanding of climate and health. *Environmental health perspectives*, **124**(4). Available at: ⅋ http://dx.doi.org/10.1289/ehp.1611410. (accessed 21 August 2019).

Bouley T, Roschnik S, Karliner J, et al. (2017). Climate-smart healthcare: low-carbon and resilience strategies for the health sector. World Bank Group, Washington, DC.

Charlesworth A, Gray A, Pencheon N, et al. (2011). Assessing the health benefits of tackling climate change. *British Medical Journal*, **343**, d6520.

Charlesworth K, Jamieson M, Butler CD, et al. (2015). The future healthcare? *Australian Health Review*, **39**, 444–7.

Charlesworth K, Jamieson, M, Davey, R, et al. (2015). Transformational change in healthcare: an examination of four case studies. *Australian Health Review*, **40**(2), 163–7. Available at: ⅋ http://dx.doi.org/10.1071/AH15041 (accessed 21 August 2019).

Charlesworth KE, Jamieson M. (2017). New sources of value for health and care in a carbon-constrained world. *Journal of Public Health*, **39**(4), 6911–7. Available at: ⅋ doi:https://doi.org/10.1093/pubmed/fdw146 (accessed 21 August 2019).

Coote A. (2006). What health services could do about climate change. *British Medical Journal*, **332**, 1343–4.

Coote A. (2008). How should health professionals take action against climate change? *British Medical Journal*, **336**, 733–4.

Crisp N. (2015). Everyone has a role in building a health creating society. *British Medical Journal*, **351**, h6654. doi:10.1136/bmj.h6654

Eckelman, MJ, Sherman J. (2016). Environmental impacts of the U.S. health care system and effects on public health. PloS ONE, **11**(6). Available at: ⅋ https://dx.doi.org/10.1371/journal.pone.0157014 (accessed 21 August 2019).

Faculty of Public Health (2019). Resources on sustainable development and climate change. Available at: ⅋ https://www.fph.org.uk/policy-campaigns/special-interest-groups/special-interest-groups-list/sustainable-development-special-interest-group/resources-on-sustainable-development-and-climate-change/ (accessed 21 August 2019).

Gill M, Stott R. (2009). Health professionals must act to tackle climate change. *Lancet*, **374**, 1953–5.

Griffiths J, Rao M. (2009). Public health benefits of strategies to reduce greenhouse gas emissions. *British Medical Journal*, **339**, b4952.

Haines A, Wilkinson P, Tonne C, et al. (2009). Aligning climate change and public health policies. *Lancet*, **374**, 2035–8.

IPCC (Intergovernmental Panel on Climate Change) (2007). AR4 climate change 2007: the physical science basis. Available at: ℘ http://www.ipcc.ch/report/ar4/wg1 (accessed 21 August 2019).

NHS Sustainable Development Unit (2009). *Forum for the future. Fit for the future. Scenarios for low-carbon healthcare 2030.* NHS Sustainable Development Unit, Cambridge.

Pencheon D. (2009). Health services and climate change: what can be done? *Journal of Health Service Research and Policy*, **14**, 2–4.

Roschnik S, Martinez GS, Yglesias-Gonzalez M, et al. (2016). Transitioning to environmentally sustainable health systems: the example of the NHS in England. *Public Health Panorama*, **3(2)**, 141–356.

Stott R. (2006). Healthy response to climate change. *British Medical Journal*, **332**, 1385–7.

Stott R, Godlee F. (2006). What should we do about climate change? Health professionals need to act now, collectively and individually. *British Medical Journal*, **333**, 983–4.

The Lancet countdown: tracking progress on health and climate change (2016). Published online: 14 November. Available at: ℘ http://www.lancetcountdown.org (accessed 21 August 2019).

Tomson C. (2015) Reducing the carbon footprint of hospital-based care. *Future Hospital Journal*, **2(1)**, 57–62.

Wilkinson P. (2008). Climate change and health: the case for sustainable development. *Medical Conflict Survival*, **24**(Supplement 1), S26–35.

References

1 Brundtland GH. (1987). *Our common future*. The Brundtland Report. World Commission on Environment and Development. Available at: ℘ http://www.un-documents.net/our-common-future.pdf (accessed 21 August 2019).

2 Costello A, Abbas M, Allen A, et al. (2009). Managing the health effects of climate change. *Lancet*, **373**, 1693–733.

3 Wang H, Horton R. (2015). Tackling climate change: the greatest opportunity for global health. *Lancet*, **386(10006)**, 1798–9. Available at: ℘ http://dx.doi.org/10.1016/S0140-6736(15)60931-X (accessed 21 August 2019).

4 Weintrobe S. (2012). Engaging with climate change: psychoanalytic and interdisciplinary perspectives. Routledge, Abingdon.

5 Costello A, Abbas M, Allen A, et al. (2009). Managing the health effects of climate change. *Lancet*, **373**, 1693–733.

6 Dhainaut J, Claessens Y, Ginsburg C, et al. (2004). Unprecedented heat-related deaths during the 2003 heat wave in Paris: consequences on emergency departments. *Critical Care*, **8**, 1–2.

7 Semenza JC, Rubin CH, Falter KH, et al. (1996). Heat-related deaths during the July 1995 heat wave in Chicago. *New England Journal of Medicine*, **335**, 84–90.

8 UNICEF (2011). *The $100 billion question: how do we secure a climate resilient future for the world's children?* UNICEF.

9 Wilkinson P. (2008). Climate change and health: the case for sustainable development. *Medical Conflict Survival*, **24**(Supplement 1), S26–35.

10 O'Donoghue D. (2010). Sustainability the seventh dimension of quality. Available at: ℘ http://renaltsar.blogspot.com/2010/05/sustainability-seventh-dimension-of.html (accessed 21 August 2019).

11 Elkington J. (1997). *Cannibals with forks: the triple bottom line of 21st century business*. Capstone, Oxford.

12 Coote A. (ed.) (2002). *Claiming the health dividend, unlocking the benefits of nhs spending*. London: King's Fund. Available at: ℘ http://www.kingsfund.org.uk/publications/claiming_the_1.html (accessed 21 August 2019).

13 Chivian E. (2014). Why doctors and their organisations must help tackle climate change: an essay by Eric Chivian. *British Medical Journal*, **348**, g2407.

14 NEF (2009). The Happy Planet Index. Available at: ℘ http://www.happyplanetindex.org (accessed 21 August 2019).

15 R. Horton, R. Beaglehole, R. Bonita, et al. (2014). From public to planetary health: a manifesto. *Lancet*, **383(9920)**, 847.

16 The Leadership Centre (2015). *The art of change making*. Curated and produced by John Atkinson, Emma Loftus and John Jarvis on behalf of the Systems Leadership Steering Group.

Available at: ॻ https://www.leadershipcentre.org.uk/wp-content/uploads/2016/02/The-Art-of-Change-Making.pdf (accessed 21 August 2019).

17 Kahneman D. (2012). *Thinking, fast and slow.* Penguin, Harmondsworth.

18 NHS Sustainable Development Unit (2009–14). *Carbon reduction strategy for NHS England.* NHS Sustainable Development Unit, Cambridge.

19 NHS/PHE Sustainable Development Unit (2014). *NHS England/PHE sustainable development strategy for the health, public health and social care system 2014–2020.* NHS/PHE Sustainable Development Unit, Cambridge.

20 Sustainable Development Unit. *Route map.* Available at: ॻ http://www.sduhealth.org.uk/policy-strategy/route-map.aspx (accessed 21 August 2019).

21 Doll R, Hill AB. (2004). The mortality of doctors in relation to their smoking habits: a preliminary report. *British Medical Journal,* **328,** 1529–33.

22 Sustainable Development Unit (2016). Securing healthy returns: realizing the financial value of sustainable development. SDU (NHS England/Public Health England). Available at: ॻ https://tinyurl.com/jf2utme (accessed 21 August 2019).

23 Sustainable Development Unit (2016). Module: creating social value. SDU (NHS England/Public Health England). Available at: ॻ http://www.sduhealth.org.uk/areas-of-focus/social-value.aspx (accessed 21 August 2019).

24 Plsek PE, Greenhalgh T. (2001). The challenge of complexity in health care. *British Medical Journal,* **323,** 625–8.

25 Levitt T. (2004). Marketing myopia. *Harvard Business Review.* July–August. Available at: ॻ https://hbr.org/2004/07/marketing-myopia (accessed 21 August 2019).

26 Haines A, Smith KR, Anderson D. et al. (2007). Policies for accelerating access to clean energy, improving health, advancing development, and mitigating climate change. *Lancet,* **370(9594),** 1264–81.

27 Dhainaut J, Claessens Y, Ginsburg C, et al. (2004). Unprecedented heat-related deaths during the 2003 heat wave in Paris: consequences on emergency departments. *Critical Care,* **8,** 1–2.

28 Public Health England (2018). Heatwave plan for England: protecting health and reducing harm from severe heat and heatwaves. Available at: ॻ https://www.gov.uk/government/publications/heatwave-plan-for-england (accessed 21 August 2019).

29 Atkinson S, Ingham J, Cheshire M, et al. (2010). Defining quality and quality improvement. *Clinical Medicine,* **10(6),** 537–9.

30 Nunes A, Lee K, O'Riordan T. (2016). The importance of an integrating framework for achieving the Sustainable Development Goals: the example of health and well-being. *BMJ Global Health,* 1, e000068. doi:10.1136/bmjgh-2016

Chapter 5.1

Sustainability of healthcare systems

Elena Azzolini, Mary Harney, and Walter Ricciardi

Objectives

Having read this chapter, you should be able to:
- define the term 'health sustainability'
- understand the importance of health sustainability to public health
- recognize opportunities and actions needed to obtain a sustainable healthcare system.

Introduction

The topic of healthcare sustainability is still a real dilemma that is increasingly debated at all levels.

If we create a ranking of the most used terms in recent years, the term 'sustainability' would probably climb the podium. We continuously hear that our system is not sustainable, that we have to act in a sustainable way, that the future sustainability of our healthcare systems can't be guaranteed, etc. Why is it a so much debated topic? Because demographic, epidemiological, and economic projections highlight that the collapse is closer than stakeholders realize. The common consequence of all the projections is the increase of healthcare demand and costs, and the urge of structural reforms able to tackle healthcare challenges resulting from the financial crisis. The need of a change is urgent, and ensuring that healthcare systems remain sustainable represents a major challenge for governments, healthcare providers, and patients. In the context of austerity policies and slow economic growth across the world, it is increasingly difficult to reconcile the growing pressure to adopt new technologies and address the complexity on healthcare services of multi-morbidity in an aging population.[1] Furthermore, sustainability issues arise even without austerity because of the hugely increased life expectancy and the rise in non-communicable diseases. Therefore, the debate about how best to achieve healthcare that is sustainable in the long term has gained traction at international and national levels in recent years.

What does health sustainability mean?

Starting from 1997, sustainability became a fundamental objective of the European Union and it has been at the centre of numerous debates and reports both nationally and globally that have analysed the various aspects of sustainability (see Box 5.1.1).

In order to simplify such a multifaceted and broad concept, the European Steering Group for Sustainable Healthcare has published a collaborative, independent, and forward-looking contribution to the sustainable healthcare debate. In this White Paper, the provided definition of health sustainability is the synthesis resulting from a debated and critical analysis of the main current definitions. Health sustainability is defined as follows: 'People centric, innovative strategies to safeguard health of individuals and society providing efficient care that fulfils and adapts to evolving health needs and leads to the highest possible level of health whilst preserving the potential outcomes of future generation.'[2]

Box 5.1.1 Sustainability profiles

- *Financial*: the contribution of the health sector to growth, employment and scientific progress, innovation and economic development;
- *Environmental*: the relationship between the development of the health sector and the ecosystems in which the person lives (see ➔ Chapter 7.6);
- *Politico-cultural*: the knowledge and the underlying values of the choices of individuals and the community with regard to health issues;
- *Social*: the factors that contribute to improving the overall health of a community;
- *Intergenerational*: the protection of health for present and future generations.

Why is health sustainability important for public health?

In almost all the industrialized and emerging countries there is in progress a demographic and epidemiological transition,[3] related to an increase in life expectancy and a reduction in the birth rate, responsible for an increase in the elderly component of the population,[4] which is associated with a progressive change in the overall picture of the main causes of death, with a substantial increase of chronic and degenerative diseases.[5] This increase of needs goes hand in hand with an increase in demand and a strong growth of the patients' or citizens' expectations with regard to health outcomes. In such a scenario, it has alas simultaneously grafted the well-known decline in human and financial resources (Figure 5.1.1).[6, 7]

These are some of the signals that individually may not be a major concern but, added together and interacting with each other, can cause catastrophic effects. To solve one of these problems, neglecting the others is not the best solution.

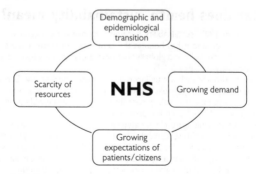

Figure 5.1.1 The changing health landscape.

Albeit briefly, we have identified the several factors that are now under-mining the sustainability of all health systems, the urgent need for a re-definition of the priorities of health systems at different levels, and an identification of specific approaches of intervention.

Across the world, notwithstanding the complexity and differences in how healthcare is funded and organised, we all face these same challenges.

What can be done to improve health sustainability?

What to do and how to ensure the sustainability of our healthcare system? How can our good ideas be turned to actions?

To obtain a sustainable healthcare system requires several changes in a multi-sectoral (and international) framework.

First, it is necessary to understand the actors involved and their goals. For example, in this scenario, policy makers and citizens would most likely be involved. For policy makers, the goal is usually to save money and it is up to public health practitioners to convey the message of the importance of investing and that health is a resource that should be considered as an in-vestment, not as an expense. For citizens, instead, the goal is to gain health. Thus, there are different perspectives and targets that need to be realigned.

Second, we should answer five questions, as listed in Box 5.1.2.

> **Box 5.1.2 Addressing five questions**
> - Which types of intervention would make the biggest difference to the health and well-being of the people?
> - What opportunities hold the greatest promise?
> - How can we prepare for the next 10 years?
> - How can we accelerate action to reduce inequalities?
> - How can we support decision-makers in their efforts to achieve better health and well-being for their people?

Health systems should be reorganized to answer to these questions ef-fectively through concrete innovative actions that are needed to make the transformation of healthcare systems a reality, from acute care to chronic care, from medical paternalism to citizen empowerment, from hospital de-pendency to integrated care across all levels of health systems, from ad hoc data collection to systematic surveillance and monitoring, as well as from cost and volume to value and outcome.[2]

From acute care to prevention and early intervention

Healthcare systems should be assessed on the basis of 'diseases avoided' rather than 'diseases treated'.

A truly sustainable healthcare model should place greater emphasis on re-ducing the incidence of avoidable diseases, such as diabetes, stroke, respira-tory disease, and certain cancers that are also major drivers of healthcare expenditure.[8] Effective prevention often delivers the best outcome and value. Efforts need to be focused on prevention and earlier intervention to delay the onset and progression of disease and disability.

From medical paternalism to citizen empowerment

Every citizen eventually becomes a patient. We need to ensure that they are empowered to play a central role in the management of their own health and to take responsibility for behavioural changes.[9] This requires equipping them with the skills needed to critically assess and interpret appropriate and informed health information so that they can make the necessary decisions to maintain a healthy lifestyle.

Health information and literacy are key drivers in making lifestyle decisions. Disease understanding is an important factor in self-management of conditions, treatment decisions, and adherence to treatment. If individuals participate in proactively managing their health, outcomes will be improved.[10] Of course, this is only possible for those who have the capability to make these choices. This caveat highlights the need for these measures to be embedded in broader policies to alleviate poverty, promote economic security, and foster inclusive and participative societies based on social, economic, and political rights.

From hospital dependency to integrated care

Many aspects of healthcare systems will need to be restructured if they are to continue to deliver high-quality, equitable, and affordable services.

The reorganisation of care delivery requires a paradigm shift and the adoption of three intertwined principles, namely: patient-centric integrated care, improved hospital efficiency, and interventions in an optimal setting, either in hospitals, at home or in communities.

By putting patients' care pathways at the centre of the system design, integrated care systems can deliver improved and tailored health outcomes while creating efficiencies in settings where they are delivered. Therefore, in the future, the emphasis should shift from the acute hospital to outpatient, community, and home settings. This would result in a much more cost-effective system with better health outcomes and higher patient satisfaction.[11,12]

From ad hoc data collection to systematic surveillance and monitoring

Healthcare systems generate huge amounts of data. This data offers considerable potential for policy makers, healthcare professionals, and patients if gathered and used appropriately. It could inform and improve prevention policies and strategies, allow better planning of treatment and care, and empower citizens and patients. However, in most countries, the collection, organisation, and deployment of data is not effectively set up and used. Issues such as patient confidentiality, civil liberties and the complexity of datasets across organisations and systems must be addressed. The challenges have become much greater as a consequence of recent revelations on the scale of surveillance undertaken by some states and the resulting loss of public trust. Concerns about the commercial use of data also pose a challenge. Addressing these challenges will unlock the huge potential presented by healthcare information and technology.

From volume to value-based payments

Health is a value in itself. It is also a precondition for economic prosperity. The health of individuals influences economic outcomes in terms of productivity, labour supply, human capital, and public spending. Some health expenditure is an investment in society that is growth-friendly. Policy makers need to ensure that short-term cost saving is not detrimental to long-term sustainability.

The financing of innovation and decisions around therapy funding both need forward thinking, where value and benefits are both rewarded and widely diffused.

As in all innovation, great value will rightly attract great reward. Truly transformative innovation creates societal value way beyond the innovator, the therapy, the device, or the price. For patients, the value of lives transformed and lives saved by innovative therapies can never be fully reflected in a price. The widest diffusion of innovation, and the creation of greatest value, happens when we adapt to the great variety of purchasers' needs and constraints. With due reward, innovation is best supported by facilitating its widest diffusion, spreading and sharing the value created.

Key messages

- Smart health expenditure can be an investment rather than a cost: investment in prevention and early intervention are essential for healthcare sustainability and socio-economic development and stability.
- Empowered and responsible citizens are the main players contributing to healthcare sustainability.
- Integrated care based on patient pathways, as well as shifting care delivery from hospitals to communities and homes, fosters greater efficiencies and better health outcomes.

What are the potential pitfalls?

The concept of sustainability is often reduced to a purely financial issue. It is wrong because an increased availability of resources does not solve five critical issues that are extensively documented in industrialized countries:[13]

- The extreme variation in utilization of healthcare services that cannot be explained by variation in patient need or patient preferences.
- Adverse effects caused by excessive medicalization, particularly over-diagnosis and over-treatment.
- Inequalities resulting from under-utilization of services—in particular, high-value services;
- The inability to implement effective prevention strategies.
- Waste, which nests at all levels.[14]

In industrialized countries, there is no evidence showing a direct relationship between the size of investments in health and improvement of population health outcomes,[15] a concept already known for decades. Indeed, according to Avedis Donabedian, increasing the resources introduced in a health system leads to benefits growing rapidly in the initial stage and then gradually flattening out. However, whereas the risks increase in a linear way, there is a trade-off beyond which further additional resources may even worsen the population health outcomes.

Thus the challenge for modern health systems consists in identifying this trade-off in the clinical areas, ensuring the highest health return compared with the invested resources.

Four important lessons

There are four fundamental points that must be remembered.
- Quite often the best ideas come from the bottom up: therefore, we must encourage those who are face to face with patients, their families and carers to share their best practices and to drive change by putting their experience and knowledge to use.
- Health is wealth: supporting healthy citizens to have access to high-quality care must remain a top priority for countries. We must never lose sight of our primary goal: ensuring the well-being of citizens and securing healthcare systems for those who need them.
- There is no one-size-fits-all solution: rather than wait for the one magic formula or solution, governments and policy makers should actively encourage and support innovative initiatives, reward excellence, and achievement, and scale up successful projects.
- Failures can teach as much as successes: not every idea will work in every country; however, every country can and should contribute its own ideas, pilot programmes, and innovations to the larger conversation. Exchanges between different countries on successes and lessons learned will lead to broader positive impacts across all healthcare systems.

Conclusions

The increase in healthcare demand and costs makes sustainability a major concern for all governments. There is much debate on the sustainability of healthcare systems and on how best to respond to budgetary pressures. This debate often continues to be dealt with in a distorted way by the various categories of stakeholders, looking at a short-term horizon, and remaining stalled on how to find the resources to maintain the status quo, instead of discussing how to reorganize the health system to ensure its survival. The hope is that national and international institutions, along with all the key stakeholders of the public and private sectors, will be motivated to contribute to the implementation of the mentioned opportunities and to translate into reality the concept of sustainability of health care.

We can no longer afford to keep our heads in the sand.

Further resources

Further reading

Baicker K, Cutler D, Song Z. (2010). Workplace wellness programs can generate savings. *Health Affairs*, **29**(2), 304–11.

European Commission (2013). Investing in health. Available at: ℘ https://ec.europa.eu/health/sites/health/files/policies/docs/swd_investing_in_health.pdf (accessed 21 August 2019).

Guthrie B, Saultz JW, Freeman GK, et al. (2008). Continuity of care matters. *British Medical Journal*, **337**, a867.

Harvey B. (2014). The case for prevention and early intervention. Promoting positive outcomes for children, families and communities. Prevention and Early Intervention Network, Dublin.

International Alliance of Patients' Organisations. (2014). Patient empowerment: for better quality, more sustainable health services globally, All Party Parliamentary Group (APPG) on Global Health, London.

Marmot M. (2010). *The Marmot Review: fair society, healthy lives: strategic review of health inequalities in England post 2010*. University College London: London.

McKee M, Chow CK. (2012). Improving health outcomes: innovation, coverage, quality and adherence. *Israeli Journal of Health Policy Research*, **1**, 43.

Stuckler D. (2008). Population causes and consequences of leading chronic diseases: a comparative analysis of prevailing explanations. *Milbank Quarterly*, **86**, 273–326.

World Economic Forum (2013). *Sustainable health systems. Visions, strategies, critical uncertainties and scenarios*. A report from the World Economic Forum prepared in collaboration with McKinsey & Company.

World Health Organization. (2005). *Preventing chronic diseases: a vital investment*. WHO, Geneva.

References

1 Barnett K, Mercer SW, Norbury M, et al. (2012). Epidemiology of multimorbidity and implications for health care, research, and medical education: a cross-sectional study. *Lancet*, **380**(9836), 37–43. Available at: ℘ http://www.thelancet.com/pdfs/journals/lancet/PIIS0140-6736(12)60240-2.pdf (accessed 21 August 2019).

2 European Steering Group on Sustainable Healthcare (2015). *Acting together – roadmap for sustainable healthcare*. European White Paper.

3 Damiani G, Azzolini E, Silvestrini G, et al. (2014). Features and developments of primary care in a public health perspective. [Article in Italian]. *Iegine e Sanita Pubblica*, **70**(5), 509–26.

4 United Nations (2015). World population ageing 2015. Available at: ℘ http://www.un.org/en/development/desa/population/publications/pdf/ageing/WPA2015_Report.pdf (accessed 21 August 2019).

5 Busse R, Blümel M, Scheller-Kreinsen D, et al. (2010). Tackling chronic disease in Europe. Strategies, interventions and challenges. *Observatory Studies Series*, **20**. WHO, Geneva.

6 Campbell J, Dussault G, Buchan J, et al. (2013). A universal truth: no health without a workforce. Forum Report, Third Global Forum on Human Resources for Health, Recife, Brazil. Geneva. Global Health Workforce Alliance, WHO, Geneva.

7 Crisp N, Chen L. (2014). Global supply of health professionals. *New England Journal of Medicine*, **370**(10), 950–7.

8 World Health Organization (2011). *Global status report on non-communicable diseases 2010. Reducing risks and preventing disease: population-wide intervention*. WHO, Geneva.

9 *Lancet* (2012). Patient empowerment-who empowers whom? *Lancet*, **379**(9827), 1677.

10 Active Citizenship Network (2014). best practices on chronic patients and organisations' empowerment. Available at: ℘ http://www.activecitizenship.net/files/patients_rights/8th_european_patients_rights_day_conference_materials/bp-chronic-patients-organizations-empowerment.pdf (accessed 21 August 2019).

11 World Health Organization (2004). *What are the advantages and disadvantages of restructuring health care system to be more focused on primary care services?* WHO Regional Office for Europe, Copenhagen.

12 The King's Fund (2011). Integrated care: our work on joined-up health and care services. Available at: ℘ http://www.kingsfund.org.uk/topics/integrated-care (accessed 21 August 2019).

13 Muir Gray JA. (2011). *How To Get Better Value Healthcare*, 2nd edn. Offox Press Ltd., Oxford.

14 Berwick DM, Hackbarth AD. (2012). Eliminating waste in US health care. *JAMA Internal Medicine*, **307**, 1513–6.

15 Hussey PS, Wertheimer S, Mehrotra A. (2013). The association between health care quality and cost: a systematic review. *Annals of Internal Medicine*, **158**, 27–347.

Planning health services

David Lawrence

Objectives and summary

This chapter shows you how to contribute to planning health services successfully at strategic and operational levels.

It first explains what health service planning is and the nature of health services as mainly 'soft' systems. It provides a conceptual framework for planning and then goes through steps and tasks in planning.

It then suggests some ways of overcoming pitfalls, notes some common fallacies about planning, and provides a real planning case study with its successes and failures. Finally, it notes ways to assess how well you are doing.

What is health services planning?

A plan has been defined as 'the way it is proposed to carry out some proceeding.'[1] Planning is the process by which a plan is put into action. All organizations that have aims—governments, armies, for-profit corporations, not-for profit community interest companies, or public service organizations—plan, whether in public service environments or in competition-based marketplaces.

The main aims of health services are:

- to prolong life
- to improve patients' clinical condition and 'health utility', which is defined here as health-related quality of life as valued by patients
- to minimize clinical morbidity and patient health dis-utility (i.e. reduce risk of mortality, pain, and distress). A secondary aim is to make the *process* of healthcare as convenient and pleasant for the patient as possible.

Health services planning is a *continual* process that converts health policy aspirations into organized practical efforts to make health services more effective and efficient.

Two overarching aspects of planning can be categorized as follows:

- Technical: e.g. effectiveness, cost-effectiveness, and optimal location and function of primary, secondary, and tertiary care units.
- Organizational: e.g. effective management, finance, training, workforce planning, and involving concerned groups, especially patients.

Planning aims to deliver specified health improvement objectives by examining options for change and choosing a prioritized course. Therefore, among other things, planning is about decision making and one important and very useful approach is to use what are called analytical models for decision making,[2] which bring together the above technical and organizational aspects. For example,

- in assessing how many residential facilities are required for people with health and care problems, 'balance of care' (between home and residential care) models have been developed that estimate the number of people with various degrees of disability, and the mix of resources and their costs needed to care for them.[3]
- Cognitive mapping[2] helps to elucidate various people's views and possibly bring about a consensus or at least make disagreement clear.

Planning takes place at various levels—whole society through to local. Strategic planning is an overall approach for achieving policy objectives. It typically involves whole or large parts of health service systems and time-scales of years. Operational or management planning is concerned with the specific tasks that will deliver a strategy. Usually these plans are shorter term and cover smaller units and individual departments of organizations.

Planning and the social/political context

So that your planning efforts will yield benefits, you must understand not only how a health service operates but also its cultural and society context. Planning within a wider context for a whole country or state is the subject of health policy.[4]

The planning process will vary depending on a country's healthcare funding arrangements and the political/economic culture. Healthcare funding may come from:

- public/social funding:
  - national and/or local taxes
  - subscription-based regulated social insurance, where services are usually 'clinical need'-based, free (or with a small co-payment) at the point of use.
- commercial, risk-based insurance or private fee for service, where access to services is partly or wholly on ability to pay.
- a mixture of these.

Publicly funded or social insurance-based services often have a community needs-based planning process. Conversely, commercially based/private funding systems usually have a demand-based market process.[5] In many countries there is a mixture of the two. Although these two approaches may differ fundamentally at the whole-country level, and different political values underpin them, practical planning processes at the local level often have common elements. The political context affects the way planning is carried out, but not the need for it.

Health services as systems

A health service is a system, which is a set of interconnected elements, where what happens in one part of the system affects the rest, so that they act together as a whole.[6] System approaches to planning are essential to understanding how health services function and for making useful changes.

A health service is a complex economic input–output system. Patients with a need for care 'demand' (in economics usage) a service and are (together with professionals, healthcare buildings and equipment) the 'inputs'. Primary planning outputs are health outcomes: changes in patients' health utility.

Health services differ from most other economic systems in important ways that will affect your ability to plan successfully:[7, 8]

- The usual pyramidal power hierarchy is inverted: doctors and other frontline healthcare professionals are numerous, wield political and managerial power, and effectively control resource use in the system.
- Most users of healthcare have relatively little medical knowledge and so 'consumer sovereignty' is limited and providers, especially clinicians, lead as patients' agents in making clinical decisions.
- Healthcare has a special political and social position in most societies.

Another way in which healthcare systems differ from usual economic systems is in defining 'productivity'. In, for example car production, productivity could be defined as the number of usable cars produced (which meet defined quality standards) divided by the amount of resources used to produce them (including resources used to produce cars not meeting the quality standards). In healthcare systems, productivity could be defined as the amount of all patients' net increase in health utility produced, divided by the resources used on all patients using the health service.

Conceptual frameworks for planning

One framework for healthcare planning is a rational system framework:[9]
- Identify a future desired state.
- Compare it with the present state.
- Identify possible pathways from one to the other (options).
- Implement the most cost-effective pathway.

This 'hard' system approach works best where there are well-defined, structured and easy-to-control systems, with easily identifiable objectives—for example, in car manufacture. Health services are 'soft' systems: people-based, with complex difficult-to-define detailed processes and objectives. Here, 'soft' systems planning is likely to be more successful.[6] This approach includes:
- intervention in an iterative cycle (with integral evaluation)
- recognizing cultural constraints
- participation in planning by most or all parties affected by the system.
- approaching the problem using both systems and 'real world' (pragmatic or 'corporate') thinking.[6]

Table 5.2.1 shows various conceptual frameworks for healthcare 'soft' systems compared to car manufacture, a 'hard' system.

Table 5.2.1 Models and examples of input–output systems

Input–output model	Input	Input	Output 1	Output 2	Output 3
'Medical care' model[a]	Need	Demand	Activity	Health utility increase	Process satisfaction
Donabedian model	Structure	Process	Process	Outcome 1	Outcome 2
Health services example: ophthalmology	Cataract patients, doctors, optometrists etc., managers, plant	Appointments requested for eye examination	Cataract extractions/ lens implants performed	Change in visual functioning	Vision-related quality of life. patient utility
Commodity production example: car manufacture	Workers, managers, materials, plant	Producers' decisions to manufacture	Cars produced	Cars sold	Cars used. User utility

a) Logan, RFL, Ashley JSA, Klein, RE, Robson, DM (1972) *Dynamics of medical care: the Liverpool study into use of hospital resources* London School of Hygiene & Tropical Medicine, London, Memoir 14, xvi+152.

What are the tasks in planning?

What planning approaches do you need?

Consider two policy-making approaches: 'rational satisficing'[10] is akin to 'hard' systems planning, whereas pragmatic, incrementalist policy making[11] is akin to 'soft' systems planning. In practice, planning is usually a mixture of both approaches. One key public health skill is to judge for any given planning situation how much the rational and pragmatic strands are going to influence the planning processes and outcomes—see Table 5.2.2.

Table 5.2.2 'Rational satisficing' or 'incremental' planning—which approach will work?

Factors	Favourable to rational, evidence-based, planning	Favourable to pragmatic, incremental or 'corporate' planning
Use of technical information and quantitative modelling	Available, understood, believed, and used	Missing, not believed, and not used
Degree of concern and interest about topic from powerful groups in the society	Topic not controversial, or little concern	Topic controversial, or great concern
Degree of consensus between most pluralist groups in the society	Much consensus	Little consensus
Local or central control	Local flexibility, good local control	Central, target-driven, little local control
Type of system: nature of objectives	'Hard' well-understood system with well-defined objectives	'Soft' system with difficult-to-define objectives

Planning can be considered as a series of projects (each project having a beginning and an end.) Then:

1. a project management approach[12] may be very useful (e.g. PRINCE2 'Projects IN controlled environments'[13]

2. a project evaluation should be built in, with relevant data collected from the start of the planning process.

The order of tasks in effective planning

Your first task is working well with the people involved in planning and managing healthcare so that they ask you to help achieve their policy-planning imperatives. You can do this by showing them how you, and the tools you use, will support and improve their decisions. The most difficult part of this task is to understand people's knowledge and perceptions: it is vital to learn about the views that people have and to develop their trust in you.

You will need to work with the following:
- Managers and clinicians within organizations who are involved in purchasing (or commissioning) and providing healthcare.
- Service users and patient carers. They will have experienced most of the good and bad aspects of services. But to be effective, patients need training in the planning role, just as professionals do. Citizens' panels can be a good way to do this, but are time-consuming and expensive.[14, 15]
- There are likely to be existing planning groups—or you will need to help set them up—and to be effective you will need to work with these groups. To be really useful, these planning groups need to be part of the power structure, with authority over budgets.

The second task you will usually carry out is to develop specific options for implementing policy, including new 'models of clinical care', involving changes to inputs or processes. Your role is to brief those involved in planning the healthcare, on a) the effectiveness of relevant clinical interventions,[16] and b) changing ways of organizing clinical work and new knowledge of the way healthcare systems work. Writing a business case often falls on public health professionals and includes considering finance, project management, and organizing effective meetings.

The third task is providing quantitative and qualitative information for planning.[17, 18] This includes quantifying how the new arrangements will affect health service patterns of provision, activity, budgets, and outcomes. Analytical models mentioned are useful for this,[2, 19] especially when various scenarios are tested (sensitivity analysis) and supported by decision analysis. The output from the above tasks is usually an implementation plan for a strategy or project proposal.

The fourth task is to work through the implications of the policy options produced in earlier tasks, including evaluation of actual changes, which should be an integral part of the planning process: see the case study in Box 5.2.1.[20]

The planning cycle then begins again, with monitoring and evaluation determining what effect planned changes are having on the health system.

Box 5.2.1 Planning integrated care in Southwark and Lambeth, London

This case study illustrates many important technical and organizational aspects of planning in healthcare—for example, the requirement for sufficient and relevant information, and the need to involve all interested parties and get their trust and agreement to planning proposals, both for process and intended aims.[a]

Aims and objectives of planning

'Southwark and Lambeth Integrated Care' (SLIC) was a planning programme whose aim was to get ' ... local health and social care systems to work in partnership to improve the way care is provided in Southwark and Lambeth'.[a]

Box 5.2.1 *(Contd.)*

Its objectives were: 1. to identify and address care needs at an early stage. 2. Join up care around people and across providers. 3. Provide care in the most appropriate setting. Further, ' ... to do this within tough financial constraints. To succeed required more than just 'joining up' services: the partnership knew it would need to bring about a fundamental culture change, radically redesigning models of care and commissioning approaches, and breaking down silos'.[a]

Methods

The programme began by focusing on the needs of people over 65, supporting them to remain independent in their own homes.

It developed a holistic, coordinated approach to supporting people and came to the realisation that the delivery of care could not be integrated unless the systems underpinning it were also integrated.

Successes

There were many, including the following:
- The project vision united people from the various organizations to achieve a common goal.
- The range of interventions, including simplified [hospital] discharge, falls pathways, integrated care managers, holistic assessments, and community multidisciplinary teams were well thought of.
- Hospital and social care activity rates stayed flat over time when neighbouring areas saw a rise, although the evidence was not robust because of lack of data.

What worked less well

'SLIC suffered from not articulating what success looked like and how it should be measured. We learned that it is crucial to know whether you are on track, and to be able to continuously measure system progress. To do this, measurement metrics should be agreed with stakeholders at the outset'.[a]

Expected cost savings were not met.

Lessons learned and recommendations

'A systems approach to developing and rolling out services relating to integrated care is seen as feasible with an evident belief from respondents that the local health and social care system is now stronger and better placed than it would have been without the SLIC initiative. We recommend that a local systems perspective is more useful than one focused on discrete agencies, even traditionally powerful ones such as NHS FTs [hospitals]'.[a]

'Lessons learnt from the stakeholder interviews suggest that the following characteristics contribute to success:
- Design of interventions—adapt the evidence base, and be explicit when generating new evidence. Interventions should be co-designed, piloted, and iteratively developed.
- Strong clinical leadership, with adequate time and resources for innovation and planning.
- Stakeholder involvement and shared ownership.

Box 5.2.1 *(Contd.)*
- Organizational structure and governance—start small scale, simple, focused, and bottom up.
- Patients and citizens—patients/service users as partners.
- Evaluation—there is a need for inbuilt evaluation and effective data collection to enable evaluation of any future programme from different stakeholder perspectives. In order to assess 'after' effects, robust 'before' data have to be collected and data collection capacity has to be robust in practice and over time.[a]

'Future interventions are evidence based, and grounded in literature that specifies how they might improve care and outcomes'.[a]

Outcome
The SLIC project has been continued as the 'SLIC Partnership'.

a) Southwark and Lambeth Integrated Care, SLIC programme. Available at: ℳ https://www. kingshealthpartners.org/assets/000/000/690/FINAL_Full_End_of_SLIC_Report_original.pdf (accessed 3 September 2019).

Overcoming pitfalls in health services planning

Full implementation of planning decisions, especially strategic ones, usually takes years and often you will not have that time. But the framework presented here can help produce the most benefit in the time you have. To save time, you may, for example, have to use estimates from others, rather than undertake your own needs surveys. The aim of using information in planning is to show planners how changing resources will affect the system.

Planning rarely goes according to plan because circumstances and personnel change. The suggested approaches using analytical models to support decisions[2] are useful in minimizing problems. You yourself can develop relatively simple spreadsheet models to support making planning decisions as circumstances change.

The intended objectives in planning are often only partially attained and there are sometimes unintended consequences. Therefore, monitoring the effects of planning and making continual adjustments are crucial.

Fallacies about health services planning

- *Planning is rational and evidence-based*: it is usually a mix of pragmatic and rational.
- *Planning is a one-off*: planning is continual and evolves.
- *Planning stifles creativity*: planning can help creativity by facilitating orderly planning processes.
- *Planning is trying to predict the future—to give the 'right' answer*: planning is providing intelligence on what might happen in complex systems using trend models with scenario 'what ifs', so as to help more effective decision making.

An example of health services planning and lessons learned

The Southwark and Lambeth Integrated Care (SLIC) case study in Box 5.2.1 is a good example of the reality of planning. The referenced report[20] is useful reading for all planners, showing the difficulties in implementing new clinical care models.

What are key determinants of success?

- As in many areas, a key skill is to know what is feasible and to work well with people. It is essential to develop trust with all groups with an interest in the planning scheme.
- Do the technical homework, but present information and detailed evidence in a way that politicians, managers, and clinicians will understand and find useful—be simple and write plainly with any jargon explained: use a policy briefing style.[21]
- Find key authoritative evidence, but also ask advice from experienced public health and other experts.
- Be useful: for example, find information on the most pressing concerns managers and clinicians have.

How do you assess your success?

- *Monitoring and evaluation:* success is usually not absolute. Obviously there should be specific objectives and measurement of their attainment. But success, like the planning process, is often iterative—it comes little by little. That implies that integral monitoring and evaluation are essential to successful planning.
- *Feedback:* discussions with colleagues and formal evaluations, including workshops, are important.

Further resources

Further reading

Department of Health (2015). *Guide to health service planning, version 3.* Queensland, Australia. Available at: ℛ https://www.health.qld.gov.au/__data/assets/pdf_file/0025/443572/guideline-health-service-planning.pdf (accessed 21 August 2019).

Green A. (2007). *An introduction to health planning for developing health systems.* Oxford University Press, Oxford.

HealthKnowledge. Health service planning. Available at: ℛ https://www.healthknowledge.org.uk/teaching/health-service-planning (accessed 21 August 2019).

Markwell S, Beynon C. (2009, 2017). Health service development and planning. Available at: ℛ https://www.healthknowledge.org.uk/public-health-textbook/organisation-management/5d-theory-process-strategy-development/health-service-development-planning (accessed 21 August 2019).

Ozcan YA. (2009). *Quantitative methods in health care management.* Jossey-Bass, San Francisco.

References

1 The Shorter Oxford English Dictionary. Clarendon Press, 1973.
2 Sanderson C, Gruen R. (2006). *Analytical models for decision-making*. Open University Press, Maidenhead.
3 The Balance of Care Group. Available at: http://www.balanceofcare.co.uk/downloads.html (accessed 21 August 2019).
4 Buse K, Mays N, Walt G. (2005). Making health policy. McGraw-Hill/Open University Press, Maidenhead.
5 Green A. (2007). An introduction to health planning for developing health systems. Oxford University Press, Oxford.
6 Van Wyk G. (2003). A systems approach to social and organizational planning. Trafford Publishing, Victoria, BC.
7 HSJ (2007). David Lawrence offers some words of advice to Mr Brown. Available at: http://www.hsj.co.uk/david-lawrence-offers-some-words-of-advice-to-mr-brown/58956.article (accessed 21 August 2019).
8 Available at: https://files.constantcontact.com/9bc520cb001/a7ff09d0-0fc3-4eca-9a29-fe0892e7c601.pdf (accessed 20 October 2019).
9 Guy M. (2001). Diabetes: developing a local strategy. In: Pencheon D, Guest C, Melzer D, Gray JAM. (eds) *Oxford handbook of public health practice*, 1st edn, p. 559. Oxford University Press, Oxford.
10 http://en.wikipedia.org/wiki/Satisficing Last accessed 7 March 2017.
11 http://en.wikipedia.org/wiki/Incrementalism Last accessed 7 March 2017.
12 https://en.wikipedia.org/wiki/Project_management Last accessed 9 February 2017.
13 https://en.wikipedia.org/wiki/PRINCE2 Last accessed 11 April 2017.
14 Abelson J, Eyles J, McLeod CB, et al. (2003). Does deliberation make a difference? Results from a citizens panel study of health goals priority setting. *Health Policy*, **66(1)**, 95–106.
15 Church J, Saunders D, Wanke M, et al. (2002). Citizen participation in health decision-making: past experience and future prospects. *Journal of Public Health Policy*, **23(1)**, 12–32.
16 National Institute for Health and Care Excellence, Improving health and social care through evidence-based guidance. Available at: https://www.nice.org.uk (accessed 21 August 2019).
17 Ozcan YA. (2009). *Quantitative methods in health care management*. Jossey-Bass, San Francisco.
18 Bullas S, Dallas A. (2002). *Information for managing healthcare resources*. Radcliffe Medical, Abingdon.
19 Annalisa software. Available at: http://annalisa.org.uk (accessed 21 August 2019).
20 Southwark and Lambeth Integrated Care, SLIC programme. Available at: https://www.kingshealthpartners.org/assets/000/000/690/FINAL_Full_End_of_SLIC_Report_original.pdf (accessed 3 September 2019).
21 https://en.wikipedia.org/wiki/Memorandum#Policy_briefing_note. Last accessed 29 April 2017.

Comparing healthcare systems

Martin McKee and Ellen Nolte

Objectives

This chapter will enable you to:
• understand why health systems are the way they are
• describe the key features of health systems
• appreciate the opportunities and challenges involved in comparing
  health systems.

Why are health systems the way they are?

Although health professionals typically look at health systems as a means by which those in need of healthcare can obtain it, in reality, the design of health systems is often primarily a result of political rather than technical decisions. This is because, unlike with most consumer goods, the purchase of healthcare involves redistribution of resources within society on a large scale. Put simply, those who are in most need of healthcare, such as older people and those with chronic illnesses, are usually least able to afford it. Unless they are to be left to suffer and, perhaps, die, someone else must pay for their care.

This redistribution should be a core function of organised health systems. It can take many forms. Some involve redistribution across the life course of the individual, recognising that they will pay into the system during their working life when they will draw from it in childhood and old age. However, mostly, it involves redistribution from the rich and healthy to the ill and poor. As with all decisions about redistribution of resources within society, this involves political choices. Those political choices, in turn, reflect the predominant views about the relationship between the individual, the state, and other groups.

The role that these considerations play can be illustrated by looking at two of the classic models of healthcare system, the tax-funded National Health Service in the United Kingdom and the statutory insurance system in Germany. In both cases, there is a widespread public acceptance of the need for a collective response to healthcare needs. However, the two countries differ in how this is to be addressed. In the United Kingdom, it is seen as a responsibility of government. This has its origins in the Second World War, when the government created an Emergency Medical Service, bringing the previously fragmented hospital system within a single national framework. In Germany, in contrast, having emerged in the late nineteenth century, the welfare system built on a strong set of relationships between the social partners, the employers' associations and trade unions and, while it initially covered only industrial workers, it went far beyond healthcare to cover many aspects of welfare.

The situation has been quite different in the United States. Although historically there have been several attempts to introduce universal coverage, overall there has been much less acceptance that the state should play a role in healthcare. Yet, paradoxically, with about half of health expenditure coming from public sources, the state has assumed responsibility for those with most needs: people who are poor, covered by Medicaid, and elderly people, covered by Medicare.

Political considerations also influence how healthcare is organised within a country. Thus, responsibilities often follow other administrative divisions. In countries such as Spain and Italy, devolution of responsibility to regions only became possible once those regions came into being and achieved autonomy in relation to other sectors. The decentralised models of care in Nordic countries reflect a long-standing tradition of power being held at the level of the county or municipality. However, there have been moves to re-gionalize health services as part of wider reforms of local government, such as in Denmark in the 2000s, although there were sound technical reasons for organizing health services on a larger geographical scale. Thus, even when there are clear advantages to configuring health services in a particular way, this will often have to work around established political structures.

Interest in the factors that influence the development of health systems can be traced to at least the 1960s, when researchers sought to develop typologies of health systems that reflected economic development and political characteristics.[1] More recently, the inclusion of universal health coverage within the 2015 Sustainable Development Goals has prompted work highlighting a number of factors that promote comprehensive health systems. These include left-wing governments, and especially those that have the ability to raise tax revenues and strong organised labour, in the form of trade unions.[2,3] Another factor is the ethnic, religious, or linguistic make-up of the country. Countries that are divided in any of these respects seem less able to implement and progress universal health coverage and achieve better health.[4] This is consistent with evidence from the United States showing that welfare is less generous in those states with a higher proportion of African-Americans.[5]

While there are important structural drivers of health systems, the role of individuals should not be overlooked. Many important healthcare re-forms have been driven by committed individuals who were able to take advantage of the prevailing circumstances. Examples include Aneurin Bevan in the United Kingdom, Tommy Douglas in Canada, and Willem Drees in the Netherlands. All combined a deep commitment to expanding health coverage with the administrative and political ability to make it happen.

For these reasons, healthcare reform should be seen as essentially pol-itical, rather than technical. While technical considerations, such as evi-dence on the best way to provide services, may play a role, it is rarely the dominant one.

A typology of health systems?

There have been many attempts to create typologies of health systems. The earliest attempts were based on the concept of 'ideal types', most often as-sociated with the sociologist Max Weber. This involved placing each health system within a broad category, sharing many characteristics with others in that category but also demonstrating certain differences. The best-known example is the distinction between the afore-mentioned Beveridge, or tax-funded, systems, exemplified by the British National Health Service but also including systems in Spain, Italy, and Scandinavia, and Bismarckian, or statutory insurance-funded systems, exemplified by Germany, but also found in countries such as Belgium, the Netherlands, Israel, and Japan (Table 5.3.1)[6]. The limitations of this approach are obvious, and gave rise to more complex models that combined different characteristics, often in a matrix, such as the means of financing on one axis and the ownership of delivery on another. Yet, even these had many limitations. As a consequence, while recognizing that such frameworks may have some value in basic comparisons, there has been a move towards more complex systems approaches.

Table 5.3.1 Key features of the Bismarck and Beveridge models of care

	Bismarck	Beveridge
	Taxation	Statutory health insurance
Entitlement based on ...	Citizenship/residence	Contributions
Levied on ...	All income/transactions	Wages
Benefits are ...	Comprehensive in theory	Defined
Choice	Usually no choice of insurer Some choice of provider	Some choice of insurer possible Some choice of provider
Controlled by ...	State/government	Independent health insurance funds, including representatives of trade unions and employers

Source: data from Mossialos E, Dixon A, Figueras J, Kutzin J. (eds) (2002) *Funding health care: options for Europe.* McGraw-Hill, Buckingham.

Systems approaches to healthcare

In the literature on systems research, there are two types of systems. The first, hard systems, include mechanical devices in which inputs are converted into outputs—for example, by means of levers and cogwheels. In contrast, soft systems involve human beings who, even when working within a framework of laws and rules, behave in ways that are not always anticipated.[7]

Soft systems are nested within other systems. For example, as we have shown above, health systems are part of larger political and legal systems. They are also influenced by other systems, such as those for professional regulation, or, in the case of pharmaceuticals, those related to industrial policy or intellectual property. In turn, health systems contain other subsystems.

Checkland's (1981) approach provides a basis for categorizing the various elements within a health system. It involves certain activities, or Transformation, for example, collecting revenue, pooling resources, investing in and designing facilities, or recruiting and retaining health workers. This transformation is undertaken by Actors, on behalf of Customers. The overall system has an Owner. In soft systems theory, the owner is defined as whoever has the power to stop the system from operating. This is the ultimate power. Each system operates within certain Environmental constraints, such as availability of funding or particular laws. The processes are influenced by norms and beliefs, here signified by the German word *Weltanschauung*, or 'worldview'. These are captured by the mnemonic CATWOE (Table 5.3.2).

Table 5.3.2 The CATWOE framework for soft systems analysis

C	Customers	The beneficiaries of the transformation
A	Actors	Those who make the transformation happen
T	Transformation	The conversion of an input to an output
W	*Weltanschauung*	The worldview that makes the transformation meaningful
O	Owners	Those who can stop the transformation
E	Environmental constraints	Elements outside the system, which are taken as given

Reproduced from Checkland P. (1981) *Systems thinking, systems practice*. John Wiley: Chichester, with permission from Wiley and Sons.

For example, a system for training health workers would be based on a transformation of school leavers into trained professionals by means of an educational process. The beneficiaries will be the students themselves but, in many countries, will also include those responsible for the health system, thereby justifying the investment of public resources in the training. The actors are those who undertake the training while environmental constraints include salaries and working conditions of health workers that influence the career choices of school leavers. The *Weltanschauung* includes the belief that it is better to have trained rather than untrained people providing modern healthcare.

Comparing health systems

There is much that can be learned from comparing health systems. Many face common challenges, such as the increasing complexity of healthcare, with multi-morbidity and the introduction of new technologies. Other challenges include how to pay for healthcare when rising public expectations clash with a political unwillingness to raise taxes. The process of benchmarking can be particularly useful, challenging assumptions that all is well. For example, international comparisons of cancer outcomes, which showed the United Kingdom lagging behind many comparable countries, played a crucial role in driving forward a major reform of the management of cancer in the British NHS from the late 1990s. Internationally, there are many examples of innovations, both successful and unsuccessful, that offer lessons for other countries. In some cases, they might be adopted, although with appropriate adaptation to local circumstances. In others, and perhaps more often, they can prevent the same mistake being made twice.

Yet, some caution is needed, much of it related to the implications of using a soft systems approach. It will rarely be helpful to compare one entire health system with another. This is because the other systems necessary for the health system to work may lie within the health system in some countries but not in others. For example, medical education may be the responsibility of the health ministry in some countries but within the remit of the ministry of higher education in others. Moreover, as noted above, there are often parallel systems, each looking after different groups within the population. Often, they will share some systems, such as the training of health workers or procurement of technology and pharmaceuticals, while other systems, such as the delivery of primary care, may be separate. It therefore is most usual to undertake comparisons of particular functions, such as the operation of hospitals or the delivery of care for people with particular conditions.

Second, something that works in one health system may not work in another, because of differences in the environmental constraints, such as the supply of health workers or money, or in the *Weltanschauung*, or norms and values. For example, physicians in countries where there is a strong tradition of liberal professionals may reject or subvert measures that have worked in others where physicians are state employees.

For these reasons, context is very important when thinking about the transferability of policies. Leichter offers a way of looking at context that can be helpful in understanding what might work in what circumstances (Table 5.3.3).[8] From a systems perspective, situational factors typically correspond to actors and owners, structural and environmental factors correspond to the environment, and cultural factors to *Weltanschauung*.

Table 5.3.3 Dimensions of policy context

Dimensions	Definition	Examples
Situational factors	Major, but transient events	Appointment of a new Minister of health
Structural factors	Constant features of the political and economic system	Regionalization of the healthcare system
Cultural factors	Values and norms	Autonomy of the medical profession
Environmental factors	External to the particular policy arena	Natural disaster or economic crisis

Source: data from Leichter, H.M. (1979). *A comparative approach to policy analysis: health care policy in four nations*. Cambridge University Press, Cambridge.

Sources of information on health systems

Quantitative data

Information on health systems can take several forms. Most governments supply quantitative data to international agencies, such as the World Health Organization and World Bank (Table 5.3.4). These include the resources available for healthcare and, in particular, the amount of money that is spent. This can be presented in several ways but, most usually, is shown in terms of percentage of Gross National Product spent on health (Figure 5.3.1), or the absolute amount that is spent. Although there has been an enormous effort to standardize national health accounts in recent years, it is important to recognize that this data is often problematic. In particular, there are differences in what is included, with areas such as social care, research and development, and higher education being particularly problematic. There are also problems in gathering data. While it may be possible to obtain official spending figures relatively easily, it is important to capture data on out-of-pocket spending. This is collected from family budget and similar surveys, but these may be infrequent and unrepresentative. There are particular problems where there is a large informal health economy.

Table 5.3.4 Sources of health and health system data

Source	Website
World Bank, World development indicators	http://data.worldbank.org/data-catalog/world-development-indicators
Institute of Health Metrics and Evaluation, (Global burden of diseases study)	http://www.healthdata.org/results/data-visualizations
World Health Organization, World health statistics	http://www.who.int/gho/publications/world_health_statistics/en
Organisation for Economic Co-operation and Development, Health statistics 2019	http://www.oecd.org/els/health-systems/health-data.htm

In international comparisons, economic data is typically presented in US dollars. Many comparisons take account of purchasing power parity, or PPP. It is important to know whether the figures use a general PPP or one that is specific to health. In most cases, it will be the former, although this can be problematic because prices in the health sector may change in quite different ways from those in the economy in general. However, health PPPs are only estimated infrequently and are heavily dependent on tradeable goods and services, and in particular pharmaceuticals. In many countries, expenditure data is broken down by category, such as spending on pharmaceuticals.

Other data covers inputs to healthcare, such as numbers of health professionals of different types or of physicians per 1,000 people (Figure 5.3.2).

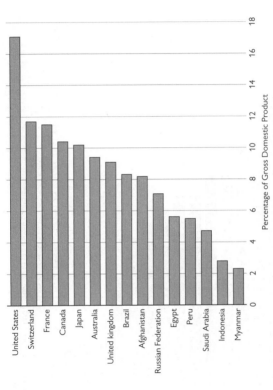

Figure 5.3.1 Percentage of Gross Domestic Product spent on health (public and private) in selected countries, 2014.

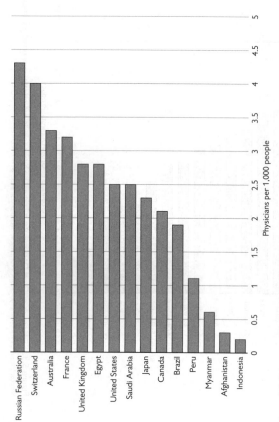

Figure 5.3.2 Physicians per 1,000 people, 2014 in selected countries.
Source: World Development Indicators, World Bank Group under a Creative Commons CC-BY 4.0 licence.

However, the categories used often reflect what can be counted rather than what is important. For example, one of the more widely used statistics is the number of hospital beds per capita even though, with the shift of much healthcare into the community and the growth of areas such as ambulatory surgery, this figure often has little meaning. Even data on health workers must be interpreted with caution. Thus, the skills profile of a nurse trained in some high-income countries, which will involve university education and include many advanced clinical roles, will be very different from that of someone entering nurse training at the age of 14 in some low-income countries.

While data on the inputs to health systems and the resources available to them can offer important insights, a comprehensive understanding should also look at the outcomes of health systems. This is discussed in much more detail in the ➲ Chapter 5.11 on evaluating healthcare systems. However, in brief, it includes measures based on the concept of mortality amenable to healthcare, which measures the number of deaths from conditions that should be avoidable with timely and effective healthcare. Health systems vary greatly in their ability to reduce these deaths.

As might be expected, data collection systems are much more comprehensive in high-income countries. Here, the Organisation for Economic Co-operation and Development has been in the forefront of efforts to develop measures of healthcare processes and outcomes, including rates of medical and surgical procedures, and outcomes of common conditions such as myocardial infarction.

Qualitative information

While numerical data can provide some insights into different health systems, a comprehensive understanding requires information on how the system is organised, who the key actors are, and how it fulfils its different functions. The European Observatory on Health Systems and Policies has pioneered work in this area, which is now also being undertaken by the North American Observatory and the Asia-Pacific Observatory.

A series of detailed health system profiles underpin much of this work. The health system in transition profiles, written by experts from the country in question and observatory staff, adhere to a common template and use standardized terminology to capture the key elements of each health system, as well as reviewing and evaluating current and planned reforms (see Box 5.3.1).

Box 5.3.1 Contents of health system in transition profiles

- Country overview.
- Organisational structure.
- Finance and expenditure.
- Healthcare delivery.
- Financial allocation.
- Reform process.

Source: European Observatory on Health Systems and Policies.

The European Observatory also undertakes numerous focused studies, looking at how health systems are responding to common challenges, such as the increasingly complex management of cancer, the threats powered by complex communicable diseases, such as drug system tuberculosis and HIV[9], or the challenges of non-communicable diseases.[10] Other studies look at how different countries have designed and implemented key health system functions, such as paying for healthcare, policies, and pharmaceuticals, or ensuring a high-quality health workforce.

Conclusion

Comparisons of health systems can be extremely valuable, challenging ideas that are taken for granted and revealing different ways of doing things. However, some caution is required. While innovations such as surgical diagnostic techniques can, in most cases, easily be transferred from one country to another, this may not be the case with more complex organizational innovations, which depend for their operation on features of the broader health system or, indeed, other systems, such as professional regulation. Consequently, while there is considerable potential for improving the delivery of healthcare by learning from best practice elsewhere, that learning should take full account of the different contexts of the countries concerned.

Further resources

Further reading

Websites

European Observatory on Health Systems and Policies Available at: ℘ http://www.euro.who.int/en/about-us/partners/observatory/about-us (accessed 21 August 2019).

References

1 Nolte E, McKee M, Wait S. (2005). Describing and evaluating health systems. In: Bowling A, Ebrahim S, eds, *Handbook of health research methods: investigation, measurement and analysis*, pp. 12–43. Open University Press, Maidenhead.

2 Reeves A, Gourtsoyannis Y, Basu, S, et al. (2015). Financing universal health coverage—effects of alternative tax structures on public health systems: cross-national modelling in 89 low-income and middle-income countries. *Lancet*, **386**, 274–80.

3 McKee M, Balabanova D, Basu S, et al. (2013). Universal health coverage: a quest for all countries but under threat in some. *Value in Health*, **16(1)**, S39–S45.

4 Powell-Jackson T, Basu S, Balabanova D, et al. (2011). Democracy and growth in divided societies: a health-inequality trap? *Social science & medicine*, **73(1)**, 33–41.

5 Alesina A, Glaeser EL. (2004). *Fighting poverty in the US and Europe: a world of difference*. Oxford University Press, Oxford.

6 Mossialos E, Dixon A, Figueras J, et al. (eds). (2002). *Funding health care: options for Europe*. McGraw-Hill, Buckingham.

7 Checkland P. (1981). *Systems thinking, systems practice*. John Wiley, Chichester.

8 Leichter, HM. (1979). A comparative approach to policy analysis: health care policy in four nations. Cambridge University Press, Cambridge.

9 Coker R, Atun R, McKee M. (2008). *Health systems and the challenge of communicable diseases: experiences from Europe and Latin America*. McGraw-Hill, Buckingham.

10 Nolte E, McKee M. (eds). (2008). *Caring for people with chronic conditions: a health system perspective*. McGraw-Hill, Buckingham.

Chapter 5.4

Commissioning healthcare

Richard Richards

Objectives

This chapter is concerned with the use of contracts and payments as a means of ensuring that care maximizes health at minimum cost. The chapter aims to cover the full range of healthcare commissioning from the simplest form, an individual patient making a private payment to an individual practitioner, through to the most complex, tax-funded, social medicine 'free at the point of delivery'.

In all healthcare commissioning, a common set of concerns arise:

- The nature of the need, including an assessment of the (cost-) effectiveness of the relevant interventions.
- Examination of the services available, including inputs, quality of care, and outcomes.
- The costs and efficiency of the care on offer.
- The development of formal commissioning agreements.

Introduction

From boom ...

In 2006, the world collectively spent $4.7 trillion on healthcare, $4.1 trillion of that by the 31 Organisation for Economic Co-operation and Development (OECD) countries and $200 billion collectively by three other countries, China, India, and Brazil.[1] It is very big business, consuming a huge proportion (9.8%) of world resources.

In terms of life expectancy, this expenditure seems to have little effect (Figure 5.4.1). Female life expectancy rises from about 30 to 70 years for up to $100 spent *per capita* (pc) on healthcare, but that spending mirrors the rise in pc gross national income GNI), resulting from the move from hunter-gatherer society to one in which the organization of society has delivered clean water, nutrition (farming), and shelter. Up to $1,000 pc spend for a further 10 years is added, but after that there is little or no upward trend in

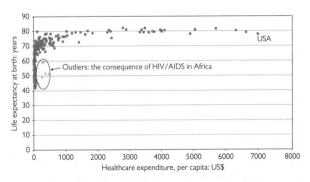

Figure 5.4.1 *Per capita* healthcare expenditure and life expectancy, 2006.

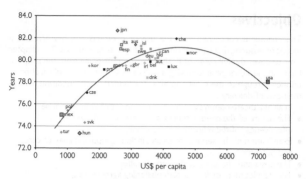

Figure 5.4.2 Healthcare expenditure and life expectancy in Organisation for Economic Co-operation and Development (OECD) countries, 2007.

life expectancy among the countries that spent that $4.1 trillion. The USA spent $2 trillion of that world total ($7,000 pc), yet had a female life expectancy less than that of Costa Rica, which spent just $400 pc. OECD data (Figure 5.4.2) paints a particularly startling situation for the USA, the highest spender, which has the seventh worst OECD life expectancy, yet the six worse countries also have the six lowest OECD pc healthcare expenditure.[2]

... to bust

250 years ago, Edmund Burke, politician and philosopher, commented that 'Frugality is founded on the principle that all riches have limits'. With the world now starting to come out from a deep economic recession, commissioning value-for-money healthcare that uses scarce resources wisely to maximize health and avoids diverting resources away from addressing the determinants of health is ever more important. Producing a marginal extension of life or improvement in quality of life in an OECD country may result, through carbon emissions and global warming, in significantly shortened lives in poorer countries.

Assessing need

For the individual, assessing need will usually require a diagnosis and often an assessment of the severity of the disease and associated co-morbidities. Often, there is much uncertainty about the patient's condition, introducing risk and limiting rational behaviour in the healthcare 'market'.

At the population level, a variety of approaches exist to assess need (see ➋ Chapter 1.4). A centrally planned healthcare system requires information on the numbers of people with each type of need to plan the extent of provision. Even entrepreneurial market systems, considered more able to change and willing to accept mistakes and failures, would first use market research to help determine the level of provision required.

Need, by definition, involves the presence of an undesirable health state plus the existence of effective interventions. In most circumstances, resources are limited, so the goal is to buy the most cost-effective care to improve health.

Complex products are typically built to plans or blueprints. Healthcare should be no different, and the equivalent is a care pathway that describes the disease progression and the interventions along that pathway: the what, when, where, and by whom of healthcare (with whys, the evidence, by way of explanation). Ideally it should be populated with probabilities (of movement between disease states as in a Markov model): the quality of life associated with each state and costs.

Inputs

The resources needed to deliver healthcare are of crucial interest both to the provider and the consumer/commissioner because they determine the *costs* to the former and the *price* to the latter. In the situation of the private consultation, an unaffordable price represents an inaccessible treatment. In the situation of a third-party payer, this condition is referred to, pejoratively, as rationing. To the consumer, be they patient or third-party payer, the input needs to be affordable and to maximize the outcomes for the available funds.

Cost containment is an inevitable goal of commissioning systems. Approaches vary from the prospective payment systems used in the US Medicare system that remove incentives remove incentives to unproductive over-activity (e.g. by placing physicians on salaries, rather than fees for service payments, and placing contracts with managed care providers. The socialized health providers in several European countries, Australia, Canada, and New Zealand operate cost containment through direct control and annual budget setting.

Inputs come in a variety of standards, quality, and availability (scarcity), which will be reflected in differences in costs and thus price. This applies to facilities, diagnostic and treatment equipment, drugs, and staff.

Quality and outcomes

The quality of healthcare has many dimensions, including the structures (staff, equipment, etc.), processes and outcomes. Commissioning should clearly state the quality expected in whatever dimensions seem necessary.

While health technology assessments can show what treatments should be given, audit will indicate whether a unit is actually providing those treatments as intended. Often units are too small and case mixes too complex to yield definitive indications of quality of care. The lack of good information on providers' quality and outcome often means that the patient/commissioner faces significant uncertainties and cannot choose rationally between providers in the way suggested by advocates of idealized market systems.

Efficiency, the ratio of costs to outcomes, provides a measure of value for money. Commissioners seek to maximize the efficiency of services, maximizing the output for the funding they give. Providers seek to maximize funding while minimizing costs: when there is a relationship between quality and higher costs, this can drive down quality for the individual patient. The profit motive can further distort incentives.

Coping with risk in healthcare commissioning

Risks take different forms. Ask a bank manager for a loan and the manager will assess the risk compared with the likelihood of profit for the bank. From the public health perspective, the 'bottom line' is not financial profit but health gain. Each commissioning decision carries a risk that the funding will not result in health gain.

Some risk, expressed as chance or probability, is purely stochastic and can be calculated in the form of statistical significance and confidence intervals of the size of benefit described in clinical trials. However, there are more problematic determinants of risk that are systematic and difficult to quantify or even note, and many result in exaggeration of benefits and thus risk un-intended inefficiencies. The most insidious of these is reflected in the term 'conflict' of interest. Such conflicts are not exclusive to research organized and funded by the pharmaceutical industry, but are seen when any inter-ested provider of care is involved in research or the secondary analysis of research data. Public health professionals, trained in epidemiology and thus aware of all the pitfalls of badly conducted research (clinical research being simply experimental epidemiology) are well placed to provide high-quality disinterested analysis and commissioning advice that can reduce those risks.

Small organizations, be they commissioners or providers, can face signifi-cant financial risks from high-cost, low-volume interventions. These occur unpredictably in any given year. Ways for commissioners to handle that risk are based on increasing these numbers to predictable levels by:

- grouping many low-volume, high-cost interventions together in one 'basket'
- collaborating with other small organizations to increase numbers, sharing costs on a weighted capitation basis
- creating a 'higher' tier (dictated by rarity of the intervention) responsible for commissioning
- any combination of these.

Commissioners and providers can share financial risk. A provider may serve a number of small commissioners and will therefore see a larger number of the rarer interventions, which will allow risks to be shared or spread.

An agreement that includes 'floors' and 'ceilings' can also be used to share risk. A range of activity around a central estimate is commissioned and paid for: no change in funding occurs within those limits. Should activity fall below the 'floor', the provider returns funding to the commissioner and, should the activity exceed the 'ceiling', the commissioner pays extra.

Agreeing costs

The amount of funding involved in commissioning a whole service depends on the concept of 'marginal' and 'step-up' cost, two sides of the same coin. Some costs to a provider are 'fixed', independent of activity levels (staff salaries, equipment, buildings, etc.). If the activity increases, these fixed costs can be spread across larger numbers of cases; the number of cases agreed determines the 'full cost' (per case) that will cover all the fixed costs.

Once fixed costs are covered, extra activity will cost marginally less, due to the use of consumables and other non-fixed costs. Conversely, lower activity will return amounts smaller than the 'full cost'.

'Step-up' costs occur when activity exceeds the capacity of the provider, despite efficient use of facilities, requiring that extra capacity be introduced. Such capacity cannot be introduced in small amounts: it is not practicable to build a one-bedded hospital ward! It is these problems that work against change in some systems, making change very expensive for commissioners.

The chosen mechanism for sharing risk will depend on circumstances and the type of commissioning arrangement in use. There are generally four types:

- *Block:* a global sum of money in exchange for a loosely defined set of services. The provider moves money between departmental budgets. The commissioner and provider negotiate differences towards the end of the financial year.
- *Cost and volume:* specified activity levels and funding at various levels of detail (e.g. surgical, medical; by specialty, procedure type, or groupings of procedures such as healthcare resource groups). Monthly plans are agreed and monitored against targets.
- *Cost per case:* each episode of care is paid for. Cost may vary depending on the level of activity, or be fixed, independent of activity levels.
- *Fee for service:* costs for individual inputs, diagnostic, or treatment activities are separately reimbursed. This system is typically used in private insurance and parts of the US health system, and is usually combined with a range of instruments to contain costs and limit coverage.

A cost per case system based on a set price ('tariff') for any provider can facilitate choice, and change through choice, but it can also stifle the creation of new capacity because providers have to carry the risk of additional marginal costs before activity levels use enough of the new capacity to generate the income needed. Despite a supposedly fixed cost, a commissioner may be forced to agree a higher price per case if extra capacity is needed.

In free markets for consumer products, increased sales typically result in lower costs, generating greater consumption as goods become more affordable, although the total amount of money spent in the market increases. In healthcare, higher volumes can also generate lower costs. However, extra consumers (patients) can only be generated by reducing treatment thresholds (to lesser severities) or treating a different condition. This will change benefit/risk and cost-effectiveness ratios, especially at the margins of this extra activity. The funding needed to cover this activity might be more effectively directed elsewhere. Commissioners need to understand the total cost and benefits, and resist simplistic claims of reduced treatment costs making a treatment more widely available.

The six basic elements of a commissioning agreement

So what would a contract or service level agreement look like? It should have at least six elements:

- *Parties to the contract:* typically one or more commissioners and a provider. A complex pathway may require several providers but this could be addressed by requiring the main provider to subcontract.
- *What treatments and services are to be provided?* Ideally, this should be described by the patient pathway and encompass 'hotel services' (nutrition, shelter, and comforts) as well as details of the diagnostic and treatment processes based on evidence of effectiveness. A good contract should be composed of many such pathways relating to the many diseases to be treated (although there are examples of providers doing a single procedure) and covering both emergency care and planned care. What is excluded may also be specified.
- *Quantity of care:* the number of patients to be treated within the contract. This may be just one or, in the case of block contracts, undetermined except by historical patterns. Ideally each pathway should have a number established by the epidemiology of incidence/prevalence and treatment thresholds. The provider will be expected to report activity levels regularly to the commissioner.
- *Standards to be achieved:* the quality of care must be clearly specified along with the mechanisms of monitoring. Such standards could and should include nutrition ('five portions of fresh fruit or vegetables a day', free access to fluids), the environment (clean; non-smoking; optional 'entertainments', and access for visitors, especially important in paediatrics), as well as the skills and knowledge of staff, equipment, devices, and drugs. For some conditions or treatments, an individual clinician and team may be designated, even named (e.g. for breast cancer), and minimum activity levels specified to maintain skills. Standards may be specified by reference to recognized clinical guidelines and protocols, such as those produced in the UK by the National Institute for Health and Care Excellence (NICE) in England and Wales and the Scottish Intercollegiate Guidelines Network (SIGN). Clinical governance (including audit) will be specified as the mechanism for maintaining standards within the provider. In some reimbursement systems, detailed standards are set for individual patient diagnosis and treatment planning. Often there are formal requirements on providers to seek permission from payers prior to starting specified forms of care. Permission procedures may involve the reporting of detailed clinical data to the payer to prove the presence of a healthcare need that is covered by the patient's insurance coverage.
- *Price:* no commissioning or purchasing agreement is complete without agreement of a price. Prices may be agreed locally or fixed by the commissioner so as to allow providers to compete on quality over and above that specified.
- *Arbitration arrangements:* things rarely go to plan and contracts are rarely exactly met as specified. Contracts should therefore specify how the parties would reach agreement should, for example, the contract not

be met, demand fail to reach (or exceed) the contract, the case mix differ in terms of severities or conditions from that anticipated, or new treatments become available (or events not covered within the contract occur, such as a major disaster).

Who should be involved in commissioning?

The commissioning process requires a broad range of skills and experience. Genuine teamwork is essential (see → Chapter 4.4). Sometimes these can all be embodied in one person, but this is rare and usually a team-based multidisciplinary process works best.

Table 5.4.1 identifies the skills, people, and tasks needed in commissioning healthcare services.

The concern over variations in clinical practice (see → Chapter 5.10) and its implications for quality of care, along with a desire to better involve the patient in decisions around the nature of the care they should receive, has resulted in a growing interest in shared decision making. The Harvard-based Foundation for Informed Decision Making has been leading the process of moving from analyses of clinical variation through research into decision making and onto translation of this research into independent, evidence-based decision aids for patients. Under these principles, patients will become informed commissioners of their own care.

Specialized services

There is no one agreed definition of specialized services. Most of what has been described above applies to specialized services but, to reiterate some important aspects, specialized services typically involve rarer conditions, thus patient numbers are *small* and *often unpredictable*.

To ensure optimum outcomes for patients (e.g. sustained training and clinical competence for specialized staff) and optimum use of resources (e.g. to ensure cost-effectiveness of provision, making the best use of scarce resources including clinical expertise, high-technology equipment, donor organs) a *critical service mass* is required at each centre and patients from a wide area must be referred to these centres to achieve minimum activity levels. As a result, the population on behalf of which services are commissioned is much larger than that of a single commissioning organization.

Specialized services may have some characteristics different from mainstream healthcare, one of which is *rapidly developing high technology services*. Services can develop very quickly and often involve high technology, where research and development need to be supported and the introduction of new technologies needs to be managed. In these situations, note that the evidence for effectiveness is often emerging rather than established, making commissioning decisions on the basis of complete evidence difficult. As the new technology becomes more widely adopted, additional clinicians can be properly trained in those centres initially established.

Table 5.4.1 Skills, people, and tasks needed in commissioning healthcare services

	Person or discipline	Tasks
Epidemiology	Epidemiologist, public health practitioner	To use data (e.g. mortality, demographic, surveys, case registers). To analyse this data to determine the actual and potential health problems in the population
Health technology assessment	Health economist, public health practitioner	To evaluate critically the (cost-)effectiveness of healthcare interventions. To highlight gaps in information where further research is needed
Negotiation and conflict management	NHS manager, all members	To negotiate skilfully, matching what the commissioner believes is required and the provider wishes to offer
Financial	Accountant, NHS manager	To handle complex finances (services are rarely costed comprehensively and in a way that readily allows comparison)
Clinical	Public health clinician, GP, specialist clinician, nurse	To understand the specialist clinical aspects of the services being offered and provided. (Beware: like any input, specialist clinical advice can be biased—more general clinical advice, e.g. from primary care practitioners, is often equally or more important. 'Experts' are almost always enthusiasts, not disinterested observers)
Experience of the wider health system	NHS manager, public health practitioner	To appreciate how the individual services fit in with the wider healthcare provision of the locality or region—experience and understanding of the wider health service is essential
Information	Information specialist, operational researcher, epidemiologist	To understand health information systems. (Information systems are complex and not always designed specifically to serve the commissioning process.) To understand issues such as case mix measurement, relationships between case mix, costs, and prices. To understand how the provision of healthcare should be matched to predictions of need
Informing and supporting patient choice	Any clinician, but also anyone appropriately trained. The patient	To provide and explain information on outcomes and quality issues to patients in a way that they can understand and will permit them to make choices that are best suited to their conditions and circumstances

Commissioning services with prominent ethical dimensions

Difficult ethical issues can arise (e.g. around equity of access), requiring commissioners of healthcare to balance the high cost needs of the minority against the needs of the majority. Examples are treatment of a variety of genetically determined diseases requiring extremely expensive genetically engineered replacement therapies, and the commissioning of very expensive secure psychiatric facilities to protect society.

Nonetheless, the general 'rules' of commissioning can and should be applied to specialized services. There is a danger that issues of cost-effectiveness are set aside. While larger populations mean that costs are a smaller proportion of the total budget and thus appear affordable, opportunity costs remain the same: the opportunity to treat the same number of patients is lost, irrespective of the population level at which services are commissioned.

There remains a reluctance to address explicitly the issues of distributive justice in these cases and costs are rising exponentially: lifetime costs for one individual can reach £10,000,000 yet deliver only marginal benefits. The principles of distributive justice must be addressed.

Further resources

Website

The Foundation for Informed Medical Decision Making. What is medical shared decision making? Available at: ℘ https://www.healthwise.org/solutions/care-transformation.aspx (accessed 21 August 2019).

References

1   The World Bank Data Catalog (2017). Health, nutrition and population statistics. Available at: ℘ http://data.worldbank.org/data-catalog/health-nutrition-and-population-statistics (accessed 21 August 2019).

2   Joumard I, André C, Nicq C. (2010). *Health care systems: efficiency and institutions*, OECD Economics Department Working Papers, No. 769. OECD Publishing, Paris.

Controlling expenditures

Thomas Rice and Chris Griffiths

Objectives

This chapter will help you understand:

- why controlling healthcare expenditures is key to achieving other public health goals
- the primary reasons for rising expenditures
- how rising expenditures have been addressed at national and subnational levels
- ways in which controlling expenditures can fit into your professional role.

A key tool in addressing rising expenditures is an understanding of health economics and you may wish to read this chapter alongside ➲ Chapter 1.6.

Why addressing rising expenditures is an important public health issue

It could be argued that expenditure control should not be a public policy issue. Such an argument might state that good health is among the most important aspects of well-being and people should have access to whatever they need—to all available medical products, devices, and procedures—to improve their health.

In fact, expenditure control is not only important but also likely to become more important as new technologies emerge and the costs of care increase. There are two reasons for this. One relates to the economic concept of 'opportunity costs'. An opportunity cost is essentially a trade-off. When we spend more money on healthcare, it means that we have less to spend on everything else, including education, housing, and social insurance. There are many compelling ways in which public resources can be productively invested and so we ought to avoid wasting resources as much as possible—all the more so when many countries are struggling with burdensome and growing national debts (see ➲ Chapter 1.6j).

The second reason is particular to the healthcare sector. There are limited resources to be devoted to healthcare so they need to be apportioned judiciously. If, for example, excessive amounts are spent on administration of health insurance, then there will be less money available for other health-related activities. Public health initiatives are often a harder 'sell' than direct medical care procedures, especially when government budgets are stressed. Focusing on rising expenditures helps ensure that we use limited healthcare resources efficiently and that we have more left for other public health activities.

In relation to both these factors, there are tensions: in the first case, this relates to pressures to reduce spending by central and local government, and in the second case to the need for public health to try to stand up to the 'healthcare delivery juggernaut'.[1] In the face of these tensions, it is important for public health practitioners to be aware of and engage with the need to prioritize and reduce expenditure.

The causes of rising healthcare expenditures

There is no agreed list of the major causes of rising healthcare expenditures. There are three reasons why this is the case. First, although much research has been done, there is a lot we do not know—understandable given the difficulty in conducting randomized controlled studies in health policy. Second, much of the analysis available is influenced by political leanings, which can lead to different interpretations of the same information. Third, means of expenditure control cannot necessarily be transferred from one country to another. What works in the United Kingdom, for example, might not work in Germany (to say nothing of the United States or India) and, even if it did, institutional and political factors often make it nearly impossible to transplant an idea from one country into another.

The following equation provides a model for the causes of rising expenditures:

$$E = P \times Q$$

where E = expenditure, P = the unit price of health services, and Q = the quantity or volume of health services consumed. The equation, while simplified in that it does not distinguish between different types of services, provides a key insight: increases in either or both price and quantity will result in increased expenditure. This means there are two approaches to addressing rising expenditures: controlling quantity or volume, and controlling prices.

Quantity of services

Increases in the quantity and intensity of services are responsible for much of the increase in healthcare expenditures.[2] This often goes under the heading of 'high-tech' medicine, and includes new and/or improved procedures and pharmaceuticals. Advances in medical technology are desirable, but concomitant expenditure increases inevitably involve an opportunity cost: unless total budgets keep growing, increasing expenditures to cover a new technology must involve cuts to other technologies and services.

The volume of services is not the same in all parts of a country. Even after controlling for the age and health of populations, there is generally a great deal of variation between different geographic regions. In the United States, for example, in 2013, *per capita* spending on Medicare (the programme for senior citizens and the disabled) averaged twice as much in the 20 counties with the highest spending versus the 20 counties with the lowest spending.[3] There is much debate about whether higher spending leads to better outcomes and healthcare processes. Although one might imagine higher spending to be associated with better outcomes, regions with higher Medicare spending also had higher mortality rates following acute myocardial infarctions, hip fractures, and colorectal cancer diagnoses.[4] Examination of such variations can be used to determine 'best practice'—within particular geographic areas or within hospital systems—that can be emulated and encouraged.

High levels of expenditure can be an unintentional outcome of fee-for-service medicine, which encourages the provision of more services as well as 'unbundling'—that is, billing for each component of care provided. While alternative methods such as capitation (paying a fixed fee over a specified time period for all the care a patient receives) and salary have their own challenges, they do not provide the same incentives to over-provide.

The appropriate use of primary care systems can be effective in controlling unnecessary use of expensive specialized services. Not only are specialist physicians paid more than generalists in most countries, they tend to provide a more intensive, expensive array of services. Countries with a primary care emphasis have been shown to have lower levels of healthcare expenditure, in large measure because primary care can prevent or manage illnesses in a more coordinated fashion.[5]

Related to this is the importance of health behaviours on healthcare costs. Cigarette smoking, poor nutrition and obesity, and lack of physical activity all contribute to rising healthcare costs. In the 40 years between 1972 and 2012, obesity rates more than doubled in the US and France (albeit France started at a very low level), and increased more than 50% in Australia and England.[6] One US study found that more than 25% of the increase in *per capita* healthcare spending over a 14-year period ending in 2001 was due to the consequences of obesity.[7]

Finally, charging patients directly for care is a way to control the quantity of services provided. This approach, called 'cost sharing', is used in most countries, often for prescription drugs but increasingly for hospital and physician services. It is often effective but is problematic for two reasons. First, patients are as likely to reduce their use of effective, necessary care as they are to cut down on unnecessary services, and this may lead to increased subsequent costs to deal with avoidable complications.[8] For example, charging more for prescription drugs cuts down on compliance among the chronically ill.[9] Second, unless designed very carefully, cost sharing is hard on people with low incomes who may have to forgo other necessities in order to afford medical care services.

Price of services

The capacity to control how much is paid to providers and for products like pharmaceuticals can have a major impact of a country's expenditure levels. As one article, exploring why the USA spends so much more on healthcare than other countries, put it: 'It's the prices, stupid.'[10]

Another thing that can raise prices is high administrative costs. Another reason the USA spends twice as much per person on healthcare as other countries is the high cost of administering a system based on private insurance. Such costs include marketing, determining eligibility for care, paperwork required for reimbursement, and profits. Organisation for Economic Co-operation and Development (OECD) reports that US administrative costs comprise 8% of health expenditures, more than twice the average of other OECD countries.[11] These factors should be considered as other countries increase their reliance on private insurance to cover healthcare costs. Further discussion of prices appears in the next section.

What can be done to control rising expenditures?

Expenditure reduction is not a goal in its own right and higher spending that brings better outcomes may be welcomed. However, over recent decades, healthcare has come to consume an increasing portion of most national incomes and this is the catalyst for most reforms that are being attempted. There are many approaches to controlling expenditures and their use varies across countries.

Most countries struggle to provide health and social services at the level expected by the population, so controlling rising national healthcare costs is generally a high priority.

We noted earlier that there are two targets—price and quantity (or volume). Regarding price, probably the most effective method is for countries or regions to take advantage of their purchasing power in bargaining prices for services and pharmaceuticals. In some countries, such as Canada, each province acts as a single payer for services. Provinces negotiate a global budget with each hospital and negotiate fees with physician representatives. The bargaining power this brings is one of the chief reasons Canada has been able to control its expenditures better than the USA.[12]

In countries with multiple payers, it is possible to control expenditures by coordinating payments made by insurers or sickness funds to providers.[13] Germany offers an example of a setting in which prices are set by negotiations between sickness funds and provider representatives. Other countries, like France, have stronger government involvement in such negotiations.

As noted, fee-for-service medicine is inherently inflationary and alternatives have been shown to be more effective in controlling spending. On the hospital side, for example, DRGs may be used. DRGs are payments for an entire hospital stay, fixed in advanced based on the patient's diagnosis, that incentivize hospitals to discharge patients sooner. For physicians, payment methods such as capitation (used for primary care in the UK) and salary (used by some health maintenance organizations in the USA) provide potential alternatives.

Many strategies have been adopted to control the quantity or volume of services. These include encouraging the training of primary care practitioners or regulating the number of specialists; developing 'practice guidelines' to provide physicians with up-to-date, scientifically verified recommendations on how to treat particular maladies; and reducing duplicated services and inappropriate prescription drugs by developing electronic medical records.

Another strategy, and our focus here, is on determining the cost-effectiveness of new technologies, services, and prescription drugs—and paying only for those found to be worth the investment. The best known is the UK's National Institute for Health and Care Excellence. Another is Australia's Pharmaceutical Benefits Advisory Committee (PBAC, see ➔ Case study).

Case study: Australia's Pharmaceutical Benefit Advisory Committee

Established in 1953 as part of the National Health Act, the Australian Pharmaceutical Benefit Advisory Committee (PBAC)[14, 15] is an independent agency that advises the Minister of Health and Ageing on which drugs should be covered by the national health benefits system. In conjunction with its sister agency, the Pharmaceutical Benefits Pricing Authority, which negotiates the price of drugs with manufacturers, it exemplifies a structure for ensuring that only cost-effective drugs are covered and that their pricing optimizes public resources. Australia was the first country to make economic analyses a prerequisite for including drugs in its pharmaceutical benefits system.

The PBAC is composed of researchers, clinicians, pharmacologists, industry, and consumers. It assesses research on both the clinical effectiveness (based, whenever possible, on evidence from randomized clinical trials) and costs of new drugs. If it concludes a new drug is more expensive than existing therapies and does not offer significant improvements in outcomes, it will either not cover the new drug or recommend its purchase only at a price comparable with existing drugs on the market—a strategy known as 'reference pricing'.

As a result of these practices, Australia pays considerably less for prescription drugs than many countries. In 2006, prices for 30 of the most commonly prescribed drugs in Australia were about half those in the USA and two-thirds what was paid in Canada and France.[16] In 2015, total per capita spending on retail pharmaceuticals was less than half as high in Australia ($427) than in the USA ($1,011).[17]

Controlling expenditures: implications for public health practitioners

You might have two reactions to this issue: first, that this is somebody else's problem; second, that there is nothing you can do about it anyway. If your reaction is the first of these, then bear in mind that rising healthcare costs tend to occur at the downstream end of healthcare, yet draw more resources away from effective upstream interventions. If we, collectively, fail to control healthcare expenditure, a likely consequence is a squeezing of public health budgets and a reduction in our capacity to address potential health problems in an equitable fashion. The more resources are drawn away from public health, the more need there will be to spend money to deal with health problems that could potentially have been avoided.

If your reaction is the second, there are a number of things you can do, depending on the role you have. If you are in a senior position and able to put in place processes to assess, and approve or reject, new expenditures, then the approaches described above (and there are others) may provide you with a suitable starting point for your organization or area of responsibility.

If you are not in a position to do this, then you may still be able to support the efforts of others trying to control expenditures. As a public health practitioner, your understanding of health systems and evidence will be of great value to those responsible for making decisions about commissioning and providing health services, including deciding what services are and are not needed, and identifying which do or do not represent value for money. Get involved in local decision-making forums and make sure that a public health voice is contributing to the discussion. Even if there is no local group that assesses effectiveness and cost-effectiveness, you can use the information produced elsewhere to inform local decisions. Just as much as more obvious issues like addressing inequity or challenging known harms to health, addressing rising healthcare expenditures is an area where public health activism is crucial.

Acknowledgement

I gratefully acknowledge Iain Lang, who co-authored this chapter with me in the previous edition of this book.

References

1 Stine NW, Chokshi DA. (2012). Opportunity in austerity—a common agenda for medicine and public health. *New England Journal of Medicine*, **366**, 395–7.
2 Smith S, Newhouse JP, Freeland MS. (2009). Income, insurance, and technology: why does health spending outpace economic growth? *Health Affairs*, **28**, 276–1284.
3 Kaiser Family Foundation (2015). *The latest on geographic variation in medicare spending: demographic divide persists but variation has narrowed*.
4 Fisher E, Goodman D, Skinner J, Bronner K. (2009). Health care spending, quality, and outcomes: more isn't always better. Dartmouth Atlas Project Topic Brief. Available at: ℳ http://archive.dartmouthatlas.org/downloads/reports/Spending_Brief_022709.pdf (accessed 3 September 2019).
5 Schoen C, Osborn R, Huynh PT. (2004). Primary care and health system performance: adults' experiences in five countries. *Health affairs*, web exclusive, 28 October, W4-497–503.
6 OECD (2014). Obesity update. Available at: ℳ http://www.oecd.org/health/Obesity-Update-2014.pdf (accessed 21 August 2019).
7 Thorpe KE, Florence CS, Howard DH, et al. (2004). The impact of obesity on rising medical spending. *Health affairs*, web exclusive, 20 October, W4-480–6.
8 Lohr KN, Brook RH, Kamberg CJ, et al. (1986). Effect of cost sharing on use of medically effective and less effective care. *Medical Care*, **24**(Supplement 9), S31–8.
9 Eaddy, MT, Look, CL, Day, K, et al. (2012). How patient cost-sharing trends affect adherence and outcomes. *Pharmacy and Therapeutics*, **37**, 45–55.
10 Anderson GF, Reinhardt UE, Hussey PS, et al. (2005). It's the prices, stupid: why the United States is so different from other countries. *Health Affairs*, **22**, 89–105.
11 OECD (2017). Tackling wasteful spending on health. Available at: ℳ https://www.oecd.org/els/health-systems/Tackling-Wasteful-Spending-on-Health-Highlights-revised.pdf (accessed 21 August 2019).
12 Evans RG. (1986). Finding the levers, finding the courage: lessons from cost containment in North America. *Journal of Health Politics, Policy and Law*, **11**, 585–615.
13 Reinhardt UE. (2011). The many different prices paid to providers and the flawed theory of cost shifting: is it time for a more rational all-payer system? *Health Affairs*, **30**, 2125–33.
14 Healy J, Sharman E, Lokuge B. (2006). *Australia: health system review. Health systems in transition*, **8**(5). European Observatory on Health Systems and Policies. Available at: ℳ http://www.euro.who.int/__data/assets/pdf_file/0007/96433/E89731.pdf (accessed 21 August 2019).
15 Morgan SG, McMahon M, Mitton C, et al. (2006). Centralized drug review processes in Australia, Canada, New Zealand, and the United Kingdom. *Health Affairs*, **25**, 337–47.

16 Squires DA. (2011). The US health system in perspective: a comparison of twelve industrialized nations. Commonwealth Fund. Available at: ℛ https://www.commonwealthfund.org/publications/issue-briefs/2011/jul/us-health-system-perspective-comparison-twelve-industrialized (accessed 3 September 2019).

17 Sarnak DO, Squires D, Kuzmak G, et al. (2017). Paying for prescription drugs around the world: Why is the U.S. an Outlier? Commonwealth Fund. Available at: ℛ https://www.commonwealthfund.org/sites/default/files/documents/___media_files_publications_issue_brief_2017_oct_sarnak_paying_for_rx_ib_v2.pdf

Using guidance and frameworks

Corrado De Vito and Paolo Villari

Objectives

After reading this chapter, you should be better able to:
- understand, appreciate, and identify issues where guidance and frameworks could help
- identify existing and relevant guidelines
- assess their validity
- support clinicians needing to integrate clinical guidelines into practice.

Why are clinical guidelines and their integration into practice important public health activities?

It has been argued that Clinical Practice Guidelines arose because policy makers and administrators needed to standardize health interventions to limit the growing healthcare costs, or, on the contrary, because physicians needed to preserve their professional autonomy against administrative pressure. Regardless of the reason, Clinical Practice Guidelines are a valuable method of regulating the quality of medical practice and a fundamental decision-making tool for doctors.

Indeed, it has been estimated that clinicians would have to read approximately 11 articles a day to keep their knowledge of the field up to date, and with this challenge increasing each year. However, clinicians simply do not have the time to read the primary research or even systematic reviews relevant to their day-to-day decision making. It has been estimated that, in practice, if clinicians cannot find the information they need within 15 seconds, they will look no further.[1]

The development of guidelines depends ultimately on the perspective from which the specific healthcare problem is approached, whether that of the individual patient, of doctors or of public health administrators. Although patients, healthcare professionals, and healthcare systems can benefit from the implementation of Clinical Practice Guidelines, flawed guidelines could lead to suboptimal, ineffective, or even harmful practices. Therefore, Clinical Practice Guidelines must be developed by a knowledgeable multidisciplinary panel using a strict methodology to avoid bias due to conflict of interests, poor methodological quality, poor writing, or ambiguous presentation.

What are Clinical Practice Guidelines?

Clinical Practice Guidelines were re-defined in 2011 by the Institute of Medicine as 'statements that include recommendations intended to optimize patient care that are informed by a systematic review of evidence and an assessment of the benefits and harms of alternative care options'.[2]

Why are guidelines essential for improvement of professional practice?

Clinical Practice Guidelines can improve the quality of healthcare by offering authoritative recommendations to clinicians. If guidelines are correctly based on a critical appraisal of scientific evidence, clinicians are properly informed of the most up-to-date and effective intervention among the many options, and can avoid those that are ineffective or potentially dangerous. This should result in evidence-based interventions overcoming outdated practices that are unsupported by good science. Many guideline clearing houses have been created to help healthcare workers retrieve and choose guidelines (Box 5.6.1).

> **Box 5.6.1 Where to find Clinical Practice Guidelines**
> - National Institute for Health and Care Excellence (NICE). Available at: ℬ https://www.evidence.nhs.uk (accessed 3 September 2019).
> - Canadian Medical Association (CMA) – CPG Infobase: Clinical Practice Guidelines. Available at: ℬ https://www.cma.ca/En/Pages/clinical-practice-guidelines.aspx (accessed 3 September 2019).
> - Scottish Intercollegiate Guidelines Network (SIGN). Available at: ℬ http://www.sign.ac.uk (accessed 3 September 2019).
> - National health and Medical Research Council (NHMRC): Clinical Practice Guidelines. Available at: ℬ https://www.nhmrc.gov.au/guidelines-publications (accessed 3 September 2019).
> - Guidelines. Available at: ℬ https://www.guidelines.co.uk (accessed 3 September 2019).
> - Guidelines International Network (G-I-N). Available at: ℬ http://www.g-i-n.net (accessed 3 September 2019).
> - Standard and Guidelines Evidence (SAGE). Available at: ℬ http://www.cancerview.ca/TreatmentAndSupport/GRCMain/GRCSAGE A (accessed 3 September 2019).

Planning guidelines

Planning objectives, formulating questions, and choosing outcomes

In the first phase of planning, it is necessary to identify the topic and key issues correctly. For this purpose, it is crucial to clarify what the scope is, who the end users of the guideline are, and why it has been decided to develop it. A preliminary search of the literature is useful, at this stage, to identify existing guidelines, systematic reviews, and/or meta-analyses and economic evaluations relevant to the topic. Once the scope of the guideline is clear, a set of background and foreground questions must be developed. It is particularly important that the foreground questions are formulated with care, because these questions will guide the evidence search, and the evidence found will underpin the recommendations set out in the guidelines.[3]

Finally, choosing the most important outcomes is crucial to the production of useful guidelines. The PICO format is an effective methodology for developing the correct questions and choosing the appropriate outcomes (Box 5.6.2).

Box 5.6.2 PICO framework

Patient problem or Population—What are the characteristics of the patients or the population? What is the condition or disease of interest?

Intervention—What is the intervention under consideration for this patient or population?

Comparison or control—What is the alternative to the intervention? (e.g. placebo, alternative drugs, surgery?)

Outcome—What are the relevant outcomes (e.g. quality of life, change in clinical status, morbidity, adverse effects, complications)

Reprinted from Egger M, Smith GD, Altman DG. (2008) Principles of and procedures for systematic reviews. In: Systematic reviews in health care. Hoboken: BMJ Publishing Group, 23–42, with permission from John Wiley & Sons.

Retrieving and synthesizing evidence

Performing a systematic review is the most effective way to ensure retrieval of the best evidence available.

The key points in the development of a systematic review are:

- developing a review protocol
- defining objectives and eligibility criteria
- performing the literature search
- selecting studies, assessing their methodological quality, and extracting data
- presenting and interpreting results.

Combining the results of relevant studies through meta-analysis, if feasible, provides more precise estimates of the effects of a particular procedure or treatment and allows potential sources of heterogeneity among studies, which could lead to contradictory results, to be explored.

Assessing evidence

After evidence has been retrieved, it must be evaluated, because clinicians and healthcare professionals 'need to know how much confidence they can place in the recommendations'.[5] One of the most useful and standardized methods of assessing the quality of evidence is the Grading of Recommendations Assessment, Development and Evaluation (GRADE) system, which considers four key elements to evaluate the quality of evidence for each important outcome: study design, study quality, consistency, and directness.

With respect to study design, randomized controlled trials (RCTs) generally provide stronger evidence than observational studies when dealing with alternative clinical management strategies. In turn, rigorously conducted observational studies provide stronger evidence than non-controlled case series. However, RCTs can be downgraded and observational studies can be upgraded depending on their methodological quality.

Consistency refers to the similarity across studies of estimates of effect. If different studies come to very different conclusions about the effect of a particular intervention, this probably reflects real differences in treatment outcomes. Variability may be due to differences among the populations considered, differences between the interventions considered, or differences in the measured outcomes. When heterogeneity exists, but a plausible explanation to support it is not found, evidence must be considered of lower quality.

Finally, directness is the extent to which people, interventions, and outcome measures are similar to those of interest. The concept of directness of evidence is perhaps best explained by describing its opposite, indirectness, of which there are three main types. The first occurs when the measured outcomes differ from those of primary interest. This is typical of so-called surrogate outcomes, whose measurement is assumed to reflect a clinically relevant end point, but which may not actually do so. This assumption leads to misleading interpretations and therefore evidence should be considered of lower quality than that provided by non-surrogate outcomes. The second type of indirectness is when indirect comparisons are made between two drugs used for the same pathology. Although RCTs might have been carried out that directly compare drug (X) with placebo and others that compare drug (Y) with placebo, there may be no studies that compare the two drugs directly. Indirect comparison of this kind is considered to have a lower quality of evidence than a head-to-head comparison. The third type of evidence indirectness includes differences between populations, interventions, comparisons, and outcomes of interest, which allow little or no information relevant to the development of the guideline to be retrieved.

Formulating recommendations

The final stage of guidelines development concerns the formulation of recommendations.

Strong recommendations must be based on high-quality evidences that allows clear conclusions to be drawn about both the beneficial and harmful effects of the intervention in question. The magnitude of the effect and the importance of the outcome must be taken into account, and an evaluation made of whether the benefits outweigh the harms. A formal economic evaluation carried out by the working group, or economic estimates retrieved during the evidence search, must drive the formulation of recommendations. The strength of the recommendations should depend on the efficacy of the interventions and the resources required for implementation.

Appraisal tools for guidelines

Evaluating the quality and reporting of guidelines is a key step in deciding on their implementation and use in clinical practice. A recent systematic review identified 40 appraisal tools currently used to assess the quality of guidelines. Which instrument to use depends on the research question, but the AGREE II appraisal tool is currently the most widely endorsed (see Box 5.6.3).[6]

Box 5.6.3 AGREE II domains and items

Domain 1. Scope and purpose
- The overall objective(s) of the guideline is (are) specifically described.
- The health question(s) covered by the guideline is (are) specifically described.
- The population (patients, public, etc.) to whom the guideline is meant to apply is specifically described.

Domain 2. Stakeholder involvement
- The guideline development group includes individuals from all the relevant professional groups.
- The views and preferences of the target population (patients, public, etc.) have been sought.
- The target users of the guideline are clearly defined.

Domain 3. Rigour of development
- Systematic methods were used to search for evidence.
- The criteria for selecting the evidence are clearly described.
- The strengths and limitations of the body of evidence are clearly described.
- The methods for formulating the recommendations are clearly described.
- The health benefits, side effects, and risks have been considered in formulating the recommendations.
- There is an explicit link between the recommendations and the supporting evidence.
- The guideline has been externally reviewed by experts prior to its publication.
- A procedure for updating the guideline is provided.

Domain 4. Clarity of presentation
- The recommendations are specific and unambiguous.
- The different options for management of the condition or health issue are clearly presented.
- Key recommendations are easily identifiable.

Domain 5. Applicability
- The guideline describes facilitators and barriers to its application.
- The guideline provides advice and/or tools on how the recommendations can be put into practice.
- The potential resource implications of applying the recommendations have been considered.
- The guideline presents monitoring and/or auditing criteria.

Domain 6. Editorial independence
- The views of the funding body have not influenced the content of the guideline.
- Competing interests of guideline development group members have been recorded and addressed.

Reprinted from Burls A. AGREE II-improving the quality of clinical care. (2010). Lancet, 376, 1128–29, with permission from Elsevier.

The Appraisal of Guidelines for REsearch & Evaluation (AGREE) Instrument[7] was developed to address the issue of variability in guideline quality. This was subsequently refined, resulting in AGREE II.[6]

AGREE II is intended for many categories of users: for example, *healthcare professionals*, who need to select guidelines to develop local healthcare paths; *organizations* that need to produce guidelines, allowing them to plan a rigorous methodology for their development, to verify that their guidelines adhere to international quality standards, and to evaluate guidelines for their potential adaptation; *managers*, who need to identify what guidelines should be used in health policy decisions; *trainers*, who need to teach a critical approach to the use of guidelines and to define the core competencies for guidelines production and reporting.

How to translate Clinical Practice Guidelines into practice

Clinical Practice Guidelines have the potential to improve the quality of care received by patients and, possibly, their clinical outcomes. However, it is well known that mere production and publication of Clinical Practice Guidelines alone does not change clinical practice. After dissemination, there are six main factors specific to healthcare providers that affect the adoption of guidelines into practice: guideline implementation, characteristics of practice, laws and incentives, patient characteristics/problems, social norms, and knowledge and skills.[8-10] In particular, integration of guidelines into practice needs a series of 'concrete activities and interventions undertaken to turn policies into desired results'[11] that constitute the core of the implementation process. This is necessary because clinicians experience a number of difficulties adhering to guidelines, such as lack of awareness, lack of familiarity, lack of agreement, lack of self-efficacy, lack of outcome expectancy, inertia of previous practice, and external barriers.

Various carefully chosen implementation strategies have been tested for their efficacy. In general, active approaches that aim to improve clinician practice and patients' outcomes have been shown to change professional performance to a greater extent than traditional passive methods. Continuing medical education strategies, including academic detailing, outreach programmes, and workshops, have been shown to be highly effective. However, non-educational methods can also improve physicians' adherence to evidence-based behaviours (e.g. integrating clinical decision support systems, reminders, and patient-mediated interventions).[8]

A specific tool, GuideLine Implementability Appraisal (GLIA), was created to assess the implementability of Clinical Practice Guidelines or, alternatively, to allow guidelines to be developed with improved implementability.[12] Version 2.0 consists of 30 items that explore eight dimensions (Box 5.6.4).

Box 5.6.4 GLIA dimensions and their characteristics

Dimension 1. Executability
Exactly what to do under the circumstances defined.

Dimension 2. Decidability
Precisely under what conditions to do something.

Dimension 3. Validity
The degree to which the recommendation reflects the intent of the developer and the strength of evidence.

Dimension 4. Flexibility
Degree to which a recommendation permits interpretation and allows for alternatives in its execution.

Dimension 5. Effect on process of care
Degree to which the recommendation impacts upon the usual workflow in a typical care setting

Dimension 6. Measurability
Degree to which the guideline identifies markers or endpoints to track the effects of implementation of this recommendation

Dimension 7. Novelty/innovation
Degree to which the recommendation proposes behaviours considered unconventional by clinicians or patients

Dimension 8. Computability
Ease with which a recommendation can be operationalized in an electronic information system

Source: data from Shiffman RN, Dixon J, Brandt C, et al. (2005). The GuideLine Implementability Appraisal (GLIA): development of an instrument to identify obstacles to guideline implementation. BMC Medical Informatics Decision Making, 5, 23. Also available at: ℛ http://nutmeg.med.yale.edu/glia/login.htm (accessed 3 September 2019).

Potential pitfalls

Leadership and management issues

The implementation of guidelines requires a strong transformational leadership committed to change and innovation in clinicians' behaviours, the environment, and the organizational infrastructure. It is essential that senior managers focus attention on organizational priorities and make resources available to encourage change. Middle managers have a key role as intermediaries between senior managers and staff members, and should be trained appropriately to facilitate the implementation of guidelines and changes in behaviour. Without a clear and explicit endorsement of the organization management, guidelines implementation is likely to fail.

Poor organization

A supportive leadership is important in any successful healthcare institution, but the implementation of Clinical Practice Guidelines also needs a high level of organization to identify and coordinate effective work practices that include clinicians. Once the leadership has created the right environment in which everyone identifies their role and understands the benefits of evidence-based medicine, it is relatively easy to promote a culture with a positive attitude towards implementation. At this stage, education is very effective at producing behavioural change—in particular, educational activities that involve the active participation of professionals, such as targeted seminars, outreach visits, and the involvement of opinion leaders.

Lack of resources

The adoption of guidelines may be constrained by lack of resources. Educational interventions, in particular, require substantial investment of resources that are beyond the reach of many groups.

Local development of guidelines

Local development of new guidelines is time-consuming and expensive. However, depending on their organizational skills, workforce and financial capabilities, groups can more efficiently choose to either adopt, adapt, or contextualize recommendations from existing high-quality guidelines.[13] In the first case, guidelines are applied entirely without changes. Adaptation refers to changes made to the recommendations to make them more adherent to the local context. Finally, one may need to contextualize guidelines by addressing implementation issues such as the local workforce, training, equipment, and/or access to services. Regardless of whether guidelines are adopted, adapted, or contextualized, attention must be paid to local empirical evidence. For example, local evidence of inappropriateness of care could be useful to highlight the need for quality improvement and to contain healthcare costs. Once a group has identified an evidence-based intervention, and improvements in the quality of care can be achieved, this must be communicated to other sections of the organization. Senior personnel should be able to repeat this cycle in other sections as long as the organization is receptive to change and any innovations introduced focus on the improvement of standards of care.

Failing to use a (rigorous) project management approach

The implementation of Clinical Practice Guidelines needs a rigorous project management approach that encompasses all aspects of the project, from budgeting to the choice of appropriate indicators for evaluating the effectiveness of the intervention. Guidelines implementation must be subjected to a rigorous assessment that determines sustainability from the outset. A project management approach can provide an initial assessment of the sustainability of guideline implementation, together with a step-by-step control of the actual implementation of the intervention and an evaluation of the actual effectiveness for subsequent reprogramming.

References

1 Moore A, McQuay H, Gray JAM. (1999). Bandolier 61: Evidence-based health care. *Bandolier*, **6**, 1–8.

2 Graham R, Mancher M, Wolman DM, et al. (eds). (2011). *Clinical practice guidelines we can trust*. Institute of Medicine Committee on Standards for Developing Trustworthy Clinical Practice Guidelines. National Academies Press, Washington, DC.

3 World Health Organization (2014). *WHO handbook for guideline development*, 2nd edn. WHO, Geneva.

4 Egger M, Smith GD. (2008). Principles of and procedures for systematic reviews. In: Egger M, Smith GD, Altman DG, eds, *Systematic reviews in health care*, pp. 23–42. BMJ Publishing Group: Hoboken.

5 Atkins D, Best D, Briss PA, et al. (2004). Grading quality of evidence and strength of recommendations. *British Medical Journal*, **328**, 1490.

6 Burls A. (2010). AGREE II-improving the quality of clinical care. *Lancet*, **376**, 1128–29.

7 AGREE Collaboration. (2003). Development and validation of an international appraisal instrument for assessing the quality of clinical practice guidelines: the AGREE project. *Quality & Safety in Health Care*, **12**, 18–23.

8 Mostofian F, Ruban C, Simunovic N, et al. (2015). Changing physician behavior: what works? *American Journal of Managed Care*, **21**, 75–84.

9 Smith WR. (2000). Evidence for the effectiveness of techniques to change physicians behavior. *Chest*, **118**(Supplement 2), 8S–17S.

10 Davis DA, Taylor-Vaisey A. (1997). Translating guidelines into practice. A systematic review of theoretic concepts, practical experience and research evidence in the adoption of clinical practice guidelines. *Canadian Medical Association Journal*, **157**, 408–16.

11 Field MJ, Lohr KN. (1992). Guidelines for clinical practice: from development to use. National Academy Press, Washington, DC.

12 Shiffman RN, Dixon J, Brandt C, et al. (2005). The Guideline Implementability Appraisal (GLIA): development of an instrument to identify obstacles to guideline implementation. *BMC Medical Informatics and Decision Making*, **5**, 23.

13 Dizon JM, Machingaidze S, Grimmer K. (2016). To adopt, to adapt or to contextualise? The big question in clinical practice guideline development. *BMC Research Notes*, **9**, 442.

Healthcare process and patient experience

Diana Delnoij, Ruairidh Milne, and Andrew Stevens

Objectives

Healthcare systems around the world aim at improving outcomes of care, such as patients' functioning or quality of life. This is important, because ultimately the value of healthcare depends on the outcomes achieved. However, research has shown that outcome is not the only thing that matters to patients. Patients also value a patient-centered process of care delivery. That is, they wish to be treated in a friendly way and with respect, they want to receive relevant information and care that is consistent and coherent across different settings, and they want to be involved in important decisions about their care. Therefore, this chapter will help you to analyse the healthcare process and, in particular, the quality of this process and its outcomes from the patient's perspective.

You will learn:
- how to measure quality of care from the patient's perspective (i.e. how to construct patient questionnaires or where to find pre-existing ones)
- how to interpret the findings in the context of the objective of your measurement (e.g. quality improvement, patient choice, pay-for-performance)
- how to take action based on the results.

This chapter provides hands-on guidance with respect to the development and implementation of surveys measuring patient experiences. However, keep in mind that this is only a first step in the quality cycle. The results of such a survey give you a 'diagnosis' of the quality of care from the patients' perspective. It does not really tell you what you should do to improve patient experiences, however. To find effective remedies for negative experiences, often you will have to do additional research.

Definitions

Healthcare process

The healthcare process is essentially a business process. A business process is defined as a complete, dynamically co-ordinated set of activities or logically related tasks that must be performed to deliver value to customers or to fulfil other strategic goals.[1] In healthcare, this process consists of all the things done for and to the patient by healthcare providers in the course of diagnosis and treatment, from the moment a patient enters the healthcare system until the moment that they are discharged, leave, or die.

Quality of care

Quality of care refers to the level of performance that characterizes the healthcare provided.[2] Measures of quality of care consist of various ingredients, including, for example, measures of effectiveness[2] and patient satisfaction or patient-centeredness (the degree to which healthcare interventions delivered are responsive to patients' needs and preferences).

Sources of information

Healthcare process

The healthcare process can be studied from various perspectives by different disciplines using different sources of information.

Economic perspective

From an economic perspective, you may want to study the healthcare process—for example, because you are interested in improving the efficiency of care provision and/or in cost control. In that case, the source of information will often consist of administrative and fiscal data. You look at the costs of care in relation to volumes provided.

Health system perspective

Health systems researchers can study the healthcare process from policy perspective—for example, designing the optimal system by strengthening primary care, or enhancing integrated care. In this case, the factors that are studied can relate to the division of tasks between the different levels in the healthcare system, such as the number of referrals from primary care to hospital care, or the number of patients discharged from hospital to nursing homes.

Operations management perspective

In operations management, the healthcare process is usually studied with the aim to redesign and improve the logistics within a healthcare facility. In that case, you would measure, for instance, waiting times at various stages in the process, auxiliary services used, the division of tasks between back office and front office, etc.

Quality perspective

From a quality perspective, the healthcare process is seen as one of the determinants of health outcomes, together with more structural factors, such as capacity (including human resources), physical equipment, and facilities. This quality perspective of looking at the healthcare process will be elaborated on in more detail in the remainder of this chapter.

Quality of care

There are two important sources of information about quality of care:
- Registration of clinical data by healthcare providers.
- Patients' reports collected through population or patient surveys.

In the scientific literature, patient reports are referred to, for example, as 'patient-reported outcome measures' (abbreviated as 'PROMs'): measures of the way patients perceive their health and the impact that treatments or adjustments to lifestyle have on their quality of life. So, PROMs include measures of patient outcomes (in terms of health or quality of life) as well as measures of patients' experiences in, or their satisfaction with, the process of healthcare delivery.

In this chapter, the focus is on the latter type of measures: patient satisfaction, or—preferably—patient experiences. In the last decennia of the twentieth century, patient satisfaction had become a frequently used outcome measure in clinical trials. In addition to that, satisfaction surveys were frequently used to measure the quality of care from the patient's perspective. However, in the second half of the 1990s, it became clear that, as a tool for quality improvement, patient satisfaction surveys were not very useful. This has to do with the fact that patient satisfaction is a multidimensional concept. Patients are satisfied if their actual experiences match or exceed their *ex ante* expectations. If you find that patients are not satisfied, it is unclear what the underlying reason is: were they given substandard care, or did they have too high expectations?

As a consequence, it was argued that in quality assurance it would be more useful to look at the underlying components of satisfaction: namely, at patients' expectations and at specific experiences. This led to the development of new types of patient survey. In these surveys, the emphasis is not on an evaluation of satisfaction but on collecting detailed reports of what actually happened to patients during a hospital stay or a visit to the doctor. Examples of these patient or consumer experience surveys are the American Consumer Assessment of Healthcare Providers and Systems (CAHPS) questionnaires, the questionnaires developed by the Picker Institute for the English National Health Service, or the Dutch Consumer Quality Index (CQ-index).

Why is this an important public health issue?

Patients have a specific kind of so-called experiential knowledge that is seen as crucial for the advancement of quality care. They know what it is to live with a specific disease and they have a lot of experience with healthcare providers and treatments. Information about patients' experiences is therefore vital. Reasons for studying patients' experiences can differ between healthcare systems. Generally, the motives vary from external accountability of healthcare providers to enhancing patient choice, improving the quality of care or measuring the performance of the healthcare system as a whole. Often, surveys of patient experiences serve multiple purposes.

Apart from that, patient experiences are an important aspect of health systems research. Since the World Health Organization (WHO) published its World Health Report 2000, the quality of care as perceived by patients has been seen as an integral part of the performance of health systems. Therefore, organizations such as the Commonwealth Fund, the Picker Institute Europe and the Organization for Economic Co-operation and Development have engaged in international comparisons of patients' experiences.

How to measure patient experiences?

There are numerous ways to gain insight into patients' experiences with healthcare. Patients share their experiences in their social network and increasingly also on social media. On websites such as PatientsLikeMe, patients share experiences with symptoms and treatments. Apart from that, patients use websites like NHS Choices for reviews and ratings of health-care providers. (See ➲ Further resources.)

Reviews and ratings shared via social media can be a valuable source of information.[3] However, depending on the purpose of measurement ,more controlled methods of data collection are preferable. Patient experiences are measured through surveys, using mail questionnaires, online question-naires, telephone surveys, and face-to-face interviews. If you want to con-duct such a survey, keep in mind the following questions.

What is the unit of analysis?

Are you interested in the performance of a healthcare system as a whole, or of specific regions within a system; in the performance of individual health-care providers; or in the experiences of patients with a certain disease or who have had a certain treatment? It is important to clearly define your unit of analysis, because it has consequences for the definition of your study population and the sampling method that you will have to use.

How do I sample respondents to participate in the survey?

Depending on your unit of analysis, you can draw samples from the gen-eral population or you can draw samples from the patient populations of healthcare providers. The latter is possible only if these healthcare pro-viders have an adequate administrative system that allows for queries of patients meeting certain criteria. Be aware of specific privacy regulations that may apply to using electronic health records for this purpose.[4]

What is an adequate sample size?

There is no ready-made answer to this question. The necessary sample size depends on factors such as the reliability of the questionnaire, the expected response rate, and the aim of the survey. In studies comparing patient ex-periences across countries, the sample sizes are usually 1,000–2,000 citi-zens/patients per country. Studies comparing patient experiences between hospitals work often with sample sizes of at least 500 patients. If the aim of your study is not to compare patient experiences in different countries or different facilities but to measure patient experiences in one facility (e.g. as part of continuous quality improvement), you can generally work with smaller samples (for example, $n = 200$). If possible, try to determine your sample size using power analysis. Beware of the fact that a power ana-lysis will give you the desired number of respondents in a survey. Your ac-tual sample size should be bigger because you will have to accommodate non-response.

How do I collect data?

You can use face-to-face interviews, telephone interviews, self-administered mail surveys, or online surveys. Which of the methods is best depends on your study population and your financial resources. Face-to-face and tele-phone interviews require more human resources than mail surveys and are therefore usually more expensive. Online questionnaires are comparatively cheap, but can only be used in populations with good access to and experi-ence with the internet. Presently, this makes online surveys less adequate for use in an elderly population.

How do I choose a questionnaire?

In several countries, there are 'families' of standardized patient experience questionnaires that you could use if they fit the topic of your study. English language questionnaires that you may want to look at are the American CAHPS surveys and the surveys developed by the Picker Institute (see ➲ Further resources).

If you are looking for instruments that measure patient-reported health outcomes, the disease-specific standards developed by the International Consortium for Health Outcome Measurement (ICHOM) may be useful (again, see ➲ Further resources).

If you cannot find an existing questionnaire in your own language, you can either translate a questionnaire that has been developed elsewhere or develop your own. There are certain scientific 'rules' for translating questionnaires. You will have to have the questionnaire translated forward and backward by different translators, and the translation should not be purely technical but also include a cultural validation and adaptation to your own healthcare system. If you need to develop your own questionnaire, follow the steps described in the next section.

Who should be involved?

Stakeholder involvement is a prerequisite for collecting information that is fit for purpose.[5] When using patient experience surveys, you should pay specific attention to the involvement of patients and patient organizations. It is essential that measurement and reporting of patient experiences takes place about those quality domains that matter most to patients.

Developing your own questionnaire

The development of these measurement instruments consists of the following phases:
• Qualitative research.
• Psychometric research.
• Analyses of discriminative power.

Qualitative research

You measure patient experiences because you are interested in the quality of care evaluated from the patient's perspective. Therefore, your measurement instrument should contain quality items that are important to patients. We already know a lot about things that are important to patients. Coulter[6] lists the following patient priorities:
• Fast access to reliable health advice.
• Effective treatment delivered by trusted professionals.
• Participation in decisions and respect for preferences.
• Clear, comprehensible information and support for self-care.
• Attention to physical and environmental needs.
• Emotional support, empathy, and respect.
• Involvement of, and support for, family and carers.
• Continuity of care and smooth transitions.

This list covers more or less what patients expect from healthcare in general. However, we also know that these priorities differ between various patient groups. For that reason, the development of an instrument measuring patient experiences should preferably start with qualitative research of the preference of the specific patient group that is studied.

You can do this through a so-called focus group: a small convenience sample of people brought together to discuss a topic or issue with the aim to ascertain the range and intensity of their views.[2] A focus group discussion leads to an operationalization of quality of care from the patients' perspective and is aimed at ensuring the content validity of the questionnaires. Ideally, some 8–12 patients should participate in a focus group and you may need more than one focus group. Ask patients how they define good quality of care, and ask them about their concrete experiences with distinct aspects of healthcare quality.

Questionnaire construction

Focus groups can result in long lists of possible questionnaire items, mostly process aspects of healthcare quality such as information, communication, and interpersonal contact. In subsequent group discussions, you try to reduce this long list of items to a short list that forms the basis of your questionnaire.

There are two ways to formulate questions about patient experiences. You can ask about:
• the degree to which experiences met quality standards
• the frequency with which experiences met quality standards.

For example:
• *Degree:* in the past 12 months, did doctors listen carefully to what you had to say (response categories e.g. yes, completely; yes, definitely; yes, to a certain extent; no)?
• *Frequency:* how often in the past 12 months did doctors listen carefully to what you had to say (response categories e.g. never, sometimes, usually, always)?

In both types, the quality of care from the patient's perspective is usually measured on a four-point ordinal scale.

From the point of view of patients, quality of care should be improved primarily with respect to aspects that are extremely important to them, but with which they have relatively negative experiences. The importance that patients attach to the various experiences can be measured by designing an 'importance questionnaire' to go along with your patient experience questionnaire. In an 'importance questionnaire', respondents are asked to score the importance of the same set of items that are also included in the 'experience questionnaire'.

For example:
• *Experience:* how often in the past 12 months did doctors listen carefully to what you had to say (response categories e.g. never, sometimes, usually, always)?
• *Importance:* how important is it that doctors listen carefully to what you have to say (response categories e.g. not important, important, very important, of the utmost importance)?

Psychometric research

After you have constructed a draft questionnaire on the basis of qualitative research, you want to examine this questionnaire more quantitatively through psychometric research. For this type of research, you need to test your questionnaire in samples that are big enough to allow for psychometric analyses. Aim for at least $n = 600$, but preferably more.

Psychometric analyses include:
- item analyses
- inter-item analyses
- analyses of the underlying structure (factor and reliability analyses).

Item analyses

Item analyses consist of, for example, looking at the skewness of the distribution of the answers to questions about respondents' experiences and problems, and looking at the non-response to questions.

Inter-item analyses

An examination of the overlap in the pattern of answers for different items. You can do that using correlation coefficients.[2] If you find considerable overlap in the pattern of answers between two different items, and if the items also deal with the same subject, this means that one of these two items could be deleted. If a correlation coefficient exceeds 0.85, there is no statistical reason to keep both items in the measurement instrument. You can delete one of the two.

Factor and reliability analyses

Factor analyses are carried out in order to estimate, describe, and measure the fundamental dimensions that underlie the observed data.[2] We advise you to carry out an exploratory factor analysis using principal component analysis with oblique rotation (because of the assumed interrelationships between the factors). After determination of the number of factors, you will have to examine the size of the factor loadings. The rule of thumb here is that an item's loading for a particular factor should be more than 0.3 if a quality aspect is to be assigned to the factor in question. If an item has factor loadings of 0.3 or more for several factors, it is assigned to the factor for which it has the highest factor loading. Furthermore, you should examine the internal consistency reliability of a measurement instrument using Cronbach's alpha[2]. A scale is sufficiently reliable if Cronbach's alpha is greater than 0.70. Typically, the scales you will find in patient experience surveys correspond to the themes listed above under patient priorities: timely access, clear information, participative decision making, etc.

Discriminative power

If the purpose of your survey is to *compare* the performance of healthcare providers with respect to patient experiences, then there is one last step that you will have to take in developing your own questionnaire—namely, you will have to assure that your questionnaire is able to detect meaningful and statistical differences between healthcare providers. An adequate way to test this is by using hierarchical analysis, also called 'multilevel analysis'.

Multilevel analysis

This is a method that allows for integration of contextual, group, or macrolevel factors with individual-level factors.[2] This method allows you to examine the variance components through the so-called intraclass correlation.[2] If the intraclass correlation is not statistically significant, this implies there is only variance on the level of patients (in other words: healthcare providers do not contribute to the variance in patient experiences). In multilevel analyses, you can compare the scores of healthcare providers on the various scales in your questionnaire through empirical-Bayes methods.[2]

Case-mix adjustment

If the purpose of your survey is to compare the performance of healthcare providers, you want to be sure that you are making a 'fair' comparison. In general, elderly people, people with a lower level of education, and people with a worse self-reported health status report more positive experiences with healthcare than younger people, people with a higher level of education, and people with a better self-reported health status. There are a number of other patient characteristics that may be systematically related to the responses in patient experience surveys. If those patient characteristics are beyond the control of healthcare providers and if the populations of the healthcare providers you are comparing vary on those patient characteristics, it is necessary to correct for systematic differences in response tendencies (so-called 'case-mix adjustment').

Analysing data and interpreting results

As mentioned earlier, the motives for measuring patient experiences vary from external accountability of healthcare providers to enhancing patient choice, improving the quality of care or measuring the performance of the healthcare system as a whole. This implies that the audience you wish to address with your findings may vary from individual healthcare consumers (patients) to health insurers or other purchasers, managers and healthcare professionals, and policy makers. These various audiences have different information needs (see Table 5.7.1). Those differences can have consequences for your analyses and the way you present your findings.

Taking action

Surveys of patient experiences often serve multiple purposes. In general, the emphasis has shifted from only using data as internal feedback for quality improvement towards also publishing this information for external accountability or to facilitate consumer choice. It is difficult to develop questionnaires that serve internal as well as external purposes. If you strive to improve the quality of care from the patient's perspective, however, it is advisable to publish the survey findings.

A review article by Fung et al.[7] suggests that individual consumers do not often use public report cards to select better-performing providers over worse-performing ones, but that publicly releasing performance data

Table 5.7.1 Information needs of different stakeholders: who wants to know what?

Who	What
Individual consumers	*Maximizers:* Who is the best provider for me (in terms of outcomes or in terms of trust)? Where can I find this provider? Do I have access (in terms of waiting times, insurance coverage, etc.)? *Satisficers:* How does my usual provider perform compared with others?
Patient/consumer organizations	Do providers meet quality standards as defined by patient/consumer organizations? Which areas of performance are lagging behind? How can we help members/patients to make an informed choice?
Health insurers	Do providers meet predefined quality standards (pay-for-performance)? Whom shall we (not) contract from the quality perspective (preferred providers)?
Healthcare providers	What are best practices? Which areas of our performance need improvement? What do patients and insurers expect from us?
Regulators	Which providers perform below a minimum quality level (and therefore need further inspection)?
National or regional policy makers	What is the overall level of quality of care and how does it develop over time?

stimulates quality improvement activity at the hospital level. Therefore, the instruments used for external accountability and consumer choice should also be useful for internal quality projects. This asks for stakeholder involvement in the development of questionnaires, the design of surveys, and the interpretation of survey findings. This is a complex and time-consuming process. However, the resulting standardization enables all stakeholders to move away from discussions about the validity of indicators and instruments towards discussions about the quality of care.

It is important that you realize that measuring patient experiences is only a first step in the quality cycle. It gives you a 'diagnosis' of the quality of care from the patients' perspective. But it does not really tell you what you should do to improve patient experiences.

To find effective remedies for negative experiences, you will have to dig deeper, for example, by:

- going back to the targeted patient population and organizing discussion groups or open interviews about the survey results, their interpretation of these results and suggestions for improvement
- identifying healthcare providers whose clients have very positive experiences, finding out what they do differently, and trying to copy that in your own organization
- looking for inspiration in improvement guides that have been developed (e.g. by the American Agency for Healthcare Research and Quality and the CAHPS Improvement Guide[8]).

Potential pitfalls

Mismatch between study purpose and information products

Various audiences have different information needs and those differences have consequences for your analyses and the way you present your findings. State-of-the art analysis methods using case-mix adjusted, empirical-Bayes methods to compare the relative performance of healthcare providers are the best way to guarantee a fair comparison between providers. However, the statistics used in this method are relatively complicated, particularly for an audience of healthcare professionals. So if you use these statistics in internal feedback reports, professionals and managers may find it difficult to understand the information and recognize the 'crude' performance data that they usually work with. If this results in distrust of the information, they will not use it for quality improvement.

How to avoid bias?

High non-response is a potential source of bias in patient surveys. Therefore, you should make sure that your method of data collection is suitable for your target population:

- Online surveys are less suitable for use in an elderly population.
- Online surveys may be inadequate tools for data collection in a population with a low level of literacy.
- Make sure you use easy, unambiguous language and short sentences in all cases.
- Resort to face-to-face or telephone interviews if you expect literacy to be a problem.
- Test your draft questionnaire among a few patients from your target population.
- Ask them to explain what they think that the questions mean and invite them to think aloud while filling out the draft questionnaire (cognitive testing).
- You can make patient surveys more inclusive by offering migrants access to questionnaires in different languages.

Ethical issues and privacy of respondents

It is not possible to measure patient experiences without the help of patients who are willing to serve as respondents in qualitative research or surveys. However, depending on the legislation in your country, you may need the approval of an ethics committee before you are allowed to send out questionnaires to patients.

Apart from that, sometimes you need to draw samples from administrative data based on medical records. If necessary, seek legal counselling to make sure that you do not violate medical confidentiality or other privacy legislation.

Further resources

Further reading

Dattalo P. (2007). *Determining sample size. balancing power, precision, and practicality*. Oxford University Press, Oxford.

Websites

NHS Choices. Available at: ℘ www.nhs.uk (accessed 3 September 2019).

PatientsLikeMe. Available at: ℘ www.patientslikeme.com (accessed 3 September 2019).

GLIA GuideLine Implementability Appraisal. Available at: ℘ http://nutmeg.med.yale.edu/glia/login.htm (accessed 3 September 2019).

International Consortium for Health Outcome Measurement (ICHOM). Available at: ℘ http://www.ichom.org (accessed 3 September 2019).

Picker Institute. Available at: ℘ http://www.picker.org/tools-resources/toolkits/ (accessed 3 September 2019).

References

1 Trkman P. (2010). The critical success factors of business process management. *International Journal of Information Management*, **30**, 125–34.

2 Porta M. (2008). *A dictionary of epidemiology*. Oxford University Press, New York.

3 Kleefstra SM, Zandbelt LC, Borghans I, et al. (2016). Investigating the potential contribution of patient rating sites to hospital supervision: exploratory results from an interview study in the Netherlands. *Journal of Medical Internet Research*, **18(7)**, e201.

4 Chung JS, Young HN, Moreno MA, et al. (2017). Patient-centred outcomes research: brave new world meets old institutional policies. *Family Practice*, **24**, pii: cmw129.

5 Delnoij DMJ, Rademakers JJDJM, Groenewegen PP. (2010). The Dutch Consumer Quality Index: an example of stakeholder involvement in indicator development. *BMC Health Services Research*, **10**, 88.

6 Coulter A. (2007). Finding out what patients want. *ENT News*, **16**, 65–7.

7 Fung CH, Lim YW, Mattke S, et al. (2008). Systematic review: the evidence that publishing patient care performance data improves quality of care. *Annals of Internal Medicine*, **148**, 111–23.

8 CAHPS (2011). Improving patient experience. Available at: ℘ https://www.ahrq.gov/cahps/quality-improvement/index.html (accessed 21 August 2019).

Health technology assessment

Chiara de Waure and Carlo Favaretti

Objectives

The aim of this chapter is to help the public health practitioner to:
- learn what health technology assessment (HTA) is in healthcare and in public health domains
- understand that HTA is a powerful tool for the governance of the healthcare systems at all their levels: macro (national and regional), meso (hospitals and healthcare services organizations), and micro (healthcare professionals)
- understand that HTA is a multidisciplinary, multidimensional and multistakeholder process
- gain knowledge about how to develop an HTA report to support decision makers in taking the best possible decisions
- know the main sources of data to base the assessment contents on evidence
- recognize the role of HTA in public health.

Public health practitioners are often requested to take decisions or to support decision makers in doing the right choices. Independently by the level, the decision-making process needs to be relied on`// evidence and data and to take into account uncertainty.

Starting from the broad concept of health technology, this chapter aims to provide the essentials of the assessment process with particular reference to public health.

The decision-making process, which involves multiple stakeholders, is not only a technical exercise. Anyway, sound technical assessments must be offered to decision makers at all levels of healthcare systems. This chapter provides guidance to develop an HTA report, using correct methods and finding the right data, and insights into its application to the public health domain.

What is health technology

Health technology can be defined as 'the application of organized knowledge and skills in the form of devices, medicines, vaccines, procedures and systems developed to solve a health problem and improve quality of lives'[1].

The notion of health technology includes almost all the tools that healthcare systems and public health are based on [2]:
- Diagnostic and treatment methods.
- Medical equipments.
- Pharmaceuticals.
- Rehabilitation and prevention methods.
- Organizational and supportive systems within which healthcare is provided.

What is health technology assessment

In general, assessment may be defined as a formal quantitative (sometimes qualitative) evaluation of a process or a system.[3] HTA is a policy-oriented comprehensive evaluation that takes into consideration several aspects from different points of view.

In fact, since its early phases in the late 1960s, the focus of HTA has shifted from the technical performance of capital-intensive technologies to diseases and clinical outcomes and, more recently, to services delivery models.[4]

Among a certain number of definitions of HTA published in the literature, the most thorough is probably that provided by the European Network for Health Technology Assessment (EuNetHTA):

HTA is a multidisciplinary process that summarizes information about the medical, social, economic and ethical issues related to the use of a health technology in a systematic, transparent, unbiased, robust manner. Its aim is to inform the formulation of safe, effective, health policies that are patient focused and seek to achieve best value.[2]

Since its inception, HTA has been used to support decisions about the introduction, diffusion, and reimbursement of new technology. In the past years, HTA methods are being used to dismiss obsolete or low-value technologies as well.

HTA can be regarded as a process or a system and five steps can be recognized:[5]

1 Identification of new technology (horizon scanning), new indications of a well-documented technology, existing technology with poor evidence.
2 Priority setting using guidelines or explicit criteria.
3 Assessment (see Hailey's assessment chain).
4 Dissemination of products as an active way of communication and transferring HTA reports and recommendations to intended audience.
5 Implementation, overcoming barriers, and setting the right incentives. In a more synthetic way, Hailey[6] termed the 'assessment chain':

1 formulation of the HTA questions
2 production of a HTA report
3 dissemination and measurement of the impact of the HTA report.

Health technology assessment as a governance tool at all levels of healthcare systems

Health, healthcare systems, and public health are adaptive complex systems 'made up of many individual, self-organizing elements capable of responding to others and to their environment'.[7] Adaptive complex systems need a high level of governance. In general, governance concerns how governments and other social organizations interact, how they relate to citizens and how decisions are taken in a complex world.[8] In the health field, two kinds of governance could be distinguished: health governance that refers to leading and strengthening health systems, and governance for health, which deals with the joint actions of health and non-health sectors, the public and private sectors, and citizens for a common interest.[9]

HTA can be considered a powerful tool for health governance. It is a multidisciplinary, multidimensional and multistakeholder technical process. Table 5.8.1 shows the main stakeholders involved in HTA and their expectations in a process of HTA.[10]

Table 5.8.1 Stakeholders involved in HTA

Stakeholders	Expectations
Health professionals	Improvement of diagnostic and clinical pathways and of clinical outcomes
Patients and citizens	Gain in health and wellness
Health and healthcare organizations	Efficiency, productivity and quality
Industries	Profitability
Regulatory bodies	Assurance of the best benefit/risk ratio

To impact on health, healthcare, and public health, technical assessments have to be followed by decisions. The political process of deciding what to do after the production of an HTA report is usually defined as appraisal: it is based on HTA but other factors are also taken into account such as local priorities, values, preferences, and resources. In some countries, assessment and appraisal are two explicitly distinct processes carried out by different bodies, but in other countries this is not the case.

Decision making following an HTA process can take place at three levels: macro, meso and micro. The macro level (national and regional) refers to political choices on planning/regulating and funding healthcare systems and public health programmes, and reimbursing health technologies. The meso level refers to organizational and managerial choices in the governance of hospitals, health authorities, primary healthcare services, etc. The micro level deals with decisions taken by health professionals to meet needs and expectations of patients and citizens and/or groups of patients.

The governance issues continue after the appraisal and the decision making: in fact, decisions must be administered to assure that the established standards of the healthcare system are reached and maintained overtime. The administration processes include decisions on disinvestment when a health technology is obsolete or of low value.[11]

Disinvestment should be based on sound approaches, such as HTA, and careful appraisal processes. Disinvestment is more complex and complicated than investment both for the number of involved stakeholders and for inputs to be assessed (see Table 5.8.2).[12]

Battista et al. gave an overview of the intersection of assessment, appraisal, and administration processes that a modern public health professional should be able to manage and lead (Figure 5.8.1).[13]

Table 5.8.2 Stakeholders and inputs in investment and disinvestment processes

Stakeholders	Inputs	Results
Payers, regulators, industries, HTA bodies	Safety Efficacy Effectiveness Value	Investment
Payers, regulators, industries, clinicians, HTA bodies, professionals, societies, patients, safety & quality bodies, employers, academia, media	Safety Efficacy Effectiveness Value and values Resistance Politics Sunk costs Disruption Loss aversion Innovation head room Uncertainty and a higher burden of evidence	Disinvestment

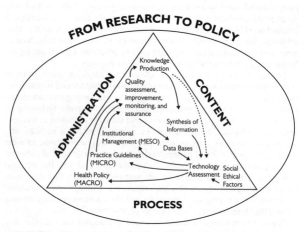

Figure 5.8.1 Steps in translating research to decision makers.

Reproduced from Battista R, Lance J-M, Lehoux P, et al. (1999). 'Health technology assessment and the regulation of medical devices and procedures in Quebec: synergy, collusion, or collision?' *International Journal of Technology Assessment in Health Care* 15(3), 593–601, with permission from Cambridge University Press.

HTA originated as a mostly centralized function conducted by government agencies and other national- or regional-level organizations. Then it evolved into a more decentralized function, both in the public and private sectors.[14, 15]

The growth in decentralized HTA activity (meso level) has arisen from the expansion of HTA programmes for particular decision-making needs, due to the increasing complexity of hospital management.

Decentralization of HTA and related functions widens the expertise available to HTA and brings broader perspectives to the process.

The EU Commission, under the 7th Framework Programme, funded AdHopHTA.[16] This project allowed the 'contextualization of HTA to a specific hospital in order to assess the choice of an available comparator, specific organizational models and patterns within the hospital, a sharper focus on the HTs of interest for the hospital, timely adjustments to the hospital context and collaboration with hospital decision-makers'.

Developing a health technology assessment report

Framing an HTA report is a tricky task. In fact, the first goal is to translate the policy question behind the report into research questions, which may be addressed through scientifically sound methods. The identification of research questions should follow predefined 'rules' to obtain a standardized evaluation. These 'rules' are described within the so-called 'EUnetHTA Core Model', which is a methodological framework for shared production and sharing of HTA information.[17] The Core Model identifies several pieces of information that need to be included in an HTA report and that cover the following domains:

- Health problem and current use of the technology: this domain provides a quantitative and qualitative description of the target condition and current management patterns.
- Description and technical characteristics of technology: this domain addresses several questions about the technology (when it was developed and introduced, for what purpose; who will use it, in what manner, for what condition, and at what level of healthcare).
- Safety: unwanted or harmful effects caused by the use of the technology are evaluated from the point of view of both individual patients and health professionals.
- Accuracy: this domain deals with the performance of diagnostic technologies.
- Clinical effectiveness: evidence that the technology works (efficacy) and works in real life (effectiveness) are provided in this domain.
- Costs and economic evaluation: starting from the description of costs, information about value for money and economic efficiency are released
- Ethical aspects: discussion on prevalent social and moral norms and values relevant to the technology.
- Organisational aspects: this domain provides information about the ways in which resources should be organized and the consequences

they may further on produce in the organization and the healthcare system as a whole.
- Patient and social aspects: this domain addresses issues relevant to individual patients, caregivers and social groups (older people, people living in remote communities, people with learning disabilities, ethnic minorities, immigrants, etc.)
- Legal aspects: rules and regulations related to the implications of the use or the dismission of a health technology are evaluated.

All the described domains are taken into consideration in the so-called full HTA report. Nevertheless, there is also another type of assessment, namely the Rapid Relative Effectiveness Assessment (REA) that covers only clinical domains and measures the medical/therapeutic added value of a technology.

Independently by the type of assessment, more specific areas of consideration are further identified in each domain. According to the definition of HTA, each assessment element has to be tackled in a systematic, transparent and reliable way. Therefore, one of the main skills that is required for an HTA doer is the knowledge of the methods of the scientific research and the capacity to apply them. Else more, because of the need to be multi-disciplinary and interdisciplinary[18, 19], HTA doers should have good team working and project management skills. All these abilities are essential in order to identify the right sources of data, to apply the proper methods to combine all the information and to end up with a final HTA report.

Source of data and methods

Doing an HTA report is a matter of searching and synthetizing evidence; using evidence in order to feed forecasting model; and collecting information for addressing and solving organizational, social and ethical issues. Methods used to do it refer mostly to the following discipline: epidemiology, health economics and qualitative research.[11]

As for epidemiology, systematic reviews and meta-analysis play an important role in addressing several domains, i.e. the health problem, the accuracy, the clinical effectiveness and the safety of the health technology.[17] In order to perform a good systematic review, HTA doers should know search engines and databases and should be able to perform a thorough literature search, a reliable assessment of the quality of articles, an unbiased extraction of data and a proper combination of them. Alongside systematic review and meta-analysis, HTA doers should be ready to consult and analyze health (services) data in order to get real-life statistics on the distribution of the health problem and its determinants, the safety, the access and the utilization of health technologies and the costs of the health problem and of the health technology itself.

Another essential method is the cost-effectiveness analysis. In fact, each technology should undergo an evaluation of the incremental cost-effectiveness ratio in comparison to the alternative(s).[11, 20] In order to do it models need to be developed and fed with reliable clinical, epidemiological and financial data in order to release an evaluation of the incremental cost for quality-adjusted life year (QALY) gained. Systematic reviews and health (service) data consultation deliver inputs for these models. At the end of the day, based on shared threshold, it is possible to define if the health technology is eventually cost-effective.

The final set of methods used in HTA is that of the qualitative research. The latter is becoming more and more used in order to catch information from key opinion leaders, the public and patients. In fact, HTA also evaluates ethical, social and organizational implications. In-depth interviews, focus groups, observations and documentary analysis all belong to the qualitative research.[20] The first two in particular are used for consensus development that is often a step of HTA.[11]

Both quantitative and qualitative methods allow HTA doers collecting and combining data and information. Nevertheless, in order to do it, sources of data and information have to be known. HTA doers should be familiar with interrogation of generic and specialized bibliographic databases, i.e. PubMed, Embase, Cochrane Library, CINAHL, as well as of databases of ongoing research and results. Furthermore, they should deeply know the requisites, the goals and the pitfalls of epidemiological study designs, which often represent the primary source of data. Finally, also registers, claims and administrative database should be handled.[11]

Health technology assessment and public health

HTA and public health have a lot in common: interdisciplinarity, methods to generate and synthesize evidence, focus on knowledge translation, issues on prioritization, complexity of the evaluation field. HTA is a policy-oriented process aimed at informing decision-making; public health is an action-oriented process with a population outlook focused on both health states and intervention.[21]

Some important trends foster convergence between them: complexity of healthcare, technological innovation, better understanding of health determinants, increased consumers' expectations.

Until recently, the majority of HTA initiatives have been focused on clinically oriented intervention, i.e. drugs and medical devices, even though from a population perspective.[22] Nevertheless, public health purpose is to respond to population health needs through organized efforts of the whole society. This means that public health should rely on organized activities aimed at preventing and managing diseases and at controlling unhealthy lifestyles and well-known risk factors for them. These activities, which are health technologies, are considered complex interventions that deserve evaluation too. The applications of HTA in this field are still limited. The most of production is on vaccination and screening programs. The production of HTA outputs more related to everyday practice public health issues and the development of more scientifically grounded decision making in public health should lead the process of convergence. Important initiatives have been launched and promoted within well-known international societies in the field of HTA applied to public health. The HTA international (HTAi), which serves as primary scientific and professional focus for all those who undertake and use HTA, has two interest groups dealing with public health issues (see ➲ Further resources). One is about the impact of public health interventions, with a special focus on nutrition, and the second is on the assessment of vaccination programmes. Similarly, a Section on Health Technology Assessment has been established within the European Public Health Association (EUPHA) with the aim of implementing the understanding, production and use of HTA in public health (again, see ➲ Further resources). Some advancement in the field has been done with a project co-funded by the European Union under the Seventh Framework Programme, namely the INTEGRATE-HTA project.[23] The project has addressed complex interventions, among them complex public health programmes, and has released several guidance on: a) the assessment of effectiveness and economic, social, cultural, legal, and ethical issues of complex health technologies; b) the elicitation of patients' preferences and patient-specific moderators of treatment; c) the way to include context, setting, and implementation in the assessment; d) choosing adequate qualitative evidence synthesis methods; e) the integration of all these issues into a patient-centred, comprehensive assessment. Within the project a case study has been developed on models of home based palliative care with and without an additional element of caregiver support (reinforced and non-reinforced home based palliative care). Table 5.8.3 provides an overview of the case study.[24, 25]

Table 5.8.3 The INTEGRATE-HTA case study on palliative care

Rationale	Albeit the availability of evidence on the effectiveness and cost-effectiveness of palliative care models, policy makers need also information about their advantages and disadvantages with respect to socio-cultural, ethical, and legal aspects, patient preferences and patient-specific moderators as well as context and implementation issues
Overall policy/ research question	'Are reinforced models of home based palliative care acceptable, feasible, appropriate, meaningful, effective, cost-effective models for providing patient-centred palliative care (compared to non-reinforced models of home based palliative care) in adults (defined as those aged 18 years old and over) and their families?'
Framework for the evaluation	Five step model • Definition of the HTA objective and technology • Creation of a logic model to define evidence needs • Evidence assessment • Mapping of the evidence for informing specific assessment criterion (effectiveness, economics, acceptability, meaningfulness, feasibility and appropriateness) • HTA conclusion

Table 5.8.3 (*Contd.*)

Methods	Systematic reviews and meta-analyses Review of reviews
	Qualitative systematic reviews
	Stakeholders consultation
	Elicitation of experts' judgment during stakeholder workshops and telephone based interviews
	Appraisal checklist tools
	Rapid applicability assessments
	Multiple Criteria Decision Analysis
Key results	• Scant evidence on the efficacy/effectiveness on patients' and caregivers' outcomes.
	• Professional stakeholders highlight that support for the lay caregiver is important.
	• From the economic point of view, home based models of palliative care may be cost saving, mostly because of an expected reduction in hospitalization.
	• Patients prefer quality instead of quantity of life. Nevertheless patients 'without caregivers; with uncontrollable physical symptoms; where physicians may not be available or where concerns exist about responding to sudden changes are less likely to die at home'.
	• There are some concerns in terms of acceptability for informal caregivers because of changing roles and relationships and caregiver's burden.
	• Other concerns refer to the relief of caregiver's burden and the availability, accessibility and equity of palliative care.
	• There are some barriers and facilitators to the implementation of home based palliative care, which are linked to the provider, the organization, the structure and the micro-context of the family and home.
	• There are differences in palliative care provision across Europe that call for caution in the evaluation of transferability of results.

Conclusion

HTA is a policy-oriented process aimed at informing decision making. It is a multidisciplinary, multidimensional and multistakeholder process that can be used at all levels of the healthcare system to assess any kind of health technologies. Its final aim is to help decision-makers to introduce, reimburse, disseminate and dismiss health technologies.

HTA is a well-known approach used to evaluate health technology mainly used in the clinical/therapeutical field (i.e. drugs and devices), but efforts have still to be made to strengthen HTA in public health.

Some very important challenges are facing the future of HTA in public health. They can be summarized as follows.

Methodological challenges

- Health technologies used in public health are mostly complex interventions that are put in place across different health and healthcare settings. Methods for setting priorities[26] and assessing complex interventions are being implemented in order to allow taking into account it.
- The evaluation of real world data should be integrated in HTA processes, in particular with respect to the evaluation of the effectiveness and the decision on disinvestment.
- Albeit a well-established process, HTA needs to be implemented in terms of transferability of results.

Strategical challenges

- HTA is a multistakeholder process but the involvement of stakeholders is still suboptimal in most assessments.
- Legal and ethical constraints in the access to individual data should be overcome in order to make it possible to use data.
- A strong commitment from national institutions should strengthen the role of HTA.
- The integration of the assessment and the appraisal phases should be pursued.

Further resources

Websites

The impact of public health interventions: Available at: ℛ http://www.htai.org/interest-groups/impact-of-public-health-interventions.html (accessed 3 September 2019).

The assessment of vaccination programmes: Available at: ℛ http://www.htai.org/interest-groups/assessment-of-vaccination-programs.html (accessed 3 September 2019).

EUPHA Section on Health Technology Assessment: Available at: ℛ https://eupha.org/health-technology-assessment (accessed 3 September 2019).

References

1 World Health Organization. Health technology assessment. Available at: ℛ http://www.who.int/health-technology-assessment/about/healthtechnology/en (accessed 21 August 2019).

2 EUnetHTA. Common questions. Available at: ℛ https://5026.makemeweb.net/faq/Category%201-0#t287n73 (accessed 21 August 2019).

3 Last JM. (2007). *A dictionary of public health*. Oxford University Press, New York.

4 Battista RN. (2006). Expanding the scientific basis of health technology assessment: a research agenda for the next decade. *International Journal of Technology Assessment in Health Care*, **22**, 275–80.

5 Banta HD, Luce B. (1993). *Health care technology and its assessment: an international perspective*. Oxford University Press, London.

6 Hailey D. (2003). *Elements of effectiveness for health technology assessment program*. HTA initiative #9. Alberta Heritage Foundation for Medical Research, Edmonton, Canada. Available at: ℛ http://www.inahta.org/wp-content/themes/inahta/img/AboutHTA_Elements_of_Effectiveness_for_HTA_Programs.pdf (accessed 21 August 2019).

7 Miller G, Gemar M, Campsie P, et al. (2003). *A toolbook for improving health in cities: a discussion paper*. The Caledon Institute of Social Policy, Ottawa, Canada. Available at: ℛ https://maytree.com/publications/a-toolbox-for-improving-health-in-cities-a-discussion-paper (accessed 21 August 2019).

8 Graham J, Amos B, Plumptre T. (2003). *Principles for good governance in the 21st century*. Policy brief 15. Institute on Governance, Ottawa, Canada. Available at: ℛ http://unpan1.un.org/intradoc/groups/public/documents/UNPAN/UNPAN011842.pdf (accessed 21 August 2019).

9   Kickbusch I, Gleicher D. (2012). Governance for health in the 21st century. World Health Organization Regional Office for Europe, Copenhagen. Available at: ℘ http://www.euro.who.int/__data/assets/pdf_file/0019/171334/RC62BD01-Governance-for-Health-Web.pdf (accessed 21 August 2019).

10 Omachonu VK, Einspruch NG. (2010). Innovation in healthcare delivery systems: a conceptual framework. *Innov Journal*, **15**(1).

11 Goodman CS. (2014). *HTA 101: introduction to health technology assessment*. National Library of Medicine (US), Bethesda, MD. Available at: ℘ https://www.nlm.nih.gov/nichsr/hta101/HTA_101_FINAL_7-23-14.pdf (accessed 21 August 2019).

12 Elshaug AG, Hiller JE, Tunis SR, et al. (2007). Challenges in Australian policy processes for disinvestment from existing, ineffective health care practices. *Australia and New Zealand Health Policy*, **4**, 23.

13 Battista RN, Lance JM, Lehoux P, et al. (1999). Health technology assessment and the regulation of medical devices and procedures in Quebec. Synergy, collusion, or collision? *International Journal of Technology Assessment in Health Care*, **15**(3), 593–601.

14 Goodman CS. (1998). Healthcare technology assessment: methods, framework, and role in policy making. *American Journal of Managed Care*, **4**, SP200–14.

15 Rettig RA. (1997). *Health care in transition: technology assessment in the private sector*. RAND, Santa Monica CA, Available at: ℘ http://www.rand.org/content/dam/rand/pubs/monograph_reports/2007/MR754.pdf(accessed 21 August 2019).

16 Sampietro-Colom L, Lach K, Cicchetti A, et al. (2015). The AdHopHTA handbook: a handbook of hospital-based Health Technology Assessment (HB-HTA), p. 20. Public deliverable; The AdHopHTA Project (FP7/2007–13 grant agreement nr 305018). Available at: ℘ https://www.researchgate.net/publication/287201164_The_AdHopHTA_handbook_a_handbook_of_hospital-based_Health_Technology_Assessment_HB-HTA/link/5672c71608aedbbb3f9f6a50/download (accessed 21 August 2019).

17 EUnetHTA (2016). Joint Action 2, Work Package 8. HTA Core Model® version 3.0 (pdf); Available at: ℘ https://www.eunethta.eu/wp-content/uploads/2018/03/HTACoreModel3.0-1.pdf (accessed 21 August 2019).

18 Banta D, Behney CJ, Andrulis DP. (1978). *Assessing the efficacy and safety of medical technologies*. Office of Technology Assessment, Washington.

19 Velasco Garrido M, Busse R. (2005). *Health technology assessment. An introduction to objectives, role of evidence and structure in Europe*. World Health Organization Regional Office for Europe, Copenhagen.

21 Swedish Agency for Health Technology Assessment and Assessment of Social Services (2014). *Evaluation and synthesis of studies using qualitative methods of analysis*. SBU, Stockholm.

22 Battista RN, Lafortune L. (2009). Health technology assessment and public health: a time of convergence. *European Journal of Public Health*, **19**(3), 227.

23 Holland WW. (2004). Health technology assessment and public health: a commentary. *International Journal of Technology Assessment in Health Care*, **20**(1), 77–80.

24 Gerhardus A. on behalf of the INTEGRATE-HTA project team (2016). Integrated health technology assessment for evaluating complex technologies (INTEGRATE-HTA): an introduction to the guidances. Available at: ℘ https://www.integrate-hta.eu/wp-content/uploads/2016/02/INTEGRATE-HTA-An-introduction-to-the-guidances.pdf (accessed 21 August 2019).

25 Brereton L, Wahlster P, Lysdahl KB, et al. on behalf of the INTEGRATE-HTA project team (2016). Integrated assessment of home based palliative care with and without reinforced caregiver support: 'A demonstration of INTEGRATE-HTA methodological guidances' – executive summary. Available at: ℘ http://www.integrate-hta.eu/downloads (accessed 21 August 2019).

26 Specchia ML, Favale M, Di Nardo F, et al. (2015). How to choose health technologies to be assessed by HTA? A review of criteria for priority setting. *Epidemiologia e Prevenzione*, **4**(Suppl. 1), 39.

Chapter 5.9

Improving equity

Sharon Friel and David Melzer

Objectives

After reading this chapter you will:
- be familiar with the concept and extent of health inequity in high- and middle- income countries
- understand how the healthcare system can be both a cause of health inequities and a mechanism by which to improve health equity
- recognize how to address the social determinants of health inequity
- begin to systematically apply an equity lens to your daily professional practice.

Definitions and key terms

- Health inequities are avoidable inequalities in health outcomes.
- Health equity is not only about health outcomes but also about equitable exposure to factors that affect health; and prevention of disadvantage due to ill health.
- Social determinants.
- Community empowerment.
- Health literacy.

Why improving equity is an important public health issue

Despite the increase in global average life expectancy of more than 20 years since 1950 and improvements in health more generally, some startling differences in health experience exists between and within countries. Improving health equity requires attention to the underlying social causes in addition to more equal access to appropriate levels of quality healthcare. Health inequities can be best reduced through needs-based universal primary healthcare and intersectoral action, action that requires leadership by public health professionals.

The extent of health inequities

The World Health Organization Commission on Social Determinants of Health (CSDH) shone a global spotlight on the marked inequities in health conditions between countries and population groups.[1] For example, premature death among adults remains a major health issue in countries rich and poor, but the rates differ enormously—for example, Australia 76 per 1,000 compared with Papua New Guinea 380 per 1000.[2]

If there is no biological reason for the systematic differences in life expectancy or health conditions between different regions and countries, then they are not inevitable and need not exist. These avoidable health inequities occur not just between countries, but also within countries. For example, an assessment of socio-economic inequities in mortality and prevalence of health risks among 22 countries in all parts of Europe demonstrates persistent and large inequities in health conditions within developed countries in the region. People with the lowest level of education were found to be consistently at higher risk of poor health compared with those with the highest levels of education (see Box 5.9.1).[3]

> Box 5.9.1 Social inequities in health: more than one measure
>
> Differences in health within countries are stratified along lines of ethnicity, gender, age, education, occupation, income, and class. Many studies (and policy and practice) concentrate on only one of these social dimensions at a time, but it is important to recognize that real people are simultaneously positioned in terms of many social strata. For example, an 18-year-old working-class urban Anglo-Australian girl behaves in particular ways, is engaged in certain social relationships, and attracts distinct social responses because of all those elements of who she is.
>
> Inequities in health are not just about differences between the top and the bottom of the social ladder. There is a social gradient in health that runs from top to bottom of the socio-economic spectrum, making health inequities a whole of population issue.

The causes of health inequities

The social determinants of health inequities

Perhaps you are a primary care physician, a tobacco cessation officer or a community health worker? When a person walks through your door, you are aware of at least two things:

- *Many factors have brought the person to this meeting*: factors positively and negatively affecting health, experienced in the immediate moment and over the course of a lifetime.
- *If in a healthcare setting*: behind the patient are many others who do not make it to your door.

By now you should be asking what it is about society that is causing such unfair differences in health outcomes (see Box 5.9.2). For health in general, people need the basic material resources for a decent life, they need to have control over their lives, and they need voice and participation in decision-making processes. The level of material, psychosocial, and political resource among different social groups is influenced by the social determinants of health and health inequities. The social determinants refer to the distribution of power, income, goods, and services, globally and nationally, and immediate circumstances of people's lives—for example, their access to healthcare and education, their conditions of work and leisure, their homes, communities, towns, or cities.[1]

Healthcare systems: a determinant of, and solution to, health inequities

International, national, and local healthcare systems are both determinants of health inequities and powerful mechanisms to reduce inequities.[4] Given the high burden of illness particularly among the socially disadvantaged groups, it is urgent to make healthcare systems more responsive to population needs.

Box 5.9.2 From social determinants to health inequities, in brief

- The global context affects how societies prosper through its impact on international relations and domestic norms and policies.
- These in turn shape the way society, at national and local levels, organizes its affairs, giving rise to forms of social position and hierarchy. Most societies are hierarchical, stratified generally along lines of ethnicity, gender, age, education, occupation, income, and class. Where people are in the social hierarchy affects their health differently.
- Economic and social policies generate and distribute political power, income, goods, and services. These are distributed unequally among different social groups.
- This, is turn, affects the nature of the conditions in which people grow, learn, live, work, and age. This means that different social groups have different exposure to, for example, quality healthcare and education, conditions of work and leisure, and quality of housing and built environment.
- Together these structural factors and daily living conditions constitute the social determinants of health.
- The social determinants of health can empower or dis-empower individuals, communities, and even nations through their influence on material resource, psychosocial control, behavioural options and political voice afforded to different groups along the social hierarchy.
- Inequities in each of these contribute to inequities in health risks and vulnerability to ill health, and to the consequences of ill health.

Inequities in healthcare are systematic differences in the use or receipt of quality primary, secondary, and tertiary healthcare services, including hospitalizations, diagnostic tests, surgical procedures, physicians' visits, allied health services, medications, and health promotion programmes. Gender, education, occupation, income, ethnicity, disability, and place of residence are all linked to access, experiences of, and benefits from healthcare.

The inverse care law, initially identified by Tudor Hart, in which the poor consistently gain less from health services than the better off, is visible in every country across the globe. Out-of-pocket expenditures for healthcare contribute to health inequities, tending to deter poorer people from using both essential and non-essential services, leading to untreated morbidity. In OECD countries, the cost of most doctors' visits are subsidized and there are provisions to limit out-of- pocket costs for a given level of need. In these countries, socio-economically advantaged groups (high-income groups) are more likely to use specialist medical and dental services than less advantaged groups.[5] These inequities in access and use of a range of healthcare services, not just the doctor, are particularly concerning in the context of chronic disease where optimal care includes use of multidisciplinary services.

However, inequities in access and utilization of healthcare are not only financial—inequities play out by race, gender, age, and location. In spite of near universal coverage for antenatal visits in Pelota, Brazil, the quality of care was consistently higher among women of white skin colour and high socio-economic status women than among black and poor women.[6]

Key messages
- Healthcare systems are socially determined and are determinants of health and health equity.
- The healthcare system, whether publicly or privately supported, should promote health equity and contribute to wider efforts to reduce health inequities.

What can be done to improve equity

Primary healthcare systems

Appropriately configured and managed health systems provide a vehicle to improve people's lives, protect them from the vulnerability of sickness, generate a sense of life security, and build common purpose within society. Healthcare systems contribute most to improving health equity when the institutions and services are organized around the principle of universal coverage (extending the same scope of quality services to the whole population, according to needs, regardless of ability to pay), and when the system as a whole is organized around primary healthcare (PHC), including both the model of locally organized action across the social determinants of health and the primary level of entry to care with upward referral if necessary.

Levels of care

Within each level of care, there are opportunities to improve health equity. Secondary and tertiary levels of care are concerned, mainly, with the progression from disease to death. How these types of care are set up can make an important contribution to health equity.

There are four main characteristics of primary care practice: first-contact healthcare, person-focused care over time, comprehensive care, and coordinated care, as well as family and community orientation. In a comparison of the supply and adequacy of primary care characteristics across 13 industrialized countries, Starfield and colleagues found that the stronger a country's primary care orientation, the lower the rates of all-cause mortality, all-cause premature mortality, and cause-specific premature mortality from asthma and bronchitis, emphysema, and pneumonia, cardiovascular disease, and heart disease.[7] In state-level analyses in the USA, there were fewer differences in self-rated health between higher and lower income-inequality areas where good primary care experiences were stronger. Evidence of success of primary level services in reducing health inequities is also available from Africa (Liberia, Niger, Zaire), Asia (China, Kerala in India, Sri Lanka) and Latin America (Brazil, Cuba).[7]

Key messages
- Strengthen geographical access to care (particularly for remote rural communities).
- Remove financial barriers (both formal and informal user fees increasing direct individual and household costs of health-seeking behaviour and treatment).
- Help poorer, less educated and other categories of socially disadvantaged patients to be aware of their rights to healthcare and to advocate for their own health needs as effectively as do patients with higher incomes.
- Ensure healthcare system working models are sensitive to cultural diversity.

A focus on prevention

As a public health practitioner, a large part of your professional remit is to prevent disease onset and promote wellbeing. A number of the inequities in health outcomes in middle- and high-income countries relate to non-communicable diseases, injuries, and accidents. Much of public health's prevention focus has been on individuals and their behaviours. Eating healthy diets, being physically active, limiting alcohol consumption and not smoking are each socially graded. For example, in high- and middle-income countries, excess body weight tends to be more prevalent among people further down the social and economic scale. Similarly, the prevalence of tobacco use decreases with increasing socio-economic status.[8] However, even if we were able to equalize lifestyle behaviour factors, health inequities are likely to persist between socio-economic groups.

A number of interventions at the individual and community level, such as screening, healthy eating advice, smoking cessation and statin prescribing, have been shown to widen socio-economic inequities.[9, 10] A more upstream systems approach would involve, for example, legislating smoke-free public spaces or banning dietary trans fats. Similarly, obesity prevention interventions that focus on behaviour change through personal skill development, information, and social marketing campaigns may perpetuate socio-economic inequities in obesity rates, given that the uptake of the message is generally greater in higher social status groups.

Obesity prevention requires approaches that ensure an ecologically sustainable, adequate, and nutritious food supply; material security; a built habitat that lends itself towards easy uptake of healthier food options and participation in both organized and unorganized physical activity, and a family, educational, and work environment that positively reinforces (see Box 5.9.3) healthy living and empowers all individuals to make healthy choices.[11, 12] Very little of this action sits within the capabilities or responsibilities of the health sector. We will return to this point later.

A central component of health promotion and disease prevention is community empowerment. Restricted participation results in deprivation of fundamental human capabilities, setting the context for differentials in, for example, employment, education, and healthcare. Health equity depends vitally on the empowerment of individuals and groups to represent strongly and effectively their needs and interests. Evidence from interventions for

---

Box 5.9.3 Some success stories

The Brazilian population-wide Agita Sao Paulo physical activity programme successfully reduced the level of physical inactivity in the general population using a multi-strategy approach including the construction of pathways, the widening and removal of obstacles on paths, walking/running tracks with shadow and hydration points, green areas and leisure spaces in permanent maintenance, bicycle storage close to public transport stations and at entrances of schools/workplaces, and private and public incentive policies for mass active transport. A whole community intervention in the town of Colac in Victoria, Australia, not only reduced unhealthy weight gain in children but also did so preferentially in those from lower socio-economic households.

youth empowerment, HIV/AIDS prevention and women's empowerment suggests that the most effective empowerment strategies are those that build on and reinforce authentic participation ensuring autonomy in decision making, sense of community and local bonding, and psychological empowerment of the community members themselves.

Integrated healthcare

The public health practitioner is a key person within a primary healthcare system, playing an important role in helping to ensure fair access and use of quality healthcare services, from health promotion through to tertiary care. Take child, adolescent, and maternal health, for example. Liu and colleagues demonstrated that linking communities and facilities in a continuum of care is more effective in reducing maternal and newborn deaths than is focusing on either community or facility alone.[13] In the case of child and maternal health, this lifecycle integrative approach to health requires primary and community healthcare workers to engage in various levels of care including:

- health promotion and community mobilization (e.g. infant and young child feeding; school health; special programme areas such as HIV)
- outpatient services (e.g. family planning; malaria prevention such as bed nets)
- case management and care (e.g. childbirth; malnutrition care and rehabilitation)
- health system tasks (e.g. essential drugs supply and logistics; data monitoring; financing such as issuing vouchers for healthcare).

A social determinants approach through intersectoral action

A critical starting point for health equity is within the health sector itself. However, to make a fundamental improvement in health equity requires not only technical and medical solutions but also action in the immediate and structural conditions in which people are born, grow, live, work, and age. As a social determinants lens on health equity illuminates, good health for all is not only a matter for the health sector but must also involve sectors such as agriculture, urban planning, employment, and education.

Effective action on health equity therefore depends vitally on cross-sectoral coordination. This is manifested in a dynamic inter-relation between the health system and the wider system of governance through which inequity in health outcomes is produced. Through your role as a public health practitioner, you can bring together the benefits of primary healthcare and action in the social determinants of health. This will promote health equity through attention to the needs of socially disadvantaged groups and help provide leadership in promoting coherent policies and practices in different sectors.

Let's take mental health as an illustrative case study. Promoting equitable mental wellbeing and reducing inequities in the causes and treatment of mental illness requires an intersectoral approach as outlined in Table 5.9.1 below.[14]

Policy making at macro, meso, and micro levels of governance and across sectors plays a key role in influencing mental health outcomes, acting on social determinants of inequalities.[15]

Table 5.9.1 Intersectoral action in relation to equity in mental health

Determinant	Intervention
Violence/crime	Violence/crime prevention programmes
Substance abuse	Alcohol and drugs policies
Social fragmentation	Promoting programmes building family and wider social cohesion
Stigma	Mental health promotion programmes
Natural disasters	Trauma and stress support programmes
Inadequate housing	Housing improvement interventions
Work stress	Protective labour policies (e.g. restrictions on excessive shift work): workplace health promotion programmes
Unemployment	Employment programmes, skills training
Financial insecurity	Welfare policies that provide a financial safety net
Social protection	Economic policies to promote financial security, and adequate funding for a range of public sector services (education, health, housing)
Lack of available health services	Improving availability of mental health services through integration into primary healthcare
Unacceptable health services	For example, ensuring that mental health staff are culturally and linguistically acceptable
Economic barriers to healthcare	Providing financially accessible services
Mental health policy and legislation	Strengthening mental health policy; legislation and service infrastructure
Differential vulnerability	Intervention
Early developmental risks	Promote early childhood development programmes
Early developmental risks, maternal mental illness, weak mother–child bonding	Mother-infant interventions, including breastfeeding
Developmental risks for adolescence	Depression prevention programmes targeting adolescents
Development risks for older adults	Education and stress management programmes; peer support mechanisms
Inaccessibility to credit and savings facilities	Improve access to credit and savings facilities for poor people
Financial consequences of impact of depression on productivity	Support to caregivers to protect households from financial consequences of depression; rehabilitation programmes
Social consequences of depression	Anti-stigma campaigns; promotion of supportive family and social networks
Financial consequences of depression treatment	Reduce cost
Lifestyle consequences of depression	Mental health promotion, including avoidance of substance abuse

Improving equity: implications for public health practitioners

There are three key areas in which public health practitioners can helpfully focus their attention in such a way that will improve health equity. What follows is not an exhaustive list, but rather an illustration of different types of action that can be taken by public health practitioners.

Evidence-informed practice

As a public health practitioner, using sound evidence to inform your daily practice offers the best hope of tackling health inequities. Evidence-informed practice requires good data on the extent of the problem and up-to-date evidence on the causes and on what works to reduce health inequities. It also requires an understanding of the evidence such that the causes of health inequities are acted on. Routine data collection and monitoring systems that collect socially stratified health information are essential for knowing the magnitude of the problem, understanding who is most affected and whether health equity is improving or deteriorating over time, and for assessing entry-points for intervention and evaluating the impact of practice.

Practical action

• Develop a national/local health equity action plan that is fully supported by an effective health equity monitoring system.
• Build up, and systematically use, an information system that collects health outcome data stratified by different social groups (including sex, income, education, occupation, age, and ethnic group).
• Incorporate measures on the determinants of health inequities into the health monitoring system.

Action on the determinants of health inequities requires a rich and diverse evidence base, not just a quantitative monitoring system. Collaborative knowledge production between researchers and public health professionals is needed to elucidate what works to reduce health inequities in what circumstances, and how best to implement interventions, such that they contribute to a reduction in these inequities.

Practical action

Commit appropriate amounts of public health research funding into understanding how to improve health equity through action in the social determinants and healthcare systems, and proactively engage with relevant researchers (see Table 5.9.1).

People-centred practice

All members of society, including those most disadvantaged and marginalized, are entitled to participate in the identification of priorities and targets that guide deliberations underlying public health practice. That focus is stimulated by, and feeds into, local conditions of inclusion and fair representation.

Practical action
- Promote the inclusion of all groups and communities in decision making that affects health, and in subsequent programme and services delivery and evaluation.
- Develop a statutory local health equity action plan that is regularly monitored and reviewed, and provide statutory funding to support community engagement and participation in the processes.
- ensure annual monitoring and reporting against a set of specific health equity-focused outcomes.

Health literacy is a critical empowerment strategy to increase people's control over their health and their ability to seek out information. The understanding of health inequity and its causes needs to be improved as a new part of health literacy. Health literacy is not just about the individual's ability to read, understand, and act on health information, but also the ability of public health professionals to communicate health-related information in relevant and easy-to-understand ways.

Practical action
- Raise awareness among the public about health inequity and its causes.
- Improve knowledge among socially disadvantaged groups about health and healthcare rights.
- Improve awareness and knowledge among health professionals of health equity literacy.

Prevention-focused practice
Action within the health sector
If public health practitioners are to improve health equity through the healthcare system, this means a refocusing of activities towards the removal of barriers to access and use of quality primary healthcare, and on the conditions in which people grow, live, work, and age.

Practical action
- Expand programmes in health promotion, disease prevention, and primary healthcare to include a social determinant of health approach. This means prioritizing services that prevent or ameliorate the health damage caused by living and growing up in disadvantaged circumstances, rather than on behaviour change and social marketing.
- Focus on developing and improving good-quality, integrated local services co-produced with the public to achieve needs-driven outcomes.

Intersectoral action
Bureaucratic structures, statutory requirements, limited funding and traditional disciplinary boundaries can act to impede intersectoral action. However, it is imperative that you act as a champion and facilitator to influence other sectors to take action to reduce health inequities.

Practical action
- Make the argument for intersectoral action to reduce health inequity using regularly updated evidence and increasing the visibility of social determinants of health issues.

- Map all public sector mechanisms (e.g. internal and external committees) that have relevance for health equity, thereby identifying points of potential overlap and collaboration.
- Sensitize colleagues in non-health sectors to the relationship between what they do and the effect on health equity (e.g. through knowledge sharing, seminars, one-to-one briefings).
- The health equity implications of actions by other sectors need to be routinely considered. Health equity impact assessment is one tool that can be used to systematically assess the potential impact of policies, programmes, projects, or proposals on health equity in a given population.

Competencies needed to achieve these tasks

A competent health workforce with the necessary specialized knowledge, skills, and abilities to translate policy and current research into effective action is vital for health equity. Public health professionals need to understand how the healthcare sector—depending on its structure, operations, and financing—can exacerbate or ameliorate health inequities. The healthcare sector has an important stewardship role in intersectoral action for health equity. This requires an understanding among professionals in the healthcare sector of how social determinants influence health equity.

Practical action

- Commit time and financial resources to the development of relevant skills and capacity among the health workforce, and provide reward structures for intersectoral working.
- Explicitly integrate equity values into public health workforce competencies.

References

1 Commission on Social Determinants of Health (2008). *Closing the gap in a generation: health equity through action on the social determinants of health.* Final report of the CSDH. World Health Organization, Geneva.
2 Rajaratnam J, Marcus J, Levin-Rector A, et al. (2010). Worldwide mortality in men and women aged 15–59 years from 1970 to 2010: a systematic analysis. *Lancet*, **375**, 1704–20.
3 Mackenbach JP, Stirbu I, Roskam AJR, et al. (2008). Socioeconomic inequalities in health in 22 European countries. *New England Journal of Medicine*, **358**, 2468.
4 World Health Organization (2013). *Closing the health equity gap: policy options and opportunities for action,* WHO, Geneva.
5 Organisation for Economic Co-operation and Development (2015). *Health at a glance 2015: OECD indicators.* OECD Publishing, Paris.
6 Victora C, Matijasevich A, Silveira M, et al. (2010). Socio-economic and ethnic group inequities in antenatal care quality in the public and private sector in Brazil. *Health Policy Plan,* **25**, 253–61.
7 Starfield B, Shi L, Macinko J. (2005). Contribution of primary care to health systems and health. *Milbank Quarterly,* **83**, 457–502.
8 World Health Organization (2009). *Global health risks: mortality and burden of disease attributable to selected major risks.* WHO, Geneva.
9 Capewell S, Graham H. (2010). Will cardiovascular disease prevention widen health inequalities? *PLoS Medicine,* **7**, e1000320.
10 McGill R, Anwar E, Orton L, et al. (2015). Are interventions to promote healthy eating equally effective for all? Systematic review of socioeconomic inequalities in impact. *BMC Public Health,* **15**, 457.
11 Friel S, Chopra M, Satcher D. (2007). Unequal weight: equity oriented policy responses to the global obesity epidemic. *British Medical Journal,* **335**, 1241–3.

12 World Health Organization (2014). *Obesity and inequities. Guidance for addressing inequities in overweight and obesity*. WHO Regional Office for Europe, Copenhagen.
13 Liu L, Oza S, Hogan D, et al. (2015). Global, regional, and national causes of child mortality in 2000–13, with projections to inform post-2015 priorities: an updated systematic analysis. *Lancet*, **385**(9966), 430–40.
14 World Health Organization (2010). *Equity, social determinants and public health programmes*. WHO, Geneva.
15 World Health Organization (2014). *Social determinants of mental health*. WHO, Geneva.

Chapter 5.10

Improving quality

**Nick Steel, John Ford, Iain Lang, and
Bernadette Khoshaba**

Objectives

This chapter will help you understand the common approaches taken to improving quality and the competencies required of organisations, teams, and individuals to improve the quality of healthcare delivered.

Why is improving quality in healthcare an important public health issue?

- Healthcare improves outcomes: about half of the 7.5 years of the increase in life expectancy seen in the USA and UK in the second half of the twentieth century can be attributed to healthcare improvements.[1]
- Healthcare is not inherently safe: an estimated 210,000 to 400,000 people die annually from preventable harm in hospitals in the USA.[2]
- People with common chronic illnesses receive only half the health care they need.[3]
- Healthcare is expensive, and spending can vary without improving quality of care. The USA spends 50% more of its gross domestic product on healthcare compared with Japan, but has worse quality in 10 out of 11 Organization for Economic Co-operation and Development (OECD) quality indicators (see ➡ Further resources).
- Patients and members of the public want better quality.[4] (See also ➡ Chapter 5.6.)
- Quality is often difficult to improve because of financial constraints, population needs, workforce limitations, and policy changes.[5]

Definitions and dimensions

Quality has been defined as 'the degree to which health services for individuals and populations increase the likelihood of desired health outcomes and are consistent with current professional knowledge'.[6]

Dimensions of quality

The dimensions of quality relate to doing the right thing to the right person in the right place at the right time in the right way at the right cost. The first stage in any attempt to measure quality is to think about what dimensions of quality should be measured, and what groups of people value those dimensions. Donabedian distinguished between measures of the 'structure, process and outcome' of healthcare:

- Structure refers to the characteristics of such resources as hospitals, clinics, and qualified staff members.
- Process measures consider the care delivered.
- Outcome is the resulting change in health status.[7]

The Institute of Medicine has proposed six key dimensions of quality healthcare: safe, effective, patient-centred, timely, efficient, and equitable.[6]

Table 5.10.1 gives examples of quality measures adapted from a chartbook on quality in the UK National Health Service.[8]

Table 5.10.1 Examples of quality measures in different dimensions of quality

Measure of quality	Donabedian dimension	Institute of Medicine dimension
Cancer mortality rates	Outcome	Effectiveness
Appropriateness of coronary revascularisation procedures	Process	Effectiveness
Practising physicians per 1,000 patients	Structure	Efficiency/capacity
Adverse events	Process/outcome	Safety
Waiting times for elective surgery	Process	Timeliness
Variation in life expectancy	Outcome	Equity
Variation in low birth weight	Outcome	Equity
Involvement in decision making	Process	Patient-centredness

How should quality be measured?

Measuring outcomes for quality improvement

The different dimensions of quality mentioned above require different approaches to measurement and specific quality indicators. Using process measures has the following advantages over outcome measures:

• Numerous factors lead to changes in outcome and, while adjustment can control for some of these, this is challenging and often unsatisfying.
• Processes measures can be clearly linked to specific actions, increasing their sensitivity.[9]

The process measures chosen should be based on evidence (when it exists) to establish a link between the healthcare intervention and improved outcomes (See also ➲ Chapters 4.2, 4.4, and 7.5.) When adequate evidence is lacking, a formal consensus of experts that delivering the indicated care will lead to improved health outcomes should be considered.[10]

Within health systems, quality is typically assessed with quantitative measures of the rates of delivery of effective healthcare processes. Delivered healthcare is compared with the healthcare that should have been delivered, sometimes referred to as 'indicated care' or 'quality standards' (see Box 5.10.1 for an example). Standards can be set out in guidelines such as those published by the National Institute for Health and Care Excellence (NICE), the Scottish Intercollegiate Guidelines Network (SIGN) in the UK, and the US Preventive Services Task Force (USPSTF) in the USA (see ➲ Further resources). In addition to guidelines, NICE has developed over 140 topic-specific quality standards. These are specifically aimed at commissioners, providers, practitioners, and regulators (again, see ➲ Further resources).

Box 5.10.1 The RAND/UCLA appropriateness method

An example of how standards of care are developed is the RAND/UCLA (RAND Corporation/University of California, Los Angeles) appropriateness method.[a] This method was developed to combine the best available research evidence with expert opinion. 'Appropriate' describes a healthcare intervention for which the benefits are expected to outweigh the risks. The method involves:

- identifying clinical area(s) of care for quality assessment
- systematically reviewing the literature on care in the relevant area(s)
- drafting quality indicators
- presenting draft quality indicators and their evidence base to a clinical panel of 6–15 specialists for a modified Delphi process
- asking panel members to anonymously rate the draft indicators for validity over at least two rounds, with or without face-to-face discussion between rounds
- approving a final set of indicators.

The indicators can then be used to measure and improve quality.

a) Shekelle P. (2004). The appropriateness method. Medical Decision Making, 24(2), 228–31.

Structured approaches to quality improvement

Initial steps

- Define the problem or quality gap. What is the topic and which dimension(s) of quality is affected? Information on effective care is available from, for example, the Cochrane Effective Practice and Organisation of Care group (see ➔ Further resources).
- Specify the health outcomes that need to change and clarify who wants them to change.
- Obtain the support of senior leaders and build a team.
- Decide on the approach (see below for more detail).
- Identify data to establish baselines, monitor progress, and measure outcomes over time.
- Quality improvement activities have a cost and a business case should be considered.

Clinical audit

Clinical audit followed by performance feedback has constituted the dominant approach for health professionals (see also ➔ Chapter 7.1). It has produced small to moderate effects on quality improvement[11] although some projects have failed to complete the audit cycle.[12]

Plan-do-study-act

Deming's Plan-do-study-act (PDSA) cycle (see Figure 5.10.1) takes audit one stage further and has been widely used in healthcare. The PDSA cycle has four stages: first, develop a plan and define the objective (plan). Second,

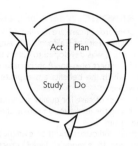

Figure 5.10.1 The plan-do-study-act cycle.

carry out the plan and collect data (do), then analyse the data and summarize what was learned (study). Finally, plan the next cycle with necessary modifications (act).

In the USA, PDSA has been used in 'breakthrough collaboratives', developed by the Institute for Healthcare Improvement (see ➋ Further resources). Collaboratives involve teams working together in a structured way for 12 to 18 months to improve healthcare in a particular area.

Statistical process control

Statistical process control (SPC) charts can be used to map baselines and evaluate whether projects are changing the chosen outcome measure. SPC charts add upper and lower control limits to a simple run chart to help identify unacceptable variation where there may be potential for improvement. For more information on SPC charts, including examples, see ➋ Chapter 4.3.

Six sigma and Lean

Six sigma is a process improvement approach originally developed by Motorola and more recently used in healthcare. It aims to reduce variation in the customer's measure of quality using statistical techniques.[13] It has been combined with Lean, which is a set of principles developed from Toyota's approach to car manufacturing. Lean involves continuous problem solving and improvement, development of people as partners, and eliminating all forms of waste in the system.[13]

Payment for performance

Pay-for-performance programmes are increasingly common in healthcare, and there is limited evidence that they can improve healthcare.[14] Perhaps the largest quality improvement initiative anywhere is the contract entered into in April 2004 between family practitioners (GPs) and the government in the UK (Box 5.10.2).

Box 5.10.2 Improving quality in UK general practice

A new contract between UK general practitioners and the government came into effect on 1 April 2004. Substantial financial rewards (more than £1 billion) were linked to performance against indicators of the quality of clinical and organizational care. The aims of the contract were to reduce variations in provision of effective care and improve quality of care for ten chronic conditions.

For each condition, quality indicators described specific clinical interventions intended to improve quality of care. Financial rewards were attached to achievement of the indicators.

Example indicators for diabetes were:
- the percentage of patients who had had influenza immunization in the preceding 12 months
- the percentage of patients in whom the last IFCC-HbA1C result was <=64 mmol/mol in the past 12 months.

Beyond structured approaches

Getting the right people involved

Quality improvement usually involves lots of different people all pulling towards the same goal. Understanding different perspectives and establishing commitment to a common objective is crucial. 'Desired health outcomes' may be different for managers (who focus on efficiency and maximizing the population health gain from a limited budget), clinicians (who focus on effectiveness and on what works for their patients), and patients (who focus on what works and how it is delivered). In addition to representatives from these three groups, a quality improvement team may require input from academics or policy makers. (See ➔ Chapter 7.4 for more on working on teams.)

Leadership and culture

Quality improvement needs strong leadership, engagement at senior levels within the organisation, and an organizational culture committed to improving quality.[15] An early task in quality improvement is to show that the existing situation is a 'burning platform', and that change is essential. Interpersonal skills to engage patients, clinicians, and managers and to build a team are fundamental.

Comparing with other regions

Care needs to be critically evaluated and benchmarked against practice in other places. Healthcare systems and healthcare activity can be compared using, for example, Donabedian's framework and/or costs, if these are available. However, caution is needed because more frequent care does not generally improve population health.

Potential pitfalls

Systems thinking: Berwick's law of improvement states that 'every system is perfectly designed to achieve the results it achieves', shifting our understanding of performance from effort to design.[16]

Ensuring equity

Equity is an important dimension of quality but can suffer when new healthcare interventions are introduced. Disparities in access to healthcare are a problem in all countries and quality improvement programmes may worsen disparities unless the improvement has proportionally greater benefit for the relatively disadvantaged population. Is it acceptable to trade off a degree of equity for excellence?

Higher quality does not always mean higher cost. In fact, when waste is eliminated, better care can also be cheaper. However, there will be times when higher costs need to be weighed against higher quality, and vice versa.

Tackling unwanted variation

If measurable outcomes are not chosen and monitored, it will be impossible to know whether quality has improved. Good intentions and hard work are not enough: faith in an intervention needs to be backed up by data, and rigorous data collection needs to be followed up with action to improve health. Analysis of variations in healthcare requires a systems approach that accepts that clinicians are influenced by the capacity of the healthcare system, and that supported patient choice in preference-sensitive conditions can lead to better outcomes. Box 5.10.3 lists some questions to ask when you encounter activity variations.

> **Box 5.10.3 Questions to ask about activity variations**
> - Are they due to recording or classification errors?
> - Do they reflect differences in need in the populations served?
> - Are they due to unwarranted care (i.e. a pattern of care inconsistent with patients' preferences or unrelated to underlying illness?)
> - Are they due to scientific uncertainty or to medical errors and system failures?
> - Are they due to differing treatment preferences? If so, does this relate to informed patient choice or physician-dominated decisions?
> - Are they driven by supply of facilities? Is there an unwarranted assumption that more activity is better?

Key determinants of success

- Adequate capacity to deliver quality improvement, including organizational support, team leadership, and interpersonal skills.
- Collection, analysis, and dissemination of data to show effects of the quality improvement activity.
- Alignment of quality improvement activities with the direction of change in the healthcare system.
- Sustained commitment.

Quality improvement is complex and there is no single simple solution. Most tested approaches work some of the time, and none of them are guaranteed to work all the time. Walshe and Freeman pointed out that the particular technique chosen is probably much less important than the perseverance of the people involved: 'Rather than taking up, trying, and then discarding a succession of different quality improvement techniques, organisations should probably choose one carefully and then persevere to make it work.'[17]

Key points of this chapter

- Many people experience healthcare that falls short of agreed quality standards.
- Healthcare can improve population health outcomes.
- The different dimensions of quality are valued differently by different people.
- There are many approaches to improving quality and no one approach is always successful.
- Quality improvement occurs with clear goals, sustained organizational commitment, leadership, and a team capable of delivering.
- Involvement of different groups (e.g. patients, clinicians, and managers) is vital—user involvement is a growing force.
- The risks of quality improvement should be considered. What are the opportunity costs of quality improvement? Do the benefits outweigh the costs?

Further resources

Websites

Cochrane Effective Practice and Organisation of Care group. Available at: ℘ http://onlinelibrary.wiley.com/o/cochrane/clabout/articles/EPOC/frame.html (accessed 21 August 2019).

Institute for Healthcare Improvement Available at: ℘ http://www.ihi.org/IHI/Programs/Collaboratives/ (accessed 21 August 2019).

Organisation for Economic Co-operation and Development (OECD). Available at: ℘ http://www.oecd.org/els/health-systems/health-data.htm (accessed 6 January 2017).

National Institute for Health and Care Excellence (NICE). Available at: ℘ http://www.nice.org.uk/ (accessed 21 August 2019). NICE has developed over 140 topic-specific quality standards. Available at: ℘ https://www.nice.org.uk/standards-and-indicators (accessed 21 August 2019).

Scottish Intercollegiate Guidelines Network (SIGN). Available at: ℘ http://www.sign.ac.uk/

US Preventive Services Task Force (USPSTF). Available at: ℘ www.ahrq.gov/clinic/uspstfix.htm (accessed 21 August 2019).

References

1 Bunker JP. (2001). The role of medical care in contributing to health improvements within societies. *International Journal of Epidemiology*, 30(6), 1260–3.

2 James JF. (2013). A new, evidence-based estimate of patient harms associated with hospital care. *Journal of Patient Safety*, 9(3), 122–8.

3 Steel N, Bachmann M, Maisey S, et al. (2008). Self-reported receipt of care consistent with 32 quality indicators: national population survey of adults aged 50 or more in England. *British Medical Journal*, 337, a957.

4 Coulter A. (2005). What do patients and the public want from primary care? *British Medical Journal*, 331(7526), 1199–201.

5 Fisher E, O'Dowd NC, Dorning H, et al. (2016). *Quality at a cost*. The Health Foundation and Nuffield Trust, London.

6 Institute of Medicine Committee on Health Care in America (2001). *Crossing the quality chasm: a new health system for the 21st century*. National Academy Press, Washington DC.

7 Donabedian A. (1980). *Explorations in quality assessment and monitoring. Vol 1. The definition of quality and approaches to its assessment*. Health Administration Press, Ann Arbor, MI.

8 Leatherman S, Sutherland K. (2005). *The quest for quality in the NHS. A chartbook on quality of care in the UK*. Radcliffe, Oxford.

9 Lilford RJ, Brown CA, Nicholl J. (2007). Use of process measures to monitor the quality of clinical practice. *British Medical Journal*, **335(7621)**, 648–50.

10 Shekelle P. (2004). The appropriateness method. *Medical Decision Making*, **24(2)**, 228–31.

11 Jamtvedt G, Young JM, Kristoffersen DT, et al. (2012). Audit and feedback: effects on professional practice and health care outcomes. *Cochrane Database of Systematic Reviews*, **(2)**.

12 Gnanalingham J, Gnanalingham M, Gnanalingham K. (2001). An audits of audits: are we completing the cycle? *Journal of the Royal Society of Medicine*, **94(6)**, 288–9.

13 Boaden R, Harvey G, Moxham C, et al. (2008). *Quality improvement: theory and practice in healthcare*. NHS Institute for Innovation and Improvement, Coventry.

14 Christianson J, Leatherman S, Sutherland K. (2007). *Financial incentives, healthcare providers and quality improvements. A review of the evidence*. The Health Foundation, London.

15 The Health Foundation (2010). *Quality improvement made simple*. The Health Foundation, London.

16 Berwick DM. (1996). A primer on leading the improvement of systems. *British Medical Journal*, **312(7031)**, 619–22.

17 Walshe K, Freeman T. (2002). Effectiveness of quality improvement: learning from evaluations. *Quality and Safety in Health Care*, **11(1)**, 85–7.

Chapter 5.11

Evaluating healthcare systems

Martin McKee, Marina Karanikolos, and Ellen Nolte

Objectives

- Understand the importance of defining the boundaries of a health system in a given country.
- Be able to explain the functions of a health system and how these relate to one another.
- Be able to describe the goals of a health system and how to evaluate progress towards them.
- Be aware of the major contemporary initiatives to assess health system performance internationally.
- Recognize the limitations, including the scope for abuse, of health system comparisons.

Defining the health system and its goals

There are two first steps in evaluating healthcare systems:
- Define the boundaries of a system.
- Agree on what it is seeking to achieve.

Defining a system's boundaries is complicated by the frequent existence of multiple systems for delivering healthcare. Perhaps the most extreme example is in the USA where even the public sector is divided among Medicare, Medicaid, the Veterans Administration, and others. However, nearly all countries have some form of private provision alongside the statutory public system, as well as systems to care for groups such as prisoners, the armed forces, or other occupational groups. Other definitional challenges relate to:
- generation of inputs to the health system, such as research and development and training
- managing the indistinct boundary between health and social care.

Defining the goals of a health system and how to measure its performance are equally challenging. For investors on the world's stock markets, health systems provide just another investment opportunity, with performance assessed as return on capital. In contrast, campaigners for social justice may assess performance in terms of the ability to protect the poor from financial ruin in the face of illness. Manufacturers of pharmaceuticals or medical technology may see performance as the ability to deliver, at least to some, advanced technology they have been working so hard to develop. Health professionals may view performance in terms of a supportive and rewarding environment for professional development. And patient groups may view performance in terms of the system's ability to respond rapidly and humanely to their physical and emotional needs.

One important advance of looking at the goals of health systems and their performance was proposed by the 2000 World Health Report,[1] which sought to create a means by which all the world's health systems could be compared using common metrics.

The health system was defined as 'all activities whose primary purpose is to promote, restore or maintain health'[1] (p.5). This was intentionally broad and includes many activities that would commonly be seen as lying outside the health system, including certain components of health promotion, although it did exclude activities, such as the promotion of female literacy, which have many other goals of which better health is only one. It also included 'selected inter-sectoral actions in which the stewards of the health system take responsibility to advocate for improvements in areas outside their direct control, such as legislation to reduce fatalities from traffic accidents.'[2]

Within the health system, a number of functions were identified, each contributing to the goals of the system. The functions were:
- financing (revenue collection, fund pooling, and purchasing)
- resource generation (human resources, technologies, and facilities)
- delivery of personal and population-based health services
- stewardship (health policy formulation, regulation, and intelligence).

The goals were:
- health improvement
- responsiveness
- fairness in financing.

The goals were operationalized to produce indicators that were then weighted and combined to create a composite measure of overall goal attainment, as well as a measure of overall performance. The latter recognised that a health system's performance would be constrained by the circumstances within which it existed, and calculated a theoretical maximum value based on a given country's level of economic and educational development with which it could compare its actual performance. On this basis, France was rated to have the best-performing health system while Sierra Leone had the least-performing system. While controversial at the time, especially because of the limited data then available, the basic principles set out in the report have stood the test of time and it provides the basis for much subsequent work on health systems performance.[3]

The remainder of this chapter builds on that work, first looking at the health system functions and then at the goals of the system, before concluding with examples of initiatives currently underway to measure and compare health systems performance.

Health systems functions

Financing a health system is complex because of the range of decisions involved, including on the collecting of funds (how much to collect and from whom; whom and what to cover); the pooling of funds (how to pool funds; how to allocate funds to purchasers); and the actual purchasing of services (from whom to buy and how to buy; at what price to buy and how to pay). At the core is the need to redistribute resources. Put simply, those who have most need of healthcare are least able to afford it. The process of redistribution occurs both within the life course of an individual (who will typically incur most expenditure around birth and death and contribute most during working years) and among individuals (from rich to poor, well to ill and, in some labour markets, males to females).

There are many different means of collecting money for health systems, most of which result from political decisions. The most common sources are:

- taxation
- statutory health insurance (where contributions are based on income)
- private insurance (where contributions are often based on risk of ill health)
- out of pocket payments.

In practice, all countries use a combination of sources, so, for example, systems operating on the basis of statutory insurance use income from taxation to cover the costs for those not in employment. Many systems also require direct payments for certain aspects of care, such as prescription drugs or dental care, from some patients.

To evaluate the elements of the financing component of health systems, it is necessary to clarify their goals. This, in turn, requires clarity about the perspective being adopted because, given the scale of resources involved, decisions will have implications for the macro-economy and employment, as well as the health system, and these may conflict.

From the perspective of the health system, the optimal means of collecting money will be the one that:

- is cheapest to administer
- has least scope for evasion
- and draws on the widest possible revenue base.

Taxation could be seen as an 'ideal' approach because it does not require a separate collection system and it draws on a wide revenue base that does not only include income but also indirect taxes and excise revenues. The important question then becomes the fairness of the taxation system, because taxes on income and capital gains tend to be progressive, taking a higher share from the rich, while taxes on sales tend to be regressive, taking more from the poor. The available research finds that, while progressive taxation is associated with better health outcomes, taxes that are regressive are associated with worse outcomes.[4] Statutory insurance systems typically draw on contributions from earned income only, which may narrow the revenue base. Also, eligibility tends to be based on employment, or linked to contributions, and may thus limit access to care for those not in employment. However, because income generated from statutory insurance is clearly earmarked for health, it is seen to be more transparent as, for example, a taxation-based system. Out-of-pocket payments and some individualized approaches, such as medical savings accounts, relate payment to utilization and may reduce overall demand for services. However, because access is related to ability to pay, direct payment may also deter use of necessary services. Importantly, out-of-pocket payments involve little or no redistribution and thus are highly regressive.

The pooling element can be judged on the basis of the transfers it brings about. Risk pools may be single, covering the entire population, or multiple, as is the case with some insurance funds. Systems that are using competing insurance funds, such as Germany or the Netherlands, have introduced systems of risk equalization.

Purchasing derives from recognition that the optimal provision of care involves something more than simply reimbursing claims, and should take account of the effectiveness and efficiency of the care provided and the extent to which it is addressing issues such as impaired access to care.[5] Strategic purchasing therefore involves assessing the needs of a population and developing appropriate models of care. This can be evaluated by observing the extent to which needs are met (for example, by assessing the experience of vulnerable and marginalized groups) and by the extent to which funders encourage evidence-based models of care.

Turning to the next core function of health systems, resource generation involves the identification, creation, and development of the resources required to produce health services and to build a sustainable and resilient health system. These include the workforce, health facilities, technology (including pharmaceuticals), and, increasingly, knowledge. Again, evaluation follows from the goals relating to each component. A health system should incorporate appropriate mechanisms for training, deployment, and, especially, retention of staff, with geographically equitable deployment of an optimal skill-mix. It should have mechanisms in place to supply modern and effective technologies, involving means of assessing their effectiveness and of ensuring their reliable distribution to where they are needed. It should deploy approaches to ensure the appropriate design, configuration, maintenance, and distribution of facilities. And, finally, it should have ways of generating, synthesizing, and distributing knowledge so that the care provided is based on the most relevant evidence.

The function of service delivery follows on from the previous activities. Services should be provided in ways that are effective, efficient, equitable, and humane. Evaluation involves a wide range of health services research methods, the choice of which will depend on the nature of the service being evaluated. It includes not only the processes by which care is delivered but the organizational context within which it is provided.

The final component is stewardship.[6] The 2000 World Health Report defined stewardship as 'the careful and responsible management of the well-being of the population'. It comprises three elements, formulating and coordinating health policy; exerting influence; and collecting and using intelligence to assure quality. Its evaluation typically involves policy research, perhaps examining the process of adopting and implementing necessary responses to a defined challenge, such as pandemic influenza or aging populations.

Improving health

Health improvement was assessed in the 2000 World Health Report as the average level of health in a given population, measured as disability-adjusted life expectancy (DALE), and the distribution of health within the population, using data on child survival.

The measure of DALE is extremely broad because it reflects, in part, the quality of healthcare delivered by the health system but also many other factors, including price, availability, and marketing of hazardous substances such as tobacco, alcohol, and junk food, exposure to vector-borne diseases, and the safety of the environment. In order to better understand the contribution of health systems to population health, the researchers introduced the measure of avoidable mortality. First introduced by Rutstein and colleagues in 1978[7] on the premise that deaths from certain causes should not occur in the presence of timely and effective care, subsequent work, by Nolte and McKee among others, has refined the concept further. Referring more specifically to the notion of amenable mortality,[8] this work has sought to reflect how advances in healthcare have rendered once untreatable conditions amenable to healthcare, as well as increases in life expectancy and, with them, changing expectations about what healthcare can do. The concept has also been refined to include differentiation of causes amenable to the healthcare system and those to public health policy, while specific causes have been partitioned into the proportion to which reductions are attributable to primary, secondary, and tertiary actions.[9]

This approach is now widely used by organisations such as the Commonwealth Fund in the USA and the European Commission, and is informing policy debates in many countries. Thus, a study showing that deaths from amenable mortality in the USA around the year 2000 had hardly changed at a time when other industrialized countries were experiencing substantial declines was cited widely in the debate on President Obama's healthcare reforms.

The concept has also been incorporated into the Global Burden of Disease study.[10] Taking advantage of the wealth of data collected within the study, it has been possible to include countries worldwide and to add a major methodological advance: standardisation for risk factors.[10] This makes it possible to differentiate more accurately the contribution of healthcare from the underlying determinants of health in a population. The resulting Healthcare and Access Quality Index (HAQI) offers considerable potential for monitoring the goal of achieving universal health coverage set out in the 2015 Sustainable Development Goals.

It is, however, necessary to step back briefly to recall how amenable mortality was initially envisaged as being used. This was indicative of aspects of care requiring more detailed examination rather than a definitive judgement on overall performance. The latter use poses a number of problems, which illustrate more generally some of the issues that arise in assessing the performance of health systems.

The first is what is measured. Clearly, premature death is only one element of the overall burden of disease in a population. However, there is little data on disability, and even less that is in any way comparable, so that most published statistics are modelled on mortality data. This is of growing importance because advances in healthcare reduce the number of deaths amenable to healthcare even further. For example, deaths from ischaemic heart disease have fallen by about half over the past three decades across Western Europe,[11] with even larger reductions in deaths arising from common surgical procedures. Once incurable cancers, such as testicular, now have survival rates of over 90%. Thus, mortality provides an increasingly incomplete measure of overall healthcare performance and, specifically, misses the marked reduction in symptoms and functioning that has occurred.

A second, related problem is that of small numbers. Even apparently common conditions may cause relatively small numbers of premature deaths, making it particularly difficult to make judgements about health systems in relatively small countries.

The third is the presence of time lags. Effective treatment of, for example, an emergency such as acute appendicitis or a cardiac arrest will save a life at once. In contrast, while effective management of a chronic disorder, such as diabetes, may save a life now, in the event of, say, ketoacidosis, it may equally prevent premature death from complications many years in the future. Hence, when investigating amenable deaths, it is necessary to ascertain when any failing in the health system occurred.

The fourth is the issue of attribution. Although there are a few situations in which death can be prevented by a 'magic bullet', as occurred when penicillin was first given to patients with severe staphylococcal infections in the 1940s or when azidothymidine (AZT now known as zidovudine) was introduced to treat AIDS in the 1980s, more often healthcare will prevent deaths through a combination of interventions that were introduced incrementally, perhaps over decades. It may be difficult to discern where the problem lies because there is surprisingly little evidence on the effectiveness of specific interventions in reducing death rates in the general population. First, randomized controlled trials often have limited external validity, because they often exclude both children and older people, those with co-morbidities and, in the past, women.[12] Second, new interventions are usually compared with best existing treatment, which is important in assessing whether the intervention should be adopted but not helpful in quantifying its effect.

Finally, it is necessary to consider the boundaries of amenable mortality. Recognising that 'everyone must die of something', deaths designated amenable have an upper age limit. However, this is arbitrary and, although it has increased over time in keeping with lengthening life expectancy, there is a danger that the use of amenable mortality distracts attention from healthcare provided for older people for whom it can be extremely effective. This criticism has also been levelled at the use of measures of premature mortality, such as that in the Sustainable Development Goals.[13]

For all these reasons, amenable mortality can be considered as a valuable indication of how a health system is performing, provoking further investigation should it appear to be lagging compared with other countries, but it should not be seen as a definitive measure.

Responding to expectations

The 2000 World Health Report assessed the responsiveness of health systems on the basis of a survey of key informants from selected countries, using a modelling approach to estimate values for the remaining ones. This was admitted to be unsatisfactory so a questionnaire-based measure was developed for use in the 2002 World Health Survey. The World Health Organization (WHO) defined responsiveness as meeting 'the legitimate expectations of the population for the non-health improving dimensions of their interaction with the health system'.[13] This explicitly excludes expectations deemed to be illegitimate or unjustified, although this clearly raises questions about cultural norms. Thus, an individual in one country may expect a hospital bed to be in a single room, with access to the internet and entertainment and to a choice of high-quality food, while someone in another country may be grateful for a bed and clean linen. In an attempt to overcome this problem, the 2002 World Health Survey used anchoring vignettes. These are standardized descriptions of encounters that are ranked by respondents as a means of calibrating their responses. However, the multi-dimensional nature of expectations meant that this was technically insurmountable.

As noted above, responsiveness was divided into two broad categories, each with a number of dimensions. Table 5.11.1 shows the weightings used to combine these dimensions in the 2000 report and the questions used to capture each of them in the later survey.

Fairness of financial contribution

Fairness of financial contribution was defined in the 2000 World Health Report as the distribution of the financial burden imposed by the health system within the population. It was measured in terms of the fraction of disposable income that each household contributes to the health system (including income taxes, value-added tax, excise tax, social security contributions, private voluntary insurance, and out-of-pocket payments).

Subsequently, it has also been operationalized in terms of existence of universal health coverage: 'quality, essential health service coverage and financial coverage—both extended to the whole population'.[15] The latter includes avoidance of catastrophic payments, in recognition that a well-functioning health system should prevent those falling ill from impoverishment, as exemplified by the observation that medical bills are the leading cause of bankruptcy in the USA. Both aspects are evaluated using household survey data, such as that provided by family budget surveys or the World Bank's Living Standards Measurement Studies.

Looking through the eyes of patients

The approaches described so far in this chapter involve the adoption of a macro-level perspective, looking at aggregate data on the overall system. They each provide valuable insights into the presence and, to some extent, the nature of problems, but are less helpful in indicating what can be done to resolve them.

The tracer methodology offers a means to do this. It involves selecting a condition whose management requires the effective operation of multiple components of the health system, and evaluating the experiences of those with that condition and their healthcare providers. Several studies have used insulin-dependent diabetes[16] because it has the advantage of ease of identification of those affected, as well as requiring well-functioning elements throughout the health system, including primary, secondary, and tertiary care, a skilled workforce, and reliable supplies of insulin and test materials, all within a framework that is responsive to needs. Others have used

Table 5.11.1 Dimensions of responsiveness as defined by the World Health Organization

Category	Dimension and definition	Weighting in the 2000 World Health Report	Questions in the 2002 World Health Survey. How would you rate...?
Respect for persons	Dignity (respectful treatment and communication)	16.7%	...your experience of being greeted and talked to respectfully? ...the way your privacy was respected during physical examinations and treatments?
	Confidentiality (of personal information)	16.7%	...the way the health services ensured that you could talk privately to healthcare providers? ...the way your personal information was kept confidential?
	Autonomy (involvement in decisions)	16.7%	...your experience of being involved in making decisions about your healthcare or treatment? ...your experience of getting information about other types of treatments or tests?
	Communication (clarity of communication)	Not included	...the experience of how clearly healthcare providers explained things to you? ...your experience of getting enough time to ask questions about your health problem or treatment?
Client orientation	Prompt attention (convenient travel and short waiting times)	20%	...the travelling time? ...the amount of time you waited before being attended to?
	Quality of basic amenities (surroundings)	15%	...the cleanliness of the rooms inside the facility, including toilets? ...the amount of space you had?
	Access to family and community support (contact with the outside world and maintenance of regular activities)	10%	...the ease of having family and friends visit you? ...your [child's] experience of staying in contact with the outside world when you [your child] were in hospital?
	Choice (of healthcare provider)	5%	How would you rate the freedom you had to choose the healthcare providers that attended to you?

Source: authors' compilation based on the World Health Survey instrument.

hypertension, which has many similar features, although with the added challenge that those affected are often undiagnosed, thereby focusing attention on the ability of the system to detect and follow up those affected.[17]

The methodology involves the use of rapid appraisal techniques, encompassing a mix of quantitative and qualitative methods, triangulating evidence from, among others, interviews with patients, providers, and policy makers, observation of facilities, assessment of supply chains, and evaluation of legislation and regulations. While its findings will be of most relevance to those suffering from the selected tracer condition, it should provide insights that are of much wider relevance. Thus, a pharmaceutical distribution system that is unable to ensure regular supplies of insulin is unlikely to be able to distribute vaccines or antibiotics.

Current developments

There are a number of important initiatives underway to take forward the methodology on health systems evaluation. The European Observatory on Health Systems and Policies is supporting the European Commission's work on understanding differences in performance of national health systems. The OECD's Health Care Quality Indicators project (HCQI) focuses on the technical quality of healthcare, using 'indicators that reflect a robust picture of healthcare quality that can be reliably reported across countries using comparable data'[18] (p.3).

These indicators must meet two conditions:
- They must capture an 'important performance aspect'.
- They must be scientifically sound.[19]

Importance is assessed on three dimensions:
- The measure addresses areas in which there is a clear gap between the actual and potential levels of health.
- It reflects important health conditions in terms of burden of disease, cost of care, or public interest.
- Measures can be directly affected by the healthcare system.

The second criterion, scientific soundness, requires indicators to be valid (i.e. the extent to which the measure accurately represents the concept/phenomenon being evaluated) and reliable (i.e. the extent to which the measurement with a given indicator is reproducible).

Uses and abuses

The increasing interest among researchers in evaluating health systems has been accompanied by a similar increase among politicians and lobbyists. Health system evaluation is an inexact science, involving choices about the goals to be pursued, the weighting to be placed upon them, the systems to be compared, and the way to present the result.

Unfortunately, this flexibility can create problems. Some comparisons have been heavily criticised on account of their lack of transparency, arbitrary choices of indicators, and the greater weighting given to different aspects of healthcare, such as choice and equity.[20]

In addition, caution is always required in interpreting existing data. One of the most studied examples is cancer registration data. This has been extremely influential in a number of countries seen to achieve less than optimal results. Yet, while cancer registration covers the entire population of some countries, it is fragmentary in others. There may also be inherent biases, as with the American SEER database, in which the poor and African-Americans are under-represented, thus tending to inflate apparent survival. It is also necessary to ensure that account has been taken of methodological traps, such as lead-time bias where screening programmes result in earlier detection of cancers but confer no ultimate benefit on mortality. These issues, collectively, account in part for the often-quoted cancer survival in the USA compared with Europe.[21]

References

1 World Health Organization (2000). *The World Health Report 2000. Health systems: improving performance.* World Health Organization, Geneva.

2 Murray CJ, Evans DB. (2003). Health systems performance assessment: goals, framework and overview. In: Murray CJ, Evans DB, eds, Health systems performance assessment, p. 7. World Health Organization, Geneva.

3 McKee M. (2010). The World Health Report 2000: 10 years on. *Health Policy Planning*, 25, 346–8.

4 Reeves A, Gourtsoyannis Y, Basu S, et al. (2015). Financing universal health coverage—effects of alternative tax structures on public health systems: cross-national modelling in 89 low-income and middle-income countries. *Lancet*, 386, 274–80.

5 Expert panel on effective ways of investing in health (2016). *Access to health services in the European Union*. European Commission, Brussels.

6 Saltman RB, Ferroussier-Davis O. (2000). The concept of stewardship in health policy. *Bulletin of the World Health Organization*, 732–9.

7 Rutstein D, Berenberg W, Chalmers T, et al. (1976). Measuring the quality of medical care. *New England Journal of Medicine*, 294, 582–8.

8 Nolte E, McKee M. (2004). *Does healthcare save lives? Avoidable mortality revisited.* The Nuffield Trust, London.

9 Tobias M, Jackson G. (2001). Avoidable mortality in New Zealand, 1981-97. *Australian and New Zealand Journal of Public Health*, 25, 12–20.

10 GBD 2015 (2017). Healthcare access and quality collaborators. Healthcare access and quality index based on mortality from causes amenable to personal healthcare in 195 countries and territories, 1990–2015: a novel analysis from the Global Burden of Disease Study 2015. *Lancet*, doi. org/10.1016/S0140-6736(17)30818-8

11 Kesteloot H, Sans S, Kromhout D. (2006). Dynamics of cardiovascular and all-cause mortality in Western and Eastern Europe between 1970 and 2000. *European Heart Journal*, 27, 107–13.

12 Britton A, McKee M, Black N, et al. (1998). Choosing between randomised and non-randomised studies: a systematic review. *Health Technology Assessment*, 2(13), 1–124.

13 Lloyd-Sherlock P, McKee M, Prince M, et al. (2016). Institutionally ageist? Global health policy in the 21st century. *British Medical Journal*, 354, i4514.

14 Anand S, Ammar W, Evans T, et al. (2003). Report of the Scientific Peer Review Group on Health Systems Performance Assessment. In: Murray CJ, Evans DB, eds, Health systems performance assessment, p. 844. World Health Organization, Geneva.

15 World Health Organization, World Bank (2016). *Tracking universal health coverage: first global monitoring report.* WHO, World Bank.

16 Nolte E, Bain C, McKee M. (2006). Chronic diseases as tracer conditions in international benchmarking of health systems: the example of diabetes. *Diabetes Care*, 29, 1007–11.

17 Risso-Gill I, Balabanova D, Majid F, et al. (2015). Understanding the modifiable health systems barriers to hypertension management in Malaysia: a multi-method health systems appraisal approach. *BMC Health Services Research*, 15, 254.

18 Kelley E, Hurst J. (2006). *Health care quality indicators project.* Conceptual framework paper. OECD health working papers no.23.

19 Carinci F, Van Gool K, Mainz J, et al. (2015). OECD Health Care Quality Indicators Expert Group. Towards actionable international comparisons of health system performance: expert revision of the OECD framework and quality indicators. *International Journal for Quality in Health Care*, **27**, 137–46.

20 Cylus J, Nolte E, Figueras J, et al. (2016). What, if anything, does the EuroHealth Consumer Index actually tell us? *British Medical Journal*. Available at: 🔗 http://blogs.bmj.com/bmj/2016/02/09/what-if-anything-does-the-eurohealth-consumer-index-actually-tell-us (accessed 21 August 2019).

21 Desai M, Rachet B, Coleman M, et al. (2010). Two countries divided by a common language: health systems in the UK and USA. *Journal of the Royal Society of Medicine*, **103**, 283–7.

Value-based healthcare

Muir J.A. Gray and Walter Ricciardi

THE MEANINGS OF VALUE

The meanings of value

The term 'value' has a different meaning in the singular and plural. Values, in the plural, may be regarded as a synonym for principles as in the statement that 'this hospital's values are compassion combined with excellence'. In the singular, the term has more of an economic meaning with four aspects.

First, personalised value is determined by the value each individual places on the probability and the magnitude of the benefits and the harms attached to the choice they have to make, and on the outcome of treatment.

Second, from a population perspective, there is also the concept of allocative value, or 'allocative efficiency' as economists term it, with the aim being to allocate resources to different geographical populations or to different subgroups optimally within each geographical population optimally. By this is meant allocated in a way that optimises value to the population as a whole.

Third, it is customary to distinguish the value derived from optimal allocation from the value derived from the use of resources once allocation decisions have been made, and economists have a number of terms covering this third meaning. First, there is 'productivity', a long-established economists' term relating outputs to inputs—for example, the proportion of cases in which treatment was provided as a day case, or the proportion of drugs that are prescribed as generics. The term 'efficiency' is a broader concept relating outcomes to the resources used—for example, by measuring the proportion of people who have had a hip replacement and report that the intervention significantly improved the problem that was bothering them most. It has become common in the United States literature to read reports of 'value-based payment systems' in which the outcomes of the patients treated are related to the resources used, and this is termed 'value' in the United States. However, in countries in which the population as a whole has to be covered by a finite budget, this is not an adequate definition of value because the person responsible for managing the budget for the population has to consider the possibility that:

- there are people not being treated who would benefit greatly
- there are people who are being treated who are gaining little benefit.

Furthermore, those who are not being treated may be being discriminated against unfairly: an example of inequity. Therefore, the concept of value in a country committed to covering the whole population has to include not only the efficiency with which those patients who reach the service are treated but also the possibility of underuse and overuse in the population served. This is sometimes termed 'utilisation value' or technical value to distinguish it from allocative value.

The concept of overuse, and indeed the whole concept of value, can be understood and measured only if the denominator chosen is the whole population in need and not just the patients who have been treated. This was first described by Avedis Donabedian in Explorations in Quality Assessment and Monitoring, published in 1980.[1] Donabedian described his 'unifying model of benefit, risk and cost'. The power of this model is that it described for the first time the relationship between the level of resources invested in healthcare and the amounts of benefit and harm obtained from that level of investment. Donabedian showed that, as healthcare resources are increased, benefit increases initially but the increase then flattens off, illustrating what some people have called the law of diminishing returns.

In contrast to the trajectory of benefit obtained in relation to investment, the amount of harm done increases in direct proportion to the resources invested. For each increase in resource, there is an increase in the volume of care and, as a consequence, a unit increase in the amount of harm done. In fact, there may be a progressive increase in the amount of harm done if, with each unit increase in the availability of care, patients who are less fit and more at risk of harm are covered by the service. This is shown in his classic diagram as shown in Figure 5.12.1.

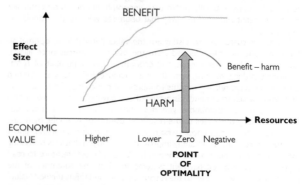

Figure 5.12.1 The relationship between the level of investment of resources, benefit, and harm, illustrating the Point of Optimality.

There are many examples of overuse in a modern health service. Antibiotic prescribing is an obvious one but others include the rising numbers of laboratory tests and imaging, inappropriate care for people in the last year of life, and even elective surgery.

The fourth aspect is called the social or societal aspect in the European Union Expert Panel report on Value based healthcare. This requires a health service to think more broadly and to ask if they could do more for their local community. For example instead of giving a catering contract to a multinational solely on the basis of short term price advantage a hospital could award the contract to a local consortium supplied by local farmers who were employing local people, many of them having health problems. In the United Kingdom there is an Act of Parliament called the Social Value Act which requires local government services to do this.

The meaning of resources

Value-based healthcare is preoccupied with outcomes and resources and it is important to emphasize that the term 'resources' means more than money.

In the NHS in England, every hospital has a carbon budget and healthcare professions are often motivated to take action to reduce the carbon footprint from their hospital when appeals to reduce its financial overspend meet with little response. Another key resource is time. The time of clinicians is finite and even the investment of more money does not bring an increase in the time available so it is important to measure waste, the opposite of value, resulting from, for example, fruitless clinical visits because the results relevant to a particular patient are not available. Increasingly, the time of patients and carers is also taken into the equation. The concept of the burden of treatment, as distinct from the burden of disease, is increasingly used particularly to assess the value of service provided to carers who may have to take a day off work to bring an elderly parent to a clinic visit that appears to have little impact upon the care of that individual or their degree of independence.

How can value be increased?

Four activities have dominated the management of healthcare in the past 20 years—prevention, evidence-based decision making, quality improvement, and cost reduction. All these are important in value improvement but it is important to remember that:

- although low-quality care is of low value, high-quality care is not necessarily high value—for example, imaging may be delivered at high quality but be of little or no value to the patients who have had the investigations.
- interventions of unnecessarily high cost are of lower value but, even when the cost is reduced, value is not necessarily increased unless that intervention produces outcomes of relevance to the people treated.

There is now a new population health management agenda developing that is:

- ensuring that every individual achieves high personal value by providing people with full information about the risks and benefits of the intervention being offered and relating that to the problem that bothers them most and to their values and preferences
- shifting resource from budgets for subgroups of the population defined by need where there is evidence from unwarranted variation of overuse of lower value interventions to budgets for other sub groups of the population defined by need in which there is evidence of underuse and inequity for example shifting resources from the budget for people with cardiovascular conditions to the budget for people with musculo skeletal problems, or *vice versa*
- creating population-based systems that ensure that
  - the service is of high quality with no waste

- there is faster implementation of high-value innovation to improve outcome, funded by reduced spending on lower-value interventions for that population
- there are increased rates of higher-value intervention within each system (e.g. helping a higher proportion of people to die well at home funded by reduced spending on lower-value care in hospital).
- deliver the service equitably through networks ensuring that those people in the population who will derive most value from a service reach that service
- create a culture of stewardship in which every clinician feels a sense of collective responsibility to the population served as well as a sense of clinical responsibility to each patient

Ensuring individualized value

Even interventions with strong evidence of effectiveness and cost-effectiveness may not add value to the life of an individual unless they address the problem that is bothering that person most and unless the decision is made in line with the individual's understanding of both the benefits and the risks of intervention.

Personalized value and population value are two sides of the one coin and, as the amount of resource in the particular service is increased, the type of patients offered treatment changes with people who are less severely affected being offered the intervention. For them, the best possible benefit is less but the probability and magnitude of harm are constant as shown in Figure 5.12.2.

In developing population healthcare therefore, it is essential also to develop personalized decision making.

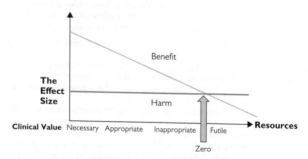

Figure 5.12.2 A graph to show how—as resources are increased—people with less severe need in the population are offered treatment, and for each individual the maximum benefit possible declines while the size of harm remains constant.

Ensuring that allocation is optimal

Whether the health service is tax-based or insurance-based, those responsible for the finance available for a population have to think about ways in which decisions are made to allocate or reallocate resources to programme budgets—for example, to
- the programme for people with cancer, or
- the programme for people with respiratory disease, or
- the programme for people with multiple morbidity.

The aim is to achieve optimal allocative value, the distribution of resources at which it is impossible to get more value by reallocation of even a single euro. This is sometimes called the 'point of indifference' by health economists.[2]

Once the resources have been allocated to each programme, then of course there is a second level of allocation—for example, within the programme for people with respiratory disease, there is further allocation to the three main population groups within that programme: namely, people with asthma, people with chronic obstructive pulmonary disease (COPD) and people with sleep apnoea.

Optimizing value from the allocated resources

The term 'population healthcare' is sometimes used to describe healthcare that is focused not only on bureaucracies and on the different levels of care but also on the population in need. The definition may refer to a symptom such as breathlessness or back pain, or a condition such as epilepsy or rheumatoid arthritis, or a common characteristic like having multiple health problems or being in the last year of life. The interaction of these three different approaches to healthcare is shown in Figure 5.12.3.

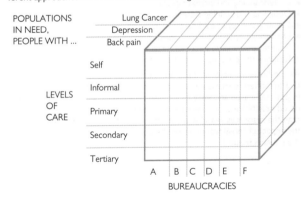

Figure 5.12.3 3D healthcare, with the populations defined by need being the third dimension.

Having developed a system—namely, a set of activities with a common set of objectives for a subgroup in the population (e.g. people with atrial fibrillation [AF]), the next step is to agree the outcomes for each objective. An example of a set of system objectives is shown below:

- To identify people with AF.
- To assess risk accurately in all people known to have AF.
- To treat people safely and effectively.
- To phase out ineffective treatment with aspirin.
- To ensure that people with AF make a well-informed decision that takes their values into account.
- To make the best use of resources.
- To promote and support research.
- To create a powerful community of practice and develop staff both as individuals and teams.
- To produce an annual report for the population served and to support quality improvement.

Having set up the system, steps can be taken to optimize value in three ways, in addition to providing high-quality care without waste, by ensuring that:

- the right patients are being seen
- high-value innovations are quickly adopted, funded by reducing expenditure on lower-value interventions for that population group
- there is the right distribution of resources along the whole of the pathway from prevention to long-term care.[3]

The new skill set

The types of skills needed to organize and deliver population healthcare, as distinct from the skills needed to manage an institutionally based service, are listed below:

- Understanding and increasing value.
- Designing and building systems and networks.
- Creating the right healthcare culture.
- Delivering population-based healthcare.
- Ensuring personalized decision making.
- Realizing the potential of the internet and digital services.

As can be seen, many of these are the skills of public health professionals and this offers a tremendous opportunity for public health professionals. In both tax-based and insurance-based health services, the move to value-based healthcare as a consequence of need and demand increasing faster than the resources available means that decisions will have to be based on the impact of those resources on the population as a whole and not just on the patients treated.

References

1 Donabedian, A. (1980). Explorations in quality assessment and monitoring (3 vols.) Health Administration Press, Chicago, IL.
2 Rice, T. (1998). *The economics of health reconsidered*. (1998). Health Administration Press, Chicago.
3 Gray JAM, Cripps M, Bevan RG. (2013). How to get better value healthcare, 3rd edn. Offox Press, Oxford.

References

Personal effectiveness

Developing leadership skills

Fiona Sim

Objective

This chapter should help you to acquire the leadership competencies that are necessary to turn excellent public health technical practice into *effective* public health practice.

Definitions

Leadership

Great leaders are usually characterized as highly charismatic, high-profile individuals, (e.g. Caesar or Mandela). Leaders have great power to influence, communicating a clear vision that is attractive to their followers, with the ability to deliver that vision.

Additional to this stereotype, in your workplace or community, you could probably identify someone, not necessarily charismatic, extroverted, or even very senior, who has been the architect of a substantial change and made it happen.

Public health leadership

Public health leadership is the application of leadership characteristics to the cause of improving the health of a given population or community.[1–3] Where this leadership sits organizationally is subject to political decision. For example, embedding leadership for health improvement in local government was a core proposal in English policy reform in 2010[4] and has been the reality since 2013.[5]

A former chief medical officer for England[6] described leadership as:

- 'knowing where you want to go and setting the direction of travel
- taking people with you on the journey in spite of their differences in views and methods, working background, and rates of travel
- giving sufficient time and energy to the process of changing things for the better—learning to do things in a different way.'

Public health leadership should produce:

- attributable improvement in the health of a population, community, or service
- better collaboration at organizational and individual levels
- a higher profile for public health
- greater efficiency in health decision making.

Is leadership different from management?

Leadership complements and differs from management in some important respects. While an effective manager requires planning and problem-solving skills to produce largely predictable, desirable results, a leader will go further to *establish the vision* and take it forward, usually by motivating and developing others, to produce significant, sometimes dramatic, change. Table 6.1.1 illustrates these distinctions.

The relationship between management and leadership is suggested by adapting the distinction between logic and imagination made by Einstein: 'Logic (or management) will take you from A to B. Imagination (or leadership) will take you everywhere.'

Table 6.1.1 Distinctions between managers and leaders

Manager	Leader
Coping with complexity	Coping with change
Ensuring order and consistency	Delivering change
Planning and budgeting	Setting direction—developing a vision
Organizing and staffing to accomplish objectives	Aligning people
Problem solving	Motivating and inspiring

Source: data from Kotter J. (1996). Leading change. Harvard Business School Press, Boston

Why is leadership an important public health attribute?

For a public health practitioner to be effective, technical skills and knowledge are essential but not sufficient. Knowing all the facts in this handbook alone will not be adequate to ensure that you are able to articulate and implement your sound professional advice, especially in the face of opposing views. It will be your leadership that prevails in ensuring your effectiveness.

In public health, as in other areas of work, it is not only those in formal leadership roles who can lead—any member of a team can adopt situational leadership if appropriate, as noted by the NHS Leadership Academy.[7]

Competencies needed by a public health leader

Virtually any piece of work in public health lends itself to scrutiny of the leadership element. For example, you are asked by the local authority to undertake a health impact assessment (HIA) in relation to a proposal to set up a waste incineration facility in your locality. Review of this task, which requires you to adopt a project management role, will reveal aspects for which your leadership skills are needed:

- Clear vision as to the nature of the task and its objectives and desired outcomes.
- Working across organizational boundaries to ensure engagement of all stakeholders through appropriate, effective communication.
- Gaining the trust of those who may be threatened by the proposal, such as employees of existing services likely to be adversely affected by the building of the new facility.
- Perseverance to complete the task despite strong opposing factions—in particular those who fear they may be disadvantaged by the HIA's conclusions.
- Professional integrity—and moral courage to present your final recommendations strongly, in support of the population's health.

The evidence base for effective public health leadership is underdeveloped. Looking more widely, and with the exception of military leadership, most modalities of leadership have little firm evidence. Research on personality type (using the Myers Briggs Personality Inventory [MBTI]) shows that leaders are more likely to have certain personality characteristics than others, but there is no evidence for a causal association between personality type and leadership ability. As pointed out in relation to health services,[8] leaders are involved in enthusing, negotiating, and pacifying, and must therefore have these competencies, as well as any more tangible qualifications for the job.

Box 6.1.1 shows competencies usually associated with effective public health leadership.

The leadership qualities adopted by the English NHS comprise personal, social, and cognitive qualities, arranged in three clusters:

Personal qualities, setting direction, and delivering the service

These qualities may be applied in public health (Table 6.1.2) as in healthcare more generally.

The NHS Leadership Academy[9] introduced a further refinement of the model in 2013, comprising nine dimensions of leadership behaviour (Box 6.1.2). Once again, these attributes are designed with healthcare leaders in mind, but the Academy emphasizes its role in promoting leadership across the whole health system.

Box 6.1.1 Competencies usually associated with effective public health leadership

Knowledge

Good grasp of the core knowledge base required for public health practice

Skills

- Ability to define and articulate a clear vision.
- Ability to share the vision so that others are influenced to adopt it.
- Resilience and perseverance towards the vision despite difficulties.
- Maintenance of professional integrity.

Attitudes

- Self-esteem combined with critical self-appraisal.
- A degree of humility to allow one to acknowledge that someone else is right.
- An understanding and respect of others' beliefs and perceptions, which may differ from yours.
- Personal values including a 'passion' for public health.

Table 6.1.2 Leadership qualities and capacities

Personal qualities	Setting direction	Delivering better population health
Self-belief	Seeing/sizing the future	Leading change through people
Self-awareness	Intellectual flexibility	Holding to account
Self-management	Broad scanning	Empowering others
Drive for improvement	Political astuteness	Effective and strategic influencing
Personal and professional integrity	Drive for results	Collaborative working

Source: data from NHS Leadership Qualities Framework, NHS Institute for Improvement & Innovation, 2006.

Box 6.1.2 **The nine dimensions of leadership behaviour**
- Inspiring shared purpose.
- Leading with care.
- evaluating information.
- Connecting our service.
- Sharing the vision.
- Engaging the team.
- Holding to account.
- Developing capability.
- Influencing for results.

Source: data from NHS Leadership Academy (2013) Healthcare Leadership Model.

Potential pitfalls

- Recognizing a public health challenge and producing a technically competent project plan to address it is necessary but not enough.
- Neither vision nor professional expertise alone will lead to change—political skills including diplomacy, communication, and timing are just as important.
- Leadership may not always be from the front. Different styles of leadership are needed for different situations—for example, in leading an outbreak control team, getting a local company to take workplace health seriously, leading evidence-based redesign of public health or healthcare provision, or introducing sustained changes to clinical practice.
- Enthusiasm may be infectious, while piety is usually not. Remember that others may not share your vision, and may need an explanation of the evidence—as distinct from the faith—on which it is based.

Dogma, myths, and fallacies about leadership

- 'Leaders are born and not made': there is no evidence for this statement, although aptitude, intelligence, and enthusiasm are helpful attributes. An ability to learn from every situation is central for effective leadership— as President Kennedy pointed out: 'Leadership and learning are indispensable to each other.'
- Leaders are tall or attractive or have significant physical presence: there are plenty of high-profile examples to refute this. Having said that, appearance can be important and leaders on occasion win hearts and minds by dressing respectfully for their audience.
- Extroverts make the best leaders: while there is evidence that leaders are more likely to be extrovert personalities (using the MBTI), there is no evidence that other types make inferior leaders. Leaders have to deploy the most appropriate attributes at the right time.
- 'What is your leadership style?' may be asked of applicants at interview, but the fact is that effective leaders have to use a range of styles to suit different situations—although most of you will have one or two preferred styles, typically on the spectrum of supportive—directive and autocratic— participative.
- Leadership is a fancy term for management: no, leadership and management should be considered as distinct. It is helpful for leaders to have an appreciation of management.

Examples of success and scope for improvement

National management of the 2009/10 influenza pandemic has been independently reviewed in a number of countries. A good published example comes from Canada[10], which made particular reference to the importance of effective leadership and collaborative working across many organizations and government departments, as well as translation of the strategy to local levels for grass roots implementation. Closer to home, the 2017 peer-to-peer evaluation of Public Health England highlighted its leadership role and includes recommendations for strengthening its impact, including a major focus on the importance of partnership working in public health leadership, both nationally and internationally.[11]

Key determinants of success

Clarity of vision, the energy to persevere despite barriers and the humility to recognize when to adjust the vision, are all necessary. Taking people with you on the journey through implementation is essential. The successful public health leader has imagination and energy as well as professional integrity, technical knowledge, and skills. And if you have passion for your subject, that will be apparent in your dedication and commitment: Barack Obama was credible to many when he said, 'Yes we can'.

How will you know if you have been successful?

Change in a public health context can take many years, although your vision would have been supported by a plan for implementation including measurable indicators of progress. These might comprise quantitative and qualitative measures, the latter including the extent of engagement of partner organizations, positive media coverage, or knowledge of the initiative in the local community.

However, to know if you, as a leader, have been successful, you will probably need to ask other people. You don't have to wait to do this. The concept of multi-source feedback (MSF) is now well established and the use of a validated MSF tool can provide valuable feedback about your performance. In the UK, MSF has been an integral part of the evidence required for the revalidation of public health medical professionals since 2013.[12]

Emerging issues

Public health increasingly requires interagency collaboration so that effective leadership across organizational boundaries is often essential (see ➜ Chapter 7.5). So is the ability to work through others—teachers, pharmacists, town planners, for example—, whose job specifications rarely indicate public health content. To be a successful public health leader, it is worth exploring the professional practices and workplace cultures of people in quite different jobs to be able to harness their enthusiasm and energy to your common cause.

The practicalities of acquiring leadership skills

In your personal development plan, consider:

* *Taking a course in leadership development:* in England, the NHS Leadership Academy is accessible online and, in addition to online resources, offers a range of programmes for people at different stages in their health and healthcare careers.[10] In the US, the Public Health Leadership Institute has been running since 1991 and evaluation has demonstrated its impact.[13]
* *Ensuring you understand your own personality type and appreciate the potential impact of others:* you can study this alone,[14] although you may want to consult a personal development consultant to take this further.
* *Getting to know and learning how to work with the mass media* (see also ➜ Chapter 6.4). The media are very effective at conveying both positive and negative health messages to the general public. Having the media, including local media, on-side for advocacy can reap rewards. Establishing a good rapport with local or national reporters can mean that, next time a public health issue comes along, the story is more likely to be covered fairly and without bias. Media training is available from many sources and your organization's press office would usually be a good starting point.
* *Developing your communication skills:* different audiences will respond to different modes of communication, so it is worthwhile becoming familiar with techniques not often yet taught to professionals, such as storytelling. Humility is valuable: arrogance has no place in public health practice.
* *Knowing and respecting partners within and outside your organization:* it could be just as important to engage a key internal budget holder as to form an alliance with a Chief Executive of another body or a community leader: there is always a need for partnership working 'inside and out'.
* *Reviewing your public health competencies systematically:* for greater understanding of the local scene, not only its demography and epidemiology, but also its key players, culture, politics, and priorities, of which health is but one. All this is needed for good practice—the scope of this book.

Further resources

Further reading

Adair J (1993). *Effective leadership*. Pan Books, London.

BBC World Service. BBC Learning English *The Handy Guide to the Gurus of Management, Programme 5, Warren Bennis* © BBC English/Charles Handy. Available at: ℘ http://downloads.bbc.co.uk/worldservice/learningenglish/handy/bennis.pdf (accessed 23 August 2019).

Hunter D, Rayner G. (2004). Guest editorial: UKPHA and WFPHA Conference Plenary Presentations. *Public Health*, **118**, 461–87.

Heartland centers, St Louis Univ. Public Health and crisis leadership competency framework.(2009). Available at: ℘ https://www.slideshare.net/Nostrad/networks-competency-framework (accessed 17 December 2017).

Wright K, Rowitz L, Merkle A, et al. (2000). Competency development in public health leadership. *American Journal of Public Health*, **90(8)**, pp. 1202–7. Available at: ℘ doi/10.2105/ajph.90.8.1202 (accessed 24 August 2019).

Rowitz L. Public health leadership: putting principles into practice, 2nd Ed, Jones & Bartlett, Mass., USA, 2009.

References

1 Acheson D. (1988). Public health in England: the report of the Committee of Inquiry into the future development of the public health function, Cm 289. HMSO, London.

2 Wanless D. (2004). Securing good health for the whole population. Final report. HM Treasury, London. Available at: http://webarchive.nationalarchives.gov.uk/+/http://www.dh.gov.uk/en/Publicationsandstatistics/Publications/PublicationsPolicyAndGuidance/DH_4074426 (accessed 17 December 2017).

3 Department of Health (2004). Choosing health: making healthy choices easier. HMSO, London. Available at: http://webarchive.nationalarchives.gov.uk/+/http://www.dh.gov.uk/en/Publicationsandstatistics/Publications/PublicationsPolicyAndGuidance/DH_4094550 (accessed 17 August 2017).

4 Departments of Health (2010). Liberating the NHS: increasing democratic legitimacy in health. Available at: http://webarchive.nationalarchives.gov.uk/+/http://www.dh.gov.uk/en/Consultations/Closedconsultations/DH_117586 (accessed 3 January 2018).

5 Department of Health. (2013) Directors of Public Health in Local Government: Roles, responsibilities and context. Available at: https://www.gov.uk/government/uploads/system/uploads/attachment_data/file/249810/DPH_Guidance_Final_v6.pdf (accessed 10 December 2017).

6 Calman K. (1998). Lessons from Whitehall. *British Medical Journal*, 317, 1718–20.

7 NHS Leadership Academy. Available at: www.leadershipacademy.nhs.uk (accessed 17 December 2017).

8 Bohmer R. (2010). Leadership with a small 'l'. *British Medical Journal*, 340, c483.

9 NHS Leadership Academy. (2013). Healthcare Leadership Model. Available at: https://www.leadershipacademy.nhs.uk/wp-content/uploads/2014/10/NHSLeadership-LeadershipModel-colour.pdf (accessed 10 December 2017).

10 Eggleton A, Chair. Standing Senate committee on social affairs, science and technology. Canada's response to the H1N1 influenza pandemic. December 2010. Available at: https://sencanada.ca/content/sen/Committee/403/soci/rep/rep15dec10-e.pdf (accessed 17 December 2017).

11 IANPHI. Public Health England: Evaluation and recommendations. November 2017. Available at: https://www.gov.uk/government/uploads/system/uploads/attachment_data/file/661350/PHE-Evaluation_and_Recommendations.pdf (accessed 17 December 2017).

12 General Medical Council (UK). Supporting information for appraisal and revalidation (2012). Available at: https://www.gmc-uk.org/static/documents/content/RT___Supporting_information_for_appraisal_and_revalidation___DC5485.pdf_55024594.pdf (accessed 17 December 2017).

13 Umble KE, Diehl SJ, Gunn A, et al. (2007). Developing leaders, building networks: an evaluation of the National Public Health Leadership Institute—1991–2006. North Carolina Institute for Public Health, Chapel Hill. Available at: https://sph.unc.edu/files/2015/03/nciph-phli-evaluation.pdf (accessed 17 December 2017).

14 Myers Briggs I, Myers P. (1980). Gifts differing, understanding personality type. Davies-Black, Palo Alto, Ca.

Chapter 6.2

Effective meetings

Edmund Jessop

Introduction

All meetings are negotiations. Whether it is a 10-minute meeting with your boss, a regular meeting with colleagues or a 20-minute presentation to a committee, you are trying to change what someone else thinks.

So there are two essentials for any meeting:

- **You**—know what you want to achieve from the meeting.
- **Them**—find out as much as you can about them.

Before the meeting

Think about your aims

Public health is about changing the way other people think. The best way to do that is face to face. Most people hate meetings—because they see meetings as a chore, not an opportunity. Of course some, even many, meetings are tediously unproductive. But for sure a meeting will waste time if you go in not knowing what *you* want out of it.

Like any negotiation, sort out in your own mind beforehand:

- What would be the best result for you (opening position)?
- What is the minimum acceptable (your fall-back position)?

For example, your opening position is probably complete acceptance of your policy, but what is your fall-back: partial acceptance or the decision deferred until later? What points are you willing to compromise on? How much you are prepared to change your views?

Research before the meeting

Find out as much as you can about the other people who will be there. It is especially important to find out:

- what other people believe
- what other people want to achieve.

Of course, you need to ask these questions of yourself first.

If you are attending an unfamiliar meeting, find out about the people who will be there. Do they like the big picture or the detail? Should you be thorough or quick? Will they be impressed by government policy or dismissive of it? Sometimes quoting the opinion of the great and good, the academy and institute, will impress; sometimes it will antagonize. Use your friends and colleagues to find out about the people who will be at your meeting.

Even if the meeting is with someone you know well, think about how they are feeling *today* about your issue.

A successful negotiation is one in which you get what you want and they get what they want—at least to some extent. Listen hard and long: find out as much as you can about what they want. You can't do that if you haven't questioned thoroughly and listened carefully.

If someone is opposing you, there must be a reason. This reason is important to them. Maybe it seems trivial, irrelevant, or outrageous to you, but it is stopping you from changing the way they think. So you need to find out what that reason is. Only then can you start to resolve the difference between you. Often the reason is fear—fear that something will happen if they agree with you. Unearth the fear and maybe you can remove it.

Sell the benefit not the proposal

Focus on how they will benefit, not what you want to do. And concentrate on benefits that are relevant to *them*. Of course you can only do this if you've already found out what they want.

Remember that differences exist in the mind, not in reality

To resolve a conflict of opinion, you need to address the other person's mind, not the 'objective facts'. Scientifically trained workers find it hard to understand why people don't respond to objective data. But if you lived next to a toxic waste dump, and your child developed leukaemia, no amount of scientific evidence on exposure, doses, and latent periods would convince you that the waste dump was safe. The same is true in any meeting, from a discussion of where to put the coffee machine to agreeing on a multimillion pound budget.

Build the relationship

Public health work takes time. The people you are meeting today will be people you have to work with again in the future:

> *The relationship is more important than any one meeting.*

So sometimes you need to lose gracefully and come back next time. As Dale Carnegie said, 'No one ever wins an argument'. If you have an argument and 'win', the other person is left feeling bruised and battered. This is always damaging to a long-term relationship. You can't afford that kind of ill will in public health work. Your success depends on other people, so you need other people to be on your side.

Setting up your own meeting

When you set up a meeting, good administration is important. If people arrive flustered, or unprepared, or can't come at all, you won't achieve your aim.

Timing

Give people plenty of notice that you want to meet them. It is difficult to generalize but four weeks' notice for a half-day meeting and 6 weeks or more for an all-day meeting is about right for senior people. People of national importance may need 6 months' notice or more.

Be aware of committee cycles: find out regular dates (e.g. budget-setting meetings). You may need to map a sequence of meetings (e.g. ethics committee before grant committee, or personnel committee before finance committee).

Venue

The venue is important, so get the best you can afford. People who are cold, sitting in uncomfortable chairs, recovering from a long, difficult journey will not be paying attention to you. Think about parking, wheelchair access, and refreshments.

Should you invite other people to your office, or go to visit them, or meet on neutral territory? For one-to-one meetings, it is more polite to put yourself out by going to them; for big meetings, you have to be the host. If conflict is severe, neutral territory works best.

If you are expecting conflict, don't sit people who are likely to disagree directly opposite each another. It reinforces the feeling that it's 'us' against 'them'. In public health, everyone is facing the shared problem of death and disease. Have everyone facing a screen or board on which the problem you have in common—an outbreak, an overspend, whatever—can be described. You can do this even in one-to-one meetings: never sit across a desk from someone.

Agenda

Send out an agenda so that everyone has the chance to prepare for the meeting. Most people *won't* prepare but, if you don't send an agenda, they *can't*.

Help people to know which are the important items, perhaps by indicating on the agenda how long you expect to spend on each one. It is wise to allow 10–15 minutes for people to settle in with small or routine items before tackling the major topic.

Focus as much time as possible on the main topics: avoid getting bogged down with updates from the last meeting. Whenever possible, find out whether people have undertaken their tasks and ask for a brief summary. Provide this as a written summary before the meeting and add anything that needs further discussion as a substantive agenda item.

It is good practice to include a verb in each agenda item (e.g. rather than writing 'Quality standards', write 'Discuss new quality standards for access to cancer services'. Other useful agenda verbs are 'decide', 'review', 'select', 'finish', or, if no action is required, 'inform'.

Even better than just having a verb in the question is to try to set as many agenda items as possible as questions (e.g. 'How can we improve access to cancer services to reduce late presentations?'). This gets people into 'discovery mode' and is more likely to be energise the group to come up with good solutions.

During the meeting

Meetings are the live theatre of public health: exciting, exhilarating, and unpredictable! Ok, so most meetings are pretty boring, but if you focus on what's going on, you can build up pictures of people and relationships. And remember:

> *Build the relationship: you'll be meeting again!*

Listen: don't speak

If you're the first to speak on a topic, human nature ensures that the next two or three speakers will oppose what you've said, if only to show that they can think for themselves. So bide your time and present your ideas towards the end of discussion on an item. Sometimes this will mean not revealing your own opinion in any briefing paper you have circulated before the meeting.

Even if you've been invited specifically to give a presentation, you need to listen first. Get there early to gauge the mood of the meeting, and find out who is asking what.

Words matter: use them carefully

You will not build a relationship by giving offence. If in doubt, find out beforehand from a colleague what terms are acceptable to your audience. Remember that some scientific words give offence to lay audiences (e.g. 'spastic' has a clear meaning in medical meetings but is a term of abuse in lay language). Is it a 'case' of meningitis or a person with meningitis?

If you've achieved your objectives, stop arguing

After you've achieved your objectives, anything else you say can *only* make things worse, so shut up! Of course this means you need to be listening hard to know when you have won. All too often, people throw away victory by continuing to argue their case and alienating people who have already been won over.

Use summary statements

With more than five people in a meeting, normal conversation is impossible and special tactics are needed. If more than eight people are present, you will not get more than one chance to speak on any topic. Often a summary statement ('soundbite')—a single phrase or sentence that puts across a message or creates an image—will be more effective than a speech in helping other people to change their minds or modify their views.

Don't read or refer to papers in the meeting

If you are reading, you are not listening. In the meeting, it is more important to concentrate hard on what is going on around you than to read some point of detail. If someone asks a detailed query, the correct response is to say, 'I'll get back to you after the meeting', and carry on with the more important business of listening hard to the discussion. If you read the papers beforehand (even if you only skim them), you won't need to read them *during* the meeting.

If you are the chair, prepare to set the tone and focus

Prepare: your role is to help the people at the meeting to come to the best collective decision they can. To do this you need to:
- know what you want to achieve and check that the agenda actually says what you want to happen
- know who will be at the meeting so you can pick up their names quickly
- know the terms of reference of the meeting.

At the meeting, welcome everyone and ensure that people are introduced. Set the tone for the meeting—its aims and how you want people to behave (e.g. getting through the agenda should be a shared endeavour not the chair battling to stop the loquacious warm to their topic while the introverts groan inwardly). Do this by setting out the purpose of the meeting to focus the group, reminding people how long has been allocated to each item and keeping your own contributions to a minimum unless you need to kick-start a discussion. Summarise regularly and repeat any decisions or actions clearly—this helps the minute taker. Check that everyone has had a chance to have their say at the end of the meeting or after each contentious item.

After the meeting

- Always follow through.
- After formal meetings, and within 24 hours, send out notes of what was decided and who agreed to take what action. Copy this to people who couldn't attend.
- Even informal meetings are worth written follow-up to ensure no misunderstanding (and no reneging on agreements!) (see Box 6.2.1).

Box 6.2.1 A 'follow-up' letter
Dear Jim

This is to confirm that Fred, you and I agreed yesterday to write a 1,500-word paper together entitled 'Waiting list solutions that work' within the next two weeks. I will let you have the statistics by Thursday, and you will do the first draft within five working days. We agreed to meet next on Wednesday 30 March at 3pm in your room.

Julie.
cc Fred

Acknowledgement

I am grateful to my colleague Hilary Guite for contributions to this chapter.

Further resources
Fisher R, Ury W, Patton B (1999). *Getting to Yes. Negotiating agreement without giving in*. Random House, London.
Webb, C. (2016). *How to have a good day. Think bigger, feel better and transform your working life*. Pan Macmillan, London.

Effective writing

Edmund Jessop

Introduction

The most important thing to remember when you write is that no one *has* to read what you write. Never think that because what you write is important people will read it: they won't. Consider for a moment how much material you have not read in the past two weeks.

If what you write is difficult to read, people will simply give up. So you must do everything in your power to make reading easy for your readers. You can't *force* people to read: you have to *tempt* them.

This chapter focuses on corporate rather than academic writing but mostly the principles are the same.

Objectives

This chapter will help you to make your writing more enjoyable to read. As a result, it will be more effective in initiating and sustaining appropriate change in others.

Writing has three stages: before, during, and after. The most important stage is before.

Before you write

Know who you are writing for

Are you writing for:
- your boss?
- co-workers?
- a committee?
- the general public?

This seems obvious, but it is the key to success. If you are going to tempt people to read, you must know who they are and what they like. Always keep the reader in mind. It is sometimes easier to think of some person you know rather than a whole group: if writing for old people, write for your aunt. If writing a committee paper, think of one typical member of the committee and write for him or her.

Give them what *they* want to read—not what *you* want to write

Never fall into the trap of thinking people *must* read what you write; they won't. Even if telling them about their own pay rise, there will always be some people who won't read your words. So give them your message in the form they want it—make it easy for them.

Most people don't want scientific methodology: so don't give it to them. If you do, they'll just give up and skip to an easier document. And if *they* have stopped reading, *you* have stopped persuading.

If your readers (e.g. a grant-giving committee) have asked you to complete a form, *complete the form*. Don't leave items out. Don't add pages of extra material. If it says do it in 12-point type, don't try to cram more in by using a smaller font. Your aim is to help them to your way of thinking; and failing to heed their instructions will not achieve that aim.

Be active in finding out what your readership wants: if writing for a committee, ask to see previous committee papers. Speak to the secretary of the committee.

Give it to them on time

Hit the deadline—even if it means your paper isn't perfect: as the journalists say to their editors, 'You want it good or you want it Thursday?' A report or paper that arrives after the decision is made is worthless. So find out when the decision will be made. And never 'table' a paper (i.e. never give the paper out for the first time at the meeting at which you want it discussed). No one can read it properly in the meeting so if you do this the only correct course of action for a chairperson is to ignore your paper completely.

To hit the deadline, allow time for all stages of writing, review, and distribution.

And remember that the formal meeting at which, say, budgets are agreed is often a formality: all details may have been sorted out long before. So you need to check whether minds will be made up *before* the formal decision.

Be aware of their constraints

The usual constraints are:
* people's attitudes, prejudices, way of life
* local regulations, law, or policy
* precedent
* available funding.

Think what each may mean for your readers. You may or may not be able to alter constraints: but, if not, you must at least show awareness of them.

Think before you write

If your thoughts are woolly, your writing will be woolly. Each piece of writing should have a single aim, and the whole structure of your piece should lead to this aim. Spend time thinking this out.

Write down your aim. Make it short and clear, for example:
* to persuade this school to adopt a no-smoking policy
* to persuade this committee to give me a research grant.

The next stage is to work out what individual messages are most likely to sell your idea. This may need further thought. For a smoking policy, it could be:
1. Smoking causes cancer in non-smokers.
2. Smoking is a fire hazard.

Message 1 may seem more important to public health workers but message 2 was what got the ban on smoking throughout the London underground transport system. Choose the message that will achieve your aim, not the one you most want to put out.

Do all your homework before you put pen to paper (or finger to keyboard)

Typically you need to research:
* some key statistics
* research literature
* law and government policy
* local precedents (what have they done before on this or similar issues?).

It's also worth finding out what your own organisation has said on this issue before (see below on 'cut and paste').

Make sure you can prove every assertion you make. You may not want to fill the text with scientific references, but truth matters: don't rely on memory! Readers increasingly want to check references online, so give an internet address (URL) when you can.

Write a framework

When you have all the facts in your head, write a framework for your piece. This needs to give:

- a major heading for each two or three pages (2,000–3,000 words)
- minor headings per half-page (500–1,000 words)
- a main point for each paragraph (100–200 words).

Start with the major headings, then fill in the minor headings, and finally the points for each paragraph. You now have a clear line of thought for your piece, be it a one-page memo or a 10,000 word report. Without a framework, your reader will find it hard to follow your line of thought and will give up trying.

Make a word budget

Make a word budget for each section. For example:

- introduction, 300 words
- evidence base, 500 words
- local situation, 500 words
- recommendations, 250 words.

Make a time budget

Most of us find writing very tiring even when all the above steps have been completed. You are unlikely to write more than 1,000 words per day, so a 10,000 word report should be planned as 10 working days FOR THE WRITING.

When you are writing

Don't write anything until you have the shape of your entire piece clear in your mind and/or sketched out on paper. I find that a pencil and paper encourage structure in a way that computers do not.

Use short words

Think what you would say in conversation: 'He had a stroke' not 'He had a cerebrovascular accident'. Sometimes the short word lacks precision— a 'heart attack' may indicate acute myocardial infarct or ventricular fibrillation. But does this distinction matter *to your readers*? If not, choose the short word.

There is one exception to this rule: don't give offence.

Don't give offence

Words such as 'leper' and 'cretin' have technical meanings but they give offence and have been replaced by 'person with Hansen's disease' and 'person with congenital hypothyroidism'. It may look odd, but if you give offence people will stop reading and your writing will not achieve its aim (quite apart from common decency).

Use short sentences

Whenever you are about to use a comma, don't. Put a full stop and start a new sentence.

Don't use abbreviations

People read word groups, not individual letters or words, so in reading (unlike speaking) readers don't get slowed up by a lack of abbreviations. Abbreviations, because they are all capitals, *are* difficult to read. If you must abbreviate, spell it out in full the first time— for example, 'acquired immune deficiency disease (AIDS)'.

Use headings and subheadings

Most people don't read: they skim. So help them to skim—use headings.

If there is a house style use it: your readers are familiar with it and any-thing different is a distraction. If there is no house style, keep to a standard format for the font size, underlining, and so on.

Structure your piece

A good general structure for a briefing paper is as follows:

1. Table of contents (if more than 10 pages long).
2. Summary.
3. Purpose or aim.
4. Background.
5. Precedent or local/national policy.
6. Current issues (i.e. why now?).
7. Options including implementation.
8. Cost.
9. Politics.
10. Recommended option and why.
11. Document control—authorship, reason (for info, action …) sent to whom, date, version …

You should number the paragraphs in your document—this helps readers refer to particular passages in meetings or correspondence.

Use lists

Lists are easy to skim. More than three of anything demands a list. Use bul-lets for three or four items, but for more than that use numbers.

Cut and paste?

Cut and paste is dangerous. Used simply out of laziness, it distorts your writing away from your key message. But sometimes cut and paste is the right thing to do. Lawyers and lobby groups seize on slight differences in wording with glee, so if your organization has standard text about an issue, use and re-use it. Of course you need to avoid plagiarism and avoid breach of copyright.

Use graphics

Try to put a chart, graph, or picture in to break up the text. Newspapers do it to attract readers—so should you. It is easy enough to insert graphics into text with modern software, although considerable effort may be needed to generate a good graphic.

The guru of graphics, McCandless (2009), says: start with the data to find the story, then sketch your graphic and lastly add design. Get the right look to get your main message across.

Electronic mail

With email, the message header may be the *only* thing people read, so use the header for your message not the topic. Try this sample:

- 'Read your papers before tomorrow's meeting' versus 're: Tomorrow's meeting'.
- 'Home called: no dinner tonight' versus 'Telephone message for you'.
- 'Teenage pregnancy rate lowest ever' versus 'Latest health statistics'.

After you write

Don't send it off

Once your paper is written, mull it over. Never send a paper out as soon as it is written: even with the most urgent deadline, walk away for an hour or so. Better still, leave it overnight or over a weekend. Then come back with a fresh eye and reread your work. You will always see something that could have been said better!

Get some feedback

Always ask a colleague to read your document. Make clear that you want comments on big issues not minor errors of spelling or grammar. Ask specifically for:

- material that just looks wrong (e.g. statistics for circumcisions that exceed the number of male births in your locality)
- important issues that have been missed (e.g. abortion clinics as well as maternity units in a study of conception).

If possible, although this is often difficult, ask someone like the intended reader to review it for clarity. Don't get defensive when people point out errors and inconsistencies. Be grateful.

Consider the distribution list carefully

Send it to your intended readership, but also think 'Who else should see this?' This is particularly important for correspondence. Do a mental check of people in your own organization and in other agencies. Other organizations won't distribute it internally to everyone you think should see it, so mail them directly. In general, anyone who will be affected by what you write should see it.

Offer to meet the individual or group you have sent it to

Offering your time shows your commitment to the cause, as well as giving an opportunity to lobby, and to remove any misunderstandings.

Summary

These rules may seem daunting, but as with so much in life they become easy with practice. Writing well is one of the best ways to improve your personal effectiveness.

Acknowledgement

I am grateful to my colleague, Hilary Guite, for her contributions to this chapter.

Further resources

Easy reading

Cutts M. (2013). *Oxford Guide to Plain English*. Oxford University Press.
Tim Albert, writer and trainer. Training. Write effectively. A quick course for busy health workers. Available at: ✆ http://www.timalbert.co.uk (accessed 13 March 2017).

Reference works

Butterfield J. (2015). *Fowler's dictionary of modern English usage*, 4th edn. Clarendon Press, Oxford.
Strunk W, White EB, Angell, R. (2019). *The elements of style*, 4th edn. Pearson. Available at: ✆ http://www.bartleby.com/141 (accessed 13 March 2017).

Writing for publication in the medical literature

Albert T. (1996). Publish and prosper. British Medical Journal, **313**(7070), classified supplement.
Albert T. (2000). *A–Z of medical writing*. BMJ Books, London.
Albert T. (2000). *Winning the publications game*, 2nd edn. Radcliffe Medical Press, Oxford.

How to do graphics

McCandless D. (2009). *The beauty of data visualization*. Collins. Available at: ✆ http://www.ted.com/talks/david_mccandless_the_beauty_of_data_visualization (accessed 28 March 2017).
Tufte E. (1983). *Visual display of quantitative information*. Graphics Press, Cheshire, CT.

Chapter 6.4

Working with the media

Alan Maryon-Davis

Objectives

After reading this chapter you should be able to:
- develop a strategy for working with the media, either as an individual practitioner or as a representative of your team or organization
- review and strengthen your strategy, if you already have one in place
- undertake simple media tasks, such as writing a press release or being interviewed by a journalist, with more confidence
- make creative use of social media to highlight and reinforce your messages.

This chapter addresses the basics of working with the print, broadcast, and social media. More provocative engagement with the media is described elsewhere in this handbook.

Working with confidence

As health professionals, we tend to be rather wary of working with the media. Like fire, publicity can be a great source of light—but can also be erratic and risky. Besides, it often takes an awful lot of matches just to get it started. Yet the media's influence and reach are invaluable to us. We need to engage large numbers of people and convey information, change attitudes, and trigger actions for health improvement. We must therefore learn how to make the most of this potential with a few basic skills and a coherent approach.

We talk of 'the media' as a single entity. In reality of course, it is very plural, not only in terms of its various modalities, like print, radio, television, online or social media, but also because it comprises a diverse collection of individual journalists, web editors and programme makers all trying to attract readers, listeners, viewers or page hits. Fortunately for us, health issues make good copy, and media professionals need us as much as we need them. This makes our task a little easier.

Developing a media strategy

There are generic and specific elements to a media strategy.

Generic elements comprise the following
- *Knowing and cultivating your media:* print, broadcast, or web-based, understanding how they can help you in your work across the board, how they operate, who they reach, what their constraints and limitations are, and what risks are attached.
- *Developing media skills:* learning how to frame a story, write a press release, use the different media in combination (media mix), be interviewed, take part in a studio discussion, and make best use of social media, and building a team of people who can do these things with confidence.
- *Providing media back-up:* anticipating the information or materials that might be needed by your media journalists, researchers, and producers, and being prepared to provide these at short notice.

Specific elements concern the issue you are planning to promote. These involve being clear about what you're trying to achieve and asking yourself the following:

- What am I trying to say? (messages)
- Who am I trying to say it to? (target audience)
- How best can I get it across to them? (media mix).

To which should be added
- What support or follow-up should I provide?
- What parallel approaches should I adopt?
- How will I know whether I have succeeded?

Simple clear messages, tailored to your target group, delivered through an appropriate media mix, make for success. If you can back that up with support (e.g. by providing a helpline or website address) and ensure that the relevant services are primed and ready to respond to increased demand, your intervention is likely to be even more effective.

Be clear about your messages

The fewer key messages the better—a maximum of five, preferably no more than three. These should be:

- topical and newsworthy (the 'hook')
- meaningful and relevant to the target audience (the 'angle')
- informative or motivating
- in plain language and jargon-free
- accurate, valid, and backed up by reliable evidence
- agreed by your partners or managers.

Understand your target audience

Be clear whom you are trying to reach and what their needs and interests are likely to be. This is crucial for framing your story and finding the right angle. If possible, meet and talk to service users themselves to gain an understanding of how they receive messages through the media—what issues they are interested in, papers they read, radio programmes they listen to, TV programmes they watch. You need to understand how to 'grab' their interest and enthusiasm, what is the best mix of media to use, and at what level to pitch your messages.

Cultivate the media

Be familiar with their output and look for opportunities. Talk to and, if possible, meet with reporters and producers. Focus on those who usually cover health stories. Explain what you're trying to do and what you can do for them. Try to be available if they need instant public health advice or information. By and large, they want to get it right.

For each issue, event, or campaign, write a well-constructed press release (see ➔ Writing a press release) and follow this up with a personalized email or phone call to 'sell' your story to the appropriate editor—news editor, health editor, features editor, or programme editor. Be clear and succinct about the hook, angle, and messages. Mention any launch event or photo opportunity. Whenever possible, try to tie the story to something happening locally or nationally.

Make use of available help

Use your organization's press officer or communications manager. They can advise you on how to frame your messages and which media are best for reaching the target group. More importantly, if you don't use your organization's press officer, not only will you not be availing yourself of quality advice but your messages may be out of step with your organization's current policy.

Always be clear, to the press and others, on whose behalf you are speaking. Even if you claim to be speaking as an individual, it may be thought more newsworthy by journalists if they forget this. Your organization's press officer will usually have a working relationship with key journalists and producers, and perhaps a budget that can be used to set up a press conference, or pay for an 'advertorial' in the local paper. If you don't have this level of support, try to link in with a partner organization that does.

Using spokespeople and case studies

People bring news stories and features to life. The audience can identify with them and they help 'sell' your story to the editors. The spokesperson may be yourself, a colleague, or someone working for the initiative, project, or service you're promoting. You may need more than one spokesperson if there are many media slots to cover, in which case it is important to make sure that they convey the same key messages. They might also benefit from the practical interview guidance below.

The case study might be a member of the general public or particular community group, or a patient, client, or other representative of the target group you are trying to reach. They, too, should be clear about the key messages and must have given their permission to be interviewed or featured. Check whether they are happy to use their real name or would prefer a pseudonym. Also make sure they agree with any details about their condition or history that you intend to disclose. If you are holding someone else's personal information, for instance on your computer, make sure it is locked and password protected. Always follow your organization's confidentiality and data security procedures.

In lining up your spokesperson or case study

- Brief them thoroughly on the purpose of the exercise.
- Agree what their particular contribution should be and the salient points to mention.
- For radio or TV, remind them to be succinct.
- Check their availability against the media slots you are trying to fill.
- Give them copies of any fact-sheets, campaign or follow-up materials.
- Note their phone number in case of last-minute snags.
- Do not give this phone number to the media without permission—instead ask your spokesperson or case study either to make contact with the journalist/researcher/producer themselves or agree to be contacted by them.

Photo opportunities

Newspapers and magazines often prefer to run a 'picture-story'—a picture with a brief caption containing the essential information. This can be a good way of raising awareness of an issue, campaign, or service, and can often be followed up later with more in-depth coverage. The trick is to come up with an idea that will grab the picture editor's attention—something visually interesting or amusing involving 'real' people. Using a well-known celebrity is a device that often pays off.

Infographics

Print and online media may welcome your key messages in the form of an 'infographic'—a diagram or chart to show the facts clearly and succinctly. This can be especially useful to display statistics or complex inter-relationships. Designing an engaging and accessible infographic requires skill and some newspapers or magazines may be able to convert your key data or rough diagram into a polished infographic. If so, ask if you can check their interpretation before it goes to press. Alternatively, you may have access to an infographic designer who can work direct to your specifications. Placing your infographic on your organization's website, or in a blog or social media outlet such as Facebook, Instagram or Twitter, can have a considerable impact, especially if widely shared.

Staging a press event

A tried and tested approach to capture the attention of the news media is to set up an event such as a press briefing or campaign launch that combines a few speakers to provide different perspectives on the issue, a press pack to give the essential information (background, fact-sheet, key messages, contacts) and a photo opportunity. To carry this off successfully requires skill and experience and careful attention to organizational detail. Whenever possible, seek the assistance of any communications staff you may have access to.

Writing a press release

Unlike a paid-for advertisement or advertorial, a press release does not guarantee that your story will be covered. News editors' inboxes are inundated with press releases. How can you make yours stand out?

Ten important guidelines
- Keep it short and simple—the equivalent of one side of A4 maximum.
- Devise a 'catchy' headline based on the main angle of the story.
- Use short sentences and only a few statistics.
- The introductory paragraph should summarize the whole story in a few lines—what, why, who, where, when, and how.
- The second paragraph fleshes out the detail—fuller background can be given in a 'notes for editors' section at the end.
- The third paragraph can give a direct quote from the spokesperson and a plug for any action you want taken.
- Editors are more inclined to use the story if they can lift text direct from the press release.
- Always give a contact name with daytime and evening phone numbers.
- Follow up with a phone call offering information booklets, photographs, or photo opportunities.
- Consider putting on a formal press conference with a panel of speakers and convivial hospitality.

It should be possible to cut a press release at any word count and for it still to make sense.

Responding to press enquiries

If you are rung up by a journalist

- Make a note of their name and their publication or programme.
- Be open, fair, and honest. Avoid bluster or pretending to know what you do not know.
- If they ask a question you are not sure about, say you will find out and call them back—and make sure you do.
- Avoid saying 'no comment'. Explain why you cannot answer that particular question—perhaps because of confidentiality or because the matter is sub judice.
- Avoid making 'off the record' comments—they have a habit of finding their way onto the record.

Being interviewed on radio or television

Approach each programme separately via the producer or researcher. Whether you call them or they call you, you are likely to find yourself being assessed not only on the merit of your story but also on how well you put it across. If you seem to be saying the right things in the right way, you may be invited to take part.

Before committing yourself to being interviewed, try to find out

- What is the programme's format and style?
- What sort of audience does it have?
- How are they pitching the item—what is the topical hook?
- In what capacity are you appearing—personal or representative?
- Is it a one-to-one interview, or a studio discussion? If so, with whom, and what's their angle?
- Is it live or pre-recorded?
- How long will your item be? (You need to know how to pace yourself.)
- What are the likely questions?
- Will it be in the studio, or will they come to you? (You may need to obtain permission for the recording to take place.)

When deciding what your messages should be

- Decide on a few key messages and get them clear in your head—you can use brief notes for radio, but not for TV. Make sure they are jargon-free.
- One or two real examples may add colour, but avoid using names unless you have been given permission to do so.
- Quote statistics very broadly: rather than '34.7%' say 'about a third' or 'about one in three'.
- Get your points across early—you never quite know when the item will be over.
- A light touch of humour may help, but only if appropriate. If in doubt, don't.
- Make sure that any resource you are promoting, such as a leaflet or a service, is in plentiful supply and someone is primed to provide it.

Radio interviews or phone-ins

Radio is a cosy, intimate medium so just talk naturally with the interviewer. Remember that the listeners are usually doing something else at the same time, so be upbeat, friendly, and plain speaking. If you find yourself taking part in a phone-in, here are a few more points to bear in mind:

- Agree the ground you want to cover with the anchor-person so that callers are kept to the subject.
- Write each caller's name down so that you can personalize your replies.
- Talk directly to the caller as if you were giving one-to-one advice.
- Avoid rambling on too long with each call—keep moving on to the next.

Television interviews

Dress simply and plainly. No glinting jewellery or jarring patterns. Avoid white, bright red, green, or blue, which can 'flare' on the screen. Go for gentle, muted colours instead.

When you are in front of the camera:

- Sit up, look alert and engaging.
- If your mouth is dry, have a sip from the water on the table.
- Maintain eye contact with the interviewer to avoid looking shifty.
- Don't fidget.

Using online and social media

Online media comprise a wide range of outlets, including websites, blogs, podcasts, apps, push emails and texts, and social media such as Twitter, Instagram and Facebook. New online platforms are appearing all the time. Traditional print and broadcast media increasingly rely on online and social media for reaction, participation, and sharing to reach wider audiences. You can use social media to engage with traditional media more effectively or as a means of reaching audiences directly.

Much of the advice above concerning print and broadcast media will apply equally to the various online media. Clarity and succinctness are usually even more important. It often makes good sense to use social media such as Twitter or Facebook to highlight, enhance, or back up your messages. Indeed, social media may be all you need to raise awareness, create a 'buzz' and spread the word, or drive people to your website. With social media, you can have more control, deciding what, when, and how to post messages or frame a debate. And using social media is relatively inexpensive. The main disadvantage is that it takes time to build up your followers to reach a sizeable audience.

When writing digital content

- Keep it brief—short, sharp, and to the point—only one or two sentences per paragraph.
- Make it lively, direct, and engaging.
- Update and refresh your content frequently.
- Use images, videos, and infographics to boost interest.
- Comment on or share media stories in your field.
- Start building your followers early—it takes time.
- Follow others, especially like-minded opinion leaders or bloggers, comment on their posts, share items of interest.
- Provide links to relevant websites.
- Include share buttons to the most popular sharing platforms.
- Check your facts—develop a reputation for reliability—become a trusted resource.

- Avoid causing offence—do not risk libel.
- Avoid plagiarism.
- Do not breach confidentiality rules.

Measuring success

Individual feedback

At the individual level, you can gauge how well you did in a radio or TV appearance by asking a few people to listen to or watch the programme and give you some honest feedback. This will be more useful if they are fairly representative of the target audience you are trying to reach. If possible, record the programme so that you can learn how to do better next time.

Media coverage

A broader assessment of the effectiveness of a press release or campaign can be obtained by auditing the coverage achieved (e.g. the number and reach of newspapers carrying the story or slots gained on radio and TV).

Web traffic

Monitor your web analytics to see how much your posts or organization's website are viewed, shared, commented on, liked, or followed up, and make any necessary changes to your media strategy.

Public response

Ultimately, the key measure is the practical response achieved in terms of take-up of whatever support materials, service, or behaviour change you are trying to promote. Requests for support materials or an increase in service use are usually easy to count and can often be directly attributed to the media coverage, but behaviour change is likely to be much more difficult to assess or attribute.

Media training

As with most things, you learn best by doing. However, you can help to avoid the pitfalls by having media training. A number of educational bodies and commercial organizations offer courses to develop basic media skills—print, broadcast, and digital media. Blogging platforms, like Wordpress and Blogger, provide free online guidance. Check to see if your organization can arrange training for you and your colleagues.

Further resources

Albert T. (2008). *Write effectively: a quick course for busy health workers*. CRC Press (Taylor & Francis), London. (A set of practical tools to help you write with more confidence in a clear, engaging way.)

Cutts M. (2013). *Oxford Guide to Plain English*. 4th edn. Oxford University Press, Oxford. (Twenty-five easy-to-follow guidelines on all aspects of the writing process: from avoiding jargon, to organizing written information in print and online.)

European Centre for Disease Prevention and Control (2016). *Social media strategy development: A guide to using social media for public health communication*. Available at: ℛ https://ecdc.europa.eu/en/publications-data/social-media-strategy-development-guide-using-social-media-public-health (accessed 10 October 2019).

Communicating risk

John Ford, Nick Steel, and Charles Guest

"Learn what people already believe, tailor the communication to this knowledge and to the decisions people face, and then subject the resulting message to careful evaluation."

M. Granger Morgan[1]

Objective

By reading this chapter, you will be able to use an understanding of risk perception to communicate about risk more effectively.

Why is this an important public health issue?

The health of the public is at risk from a wide range of factors, including harmful food or medicines, poorly controlled infectious diseases, pollutants or natural environmental hazards, and poor diet. Public health practitioners are often involved in minimizing the harm from these risks, and this requires communicating directly to the public or influencing stakeholders. There is an increasing moral and legal requirement for the public sector and private industry to inform populations about the health hazards to which they might be exposed. Risk communication is fraught with difficulty, not least because 'experts', such as policy makers, scientists, and clinicians tend to understand and perceive risks differently from the public. However, there are some predictable patterns, and an understanding of these will improve communication about risk.

Definitions

Risk

Risk is the probability that a particular adverse event occurs during a stated period of time, or results from a particular challenge.[2] It can never be reduced to zero.

- *Absolute risk* is the probability of an event in a population, as contrasted with *relative risk*, which is the ratio of the risk of an event among the exposed to the risk among the unexposed.
- *Attributable risk* is the rate of an event in exposed individuals that can be attributed to the exposure. Some people find the number needed to harm (NNH) more comprehensible than the attributable risk. The NNH is the number of people exposed that would result in one *additional* person being harmed over and above the background risk in the general population.

Risk assessment

Risk assessment is the qualitative and quantitative assessment of the likelihood and size of adverse effects that may result from exposure to specified health hazards (or from the absence of beneficial influences). It has two components, risk estimation, and risk evaluation.

Risk estimation

Relies on scientific activity and judgement. Statistics about past harmful events can be used to predict both the size and the likelihood of future harmful events, including estimates of uncertainty. It involves identifying the health problem and the hazard responsible, and quantifying exposure in a specified population.

Risk evaluation

Relies on social and political judgement. It is the process of determining the importance of the identified hazards and estimated risks from the point of view of those individuals or communities who face the risk. It includes the study of risk perception and the trade-off between perceived risks and benefits. The term 'outrage' has been used to describe the things that the public are worried about that experts traditionally ignore.[3]

Risk communication

Risk communication is the way in which information about risk is communicated to various audiences—the public, healthcare organisations, elected members, local authorities, or private companies. It is a two-way process that needs to be considered at all stages of risk management (Figure 6.5.1).[4]

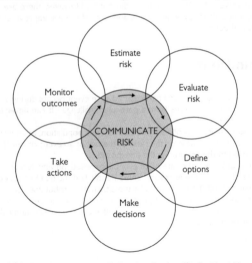

Figure 6.5.1 The risk management cycle. Based on data from The Presidential/Congressional Commission on Risk Assessment and Risk Management (1997). Framework for environmental health risk management, final report volume 1. Washington, DC.

Tasks for effective risk communication

The best strategy for risk communication will depend on the audience and size and likelihood of harm. Here we describe steps that should be considered when communicating a health risk to the public.

Identify and involve relevant stakeholders

The first step is to identify all those within the organization who will be involved, in order to:

- agree a line to take to avoid sending contradictory messages
- identify who will lead the communication process
- involve public affairs or a press office if available
- consider legal advice
- consider the timescale.

The next step is to involve external stakeholders early. These might be the media, professional groups, experts, special interest groups, the local community, patients, politicians, manufacturers, environmentalists, and health officials. Early involvement and acceptance as partners in risk communication will build trust and allow the exchange of information.

Clarify objectives

With whom are you trying to communicate? Do you want to warn, reassure, or inform? You are unlikely to resolve all conflict over a controversial issue, but may clarify disagreements, minimize conflict, and improve decision making. Extra care is needed when you wish to both reassure (the risk is tolerable) and at the same time to warn (but if, in the unlikely event that the situation changes, the following emergency action will be necessary), as sometimes required with infectious disease management. If behaviour change is desired, consider the wider influences on behaviour.

Anticipate potential pitfalls

Check the source of your information. Is it consistent with other knowledge? Is it peer reviewed? Expert overconfidence is a common cause of failure in risk communication. It can be countered by explicitly seeking to uncover uncertainties, and by seeking different views to expose assumptions about your scientific evidence. Listen to the language and signs of concern of all persons involved. Pilot messages before release:

> "One should no more release an untested communication than an untested product."[5]

Resist the temptation to offer bland reassurance where there is real uncertainty. If the news is bad, share the burden with other stakeholders.

Particular care is needed for communication with marginalized groups such as refugees, gypsies and travellers, and migrant workers. Traditional media channels such as the internet and newspapers may prove ineffective, and collaborating with a community gatekeeper or representative will help in understanding relevant communication techniques.

Post-truth culture

The concept of 'post-truth' came to prominence during the 2016 UK referendum on EU membership and USA presidential election, and puts effective risk communication in jeopardy. Post-truth is 'an adjective relating to circumstances in which objective facts are less influential in shaping public opinion than appeals to emotion and personal belief'.[11] This public fatigue with expert advice adds further challenges to communicating risk. In addition to the general principles outlined in this chapter, a post-truth environment requires an ability to:

- distinguish between scientific knowledge and value judgement, and accept that science may not change values and emotions
- advocate evidence-based decision making, directly challenging incorrect facts or 'fake news'
- present relevant facts and figures simply and clearly. Facts are meaningless if they don't resonate with an individual's lived experience, and should be placed in context.

Consider the target audience's risk perceptions

Analyse the different perspectives of, for example, politicians, the media, and scientists. Consider the relative importance of evidence from different domains, such as health and environment. Produce written materials and other information sources if needed.

Monitor and review each communication routinely

Keep records of decisions taken and the resulting outcomes, and identify learning points.

What are the competencies needed to achieve these tasks?

Effective risk communication requires:
- commitment to openness and acceptance of the need to share uncertainty
- familiarity with the language of risk
- understanding of risk perception
- recognition of the benefit of continual learning from experience.

Commitment to openness

Openness is a matter of principle that also produces practical benefits. Early and ongoing open and honest interaction is an essential component of effective and ethical risk communication, even though there may be strong disincentives to early openness.[6] Uncertainties should be addressed openly, if only because subsequent events may show that a risk prediction was flawed, or resulted in a contradictory message. People find it difficult to judge between experts when they disagree, and hard-won trust can be easily lost. Openness helps maintain trust in the source as well as the message.

The language of risk

The range of magnitudes of risk that we face is so wide that the extremes can be hard to grasp. A logarithmic scale can span this wide range and provide a basis for describing risk. Such a scale can be anchored to the size of human communities, or use the analogy of a 1m 'risk stick' in a certain distance[7] (Table 6.5.1). A potential problem of using risk comparisons is that people tend to overestimate the risk of death from dramatic causes such as lightning, and underestimate the risk from common problems such as stroke.

Table 6.5.1 Risk scales

Risk	Risk magnitude	Unit in which one adverse event would be expected ('community risk scale')	Distance containing one 'risk stick' 1m long ('distance analogue risk scale')	Example (based on number of deaths in Britain per year)
1 in 1	10	Person	1 m	
1 in 10	9	Family	10 m	
1 in 100	8	Street	100 m	Any cause
1 in 1,000	7	Village	1 km	Any cause, age 40
1 in 10,000	6	Small town	10 km	Road accident
1 in 100,000	5	Large town	100 km	Murder
1 in 1,000,000	4	City	1000 km	Oral contraceptives
1 in 10,000,000	3	Province or country	10,000 km	Lightning
1 in 100,000,000	2	Large country	100,000 km	Measles
1 in 1,000,000,000	1	Continent	1,000,000 km	
1 in 10,000,000,000	0	World	10,000,000 km	

Reprinted from Calman K and Royston G (1997) 'Personal paper: risk languages and dialects' *The BMJ* 315:939 with permission from The BMJ Publishing Group.

Risk perception

Risk perception involves people's beliefs and feelings within their social and cultural context. A particular risk or hazard means different things to different people, and different things in different contexts. An understanding of risk perception underpins all effective risk communication.

Framing

The way information about risk is presented affects the choices that will be made. For example, both patients and doctors prefer treatment with a 90% *survival* rate to treatment with a 10% *mortality* rate, although the measures are equivalent.[8]

Absolute and relative risk

It is important to distinguish between absolute and relative risk. The anxiety generated in the UK over the doubling of the relative risk of venous thrombosis with third-generation oral contraceptives compared with second-generation ones obscured the message that the absolute risk was minimal.[9] Estimated reduction in relative risk gives a more favourable impression of the benefits of medical treatment than reduction in absolute risk.

Acceptability

It cannot be assumed that a risk is acceptable just because it is smaller than another risk that people already take. The qualitative aspect is more important than the quantitative aspect in risk perception. Risks are usually considered less acceptable if they:

- are involuntary (e.g. genetically modified food or pollution) rather than voluntary (e.g. skiing or smoking)
- arise from a novel or human-made source
- cause hidden damage, perhaps through onset of illness many years after exposure
- pose a danger to small children or pregnant women
- are poorly understood by science
- damage identifiable rather than anonymous victims
- are close—concern diminishes with distance
- threaten a form of illness arousing particular dread (e.g. death from cancer rather than a sudden heart attack).[10]

Working with the media

Journalists are constrained by the nature of their work to convey complex information about health risks simply, unambiguously, and dramatically: 'terribly dangerous' is more newsworthy than 'perfectly safe'.[3] Public health practitioners cannot afford to exaggerate, and need to acknowledge the uncertainty of many health risks. 'Possibly dangerous' may be nearer the truth.

The following are indicators of potential media interest:

- Questions of blame.
- Secrets and 'cover-ups'.
- Conflict (between experts or experts versus the public).
- Links to sex or crime.
- Human interest through identifiable heroes or villains.
- Links with existing high-profile issues or personalities.
- Strong visual impact.
- Signal value, or suggestion that the story is a sign of further problems.[10]

Continual learning from experience

Routine and honest review of experiences and dissemination of learning points improves future risk communication.

Examples of success and failure in risk communication

Success

Singapore showed good risk communication during the outbreak of severe acute respiratory syndrome (SARS) in 2003, when the Prime Minister acknowledged that it made sense for other countries to restrict travel to Singapore until SARS was under control. In contrast, China urged people not to cancel trips to Guangdong Province, Hong Kong asserted that Hong Kong was absolutely safe and did not have an outbreak, and Toronto was slow to take action. Singapore also communicated well over the decision to close schools, which a minister explained was not on medical grounds but because teachers and doctors reported that parents were concerned about risks to their children.[12, 13]

Failure

The World Health Organization (WHO) was accused of a lack of transparency in its decisions about the swine (H1N1) flu pandemic in 2009–10, with some loss in the credibility of the organization and trust in the global public health system.[14]

Success and failure

The complex saga of bovine spongiform encephalopathy (BSE) in cattle and its possible links with a new variant of the human disease Creutzfeldt–Jakob disease (vCJD) aroused considerable public concern (Box 6.5.1).[14]

Box 6.5.1 Communicating the BSE–CJD epidemic in the United Kingdom and Australia

United Kingdom

The Ministry of Agriculture was perceived to be secretive, and was criticized for denying the possibility of a link between bovine spongiform encephalopathy (BSE) in cattle and Creutzfeldt–Jakob disease vCJD in humans. The Minister of Agriculture denied risks of human infection from BSE, but later a group of 'eminent scientists' reported that they had stopped eating British beef. Articles in the press contained estimations of wildly differing numbers of people who may have contracted vCJD.

Australia

The government provided easy access to information via the media and a telephone information line to prevent the release of contradictory information and to acknowledge that there were risks involved, although small. Coordinated media liaison between government agencies helped to promote balanced reporting by the Australian media. It is not possible to say whether the government's media strategy would have been as effective if BSE had been discovered in Australia.

Key points

Avoid secrecy, the denial of risk, and contradictory messages. Acknowledge uncertainty promptly.

How will you know if your communication about risk has been successful?

Success means reaching a shared understanding of risk with the relevant target audience. This can be assessed in terms of how close you have come to fully meeting your objectives about the purpose of the communication. Absence of outrage is usually the desirable outcome, and, as usual, this attracts little attention or gratitude!

Further resources

Further reading

Sandman PM, Lanard J. (2010). *The 'fake pandemic' charge goes mainstream and WHO's credibility nosedives.* Available at: ℜ http://www.psandman.com/col/swine-old.htm#Jun29 (accessed 24 August 2019).

Sunstein CR. (2002). *Risk and reason: safety, law, and the environment.* Cambridge University Press, Cambridge.

Zeckhauser R, Kip Viscusi W. (2000). *Risk within reason.* In: Connolly T, et al., eds, *Judgement and decision making: an interdisciplinary reader.* Cambridge University Press, Cambridge.

References

1 Morgan MG. (1993). Risk analysis and management. *Scientific American*, July, 24–30.

2 Royal Society Study Group (1992). *Risk: analysis, perception and management.* Royal Society, London.

3 Sandman PM. (1993). *Responding to community outrage: strategies for effective risk communication.* American Industrial Hygiene Association, Fairfax, VA.

4 The Presidential/Congressional Commission on Risk Assessment and Risk Management (1997). *Framework for environmental health risk management*, Final report, Vol 1. Washington, DC. Available at: ℜ https://cfpub.epa.gov/ncea/risk/recordisplay.cfm?deid=55006 (accessed 28 August 2012).

5 Morgan MG, Fischhoff B, Bostrom A, et al. (1992). Communicating risk to the public. *Environmental Science Technology*, **26**, 2048–56.

6 National Research Council (1989). *Improving risk communication.* National Academy Press, Washington, DC. Available at: ℜ https://www.nap.edu/catalog/1189/improving-risk-communication (accessed 25 August 2019).

7 Calman KC, Royston GH. (1997). Risk language and dialects. *British Medical Journal*, **315**, 939–42.

8 McNeil BJ, Pauker SG, Sox HC, et al. (1982). On the elicitation of preferences for alternative therapies. *North England Journal of Medicine*, **306**, 1259–62.

9 Calman KC. (1996). Cancer: science and society and the communication of risk. *British Medical Journal*, **313**, 799–802.

10 Department of Health. (1997). *Communicating about risks to public health: pointers to good practice.* Department of Health, London. Available at: ℜ http://www.bvsde.paho.org/tutorial6/fulltext/pointers.pdf (accessed 24 August 2019).

11 Oxford Dictionary of English (2015). 3rd edn. Oxford University Press. Oxford.

12 Sandman PM, Lanard J. (2003). Fear is spreading faster than SARS—and so it should! Available at: ℜ http://www.psandman.com/col/SARS-1.htm (accessed 6 August 2010).

13 Fung A. (2003). SARS: how Singapore out managed the others. *Asia Times*, 9 April.

14 Cohen D, Carter P. (2010). WHO and the pandemic flu 'conspiracies'. *British Medical Journal*, **340**, c2912.

Consultancy in a national strategy

Charles Guest

Objectives

This chapter introduces the steps for developing a public health strategy. It should assist you to play a constructive role as a public health consultant (see ➜ Definitions), working closely with government officials, policy advisers, and other stakeholders in the creation of a major strategy.

You will consider:

- the definition of a public health problem and the development of a strategy as a response to it
- the need to create and clarify objectives
- the need to collect and analyse relevant information
- the development of proposals and options, with appropriate balance between brevity and comprehensive detail
- the importance of a detailed study of options, which should include the case against, as well as for, the options favoured by the consultant
- consultation, one activity for improving a draft of the strategy.

Implementation and evaluation of the strategy are addressed only briefly.

Definitions

In this chapter, the word '*consultant*' is used in a general sense to indicate a provider of independent professional advice or services, on a contractual basis. An independent consultant working alongside government agencies will have a quite distinct role from that played by employees of those agencies (public servants). Also, distinguish the role played by medical specialists as salaried officers of a health service (e.g. consultants in public health medicine).

A public health strategy is an organized programme for public health activity at a local, regional, or national level. In this chapter, 'strategy' comprises the development and documentation of a specific agenda in public health. 'Policy', a more general term, refers to a course of action, expedient or prudent, that may be less adequately documented than a specific public health strategy (see ➜ Part 4).

Development of a strategy should include many of the same evidence-based steps that apply to the development of guidelines. This chapter assumes some familiarity with the latter process, and addresses additional steps and departures from the more circumscribed activity of developing guidelines.

Why is this an important public health activity?

Strategies represent tangible public health activities that often have large associated budgets. Most people are affected by a number of public health strategies. At some time, most practitioners will participate in the development or implementation of a public health strategy.

Methods, stages, and tasks of developing a public health strategy

Initial clarification

Whether or not to develop a major public health strategy is usually a decision taken at a high level in a government department after politicians, special interest groups, or journalists have moved an issue onto the national agenda. People in the public health field may have participated in that process, or their influence may have been slight. As the consultant, you should appreciate the circumstances that produced the requirement for a strategy, such as changes in:

- population health status
- health services
- perspectives in sectors other than health (e.g. environment or transport)
- financing
- economic and performance pressures
- alliances.

A potential for improvement in at least some of these variables may justify the development of a strategy. If you are contributing to early decisions about the possible development of a public health strategy, your advice should:

- provide structure to promote systematic thought and action about a major problem that has been poorly understood
- gather the minimum necessary information, with appropriate analysis
- indicate a range of options for public health action
- communicate results of this work to the client in a timely and understandable way.

Other stages may then follow

Defining the scope of the public health problem

A more formal definition will usually be required, in consultation with a reference group of senior officials and stakeholders, referred to in this chapter as the 'steering committee'. A review of the relevant epidemiology and potentially effective interventions is usually required, with reference to the current position. Public opinion survey data may be available: it should be considered early in the strategy process. (Alternatively, surveys may be planned as a research activity, noted below.)

Establishing the policy framework

This includes identifying guiding principles (including, but not restricted to, 'government policy') and appropriate key partners, and then, according to the circumstances, contributing to the:

- establishment of priorities
- definition of roles and responsibilities
- planning of research and development
- scope of intervention—tools for the strategy (e.g. guidelines, standards, regulation, legislation, grants, subsidies, tax credits)
- development of a work plan for some or all these tasks (implementation)
- planning of the evaluation (measurable achievements and other outcomes).

Consultation with stakeholders

You may play a role in the conduct of consultations, of possible relevance at several phases in the development of a strategy. These may serve to obtain critical information and to foster a receptive attitude among stakeholders to the development of a strategy. Include views from a wide range of individuals and organizations by such methods as focus groups, interviews, and written submissions.

Drafting the strategy

This will then be informed by:
- views of the government (the client) and the steering committee
- results of the consultations
- review of the literature
- your own observations.

The draft strategy is then usually subject to further consultation and revision before approval at senior levels.

Managing the strategy's development

Assemble essential resources

Influence with policy makers, peers, and the public, for any activity in public health, has to be earned and cannot be granted by fiat. You will have earned at least some influence if you play a major role in the development of the strategy. If you do not also have it, ensure that your contract[1] enables you to obtain the necessary:
- legal authority
- convening power
- information
- scientific and technical expertise (e.g. for community health assessments, epidemiology, health education campaigns, or detailed policy analysis)
- advocacy, lobbying, and public relations skills.

The development of many strategies requires simultaneous attention to inputs and process.[2]

Inputs

Management

Good management is essential for the development of a strategy, including:
- competent leadership and senior management
- effective communication of objectives and priorities by the executive to all staff
- openness that seeks positive external linkages
- performance guidelines that adequately define success and failure, with due reference to integrity and ethical standards.

Staff

Appropriately qualified and motivated staff may need to be recruited and retained. Time must be allowed for this. Training may be relevant to the development of staff in major national policy activity, but you may not have time for this during the more constrained schedule for developing a new strategy.

Information technology

Is your equipment adequate? For example, do you have enough storage and processing power and software to perform tasks efficiently in the field?

Process assessment

The public health consultant needs to rapidly identify and use networks in government (within and between portfolios) and outside it. The views of those likely to be affected should be sought actively, and carefully incorporated in the development of the strategy.

Detailed analysis should establish:
- the successes and failures of previous and related programmes
- possible consequences, intended and unintended, of options for the strategy
- the institution's capacity to implement the strategy, including the support at middle and lower levels necessary for the achievement of objectives.

Outputs

An immediate output of a strategy's development is represented by its publication. The published strategy may be accompanied by other background or technical reports.

The publication should specify:
- the problem to be addressed, with adequate analysis
- the scientific basis on which the strategy was developed
- who will do what, when.

Desirable features include:
- creative approaches to options and their implications
- coherence with other programmes and strategies
- practicality
- cogent advocacy of the preferred options.

A background report[3] could specify:
- how the need for the strategy was identified
- how the strategy was developed
- how strategy development has been funded, and the resources available for implementation
- who was responsible for development of the strategy
- who was consulted
- possible—as well as probable—outcomes of the strategy
- cost-effectiveness of solutions identified
- the time frame for evaluation.

Dissemination and implementation require much greater attention than previously accorded to many major strategies. Approaches now include:
- summaries on the internet and elsewhere
- mass media
- professional and consumer organizations
- incentives.

Engaging people in the importance of a strategy

The whole spectrum of public interests, government, and management must be engaged if a public health strategy is to achieve its goals. You should promote the development of goals that all health and other sectors can share.

As with any collaborative venture:

- seek the early involvement of partners
- identify reasons (additional to the public health concerns) for others, including representatives of industry or the private sector, to become actively involved
- expect and listen to a wide range of opinions about the development of the strategy
- obtain influential endorsements.

Potential pitfalls

Underestimating complexity

Public health strategies may require the participation of various government departments. Identify the complexity and constraints early, to ensure that resources match the task.

Inadequate communication

For example, lack of awareness and understanding of the strategy among the target population, or failure to engage all relevant professionals and sectors, may lead to people ignoring or undermining the new approach.

'We have the minister's full support'

Continued support from within government should not be assumed, even if the development of a public health strategy was the minister's initiative. Choosing not to decide about possible government projects is sometimes the preferred option for politicians and their advisers. They will sometimes go to extremes to avoid association with an initiative that could fail.

The development of a strategy distorts the political process, while the real questions remain undebated

From the citizen's perspective, this may be the worst problem. Technical issues should not be allowed to obscure political questions, while the public health consultant cannot and should not assume the responsibilities of the elected representative.

The independent consultant should avoid

- arrogance
- self-censorship (tell clients what they need to know, not what you think they want to hear)
- creating problems rather than solving them
- neglect of current clients while chasing new ones.[4]

What are the key determinants of success?

- Political support.
- Committed, adequate financial resources.
- Collaboration across sectors.
- Community participation.

How will you know when/if you have been successful?

Development of the strategy

Desirable qualities of the process and outputs of the strategy include:
- comprehensiveness
- timeliness
- responsiveness (e.g. evidence of adequate consultation with interested parties)
- clarity
- practicality
- relevance
- fairness (e.g. recommendations are balanced and equitable, as well as objective)
- cost-effectiveness (comparative costs for various solutions should be provided).

Subsequent evaluation

- Were the objectives of the strategy met?
- Did the original objectives remain in place?
- What has actually been implemented?[5]
- Has the public health problem itself changed?
- What relevance does the strategy now have?
- What were the outcomes? Were they anticipated or not?

Your role as consultant

- Was your analysis of the problem accurate?
- If the strategy was developed according to your plans, did you predict the outcome?

Also assess your efficiency (e.g. the timeliness of preparation and real costs of your input to the strategy). The measurement of effectiveness assumes a causal link between your role as a consultant and the outcome of the strategy. This will probably remain a matter only for speculation.

Conclusion

Like any project in public health, a strategy requires:
- collaboration that may be broad, while retaining sufficient focus for effectiveness
- adaptability to local and regional needs
- careful attention to the allocation and use of resources, including government and other infrastructure.

This chapter has addressed strategy as a product, while other parts of this book present strategic processes.

A parting thought

> *No matter how beautiful a strategy might be, it is wise, occasionally, to see what it achieves.*

Attributed to Winston Churchill, 1874–1965

Further resources

Further reading

Badiru AB (2012) *Project management*. CRC Press, Boca Raton.

Baylis J, Wirtz J, Gray CS, Cohen E (2007) *Strategy in the contemporary world*. Oxford University Press, Oxford.

Block P. (2007). *Flawless consulting: A guide to getting your expertise used*. Pfeiffer, Amsterdam.

Harvard Business School. (2004). *Harvard business essentials. Manager's toolkit*. Harvard Business School Press, Boston.

Kaplan R, Norton D. (2001). *The strategy-focused organization*. Harvard Business School Press, Boston.

Swayne LE, Ginter PM, Duncan WJ. (1996). *The physician strategist*. Irwin, Chicago.

Walt G. (1994). *Health policy*. Zed Books and Witwatersrand University Press, London.

References

1 Lasker RD, Committee on Medicine and Public Health. (1997). *Medicine and public health: the power of collaboration*. Academy of Medicine, New York.

2 Uhr J, Mackay K (ed.). (1996). *Evaluating policy advice: learning from Commonwealth experience*. Federalism Research Centre, Australian National University and Commonwealth Department of Finance, Canberra.

3 National Health and Medical Research Council (Australia). (2009). *A guide to the development, implementation and evaluation of clinical practice guidelines*. National Health and Medical Research Council (NHMRC), Canberra.

4 Nelson B, Economy P. (1997). *Consulting for dummies*. IDG Publications, Foster City.

5 Rist RC. (1994). Influencing the policy process with qualitative research. In: Denzin NK, Lincoln YS, eds, *Handbook of qualitative research*, pp. 545–57. Sage, Thousand Oaks.

Chapter 6.7

Effective negotiating

Leonard Marcus

Introduction

The work of public health requires frequent decision making, problem solving, and transactions among people who have different stakes in the outcome. When authority is distributed among those people—such that no one stakeholder can make a unilateral and binding decision upon others—then that outcome is negotiated.

Those negotiations involve exchanges in which the parties both contribute and glean expertise, resources, and information through the process. The tenor of the negotiation is often determined by the temperament, strategies, and desired outcomes that each of the stakeholders bring to the process. Are the negotiations collaborative or contentious? How are the parties framing the questions and issues to be resolved? What is each hoping to achieve and might there be opportunities to reap mutual benefits?

Case example

A newly elected mayor is interested in fulfilling campaign promises to develop new community-based health initiatives. The new public health commissioner is dispatched to meet with community representatives about the initiatives, programmes and support that would make a difference. A limited budget has been allocated to jump-start the process. The first meeting between the commissioner and community representatives is round one of the negotiations. Expecting a warm reception, the new commissioner is surprised by the animosity and suspicion that emerges. Promises of prior administrations were not kept. Often, small budgets made little real difference and resulted in little more than pictures and plaudits for elected officials. The community is wary of a repeat.

The commissioner listens with interest to the community representatives, recognizing that it is better to hear and work with this animosity than to dismiss it. The negotiations will be more complex than originally conceived. However, with the right approach, this could be a win for all involved.

Negotiation strategies: interest-based and positional

Broadly conceived, how one negotiates lies along a continuum, from collaborative to contentious. Often, the best strategy combines elements of both, matching tactics both to desired outcomes and the strategies and moves of other parties.

In the case example, the commissioner approaches the meeting with the intent to be collaborative, working with the community to identify priorities and develop programmes to address those health issues. By contrast, based on prior experience, the community comes with an adversarial tone. This also results from the belief that they will get more if they mount a fight, generating concern that they could politically embarrass the mayor into giving them more than they would otherwise get from the city. Strategically, it is possible to combine objectives that are ultimately collaborative with negotiative tactics that are initially contentious.

Collaborative approaches are described in the literature as 'interest-based negotiation'. This framework was originally popularized by Roger Fisher and Bill Ury in their book, *Getting to yes, OK?*, and applied to healthcare and public health in *Renegotiating health care: resolving conflict to build collaboration* (Marcus et al., 2011). When applying interest-based negotiation, the parties view one another as collaborators seeking overlapping objectives. The questions include: What are the interests of each stakeholder? What do they hope to achieve? What are their prior experiences that affect a particular negotiation? What are their concerns and fears? Recognizing the potential for achieving mutual successes, the parties discover that they each benefit by enhancing the advancement of one another. In the process, they build the confidence and the trust that can extend goodwill beyond a specific transaction.

Interest-based negotiation is particularly applicable to the work of public health and healthcare. The common overriding objective is the well-being of the community—applicable to population health objectives—or the well-being of a patient and the clinical and social criteria necessary to achieve that benefit. In the long run, integrative objectives that intend to benefit community well-being are best achieved through a process that mirrors those objectives. 'Whole image negotiation' (WIN) applies to the work and thinking of public health and healthcare. What is the big picture outcome that stakeholders hope to achieve, how can they collaborate to reach those objectives, and how do their individual interests fit together to accomplish those ends? They apply their imagination to both process and outcome, seeking agreements that reap mutual benefits.

By contrast, contentious negotiation is referred to as 'positional' or 'distributive' bargaining. In this approach, the parties stake a position and do their best to hold to that position or set of demands. They view the outcome as a win–lose distribution of resources and benefit, and their sole objective is maximizing gains for themselves and denying gains to the other sides.

Positional bargaining can prove to be toxic when applied to public health or healthcare negotiations. Yes, there are times to fight for what is right and, in those cases, the objective is to win on behalf of the population or patient. However, when the well-being of the community or clinical care is on the line, marshalling resources for the common good, prioritizing the interests of health, and seeking ways to best apply resources often results in just and balanced outcomes. When the patient or community become the battleground for the professional priorities of different specialists, professions or payment schemes, often it is the patient or community that loses and the positional professionals who gain.

Case example

How might these different methods combine over the course of a negotiation? The commissioner comes to the meeting seeking interest-based negotiation, hoping to combine the substantive and political ambitions of the mayor to support the community and the community's interests in programmes that enhance population health. By contrast, community representatives come to the meeting ready for positional bargaining, unwilling to give the mayor a political win without meaningful benefit for the community. They are ready to fight for their cause, suspicious of the commissioner and the political agenda of the mayor.

How might this negotiation be framed and reframed to find the common ground upon which the parties can achieve a mutually beneficial outcome? First, the commissioner must be ready to listen to community representatives. That listening must be sincere, open-minded and transparent. As community members recognize the genuine interest of the commissioner, they are more likely to be open to negotiating with the city to achieve heretofore unachievable initiative in collaboration with municipal officials. Once each side recognizes the potential benefits of interest-based negotiation, they commence to find how resources, services and programmes can be effectively launched with sensitivity to community concerns. By opening with a positional approach, they got the attention of the commissioner, engaged his interest and shared concerns they had about engaging with the city. By shifting toward a more interest-based and collaborative approach, they were able to open opportunities and possibilities that otherwise would have been inaccessible.

The 'Walk in the Woods': a framework for interest-based negotiation

How do you plan for, engage, and advance the processes of interest-based negotiation? One method—developed by the author and colleagues in their work with healthcare and public health complex problem solving—is the 'Walk in the woods'.

Building unity of effort among stakeholders with divergent interests requires active negotiation and, at times, conflict resolution. The 'Walk in the woods' is a systematic, iterative guide to interest-based negotiation, designed to help parties better understand their shared problem and the diverse motivations of those involved.

The 'Walk in the woods' is named for a famous case of interest-based negotiation between the US and Soviet Union during the Cold War. The intent of the process is to develop solutions that account for differing stakeholder interests. Walk participants ultimately want the outcome to succeed because they work together to understand, discover, develop, and agree to it. That shared experience generates collaborative buy-in, which is valuable when it becomes time to execute the agreement.

Conflict resolution

The 'Walk' is a four-step process for multi-dimensional problem solving, assessing interests from different angles. What is accomplished in each step prepares the stakeholders for what comes in the next step. The method guides them in finding and agreeing to a mutually beneficial solution. The differences between stakeholders can at times turn into obstructive conflict. For leaders, this conflict can limit progress toward intended outcomes. Generating agreement is key in forging progress.

- *Self-interests:* each of the parties states their objectives, purposes, experiences, and fears in a safe environment that encourages fuller disclosure. Most important: those involved genuinely *hear* one another.
- *Enlarged interests:* stakeholders list first what they agree upon and then what they disagree upon, most often finding that there is more agreement than disagreement. This reframes understanding of the issues.
- *Enlightened interests:* with the problem reframed, stakeholders brainstorm creative solutions that they had not previously pondered, opening a set of hopeful possibilities that further drives the negotiation process.
- *Aligned interests:* with a new set of options, the stakeholders negotiate toward mutually beneficial outcomes, articulating what they hope to 'get' and what they are willing to 'give' in exchange.

The 'Walk in the woods' in practice

In the case example described here, how would the 'Walk in the woods' inform the participants?

Assuming they are all aware of the methodology, in the first step, they would express and hear the interests around their negotiating table. In the self-interests step, the commissioner would hear the frustrations and experiences of the community. The community would hear the understanding of the commissioner and mayor while also beginning to understand the opportunities that could result from a partnership. With that awareness among the stakeholders, they progress to the next step: the enlarged interests. They first identify points of agreement: they all recognize the need for new programmes in the community, they agree on priorities regarding drugs, jobs, and clinical care, and they agree it is time to get beyond prior animosities. There is disagreement on specific priorities, governance, and allocations. However, there is consensus that there is enough value to warrant active exploration of new opportunities. In the enlightened interests, they brainstorm a number of new and innovative programmatic models that could engage the community, build significant community buy-in, and benchmark significant progress on health objectives shared by both the community and City Hall. In the aligned interests, they assemble together a strategic plan and timeline for moving the community health initiative forward.

In applying the 'Walk in the woods' methodology, they discovered, designed, and successfully negotiated a mutually beneficial solution that satisfied the interests of both the community and the mayor.

Negotiation and complex problem solving

What factors should you plan and account for during your negotiations?

- *Complexity:* interlocking exchanges among multiple and formally disconnected stakeholders and intermediaries. The more stakeholders, questions, and intermediaries, the more complex the negotiation.
- *Simple negotiation:* decision making that only involves and affects those directly at the table and nobody else.
- *Representational negotiation:* decisions on behalf of, or affecting, people not at the table.
- *Stakeholder map:* the web of stakeholders and their connections, people who influence, who must approve, or who are affected by the negotiation.
- *Symbolic negotiation:* what do stakeholders signify for one another around the negotiation table? If someone works for the city or lives in the community, what could that association signify for others around the table? History, experience, or the stakes involved could have symbolic value for those around the table.
- *Conflict:* an expressed difference, disagreement, or dispute among two or more people, having consequences—potentially both positive and negative—for both sides.
- *Shadow effect:* a process by which a culture of conflict or collaboration can disseminate through the management of an organization. For example, if unresolved conflict occurs at senior levels of an organization, the differences are often embedded in policies and relationships that, like a long shadow, affect working at the front lines of an organization. Conversely, when senior-level collaboration typifies relationships, it can permeate an organization, encouraging the replication of constructive working scenarios.
- *Enemy image:* this phenomena typifies highly polarized and contentious conflict. It is a conviction that the other side is out to destroy you. You, and often they, then become obsessed to defeat one another in order to avoid elimination.
- *Conflict escalation:* the growth and persistence of conflict—costs, stakes, and damage increase as the parties become increasingly obsessed with defeating the other side.
- *Framing and reframing:* the mindset that negotiators bring to the table. That mindset embodies objectives, attitudes about others, the preferred process for negotiation, and the ways that negotiators interpret and arrange new information. Often during a negotiation, the mindsets of those around the table evolve. That evolution is called 'reframing'.
- *'Expand the pie':* an expression that reflects that attitude of building a wider set of options than one side wins and the other loses. This is accomplished by adding value to the negotiation. For instance, side A gives something to side B that is high value to side B and low cost for side A (e.g. allowing side B to attend an existing seminar at no cost). In exchange, side B can introduce side A to someone who is of high value to side A. Again, this costs side B little if anything. The more added value

the parties can bring to the negotiation process, the more likely are they to find a mutually beneficial outcome.

- *'Go to the Balcony':* An expression that encourages the stakeholders to step back and watch the fray from a distance, as in a theatre, to see oneself as well as others from an objective distance and, in the process, to achieve a more objective perspective on what is really going on and how it might be reframed.
- *Best Alternative to a Negotiated Agreement (BATNA):* the point when you walk from the negotiation table, either to pursue more adversarial methods or to abandon the cause. Have your better alternative—which could include a different job offer, a different partner, or an adversarial campaign—set and ready to go when you actually walk from the table.

Conclusion

Negotiation is essential to public health practice. It is also essential to living, because we negotiate constantly with family members, colleagues, and other organizations. It is therefore both a life skill and a professional discipline worth learning and practising, both at home and at work.

Further resources

Marcus LJ, Dorn BC, Kritek P, et al. (1995). Renegotiating health care: resolving conflict to build collaboration. Jossey-Bass Publishers, San Francisco.

References

1 Fisher R, Ury W. (1981). *Getting to yes: negotiating agreement without giving in.* Penguin Books, New York.
2 Marcus LJ, Dorn BC, McNulty E. (2011). Renegotiating health care: resolving conflict to build collaboration, 2nd edn. Jossey-Bass Publishers, San Francisco.
3 Ury W. (1991). *Getting past no: negotiating with difficult people.* Bantam Books, New York.

Part 7

Organizations

Governance and accountability

Virginia Pearson

Objectives

Reading this chapter will:
- improve your understanding of the principles of governance and accountability
- help you recognize potential shortcomings in systems that may result in risk to individuals
- improve your knowledge of how to reduce risk through creating assurance that those systems are working effectively.

Definitions

Governance is the process by which an organization safeguards the interests of its stakeholders and delivers its objectives through a monitored framework of rules and procedures (from the Greek *kubernao*, to steer).

Governance may be sub-divided into different types, all commonly found within both public and private sector organizations, including:
- corporate governance
- clinical governance
- research governance
- information governance.

Each type of governance is a building block of integrated governance (see below) and assures an organization that its interests in each area are being safeguarded using tools including risk assessment and an assurance framework. Each type is described in more detail in this chapter.

Why is this an important public health issue?

To assess how well an organization is meeting its objectives, you will need to understand how those objectives are defined and how the organization assures itself that they are being met. To do this and to be able to make change and deliver improvements, you will need to know how, and how well, that organization is governed and made accountable. For example, if you are using your public health skills to assess quality of care, knowledge of the organizational approach to governance in clinical systems is essential.

As an employee of an organization, you should be aware of how your organization governs itself, how your personal work objectives contribute to the organization's, and what policies and procedures you must follow as part of your contract of employment.

Integrated governance

'Integrated governance' is a term used to describe the interlinking elements of good governance. This ensures, irrespective of the type of governance, that the underlying principle is co-ordination. One definition of integrated governance is: 'Systems, processes and behaviours by which [organizations] lead, direct, and control their functions in order to achieve organizational objectives, safety, and quality of service and in which they relate to patients and carers, the wider community, and partner organizations.'[1]

The governance function of a board or governing body relies on it defining, within the organization's overall goals, its own purpose and strategic direction. Successful integrated governance includes risk assessment and assurance, the use of 'intelligent' information, and committee structures and supporting arrangements with clear terms of reference and clarity about expected actions and behaviours.[1] Behaviours are important because the culture of the board drives that of the organization: a board-level commitment to openness, transparency, honesty, and accountability helps embed those values in the organization.

How do I assess organizational governance arrangements?

To assess how well an organization is assuring itself that it is delivering its objectives, you should check whether these core components of governance are in place:

- A defined group of people, or person, responsible for the delivery of the organizational objectives (such as a board of directors or a governing body, a chief executive officer, or an 'accountable officer').
- A written contract or similar document between the organization and its stakeholders or (for the public sector) the relevant government department (for example a Department of Health).
- Rules or procedures by which the organization operates.
- Systems for collecting, monitoring, and acting on information about the delivery of the organization's objectives.

It should be possible for any individual working within an organization to track their responsibilities through the management structure directly to the accountable officer—this is the line of accountability. When the line of accountability is unclear, an organization cannot be confident that failures in the system can be escalated to a higher managerial level, and ultimately to the board, for resolution. The process by which the board assures itself that its objectives are being delivered relies on these lines of accountability and escalation arrangements working properly.

Corporate governance

Corporate governance is the mechanism by which an organization can demonstrate that it has systems in place to manage its corporate functions, such as its financial and business processes, and its assurance systems. An example of best practice in corporate governance is contained in the seven principles of public life documented in the Nolan Report from the UK:

- *Selflessness:* holders of public office should act solely in the public interest and should not act in order to gain financial or other benefits for themselves, their family, or their friends.
- *Integrity:* holders of public office should not place themselves under any financial or other obligation to outside individuals or organizations that might seek to influence them in performing their duties.
- *Objectivity:* in conducting public business, such as making appointments, awarding contracts, or recommending individuals for rewards and benefits, holders of public office should make choices on merit.
- *Accountability:* holders of public office are accountable to the public for their decisions and actions, and must submit themselves to whatever scrutiny is appropriate to their office.
- *Openness:* holders of public office should be as open as possible about the decisions and actions they take. They should explain their decisions and restrict information only when the wider public interest clearly demands it.
- *Honesty:* holders of public office have a duty to declare any private interests relating to their public duties and to take steps to resolve any conflicts arising in a way that protects the public interest.
- *Leadership:* holders of public office should promote and support these principles by leadership and example.[2]

Putting good corporate governance in place

If you are undertaking work for an organization—for example, a health needs assessment service review, or evaluation—you should be able to define the *line of accountability* for the work through to the top of the organization.

You may need to put these structures in place to ensure adequate ownership and accountability. You will need to understand whether you or your group have *delegated authority* to make decisions. Your group could be a working or steering group that reports to a formal subcommittee of the organization's board of directors or management board. You should write *terms of reference* and include:

- the name of the group or committee
- the purpose of the group (including any delegated powers or executive function) and whether it has a defined lifespan
- membership (including who will chair the meeting)
- accountability and reporting arrangements (if the structures are complicated, a diagram may be appended to the terms of reference showing the links through to the board of directors)
- frequency of meetings
- how many members and of what type will be required to make decisions (e.g. 'three out of five members of the group, of whom one must be clinical'; this is known as the 'quorum')
- administrative arrangements (e.g. who will take the minutes; how far in advance of meetings will papers be sent out; when draft minutes will be made available after the meeting)
- when the terms of reference will be reviewed (e.g. 'annually from the date of adoption').

You should ensure that you have sufficient information to do the work required and make sensible decisions. You must also ensure that there is sufficient challenge within the group so you do not produce work that may be unduly criticized from outside.

Understanding the timescale is important because your own work plan may need to be constructed backwards from a particular date—for example, when the board receives your work. You should be clear what action you expect of board members. Will they be approving it? Does it have financial or wider service implications that need to be considered?

Good-quality minutes with clear action points will help in providing an audit trail for actions and ensuring that all tasks are completed by the deadlines set. Action points should define:

• the action to be undertaken
• who is responsible for completing the action
• the date by which the action needs to be completed.

(See also ➲ Chapters 6.1 and 6.2.)

Clinical governance

Clinical governance provides 'a framework through which [healthcare] organizations are accountable for continually improving the quality of their services and safeguarding high standards of care by creating an environment in which excellence in clinical care will flourish.'[3] Lack of effective clinical governance can have dire consequences, as shown in the two case studies below (Boxes 7.1.1 and 7.1.2).

> **Box 7.1.1 Case study A: independent inquiry into care provided by Mid Staffordshire NHS Foundation Trust, England, January 2005—March 2009, chaired by Robert Francis QC[a]**
>
> Robert Francis QC was asked by the UK Secretary of State for Health to chair an inquiry into the poor standard of hospital care at Mid Staffordshire NHS Foundation Trust during the period 2005–09. He noted that the appalling experiences of patients were the result of problems that had existed in the Trust for a long time and were known about by those in charge. A constant theme at the Trust was the perception it had lacked effective clinical governance. One comment from a witness indicates the lack of proper governance in place in the Trust:
>
> > … there was no effective governance. There was a very poor flow of information. It was very poor information anyway, there was muddled data collection, there were very complicated incomprehensible structures of committees and it was very unclear which committee reported to which or what the functions were. There were few terms of reference. I mean I could go on. (p. 244)

a) Independent inquiry into care provided by Mid Staffordshire NHS Foundation Trust January 2005 – March 2009. Department of Health, London.

> **Box 7.1.2 Case study B: The report of the public inquiry into children's heart surgery at the Bristol Royal Infirmary 1984–95, chaired by Ian Kennedy[a]**
>
> It is an account of a time when there was no agreed means of assessing the quality of care. There were no standards for evaluating performance … and it is an account of a system of hospital care which was poorly organised. It was beset with uncertainty as to how to get things done, such that when concerns were raised, it took years for them to be taken seriously.
>
> a) Kennedy I. (Chair) (2001). The report of the public inquiry into children's heart surgery at the Bristol Royal Infirmary1984–1995. CM5207(I). HM Government, London. Available at: ⌕ https://webarchive.nationalarchives.gov.uk/20090811143822/http://www.bristol-inquiry.org.uk/final_report/the_report.pdf (accessed 21 August 2019).

Good clinical governance, just like good corporate governance, relies on clarity of strategic direction, effective leadership, and reliable systems. Clinical governance has a number of components:

- Clinical effectiveness.
- Clinical audit.
- Serious incident investigation, significant event audit, and root cause analysis.
- Risk management (including learning from incident reports and complaints).
- Continuing personal development.
- User/patient experience.
- Value for money.
- Research and development.

Quality can drive change and, for healthcare organizations, clinical governance sits at the heart of the integrated governance agenda.[4] Some components of good clinical governance involve monitoring or supervision to ensure that the quality of services is measured, such as assessing the nature of the interventions, the performance of the staff carrying out those interventions, and the environment in which interventions are delivered. It should be possible to detect both good and poor performance through data monitoring. Structure, process, and outcome measures can all be useful, but you should remember that some of the most significant failures in clinical governance occur when insufficient emphasis is placed on outcome monitoring.

In addition to regular monitoring, there is a developmental aspect to clinical governance that applies the principles of continuous quality improvement to the system. The cycle of improvement occurs when repeated learning is applied to the system. This includes staff members demonstrating improvements in their own practice.

Clinical effectiveness

Clinical effectiveness is the application of evidence-based practice and relies on an understanding by the practitioner of the quality of evidence for a particular intervention or technology, and its generalisability from existing research evidence to that particular setting. Whether in the form of guidelines or otherwise, quality standards form the basis of expected good practice by professionals.

Clinical audit

Clinical audit is the process of measuring clinical practice against a given set of standards for clinical care. The audit cycle is the mechanism by which adjustments are made to achieve these standards and re-measurement can occur to demonstrate the improvement in care. Clinical audits are related to health equity audits, which measure, on a regular basis, the closure of the gap in unmet need to achieve equity in health status as defined by a health needs assessment (see ➋ Chapters 5.9 and 1.4, respectively).

Continuing personal development

Continuing personal development (CPD), which is related to clinical audit, is the process by which professionals or practitioners are able to apply their learning to ensure safe practice and drive improvements in quality. CPD includes incorporating training, education and learning from incidents or complaints. CPD, along with personal reflection and peer review, forms the basis of professional revalidation.

User/patient experience

No assessment of quality of service provision is possible without an understanding of the perception of the customer (see also ➋ Chapter 5.7). Dimensions that should be assessed include being treated with respect, being given sufficient information about the service, and whether expectations have been met in relation to the intervention and any personal care received. There are standard tools available for the measurement of patient experience, such as those produced by the Picker Institute (see , whose principles for patient-centred care are:
- respect for patients' values, preferences, and expressed needs
- coordination and integration of care
- information, education, and communication
- physical comfort
- emotional support, and alleviation of fear and anxiety
- involvement of family and friends
- continuity and transition
- access to care.

Value for money

Any judgement about the quality of a service must take into account value for money. An integrated governance approach links this directly to financial objectives.

Research and development

As part of a quality improvement process, research and development add to the knowledge base and influence future practice, improving the quality of care. Research is subject to its own governance arrangements, because there is an ethical dimension to it that requires additional safeguards (see the next section).

Research governance

Research governance involves a series of principles, requirements, and standards for research and covers how those standards will be monitored and assessed. The intention of research governance is to safeguard the public and researchers by enhancing ethical standards for research; reducing the number of adverse incidents; generating learning opportunities; promoting good practice; and forestalling any problems that might arise through poor performance or misconduct.[5]

Information governance

Information governance provides safeguards and systems for personal and patient information, and has four main components: management of information governance and assurance of

- confidentiality and data protection
- information security
- information quality.

Information governance incorporates legal frameworks for the use of information and is defined in codes of practice governing how that data is managed and accessed. It includes the storage and handling of personal and patient information, on paper or electronically, including the transfer of information by email.

Confidentiality is essential to the management of health records. Personal and private information should only be shared on a 'need to know' basis—see Box 7.1.3 for an example of how this has been handled within a health system.

Box 7.1.3 Ensuring confidentiality in the English NHS: Caldicott Guardians

In 1997, Dame Fiona Caldicott chaired a committee that made recommendations for regulating the use and transfer of person-identifiable information between NHS organizations in England and to non-NHS bodies.[a] Health organizations must have a board member (known as a 'Caldicott Guardian') who has a specific responsibility for ensuring that patient confidentiality is safeguarded. The Caldicott Guardian works strategically to support the sharing of information where it is legally and professionally appropriate to do so.[b]

The updated *Caldicott principles* are:

- justify the purpose(s) of using confidential information
- don't use personal confidential data unless absolutely necessary
- use the minimum necessary personal confidential data
- access to personal confidential data should be on a strict need-to-know basis
- everyone with access to personal confidential data should be aware of their responsibilities
- understand and comply with the law
- the duty to share information can be as important as the duty to protect patient confidentiality.

a) Caldicott F. (1997). Report of the review of patient-identifiable information. Department of Health, London.
b) Caldicott F. (2013). Caldicott review: information governance in the health and care system. Department of Health, London.

Risk and assurance

When setting organizational objectives, the responsible body—for example, the board of directors—should regularly review the risks to achieving those objectives. Risks may be strategic or operational. For the purposes of review, a process of risk assessment is used in which a judgement is made about the level of risk. This level of risk is assigned a numerical value by multiplying the likelihood and impact of the event. For example, being hit by a car when crossing a road as a pedestrian has a low probability but, if it were to happen, the impact would be high: it could result in death or serious injury. On a scale of 1–5 (where 5 represents the greater likelihood or impact), a probability of 1 and an impact of 5 would give us an overall risk score of 5.

Risk register

A risk register contains all the risks identified in relation to a project or an organization's functions. It can be ranked according to the product of the likelihood and the impact. The higher the risk score, the more important it is to put in place measures to manage or mitigate that risk. Not all risks on the risk register need to be reviewed by the highest level in the organization—it is common for a board of directors to only review risks that fall into a category of high or very high risk, relying on managers within the organization to review other risks on a regular basis and increase the risk score if necessary. This then escalates the risk to the appropriate level within the organization for review and, if necessary, management action. Effective systems of incident reporting and monitoring are also an important component of risk assurance.

Assurance framework

An assurance framework contains information about controls and mitigating factors that reduce either the likelihood or impact of a risk. An organizational control describes the part of the governance framework in place to help manage the risk, such as a monthly report to the board of directors. A mitigating factor is something that diminishes the risk (such as the installation of a pedestrian crossing). A further assessment of risk can then be made according to the revised assessment of the controls and mitigating factors of the original risk. This is defined as the residual risk, and it is the residual risk that indicates the significance of the risk to the organization. The risk threshold is the level at which risks are escalated and each organization can define its own threshold depending on how risk averse it is.

Audit committee

Audit committees are a cornerstone of good governance. They are the place where the assurance framework is reviewed, including both the risks to the organizational objectives and the management action in place to control and mitigate the risks. Internal and external auditors scrutinize aspects of the organization's functioning and produce independent assessment of compliance with legal or organizational duties and standards of conduct.

What questions should I ask about governance?

To assess governance arrangements, you can ask specific questions about an organization, service, or function:

- To which organizational objectives does the service relate?
- Where does responsibility lie, and what are the lines of accountability up to the highest level in the organization?
- How does the board assure itself that it knows what the service is doing and how well it is doing it?
- How is the service managed?
- What types of data are being reviewed?
- How reliable is this data and what does it really tell us about the service? Does it focus sufficiently on outcomes?
- How regularly does the board see this information?
- Is additional data available but not routinely reviewed, such as comparative data from elsewhere (benchmarking) or other points in time (trend analyses)?
- Have there been internal or external audits of the service, or peer reviews, that add to the knowledge we have?
- How is user or customer feedback about the service obtained, and how is this taken into account in the board's assessment of the service?
- Does the organization regularly review the risks in this area? How does it do this?
- What evidence is there of action taken by the organization to control or mitigate (that is, reduce) risks? Are they effective?

Further resources

Further reading

International Health Care System Profiles (2018). What are the key entities for health system governance? The Commonwealth Fund. Available at: ஃ https://international.commonwealthfund.org/features/governance (accessed 21 August 2019).

Kickbush I, Gleicher D. (2012). Governance for health in the 21st century. World Health Organization Regional Office for Europe: Copenhagen. Available at: ஃ http://www.euro.who.int/__data/assets/pdf_file/0019/171334/RC62BD01-Governance-for-Health-Web.pdf (accessed 21 August 2019).

Lewis M, Pettersson G. (2009). Governance in health care delivery: raising performance. World Bank policy research working paper 5074. Available at: ஃ http://documents.worldbank.org/curated/en/792741468330936271/pdf/WPS5074.pdf (accessed 21 August 2019).

NHS Leadership Academy (2013). The healthy NHS board 2013: principles for good governance. Available at: ஃ https://www.leadershipacademy.nhs.uk/wp-content/uploads/2013/06/NHSLeadership-HealthyNHSBoard-2013.pdf (accessed 21 August 2019).

Pickering Institute (tools for measuring patient experience). Available at: ஃ www.pickerinstitute.org (accessed 21 August 2019).

USAID Leadership, Management, & Governance Project (2014). Continuous governance enhancement for health systems strengthening. Series of guides for enhanced governance of the health sector and health institutions in low- and middle-income countries. Available at: ஃ http://www.lmgforhealth.org/sites/default/files/Continuous%20Governance%20Improvement%20Guide%20English.pdf (accessed 21 August 2019).

References

1 Department of Health (2006). *Integrated governance handbook: a handbook for executives and non-executives in healthcare organizations*, Gateway reference 5947. Department of Health, London. Available at: ♒ http://webarchive.nationalarchives.gov.uk/+/www.dh.gov.uk/prod_consum_dh/groups/dh_digitalassets/@dh/@en/documents/digitalasset/dh_4129615.pdf (accessed 23 August 2019).

2 House of Commons Library. (2018). Briefing paper number 04888, 21 December, page 5. Available at: ♒ https://researchbriefings.files.parliament.uk/documents/SN04888/SN04888. pdf (accessed 23 August 2019).

3 Scally G, Donaldson LJ. (1998). Clinical governance is here to stay. *British Medical Journal*, **317**, 61–5.

4 Francis R. (Chair) (2009). *Independent inquiry into care provided by Mid Staffordshire NHS Foundation Trust January 2005 – March 2009*. Department of Health, London.

5 Department of Health (2005). *Research governance framework for health and social care*. Department of Health, London.

Programme planning and project management

John Fien

Objectives

Programme management, the coordinated development, implementation, and evaluation of a series of related sub-programmes or projects, is central to the efficient delivery of all public health services. This chapter draws from the project management and programme and project evaluation fields to provide a practitioner's guide to programme planning and project management. You may find it useful to read this chapter alongside ➔ Chapter 7.3.

This chapter covers:
- the relationship between programmes and projects
- the components of effective programme and project planning
- how to develop a programme theory and logic model for a project and how to implement it
- ways of developing an evaluation strategy
- managing projects as part of a programme
- how to be an effective programme planner and project manager.

Definitions

You may hear the terms 'project' and 'programme' used to refer to any undertaking that requires people to plan tasks and organize themselves to achieve specific objectives. Indeed, 'project' and 'programme' are often used interchangeably. Here, we distinguish between them and refer to a project as a smaller and more discrete activity than a programme, which is a set of activities or projects, usually with multiple levels and work across two or more organizations. In a public health context:
- a *project* has objectives for a particular group of people in a particular place in relation to a particular health target, often using a specific strategy
- a *programme* comprises an integrated suite of related projects for a wider group of people and often across a wider region, over a longer period of time, and involving multiple strategies and projects.

A programme may have a series of projects within it, and each project may need to have its own set of objectives and activities to ensure that it is planned well and implemented effectively. Table 7.2.1 compares the features of programme and project management.

Table 7.2.1 A comparison of programme and project management

Programme management	Project management
Whole-of-organization focus	Section or department focus
Aligned to organizational strategic vision and goals	Aligned to the strategy and objectives of the programme
Focus on interdependencies between projects, and complementarity and scheduling of deliverables across projects	Focus on deliverables, milestones, and activities of a single project
Ensure consistent use of common processes across projects	Focus on application of programme processes within a single project
Risk spread across projects	Risk contained within a single project
Broad range of management, leadership, and project management skills needed	In-depth project management skills required

Programme planning

Programme planning is key to successful public health campaigns. It involves identifying the most important needs of stakeholders and partners, and determining priority responses to them. This could be a consequence of a health needs assessment (see ⮞ Chapter 1.4). When involved in such priority setting, you need to decide:

- what are the most important activities to undertake
- how to complete these activities, and the steps involved
- how much time to spend on them
- what staff, financial, and other resources will be allocated to them.

After priority setting

Following needs assessment and priority setting, the basic steps in programme planning are:

- *preparing a rationale or business case* for the programme
- *developing a goal statement or aim* for the programme
- *determining objectives* by analysing the goal statement and breaking it down into workable 'chunks' around which projects and activities can be organized; objectives describe the intended results for the targeted need and, as far as possible, should be measurable
- *designing projects* by developing and resourcing specific methods and activities for projects that will produce the desired results
- *scheduling projects:* normally the responsibility of individual project managers but programme managers are responsible for coordinating the development of project implementation plans to complement each other—the outputs and outcomes of one project can be the inputs to a related or subsequent project
- *evaluating the programme:* making plans to monitor and evaluate the programme on four levels (and sometimes more): (i) as an ongoing process within each project; (ii) as a summative or concluding assessment of each project; (iii) as an assessment of whether the

outcomes and impacts of the projects have delivered the programme goal; and (iv) as a synthesis of the appropriateness of all projects and activities in the programme.

Managing a programme

Effective programme management structures and processes enable programme directors to support project managers.[1] The first step in programme management is programme planning. Other aspects of programme management include:

- *governance:* defining roles and responsibilities; ensuring an appropriate culture across the programme team; coordinating oversight and feedback (see ➲ Chapter 7.1)
- *administration:* ensuring appropriate and rigorous processes for documenting all programme and project activities
- *financial management* and accountability
- *personnel management and programme team culture* (see ➲ Chapter 7.7)
- *infrastructure:* ensuring appropriate workspaces, technology, and related facilities are available to support the programme effort.

You will find these fundamentals of programme management discussed in more detail in programme management textbooks and other resources (see ➲ Further resources). You may find the *Gateway Review* materials produced by the UK Office of Government Commerce particularly useful.[2]

Project management

The logic of a project

Project management begins with the development of a logic model—or theory—of what will make the project work. Figure 7.2.1 shows the logical links between the original problem, your inputs, and the outputs, outcomes, and impacts you seek.

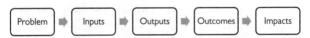

Figure 7.2.1 Steps in the logic of a project.

You need to think about evaluation at the same time you plan a project because this helps clarify:

- *inputs:* the resources of time (labour), funds, and other resources you have to invest in a project
- *outputs:* the activities you plan and implement to achieve your results and the participation level needed
- *outcomes:* the short- and medium-term results you seek. *Short-term* outcomes are usually expressed in terms of what people will learn from their participation in activities; *medium-term* outcomes are usually

expressed in terms of changes in what participants will be able to do following their learning
• *impacts:* the long-term goals you seek to attain through the project. These are usually achieved at the programme level rather than the individual project level because impacts take longer to achieve (and may not be realized during the lifespan of a project) and require the combined outputs and actions from several related projects (i.e. a programme).

Paying attention to these distinctions will help you ensure that the causal relationships between outputs, outcomes, and impacts are carefully thought through as a *hierarchy of objectives* that clarifies exactly what the project will need to achieve in each of its different phases and in what sequence.

These relationships are usually represented in a logic model, which is a visual or diagrammatic way of explaining why and how you believe a project will work as you plan, implement, and evaluate it. Figure 7.2.2 illustrates the 'logic' of a youth leadership project through a series of 'if-then' relationships.[3]

Constructing a logic model

Problem analysis

The most important aspect of problem analysis is distinguishing between the causes and symptoms of a perceived problem. Many projects fail because they focus on symptoms rather than causes. For example, one symptom of youth disengagement in a community—a growing concern in youth mental health—might be increased levels of anti-social behaviour (such as vandalism and petty crime). If a community perceives this as a problem and initiates a campaign to prevent anti-social behaviour, it risks failing to recognize root causes and may increase youth disengagement and anti-social behaviour.

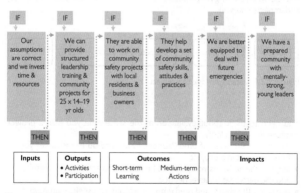

Figure 7.2.2 The 'if-then' relationships in a logic model of a youth leadership project in the area of emergency management.

Research involving social mapping, surveys, and focus groups, as well as regular and genuine community engagement, is an important tool for identifying root causes and planning activities to address them, rather than putting Band-Aids on the symptoms (see ➥ Chapter 3.4).[4, 5]

Assumptions

These logical relationships depend upon the assumptions you make about the resources available, the commitment brought by organizations and clients to a project, and your reasons for believing the planned activities will work in a particular community.

For example, the logic model in Figure 7.2.2 is for an adolescent mental health project planned in MyTown. The aim of the project is to integrate young people better into the community by engaging them in a community disaster-preparedness project. Assumptions involved include the following:

- Many adolescents in MyTown feel isolated due to the lack of opportunities for community engagement and service.
- MyTown lacks a history of organized youth volunteering despite local government surveys indicating that young people want opportunities to show community leadership.
- While MyTown is threatened by typhoons and flooding every wet season, and climate change seems to be increasing their severity, most households and small businesses lack emergency evacuation plans.
- Easily accessible, donated space can be found for project workshops and emergency services staff are available as trainers.
- Young people have time to be involved during long summer holidays.

External influences

As well as being aware of your own assumptions about a project, you need to take stock of the social, economic, and political factors in the community that can act as positive and negative external influences. This is the context of the project, and involves seeking answers to questions such as: What are the potential barriers and/or supports that might have an impact on the change you hope for? What skills and assets in the community can be drawn on? Are there policies or other factors that could affect the success of the programme?

Inputs

Project inputs include everything you need to invest in the activities essential to building the knowledge, skills and competence of participants.

Outputs

Project outputs are the staged activities for particular groups of involved people that you plan and implement. Outputs are usually expressed in terms of (i) activities, and (ii) participants. Table 7.2.2 provides examples of the wide range of activities that could be part of the outputs from a project. You can express outputs as a work plan, a set of milestones and deliverables, or a Gantt Chart. Such tools are important not only for the scoping of the project but also to facilitate effective time management by all participants.

Table 7.2.2 Project outputs: sample activities and participants

Sample activities	The range of possible participants
Survey community attitudes	Clients
Conduct a workshop	Business associations
Make a website	Service clubs
Network with others	Neighbourhood groups
Build coalitions	Government agencies
Meet with politicians	Decision makers
Train staff and volunteers	Policy makers

Outcomes and impacts

As explained above, the logic of a project requires a connection between short-, medium-, and long-term results (see Table 7.2.3). A sample logic model of the youth project described earlier is shown in Figure 7.2.3.

Table 7.2.3 The logical connections between short-, medium-, and long-term results of the youth engagement project

Short-term outcomes	Medium-term outcomes	Long-term impacts
Young people improve skills in planning, decision making and problem solving	Young people demonstrate leadership skills	We have a prepared community with mentally strong, young leaders
Young people learn about community emergency management	Young people successfully complete community safety projects	We are better equipped to deal with emergencies
Young people gain confidence in helping to protect the community	Young people are connected with, and feel valued by, their community	Community cohesion and neighbourhood social capital are developed

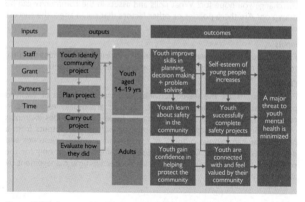

Figure 7.2.3 Logic model of the youth community engagement and emergency management project.

Project evaluation

Many people think evaluation occurs when a project has been completed. This can be the case but, to improve project and programme quality, evaluation should be planned from the outset, occur throughout the project, and provide information about progress. Projects are not linear and you need to monitor whether the logical causal links between inputs, outputs (activities and participation levels), outcomes, and impacts are performing as anticipated.

Logic models can help you to:
- match evaluation to the planned results of the project
- understand what and when to measure (e.g. are you primarily interested in process, outcomes, or both?)
- focus on obtaining important information by prioritizing where you spend your limited evaluation resources.

The purpose of evaluation is related to its focus and timing. A number of related processes can be considered part of this, including needs assessment, system evaluation, and impact assessment (see ➲ Chapters 1.4, 1.5, and 5.11).

Potential pitfalls

Several conceptual and practical issues make programme and project management more complex than you might anticipate. First, be mindful that the vernacular use of the terms 'programme' and 'project' often results in confusion when discussing specific professional activities—even books dedicated to these topics often use the terms interchangeably.

Second, a belief you should challenge is that programme planning and project management are common tasks that everyone can do. This is true in that we do use these skills every day but we are not all equally capable at planning and logistics. When you have had the benefit of working with a professional project manager a few times, you may wish you could have one as a life coach! Developing a programme theory and a logic model based on a hierarchy of objectives for a project, all held together by a strategy for evaluation, involves specialized rather than intuitive skills.

Finally, the best advice on programme planning and project management comes out of the evaluation literature. This means the most effective programme and project planning often begins with thinking first about evaluation. This is because thinking about the results you want is the only real way of planning a strategy for achieving them. As the famous baseball catcher and coach Yogi Berra once said, 'If you don't know where you're going, how are you gonna know when you get there?'

Conclusion

Getting programme planning and project management right is central to effective public health practice. Ensuring a sound and feasible hierarchy of objectives, and a logic model that relates needs assessment to inputs, activity, and participation outputs, can help achieve the desired outcomes and impacts and are logical consequences of all you do.

See ➔ Further resources for ways of using the logic model approach to project management as well as issues of project initiation and scheduling, building staff capacity for effective implementation, financial controls, process and output monitoring, and project closure.

Further resources

Further reading

Centers for Disease Control and Prevention (multiple dates) CDC evaluation resources. Available at: ℬ http://www.cdc.gov/eval/resources/index.htm#logicmodels (accessed 23 August 2019).

Watson DE, Broemeling A-M, Wong ST. (2004). *A results-based logic model for primary health care.* Centre for Health Services and Policy Research University of British Colombia, Vancouver. Available at: ℬ http://www.ncbi.nlm.nih.gov/pmc/articles/PMC2906214/pdf/policy-05-033.pdf (accessed 23 August 2019).

University of Wisconsin (2010) *Enhancing program performance with logic models.* A free introductory e-course (and downloadable PDF version also). Available at: ℬ https://fyi.extension.wisc.edu/programdevelopment/files/2016/03/lmcourseall.pdf (accessed 23 August 2019).

WK Kellogg Foundation (2017). *Step-by-Step Guide to Evaluation.* Available at: ℬ https://www.wkkf.org/resource-directory/resource/2010/w-k-kellogg-foundation-evaluation-handbook (accessed 23 August 2019).

References

1 McNamara C. (2017). *Field guide to non-profit design, marketing and evaluation.* (5th ed.) Authenticity Consulting, Minneapolis. (For more on programme planning and management, especially in public health organizations.)

2 Office of Government Commerce (OGC) (2010). *OGC Gateway Review guidance and templates.* Available at: ℬ https://www.gov.uk/government/publications/ogc-gateway-review-0-strategic-assessment-guidance-and-templates (accessed 23 August 2019).

3 WK Kellogg Foundation (2006). Logic model development guide, p.3. Available at: ℬ https://www.wkkf.org/resource-directory/resource/2006/02/wk-kellogg-foundation-logic-model-development-guide (accessed 23 August 2019).

4 Wadsworth Y. (2011). *Do it yourself social research,* 3rd edn. Allen & Unwin, Sydney/Left Coast Press, San Francisco.

5 Wadsworth Y. (2011). *Building in research and evaluation: human enquiry for living systems.* Allen & Unwin, Sydney/Left Coast Press, San Francisco.

Chapter 7.3

Business planning

Mike Gogarty

Objectives

This chapter will help you:
- understand the fundamentals of business planning
- develop an effective business case.

Why is this an important public health issue?

To be an effective public health practitioner, you need to be able to secure funding for initiatives and interventions as well as influence and support proposed developments likely to have an impact on the wider determinants of health. This includes understanding and fully participating in cross-agency corporate thinking. If public health is not central to this, it is unlikely it will be effective.

Definitions

Business planning, or operational planning, is the way an organization agrees how it will use the resources entrusted to it. The resulting plan usually covers a single financial year. New investment in the plan is often the sum of business cases that determine how and why developments should be resourced. As part of this, it is appropriate to look at opportunities for disinvestment and increased efficiencies within current spend.

What informs the content of the business plan?

An organization should have a clear strategy of which staff are aware and that has a small number of high-level outcomes defining the organization's direction of travel. Public health practitioners will ideally have contributed to the elements of this strategy that relate to public health and at the very least need to be aware of the strategy and work to secure its outcomes.

Public health teams may be part of organizations that commission services, provide services, or do both. Increasingly, they need to work through influence and in alignment or jointly with a wide range of partners. Whatever the case, business planning is crucial to determining how public health objectives are to be delivered within available, often decreasing, resources.

The business plan defines how resources will be used over the next year to deliver services, health gains, and outcomes, and is informed by:
- the strategic goals of the organization
- political considerations
- national targets, plans, and objectives the organization must deliver (mandated services)
- formally agreed prioritization that will be more or less robust
- pressures and demands arising from changing political and health needs and emerging technologies
- the resources available.

Developing a business plan

Identify 'must-do' activities

The things an organization 'must do' may arise from national political imperatives, unavoidable service pressures, or changes essential to accommodate shifting demand for services. Financial commitments made in previous years are usually considered in this growth but resource-constrained organizations need to identify non-essential areas where disinvestment may release resources for use elsewhere.

Consider the opportunity to deliver the organizational strategy

Delivering organizational strategy is of key importance but you will often find deliberate progress tempered by the need to achieve a plethora of 'must-dos' within very limited resources. Often there are few resources left to progress schemes in this area, although every effort should be made to deliver strategy and align resources. Increasingly, there is a need for public health practitioners to rethink how outcomes might be achieved. This may involve a shift from historic contracts to more joined-up approaches with other commissioners or providers, and increasingly to community-led solutions.

Work with providers/budget holders

You should share, as early as possible, information about how much money is available, what the likely cost pressures are within the system, and what developments you wish to see. A clear understanding of the organization's strategy, priorities, and financial pressure will help you develop a realistic plan. There will be a need to understand current contracts and opportunities to seek efficiencies within them or to re-procure to deliver higher-quality, innovative, and effective services.

Decide the priority of discretionary developments

The organization should have a robust, widely shared, and widely owned prioritization process that has been developed with local stakeholders. Public health is well placed to lead on this work, which will link back to the organization's strategic outcomes. This prioritization process should be applied to any proposals for development that may be funded in addition to the must-dos. These could be prioritized before you know what resources are available but often need to be revisited for a 'reality check' in the light of available funds.

Be clear about the realities of investment and disinvestment

Your business plan must be financially robust. You may encounter pressure, particularly when resources become tight, to move investment from current 'tried and trusted' (but potentially inefficient) services into more innovative cost-effective models of care. This is appropriate but you need to be clear about what resources will actually be released and how they will be used. There is a potential danger that savings will be overestimated and not realized from the service where disinvestment occurs, and that the assumptions around the promise of the new service may be optimistic. Where complex, multiple, and perhaps less-structured providers are involved, time to mobilize may be longer than initially anticipated. Similarly, in considering disinvestment opportunities, it is important that timescale and savings take into account notice periods on existing contracts.

Consult

Consulting with those likely to be involved with implementing a service change, or affected by it, is good practice. Failure to consult with the right groups or individuals may lead to barriers to or delays in the implementation and uptake of service change (see also → Chapter 7.5). In addition, consulting with stakeholders on changes in services is often required by local or national policy.

Developing a business case

Unless ideas and thoughts can be turned into health gains for the population you serve, public health will be ineffective. Skills in writing and presenting a business case are crucial to securing resources to deliver changes (see also → Chapter 6.3).

Your business case explains your proposal and why it should be funded. You will need to set out clearly how what you propose will deliver health improvement, release resources, and/or improve the quality of services. You will need to make the best case you can to secure limited resources in competition with other business cases. Your case is most likely to be successful if the following issues are addressed:

Relevance to organization

Your business case should:
- fit with the organization's strategy—and this link should be made explicit
- complement the evolving business plan in terms of delivering a national 'must-do', addressing a recognized gap in service, or improving a poor-quality service
- recognize the broader financial climate:
  - when resources are plentiful, services can be more focused on optimal target achievement and health improvement
  - when resources are tight, a focus on ideas that produce a return on investment by releasing resources elsewhere will be required.

Robustness of the case

Public health business cases should:
- define the problem to be addressed; public health practitioners are well placed to define and quantify population health needs using available data.
- be supported by evidence of effectiveness or a consideration of generalizability; this is certainly not always done and public health practitioners have a role in challenging colleagues around these issues to ensure the best use of limited resources.
- be affordable and represent value for money; this may be defined in terms of cost of adverse health events prevented or release of resources elsewhere in the system (e.g. hypertension management in older people to prevent the cost of stroke admissions to hospital or residential care).

Ownership

It is important that you have support for your case from key decision makers and opinion formers, including politicians and clinicians. The extent to which engaging with politicians plays a role in the preparation of your business case will depend on the context in which you are working. For example, much public health in England now happens in local government organizations so decisions on policy, strategy, and direction are developed and agreed by elected politicians. It is important to keep politicians, and especially the appropriate portfolio holder (in a cabinet system) and leader, sighted on the evolving thinking and developments, as well as a wider political group as appropriate. It is good practice, as well as expected, that service users are consulted, sighted, and involved in the planning, and a full and formal equality impact assessment is appropriate.

Clinical support is always helpful in developing a business case and securing funding. Depending on the subject of your business case, it may be crucial. Support may come from clinicians in primary or secondary care. You may find it helpful to identify clinical champions and ensure that they are engaged and informing the proposals.

Flexibility

To be successful, flexibility is helpful—it may be that certain points of your case require reworking, or less funding may be available than you require. Sometimes there are ways to work around such difficulties: for example, if funding is inadequate, a simple solution would be to try and negotiate a later start in the year for the full scheme with the understanding that all costs will be covered in the following financial year. You may have to consider whether reducing the size of your scheme may be possible while still realizing many of the benefits.

Content

The business case should cover:
- strategic context
- health needs
- evidence base
- objectives and benefits
- costs, capital, and revenue
- workforce implications
- timetable—what will be achieved by when
- wider impact and implementation
- evaluation and outcomes
- possible sources of funding (e.g. national bid, local funding, grants)
- risk assessment (e.g. funding, recruitment)
- procurement process
- equality impact assessment.

Appraisal of other options will also be required if major investment is undertaken.

How will you know whether you have been successful?

In the short-term, it will be clear whether you have been successful: you will have secured funding for public health work or been able to influence other proposed developments in a way likely to have a positive impact on the broader determinants of health. In the medium- or longer-term, the initiative or intervention should be evaluated in order to inform and improve future business plans.

Further resources

Bryson JM. (2018). *Strategic planning for public and nonprofit organizations: a guide to strengthening and sustaining organizational achievement*, 5th edn. Jossey-Bass, London.

De Geus A. (2002). *The Living Company*. Harvard Business Review Press, Cambridge MA.

Flanagan N, Finger J. (2003). Planning. In: *The management bible*. Plum Press, Toowong, Queensland.

Gericke C, Kurowski C, Ranson MK, et al. (2005). Intervention complexity—a conceptual framework to inform priority setting in health. *Bulletin of the World Health Organization*, **83**, 4.

Handy C. (2005). *Understanding organizations*, 4th edn. Penguin, London.

Horton C. (2018). *Healthcare: Planning and management*. Hayle Medical, London.

Orton SN, Menkens AJ, Santos P. (2011). *Public health business planning: a practical guide* (1st edn.) Jones & Bartlett Learning, New York.

Chapter 7.4

Working in teams in public health

Shannon L. Sibbald, Anita Kothari, Malcolm Steinberg, and Beverley Bryant

Objectives

This chapter will help you:
- define types, characteristics, and roles of teams in the context of public health
- identify common challenges experienced by teams
- consider strategies to foster high-performing teams
- Suggest methods to assess, evaluate, and improve team effectiveness.

Why is this an important public health issue?

Successfully tackling today's complex population and public health challenges within a context of finite resources requires specific competencies to perform effectively in interprofessional teams.[1] This can demand broad and sophisticated collaborative efforts, frequently requiring public health practitioners to work in teams beyond the health sector. Participating in teams may take you outside your domain of control and comfort zone. Collaborations may lack a common purpose and/or basis for problem solving and decision making, made more complicated by power differentials and dissimilar cultures of practice. However, research has shown that teams that work well can lead to improved client care and improved public health interventions.[2] Supportive and well-functioning teams can protect against staff exhaustion, mitigate tensions, and help manage conflicts. Cohesive and integrated teams maximize their collective efficacy so that team members experience better outcomes.[3, 4]

What is a team?

The defining characteristic of a team is that it is a group whose members share a common goal or purpose.[5] Partnerships, networks, and collaborations share a purpose or a vision but, unlike teams, do not necessarily have a shared mandate that expresses formal or informal requirements (and/or expectations) to achieve this. Team members have mutual accountability and commitment to a common purpose and the collective output.[6]

Teams allow collaboration among multiple disciplines even when members are not co-located.[7] Teams can support knowledge creation, knowledge sharing, and knowledge management. Teams are often embedded in an organizational context. As such, a team can be an arrangement within an individual organization or as part of a partnership (see ➋ Chapter 7.5), network, or collaboration.[8] Teams can be permanent or temporary (i.e. dissolve once the task is accomplished) and often indicate some formality that include terms of reference and governance procedures. There are three broad types of teams: those that recommend (task force, project), those that create or carry out tasks (operations, marketing), and those that run, direct, or guide (leadership),[6] and in public health practice you are likely to encounter all three.

Box 7.4.1 gives an example of the constitution and role of a team in public health.

> **Box 7.4.1 Introducing Peel Public Health**
>
> Peel Public Health (PPH) is a large health unit in Ontario, Canada, that provides public health programmes and services to a population of around 1.4 million people. PPH organizes most of its workforce into teams that come together to solve complex public health problems.
>
> For example, the PPH family health division looked at population-level data to understand the issues facing parents and children in the community. They developed a team, comprised of public health nurses, analysts, health promoters, and leadership staff to collaborate with epidemiologists from a centralized population health assessment group to unpack the data, analyze its meaning and consider a range of interventions. This combined team also developed knowledge translation workshops to assist all staff in family health to better understand the main findings. Using this team-centred approach, family health staff gained valuable knowledge about the population they served and built knowledge and skill in all their members.

Characteristics of teams in public health

Public health teams are complex: multiple professions, skills, service organizations, and management structures can have an impact on team development and effectiveness.[9] You may find working in interdisciplinary teams both beneficial (novel ideas, differing perspectives) and disadvantageous (different languages, valuing different forms of evidence).[10, 11] A truly public health-centred approach embraces the concept of collaboration[12] and working across systems (e.g. consider the many governance levels and stakeholders involved in work on the built environment).

While the literature on teams in public health is expanding, research has been hindered by lack of common definitions and frameworks with which to understand,[13, 14] compare,[15] and implement[16] team-based approaches. Much of what has been written about partnerships in public health has focused outward, on understanding how public health works together with other organizations,[17–21] rather than on the achievements of, and challenges faced by, public health teams in their efforts to realize shared outcomes.

In general, successful teams share common attributes including commitment to team success and shared goals, interdependence, interpersonal skills (openness, honesty, trustworthiness, supportiveness, and respectfulness), open communication and positive feedback (which includes active listening), appropriate team composition (role clarity), and commitment to team processes, leadership, and accountability.[22] A review for the US National Academy of Medicine[23] highlighted five principles that characterize the most effective high-functioning teams in health settings:

• *Shared goals:* the team works to establish shared goals that reflect shared priorities, and that can be clearly articulated, understood, and supported by all team members.

- *Clear roles:* there are clear expectations for each team member's functions, responsibilities, and accountabilities that optimize the team's efficiency and make it possible for the team to take advantage of division of labour, thereby accomplishing more than the sum of its parts.
- *Mutual trust:* team members earn each other's trust, creating strong norms of reciprocity and greater opportunities for shared achievement.
- *Effective communication:* the team prioritizes and continuously refines its communication skills and approaches; it has consistent channels for candid and complete communication that are accessed and used by all team members across all settings.
- *Measurable processes and outcomes:* the team agrees on and implements reliable and timely feedback on successes and failures in both the functioning of the team and achievement of the team's goals; these are used to track and improve performance immediately and over time.

Development of a team

Teams may be mandated by organizations or come together more organically to collaborate on a specific task or goal. Classical models of team formation suggest that teams go through stages in development (forming, norming), productivity (performing), and maintaining or sustaining (or, if the team is non-permanent and the outcome is achieved, dissembling or adjourning).[24] In practice, team formation is rarely linear and teams often enter and exit the process at any time. Challenges include team attrition (members leaving or being 'reassigned') and enculturation of new members (either required to replace previous members or to bring in skills required by the team). Optimal team size is often task dependent. When developing a team, sometimes team performance can be optimized by avoiding having too many people involved.[25] Teams working on complex tasks, such as those in public health, often benefit from a more heterogeneous mix (but this is also task dependent).[26] Furthermore, teams have been shown to make team members feel more satisfied and bolster confidence, irrespective of actual team performance.[27] Systematic and thoughtful team development can contribute to the effectiveness of the team—and bear in mind that, for some tasks, involving a team may not be the most effective approach.

Box 7.4.2 provides an example of the successful development of a public health team.

> **Box 7.4.2 A clear focus is essential to effective team development**
>
> Clear objectives are essential for effective team performance. Peel Public Health's oral health teams recently underwent significant change in both the structure and delivery of their oral health programmes and services. These changes were preceded by a thorough analysis of the characteristics of the population, identification of effective oral health interventions (e.g. the placement of dental sealants on permanent molars of children in at-risk segments of the population), and detailed consideration of how to effectively address the oral health of over 250,000 school-aged children. These decisions required staff to work together in different ways, to adapt to their new roles, and to adopt new duties outside their comfort zones. Clear goals and objectives, together with skilled leaders who addressed the interpersonal and team-level challenges of significant change, paved the way for reorganization of both the team structure and oral health programmes and services. Staff at all levels grew to feel confident in their new roles and could see how their work contributed to improving the oral health of Peel residents.

Challenges in teams and strategies to overcome them

A truly effective team functions well through team processes and team outcomes but you may find it challenging to navigate between the two. According to Millward & Jeffries (2001),[28] 'good teams monitor their performance and self-correct; anticipate each other's actions or needs and co-ordinate their actions' (p. 277). That is, a high-performing team not only successfully achieves the outcome but also succeeds in team processes as well. In contrast, a team is likely to be seen as unsuccessful if intended outcomes are not met. Challenges might come from outside (e.g. lack of support from superiors, outdated policies, and external contextual influences upon individuals) or inside (e.g. domination by powerful subgroups, hidden conflicts, and absenteeism).

Smith (2004)[29] identifies five reasons teams may fail: lack of a clear and compelling vision and purpose; team members who do not hold each other accountable; lack of shared leadership; processes that are ineffective or not well established; and too much or too little autonomy. To avoid these problems, Smith recommends seven strategies:

- Provide an inspiring, meaningful reason for working together for team members and identify clear but adaptable roles and responsibilities.
- Make building relationships a primary goal.
- Establish norms of accountability and trust and having team members openly discuss their expectations of one another.
- Create effective team processes.
- Include shared leadership in the team vision and purpose statement, and include the practice of shared leadership in roles and responsibilities,

- Put in place measurable performance objectives,
- Establish clear group norms for making decisions as a group and resolving team conflict.

Teams, and the way they are constituted, also need to be flexible and adaptable to changing circumstances. Box 7.4.3 gives an example of how this may be achieved.

> **Box 7.4.3 Ensuring teams are fit for the contemporary public health challenges**
>
> In Peel Public Health (PPH), the composition of public health teams has evolved over the past ten years: in particular, increased diversification of knowledge and skills has been essential to increase capacity across the full scope of public health practice. These transitions in team composition have required considerable attention to the development of role clarity during times of change, courageous conversations that build trust and the focus on shared goals that lead to measurable outcomes. PPH instituted specific training for change management at the level of the middle manager in order to facilitate these transitions. At every opportunity, leaders are encouraged to ask: 'What skill set does this team need in order to improve public health in our community?'

Evaluating team performance

You can evaluate team performance in three ways: (i) individual contribution to the team, (ii) team process level (or group dynamics), and (iii) team results (or outcomes). Team effectiveness is a function of team characteristics (composition and size), nature of the task (goals and interdependence) and context (culture and relationships) coupled with supporting team processes (i.e. leadership and communication).[30] Successful teams have effective leaders. Team leadership capacity requires separate competencies, essential to the success of public health teams.[31]

There are very few tools developed to specifically evaluate public health teams. There are many tools available online (for a fee, or free of charge) that have their roots in the business sector. However, most tools have not been used in healthcare settings, it is not often clear how the tools were developed because most have a weak evidence-base (if any at all), and very few have been tested for reliability or validity. Most team effectiveness tools are based on teams that work together in one setting or sector that have little fluidity or change in membership,[32] and that have the ability to assess behavioural dimensions (communication[33] or group cohesion).[34]

Most tools have limited practicability (i.e. do not explain what to do after the evaluation) and instead function to create awareness of team-based components such as structure and support.[35] While some tools provide promise for meaningful use, review caution against using any tool 'as is' and suggest more research is needed to adapt tools to meet the needs of the current team landscape.[18, 24, 36] This is especially true in the case of public health teams. However, some partnership evaluation tools offer potential for team evaluation in public health. A report investigating partnership effectiveness found 'synergy' (or the degree to which partners successfully combine perspectives, knowledge, and skills), along with the ability to identify problems and highlight strengths, as important to success.[37]

Conclusion

Working in teams presents both opportunities and challenges. When they have a clear purpose and vision alongside strong organizational support and leadership, teams can (and do) improve outcomes for clients and communities. Public health is interdisciplinary: working in teams is part of the ethos of the field and invariably we will continue to see more complex health issues requiring teamwork and inter-disciplinary contributions.

References

1 Council on Education for Public Health. (2016). Accreditation Criteria Schools of Public Health. Available at: M https://ceph.org/assets/2016.Criteria.pdf (accessed 21 August 2019).

2 Weaver SJ, Dy SM, Rosen MA. (2014). Team-training in healthcare: a narrative synthesis of the literature. *BMJ Quality & Safety*, (February), 1–14.

3 Leggat SG. (2007). Effective healthcare teams require effective team members: defining teamwork competencies. *BMC Health Services Research*, 7, 17.

4 Willard-Grace R, Hessler D, Rogers E, et al. (2014). Team structure and culture are associated with lower burnout in primary care. *Journal of the American Board of Family Medicine* (JABFM), 27(2), 229–38.

5 Salas E, DiazGranados D, Klein C, et al. (2008). Does team training improve team performance? A meta-analysis. *Human Factors*, 50(6), 903–33.

6 Katzenback JR, Smith, DK, et al. (2005). The discipline of teams. Available at: https://hbr.org/2005/07/the-discipline-of-teams (accessed 21 August 2019).

7 Allen NJ, Hecht, TD. (2004). The "romance of teams": Toward an understanding of its psychological underpinnings and implications. *Journal of Occupational and Organizational Psychology*, 77(4), 439–61.

8 Kozlowski SWJ, Bell, BS. (2003). Work groups and teams in organizations. In: Borman WC, Ilgen DR, Klimoski RJ, eds, *Handbook of psychology* (Vol. 12): *Industrial and Organizational Psychology* (pp. 333–75). Wiley, New York.

9 Nancarrow SA, Booth A, Ariss S, et al. (2013). Ten principles of good interdisciplinary team work. *Human Resources for Health*, 11(1), 19.

10 Winters S, Magalhaes L, Kinsella E, et al. (2016). Cross-sector service provision in health and social care: an umbrella review. *International Journal of Integrated Care*, 16(1).

11 Zwarenstein M, Goldman J, Reeves S. (2009). Interprofessional collaboration: effects of practice-based interventions on professional practice and healthcare outcomes. *Cochrane Database Syst Rev*, 3(3).

12 Dion X. (2004). Turning strategy into action: a multi-disciplinary team approach to public health working. Available at: https://www.ncbi.nlm.nih.gov/pubmed/15150485 (accessed 21 August 2019).

13 Körner M, Bütof S, Müller, C, et al. (2016). Interprofessional teamwork and team interventions in chronic care: a systematic review. *Journal of Interprofessional Care*, 30(1), 15–28.

14 Lemieux-Charles L, McGuire WL. (2006). What do we know about health care team effectiveness? A review of the literature. *Medical Care Research and Review*, 63(3), 263–300.

15 Reeves S, Lewin S, Espin S, et al. (2011). *Interprofessional teamwork for health and social care* (Vol. 8). John Wiley & Sons.

16 Baker DP, Gallo, J. (2013). Measuring and diagnosing team performance. *Improving patient safety through teamwork and team training*, 234–8.

17 Graham R, Sibbald, SL, Patel P. (2015). Public health partnerships. *Healthcare Management Forum*, 28(2), 79–81.

18 Hayes SL, Mann MK, Morgan, et al. (2012). *Collaboration between local health and local government agencies for health improvement*. The Cochrane Library.

19 Mitchell SM, Shortell SM. (2000). The governance and management of effective community health partnerships: a typology for research, policy, and practice. *The Milbank Quarterly*, 78(2), 241–89, 151.

20 Sibbald S, Kothari A. (2012). Partnerships in public health: lessons from knowledge transla-tion and program planning. *Canadian Journal of Nursing Research*, 44, 94–119. Available at: ℗ http:// www.ingentaconnect.com/content/mcgill/cjnr/2012/00000044/00000001/art00007 (accessed 21 August 2019).

21 Smith KE, Bambra C, Joyce KE, et al. (2009). Partners in health? Asystematic review of the impact of organizational partnerships on public health outcomes in England between 1997 and 2008. *Journal of Public Health*, 31(2), 210–21.

22 Tarricone P, Luca J. (2002). Employees, teamwork and social interdependence—a formula for successful business? *Team Performance Management: An International Journal*, 8(3/4), 54–9. doi: 10.1108/ 13527590210433348

23 Mitchell P, Wynia M, Golden R, et al. (2012). Core principles and values of effective team-based health care. National Academy of Medicine discussion paper.

24 Tuckman BW. (1965). Developmental sequence in small groups. *Psychological Bulletin*, 63(6), 384.

25 Stewart GL. (2006). A meta-analytic review of relationships between team design features and team performance. *Journal of Management*. Available at: ℗ http://journals.sagepub.com/doi/abs/10.1177/0149206305277792 (accessed 21 August 2019).

26 Balkundi P, Harrison D. (2006). Ties, leaders, and time in teams: strong inference about network structure's effects on team viability and performance. *Academy of Management Journal*, 49(1), 49–68.

27 Allen NJ, Hecht, TD. (2004). The "romance of teams": Toward an understanding of its psychological underpinnings and implications. *Journal of Occupational and Organizational Psychology*, 77(4), 439–61.

28 Millward LJ, Jeffries N. (2001). The team survey: a tool for health care team development. *Journal of Advanced Nursing*, 35(2), 276–87.

29 Smith S. (2004). The 5 reasons business teams fail. Available at: ℗ http://actionplan.com/pdf/SidSmithart.pdf (accessed 21 August 2019).

30 Fried BJ, Topping S, Edmondson AC. (2011). Teams and team effectiveness in health services organizations. In: Burnes L, Bradley E, Weinder B, eds, *Shortell and Kaluzny's health care management: organization design and behavior*, 6th edn. Delmar Cengage Learning, Clifton Park, NY.

31 Setliff R, Porter JE, Malison M, et al. (2003). Strengthening the public health work-force: three CDC programs that prepare managers and leaders for the challenges of the 21st century. *Journal of Public Health Management Practice*, 9, 91–102.

32 Brannick MT, Roach RM, Salas E. (1993). Understanding team performance: a multimethod study. *Hum Perform*, 6, 287.

33 Anderson NR, West MA. (1998). Measuring climate for work group innovation: development and validation of the team climate inventory. *J Organ Behav.*, 19, 235–58.

34 Alexander JA, Lichtenstein R, Jinnett K, et al. (2005). Cross-functional team processes and patient functional improvement. *Health Serv Res.*, 40, 1335–55.

35 Sibbald S, Kothari A. (2012). Partnerships in public health: lessons from knowledge translation and program planning. *Canadian Journal of Nursing Research*, 44, 94–119. Available at: ℗ http://www.ingentaconnect.com/content/mcgill/cjnr/2012/00000044/00000001/art00007 (accessed 21 August 2019).

36 Østergaard HT, Østergaard D, Lippert, A. (2008). Implementation of team training in medical education in Denmark. *Postgraduate Medical Journal*, 84(996), 507–11. Available at: ℗ http://dx.doi.org/10.1136/qshc.2004.009985 (accessed 21 August 2019).

37 Weiss E, Anderson R, Lasker, R. (2002). Making the most of collaboration: exploring the relationship between partnership synergy and partnership functioning. *Health Education and Behavior*, 29, 683–98.

Partnerships

Julian Elston

Objectives

This chapter should help you understand:
- what is meant by partnership
- how national and local contexts influence partnership
- what processes and interactions are key to partnership success
- how to develop partnership and achieve collaboration
- key elements of success and the signs of a faltering partnership.

Why is this an important public health issue?

Working in partnership has become central to public policy in many countries in recent years. Policy documents, directives, and dictates have encouraged, if not mandated, health organizations, local government, and the voluntary sector to work together to improve population health, reduce health inequalities, and enhance the quality of health and social care services, and partnership working has become a standard way of working in public health.[1]

Often partnership is seen as an alternative to bureaucratic or market modes of delivering services. It is seen as having the potential to improve the coordination, effectiveness, and efficiency of services while increasing their responsiveness to users' needs and, when working well, to generate novel approaches to 'wicked' public health problems. Furthermore, it is argued, such participative approaches to decision making enhance the legitimacy of solutions and provide greater local accountability.[2] (See also ➔ Chapter 3.4.)

Many organizations and agencies have an important role to play in improving population health but may not recognize their role or see it as within their remit. Services provided by government-funded agencies are often designed around the needs of those agencies rather than users or populations, with the result that services are fragmented and unresponsive. Partnership working recognizes that solutions to health problems are complex and cross-cutting in nature, so cannot be solved by any single organization.[1] It provides a means of joining up perspectives and resources from different policy arenas, organizations, professions, and communities in a coordinated and collective effort to improve health outcomes.

It is often assumed that partnership is a good thing[1] but the extent to which partnership working contributes to better population health is uncertain because there have been few well-designed evaluations that link how well a partnership is functioning (process) to its impact on health outcomes at a service user or population level, and the findings of the studies that have been done are equivocal.[3] The evidence base that does exist focuses on process (and interaction), often exploring the influence of structure and the wider context on how partnership works, and is often limited by the lack of clarity over its use of terms and concepts.[4, 5]

Definitions

Partnership

- is a mutually beneficial process by which stakeholders or organizations work together towards a common goal
- involves the joint development of structures in which decisions are made, resources shared, and mutual authority and accountability exercised.

Partnerships differ with respect to the number and type of partners involved, the centrality of common goals to member organizations, the formality of structures and governing rules, the scope and quantity of resources mobilized, the degree of information sharing and reframing of the problem under scrutiny, the type of decision making, the extent of each partner's influence over decisions and the types of outcome attained. Table 7.5.1 sets out criteria by which to distinguish different forms of partnership.

The objectives of partnership can be considered in terms of outcome and process objectives, and it is important that objectives are clear from the outset so that appropriate structures and processes are developed to support them. Failure to do so may create unrealistic expectations, lead to dysfunctional relationships, weaken commitment, and undermine performance. It has been argued that structure is less important to the success of partnership than purpose, but absence of good links between strategic and operational levels can have a negative impact on outcomes.[5]

Table 7.5.2 compares the suitability of different forms of partnership with delivery of different types of outcome and process objectives.

Table 7.5.1 Types of partnership working by key dimensions

Type of partnership	Co-existence / competition	Networking	Co-operation	Co-ordination	Collaboration
Decision-making	Independent	Consultative	Consultative	Joint (possibly unequal)	Participative (equal)
Threat to autonomy	No threat	Little threat	Little threat	More threatening	Significant loss
Resource sharing	None	Limited—on individual basis	Relatively few—requires lower grade officers	More resources involved—requires higher grade officers	Resources pooled—requires senior officers
Information/ knowledge sharing	Independent use	Some knowledge sharing	Some knowledge sharing	Sharing and joint interpretation	Sharing and reframing of problem
Rules and formality	Own rules	Informal; based on cultural norms	No formal rules	Some formalization of rules	Formal rules agreed
Structural linkages	None or market price signals	Transient, as required	Few linkages in areas	Some vertical or horizontal linkages	Stronger vertical or horizontal linkages
Goals congruity	Own goals	Own goals although some crossover	Own goals although some crossover	Overlapping goals and aligned activities	Joint goals and supporting activities
Organizational vision	Individual perceptions	Some shared perceptions	Some shared perceptions	Shared perceptions	Joint perception
Mutual activity	Non-mutual activity	Some mutual activity	Some mutual activity	More mutual activity	Novel, mutual activity

Table 7.5.2 Comparison of the suitability of different partnership forms for achieving different partnership objectives

Purpose	Partnership form			
	Networks	Cooperation	Coordination	Collaboration
Outcome objectives				
Information exchange or joint agreements	✓	✓✓	✓✓	✓✓✓
Developing a shared task or vision			✓✓	✓✓✓
Advancing a novel solution			✓	✓✓✓
Process objectives				
Empowerment and participation		✓	✓	✓✓✓
Power relationships		✓	✓	✓✓✓
Addressing conflict			✓	✓✓✓

Key: ✓✓✓—well suited; ✓✓—moderately suited; ✓—less well suited; blank—not well suited.

Types of partnership

Partnerships may be strategic or operational and typically involve individuals or service users, teams, professional groups, health and social care providers, and health and well-being organizations. They may:

- develop a project to tackle a specific health concern
- formulate a joint local health and well-being policy or strategy
- improve the coordination of information and human resources between providers
- improve the supply of goods and materials to support services
- improve service quality and responsiveness to users' needs
- coordinate and govern a number of smaller partnerships.

Motivation for partnership working

Individuals, agencies, and organizations should recognize two things before engaging in partnership:

- Their interdependence in tackling a health problem.
- The potential mutual benefit arising from working together.

Without these, commitment to working in partnership will be weak because partners cannot see the relevance to their work, only the immediate costs associated with participating. For this reason, voluntary, 'bottom-up' partnerships tend to be stronger than those mandated by government, where partners are obliged to participate.[1] Reluctance to engage can be mitigated by the provision of incentives such as funding or greater freedoms and flexibilities to act, or sanctions for non-compliance such as reduced financial autonomy.

Influence of national context on partnership

The context of partnerships is important. Health service and local government departments, for example, are subject to external influences at a national level with the potential to affect not only the structure and functioning of a partnership but also its outputs and outcomes.[5] Partners need to be aware of the impact of four influences: policy, resource flows, incentives and sanctions, and performance management.[6]

Policy

National policy is often incoherent, multi-themed, and fluid, and thus can be detrimental to working in partnership. It is not unusual for government departments to work in 'silos' (rather than in partnership) and to develop conflicting policy goals or multiple policy priorities. The focus of policy may shift as politicians respond to emerging social issues, leaving partners struggling to join up policy imperatives and targets or to decide which policies should take priority and which are no longer relevant.

Resource flows

The conditionality of resources, particularly (additional) funding, may influence the focus and outcomes of partnership. Ring-fenced funding may protect resources from redirection but restrict the funding of innovative initiatives outside the remit of what would be considered 'health'. Pressure to spend funds within a financial year may lead to hasty decision making while short-term funding may result in difficulties in recruiting and retaining suitable staff. Funding is rarely available to support partnership itself.

Incentives and sanctions

Incentives and sanctions can enhance or undermine motivation to work in partnership and distract from shared aims. Relaxing organizational statutes or providing additional resources may entice more agencies into partnership but this risks attracting partners whose only interest is getting a piece of the funding pie, may require lengthy negotiations between multiple competing interests, and can lead to tokenistic involvement.

Performance management

Following the decentralization and privatization of many state services, some governments have turned to performance management as a means to influence the implementation of their policies by local agencies (see ➜ Chapters 4.2 & 4.3). In the context of partnership working, the scope, degree, and alignment of performance monitoring by different organizations may detract resources (time, effort, and energy) away from the partnership, often at the expense of relationship building, problem solving and decision making. The pressure to report performance at set times can come at the expense of developing creative solutions.

Influence of local context on partnership

At a local level, you will find that partnerships are subject to five contextual influences that affect their development and functioning, and potentially their outputs and outcomes.[6]

Professional

Partnership working often involves multiple professional groups. Each will have its own perspective on health that shapes how its members think about an issue, what solutions are proposed, and how this fits with traditional roles. The opinions of some professional groups may carry greater weight than others in discussions because of their higher status. Initial educational work with partners may be required to ensure that partners understand why they have been invited, what they can contribute, and how they stand to benefit.

Cultural

Public, private, and voluntary sector organizations often have different cultures of management, decision making, and public involvement. Health service organizations typically a have top-down, managerial, or professional decision-making structure. Local government organizations are influenced by local politicians in relation to deciding priorities and allocation of resources. Officers involved in partnership, although more used to democratic decision-making processes, may have limited capacity to act without consultation. Political elections can also result in a change in political leadership and policies, which may or may not favour partnership or its aims. Voluntary sector organizations, on the other hand, tend to have flat decision-making structures that facilitate consultation with their memberships. Partners need to understand that decision making may be slow, referential, and protracted. Otherwise, expectations will be unrealistic and frustrations will arise.

Financial

Partners often have different financial arrangements and planning cycles. This can be challenging when determining budgets (which may be subject to different financial pressures and change) and planning actions. Larger, statutory organizations are more likely to absorb the human and financial costs of working in partnership while smaller, voluntary sector organizations may struggle, limiting their capacity to participate fully.

Relational

Besides working in partnership to tackle public health issues, local organizations may have other relationships that make them dependent on each other for resources (i.e. goods and services). The symmetry of resource dependencies can influence how partners interact. The relative size of the resource exchange to the organization and the presence of alternatives may weaken a partner's influence and lead them to avoid conflict for fear of jeopardizing future access to resources. Voluntary sector organizations may be particularly vulnerable to this influence.

Structural

Organizations have different boundaries, procedures, and financial arrangements. In some locations, these are coterminous. In others, typically rural areas, they do not coincide. This may result in many more organizations having to be involved in the partnership, each with their own priorities and timelines. This can hinder consensual decision making, particularly the development of a shared vision and joint actions.

Process in partnership

You will find that partners are constrained by their own organizational contexts and have their own priorities and interests, such as those outlined above. Understanding the outcomes of partnerships means understanding three elements of process in partnership:[7]

- *Cognitive process:* developing a joint appreciation of the problem (possibly involving reframing perspectives and understanding) and developing appropriate solutions.
- *Social process:* understanding the social order of the group (i.e. the perspectives and interests of each partner [individually, organizationally, and professionally] and the resources they bring.)
- *Managerial process:* directing group interaction in a systematic and purposeful way to achieve the aims of the partnership. This will involve jointly agreeing ground rules and governance mechanisms as well as employing problem-solving techniques (such as brainstorming or more sophisticated techniques from operational research and systems science).

The nature of interaction

To work effectively in partnership, you need to be able to influence others in relation to what should be done, who is going to resource it, and how. Understanding how partners interact and how relationships develop is key to progress. In particular, you need to understand the nature and influence of power, authority, and trust in partnership and their effects on decision-making.[5]

Power

There are three dimensions of power, each of which can be active in partnership.[8] The *first dimension* of power is influencing others to do what you want them to do, without coercion. The *second dimension* is limiting membership and/or what is discussed in partnership. The *third dimension* relates to wider social and economic forces that condition thinking about what could and should be done. Box 7.5.1 illustrates how and when power can manifest itself in partnership.

There are three elements to the first dimension of power that need to be understood:[9]

- *Formal authority:* a partner's legitimate right to convene a partnership and influence decisions crucial to the partnership without directing

---

Box 7.5.1 Examples of power in partnership

- Who is invited or excluded from the partnership?
- Who sets the agenda?
- Which issues are 'kept off' the agenda?
- How issues are conceptualized or framed and the language used.
- Who decides how resources are allocated and who does not?
- How decisions are made.
- What type of solutions are developed and whose interests are served (individual, professional, organizational)?
- How partnership arrangements evolve over time.

---

others. This is particularly evident in partnerships mandated by government.

- *Control over critical resources:* partners that provide critical resources can exert control over their use; these organizations can often dictate terms, the nature of interaction, and the type of partnership developed.
- *Discourse legitimacy:* partners that speak on behalf of others (e.g. users' organizations or community groups) often have discourse legitimacy—that is, their influence comes from being seen as a legitimate voice of marginalized stakeholders or of a specialist body of knowledge.

How partners use these elements determines the structure and process of partnership and the nature of interaction. In partnerships with diffuse resources or symmetrical resource dependencies, decision making is more likely to be marked by negotiation, compromise, and resource pooling. If critical resources rest solely with one partner or dependencies are un-balanced, debate may be biased and lead to more powerful partners dominating the agenda (rather than jointly owning it).[1] This may lead to strife, disillusionment, and withdrawal from the partnership (particularly if dependencies are unbalanced or weak).

Trust

Trust is the degree of assuredness that partners will do what they say they are going to do, and do it well. You must nurture trust for a partnership to perform.[10] Without trust, partners may fear that others will exploit them opportunistically and this can lead to defensive behaviour. Lack of certainty or ignorance about how others will behave may lead to partners taking fewer risks, and can have an impact on the development of innovation.

There is rarely a complete absence of trust between partners but levels may be low when a partnership is formed, particularly if partners have had a poor experience of working together previously.[1] However, some part-ners may bring *goodwill trust* (an open commitment to keep to promises) or *competence trust* (a willingness to accept that others will not only complete their actions but do so to a required standard). Organizational reputation is important for both but any initial baseline of trust can be diminished by poor performance, perceived lack of commitment, or inappropriate use of power.

The building and maintenance of trust is a critical, ongoing endeavour in partnership whereby small, successful outcomes reinforce trust.[12] Over time, this can encourage partners to take greater risks and can lead to innovation and synergy.[11] To achieve this, you will need not only resources but also active management of the following:

- *Purpose of partnership*: clarity of aims, objectives, and partners' roles.
- *Conflict*: skills to resolve disputes fairly.
- *Leadership*: without one party trying to taking over.
- *Time*: for relationships and understanding to develop between partners.
- *Workload*: it is shared evenly (i.e. partners do not feel exploited)
- *Commitment*: differences in levels are resolved.
- *Credit sharing for achievements*: particularly in the public sector.

You will also need shared acceptance that partnership working takes time to start delivering—typically two to three years.

Pathway to developing partnership

There are four distinct steps towards developing a partnership (see Box 7.5.2) and during each different process elements will come to the fore and need to be managed. Because partnership is a dynamic process[5], you may find that individual steps need to be revisited at different stages of the journey.

Active participation by partners in recognizing and debating the health problem from a variety of perspectives is important. Conflicting views about the issue can lead to a reframing of perspectives and the development of a *joint appreciation* of the problem—an important part of the development of novel solutions.[13] Ensuring that conflict plays a positive role in partnership requires the process of interaction to be non-judgmental so that views can be expressed openly and critiqued constructively without ridicule or opprobrium, and recognises that all members must have an equal opportunity to contribute.[7] Investing in a trained, impartial facilitator (plus administrative support) can aid this process. Conversely, abuse of power by any one partner can undermine it.

Achieving collaboration

This is the most difficult type of partnership to achieve, although potentially the most rewarding because it can lead to synergy and innovation.

Box 7.5.2 Pathway to successful partnership

- Assessing the need for partnership:
  - Identifying stakeholders
  - Recognizing common interests and developing shared goals
- Building the partnership: clarifying roles and constructing relationships (trust, commitment, empowerment)
- Managing negotiations and social relations: agreement, implementation, and delivery
- Evaluating the partnership (processes and impact):
  - Feeding back and learning from the experience
  - Termination if successful.

Role of leadership

Effective leadership is essential to partnership working, helping to forge the vision, ensuring that people know why they are there and what is expected of them, and ensuring that the process of partnership is managed effectively. Unlike organizations where leaders can use formal authority to get things done, leadership in partnership, often embodied in a 'local champion', relies heavily on drive, persuasion, passion, charisma, temperament, and interpersonal skills. Networking abilities are important. Because of the potential for disruptive personality clashes to emerge, good facilitation and agreement on ground rules are important (see also ➲ Chapter 6.1).

Third sector participation in partnership

Voluntary sector agencies, such as community organizations and user groups, are often important stakeholders and can provide insights into the nature of health (or a health condition),[14] add authenticity, and increase efficiency.[5] Most voluntary sector organizations operate on tight budgets with few resources, so power to influence decision making often resides in their discourse legitimacy. Voluntary sector participation in partnerships can be undermined by:

- lack of resources and organizational capacity to engage
- partners not responding to their input—perceived lack of action can lead to disillusionment and disengagement ('consultation fatigue')
- lack of partnership/networking skills of non-experts/lay participants
- lack of skills of other partners to recognize these limitations
- lack of a long-term, public sector strategy to develop the voluntary sector and support its involvement in partnership.

How will you know whether you have been successful?

A contribution analysis of the inputs, activities, behaviours, and processes influential in successful partnerships[5] is presented in Figure 7.5.1.[5] If your partnership is successful, you may see some or all of the following:

- Recognition of interdependence.
- Recognition of a stake in the outcome (mutual interest).
- Development of, and belief in, a shared vision and goals.
- Sense of commitment to the group and its objectives.
- Full participation and decision making by consensus.
- Open expression of feelings and disagreements.
- Free flow of information and avoidance of jargon.
- Feelings of mutual trust or dependency.
- Resolution of conflict by members themselves.
- Mutual support and problem solving.
- 'Enabling' and 'can do' approach.
- Implementation and delivery of actions to achieve outcomes.
- Critical and constructive self-evaluation.
- Improved health outcomes, greater equity, and reduced costs.

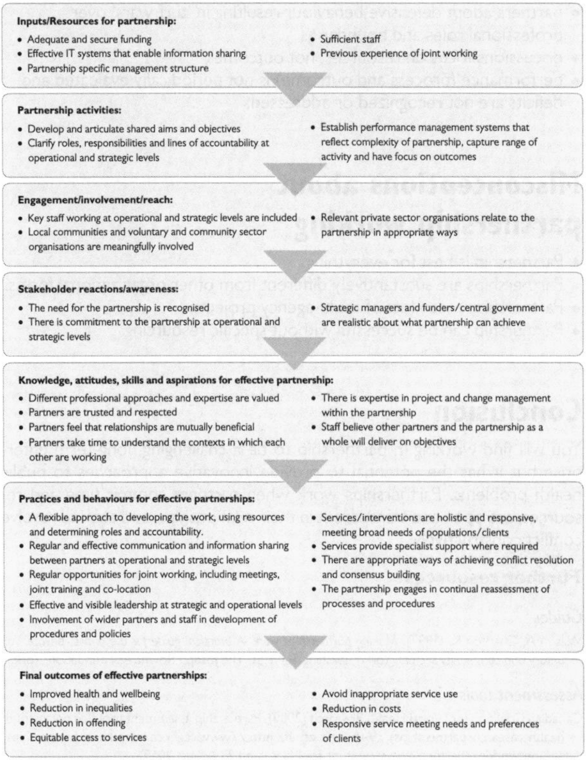

Inputs/Resources for partnership:
- Adequate and secure funding
- Effective IT systems that enable information sharing
- Partnership specific management structure
- Sufficient staff
- Previous experience of joint working

Partnership activities:
- Develop and articulate shared aims and objectives
- Clarify roles, responsibilities and lines of accountability at operational and strategic levels
- Establish performance management systems that reflect complexity of partnership, capture range of activity and have focus on outcomes

Engagement/involvement/reach:
- Key staff working at operational and strategic levels are included
- Local communities and voluntary and community sector organisations are meaningfully involved
- Relevant private sector organisations relate to the partnership in appropriate ways

Stakeholder reactions/awareness:
- The need for the partnership is recognised
- There is commitment to the partnership at operational and strategic levels
- Strategic managers and funders/central government are realistic about what partnership can achieve

Knowledge, attitudes, skills and aspirations for effective partnership:
- Different professional approaches and expertise are valued
- Partners are trusted and respected
- Partners feel that relationships are mutually beneficial
- Partners take time to understand the contexts in which each other are working
- There is expertise in project and change management within the partnership
- Staff believe other partners and the partnership as a whole will deliver on objectives

Practices and behaviours for effective partnerships:
- A flexible approach to developing the work, using resources and determining roles and accountability.
- Regular and effective communication and information sharing between partners at operational and strategic levels
- Regular opportunities for joint working, including meetings, joint training and co-location
- Effective and visible leadership at strategic and operational levels
- Involvement of wider partners and staff in development of procedures and policies
- Services/interventions are holistic and responsive, meeting broad needs of populations/clients
- Services provide specialist support where required
- There are appropriate ways of achieving conflict resolution and consensus building
- The partnership engages in continual reassessment of processes and procedures

Final outcomes of effective partnerships:
- Improved health and wellbeing
- Reduction in inequalities
- Reduction in offending
- Equitable access to services
- Avoid inappropriate service use
- Reduction in costs
- Responsive service meeting needs and preferences of clients

Figure 7.5.1 Effective partnerships process: evidence overview.

Reprinted from Cook, A. (2015) Partnership working across UK public services Edinburgh. What Works Scotland under a Creative Commons CC BY 4.0 licence.

What goes wrong with partnership working?

You may find that working in partnership is ineffective or unproductive if:
- the wrong people attend (i.e. people who cannot influence resource use in their organization or do not have a stake in the outcome)
- too many people attend, making it difficult to manage a large number of conflicting views positively
- partners lack partnership skills, such as those relating to problem solving, negotiation, and management

- partners adopt defensive behaviour resulting in 'turf wars' over professional roles and boundaries
- discussions focus on resources, not outcomes
- performance (process and outcome) is not periodically evaluated and deficits are not recognized or addressed.

Misconceptions about partnership working

- Partnership is best for everything.
- Partnerships are substantively different from other organizational forms.
- Partnerships mean lots of multi-agency projects.
- Partnership can be successful without specific resourcing.

Conclusion

You will find working in partnership to be a challenging, long-term enterprise but it has the potential to provide innovative approaches to public health problems. Partnerships work when partners commit time and resources, are open and transparent in their relationships, and seek to resolve conflict constructively.

Further resources

Guides

Wilson A, Charlton K. (1997). *Making partnerships work. A practical guide for the public, private, voluntary and community sectors*. York Publishing Services, The Joseph Rowntree Foundation, York.

Assessment tools

Canadian Coalition for Global Health Research (2009). Partnership assessment tool (for north-south health research partnerships) . Available at: ℘ http://www.ccghr.ca/resources/partnerships-and-networking/partnership-assessment-tool (accessed 23 August 2019).

Victorian Health Promotion Foundation (2016). The partnerships analysis tool, Australia. Available at: ℘ https://www.vichealth.vic.gov.au/media-and-resources/publications/the-partnerships-analysis-tool (accessed 23 August 2019).

Evaluation

Dickinson, H. (2008). *Evaluating outcomes in health and social care*. Policy Press, Bristol.

References

1 Hunter D, Perkins N. (2014). *Partnership working in public health*. Policy Press, Bristol.
2 Glasby J, Dickinson H. (2014). *partnership working in health and social care: what is integrated care and how can we deliver it?* 2nd edn. Policy Press, Bristol.
3 Smith KE, Bambra C, Joyce, KE, et al. (2009). Partners in health? A systematic review of the impact of organizational partnerships on public health outcomes in England between 1997 and 2008. *Journal of Public Health (Oxford)*, **31(2)**, 210–21.
4 Dowling B, Powell M, Glendinning C. (2004) . Conceptualising successful partnerships. *Health and Social Care in the Community*, 12(4), 309–17.
5 Cook A. (2015). Partnership working across UK public services. What works. *Scotland Evidence Review*, Edinburgh.

6 Bridgen P. (2003). Joint planning across health/social services. *Local Government Studies*, **29**, 17–31.

7 Eden C, Ackerman F. (2001). Group decision and negotiation in strategy making. *Group Decision and Negotiation*, **10**, 119–40.

8 Lukes S. (1974). *Power: a radical view*. MacMillan, London.

9 Hardy C, Phillips N. (1998). Strategies of engagement: lessons from the critical examination of collaboration and conflict in an inter-organizational domain. *Organization Science*, **9**, 217–30.

10 Vangen S, Huxham C. (2003). Nurturing collaborative relations. Building trust in interorganizational collaboration. *Journal of Applied Behavioral Science*, **39**, 5–31.

11 Jagosh J, Bush PL et al. (2015). A realist evaluation of community-based participatory research: partnership synergy, trust building and related ripple effects. *BMC Public Health*, **15**, 725–35.

12 Powell K, Thurston M, Bloyce D. (2014). Local status and power in area-based health improvement partnerships. *Health: An Interdisciplinary Journal for the Social Study of Health, Illness and Medicine*, **18(6)**, 561–79.

13 Gray B. (1989). Collaborating. *Finding common ground for multiparty problems*, Jossey-Bass, San Francisco.

14 Carnwell R, Carson A. (2009). The concepts of partnership and collaboration (Chapter 1). *Effective practice in health, social care and criminal justice: a partnership approach*, 2nd edn. Open University Press, Oxford.

Getting research into practice

Jeanette Ward and Jeremy Grimshaw

Objectives

After reading this chapter, you will be able to:
- identify and respond to situations in clinical and public health practice that require research transfer
- apply a systematic approach to research transfer, learning from the work of others and planning locally in context
- contribute to a growing body of evidence about research transfer itself

Key concepts

- Public health practitioners are well placed to facilitate implementation of research findings in clinical and public health practice.
- Systematic reviews that synthesize the totality of evidence are better foundations for conveying 'best practice' than individual studies.
- Planning local implementation strategies should incorporate insights garnered from previous implementation research, local contingencies, and available resources.
- Greater reference to theory and a systematic, disciplined approach will deliver better research transfer by building its own evidence base.

> "Evidence-based medicine should be complemented by evidence-based implementation"
>
> Grol R. (1997)[1]

Why is getting research into practice an important public health responsibility?

There is an increasing evidence base to inform and define 'best practice' in clinical and public health practice. Unless healthcare professionals and public health practitioners know and apply evidence relevant to their work consistently, the promise of health and medical research will not deliver better population health. Information overload, pressures of work, organisational culture, and other factors can result in troubling lag-times between definitive research findings and their consistent delivery in practice (Box 7.6.1).[2, 3] The population health gain inherent in more effective and efficient research transfer affords public health a unique strategic leadership role in getting research into practice wherever aspects of the health system are under-performing.

Box 7.6.1 Examples of failure in research transfer

Clinical

Many studies conducted in different countries compare current practice against best evidence. Treatments shown to improve survival are not always used in routine clinical practice. There is persistent evidence that 20–30% of patients may receive unnecessary interventions or care that might be potentially harmful with no promise of benefit. Subgroups of patients may miss out disproportionately on best-practice treatments, such as women presenting with chest pain (gender bias in care) or indigenous patients diagnosed with cancer.

Public health

In regions with endemic rates of preventable diseases, such as sexually transmissible infections, primary healthcare systems rarely achieve peak rates of disease screening despite known population benefit.

Despite a clear evidence base for 'best practice', studies of the frequency and quality of smoking cessation advice given by primary care providers to smokers in their care repeatedly show poor preventive practice.

A systematic approach to getting research into practice

A systematic approach is required to reduce the gap between achievable 'best practice' based on evidence and the care actually delivered. There are three interrelated stages to promote getting research into practice:

- *identifying* the magnitude and importance of this gap and prioritizing research transfer within your organization
- *developing* an implementation plan for research transfer with particular reference to 'research about research transfer' relevant to your circumstances
- *evaluating* the impact of research transfer and, when possible, publishing your results to help others.

Identifying and prioritizing gaps between evidence-based 'best practice' and current practice

Situations where action to improve practice through the application of research include situations in which:

- suboptimal or inequitable population health outcomes shown by surveillance, performance audits, or needs analyses by public health observatories demonstrate inadequate uptake of evidence
- critical event analysis suggests specific problems in healthcare delivery
- stakeholders or professional opinion perceive discrepancies or gaps between evidence and current practice that are confirmed

- publication of definitive new evidence, systematic reviews, or evidence-based guidelines invites accelerated improvement on documented current performance.

To prioritize efforts to get research into practice, consider a suite of screening questions as follows:
- What is the magnitude and distribution of suboptimal population or clinical outcomes? Does this arise from known knowledge not implemented in practice or other decisions in policy or resource allocation?
- Could research transfer achieve better population or clinical outcomes?
- Where is maximal health gain most likely if research transfer is effective?
- What are the agreed local, regional, or national health priorities?
- Is there sufficient momentum for local initiatives to facilitate research transfer?

Answers to these questions allow a deliberate prioritization of manageable topics for research transfer at the local level. Once prioritized, a systematic approach to implementation can proceed.

Developing a plan for getting research into practice

Creating local coalitions

From the outset, getting research into practice requires collaborative leadership, a mandate for change, and coordinated action by a range of local organizations and healthcare professionals at relevant levels.[4, 5] Creation of a local multidisciplinary coalition of stakeholders and their active engagement in planning will enhance the process. These coalitions may not already exist and will require significant commitment from public health practitioners to engender. Creative thinking with due attention to local politics, power bases, and resolute champions for 'best practice' are critical.

Developing local evidence messages

Be clear in your answer to the question, 'What is the evidence that should be transferred?' This discipline will force you to articulate the evidence-based 'best practice' that you seek to promote in a clear, compelling message. Be ready to be challenged about the level of evidence and to be interrogated about why practice needs to change. Be clear about benefits for patients and communities, sharing how you envisage successful research transfer in terms of behaviour and outcomes.[5]

Systematic reviews summarize the entire body of evidence relevant to a clinical condition or public health challenge. Diligence in finding or producing a systematic review of the evidence base to explain the need to change will pay off. You should also consider finding or producing derivative formats such as guidelines, decision aids, or actionable messages for local consumption that remain 'true' to the evidence collected as synthesized in the systematic review. Local adaptation of any given systematic review might appeal to an engaged multidisciplinary group with adequate technical and administrative support mobilized through your local coalition (Box 7.6.2).

> **Box 7.6.2 Example of a local multidisciplinary coalition to implement guidelines about referral of patients with microscopic haematuria**
>
> - General practitioners.
> - Urologist.
> - Nephrologist.
> - Anaesthetist.
> - Theatre nurse.
> - Specialist nurse.
> - Public health systems specialist.
> - Manager.
> - Patient (consumer) representative.

Identifying barriers and previous approaches relevant to your context

Thorough analysis of local barriers and facilitators alongside an enumeration and description of target audiences are needed to inform your implementation plan. By establishing the primary target audience, you will have identified the relevant professional groups whether clinicians, managers, medical officers of health, or senior health bureaucrats. Also be mindful that there are likely to be different barriers and facilitators operating at distinct levels (Box 7.6.3). Individual professionals in any target group may face different barriers and facilitators. Furthermore, different 'segments' in this target audience may need different implementation approaches. And don't forget that patients and members of the public will almost always be important to whatever it is you are trying to achieve! (See ➲ Chapter 5.7.)

> **Box 7.6.3 Barriers to evidence-based practice**
>
> Determine barriers by considering five organizational levels:
> - within the healthcare system—for example, methods of reimbursement may present perverse incentives to professionals counter to evidence-based best practice
> - within the healthcare organization—for example, inappropriate skill mix in the hospital or an organizational culture that does not embrace purposeful change
> - within local professional peer groups—for example, the desired behaviour change may be counter to prevailing norms and attitudes
> - within individual professionals—for example, individuals may not be up to date, may lack skills to perform a procedure, or may have concerns about patient safety consequent to the proposed change in practice
> - within professional–patient consultations—for example, professionals may overlook important items of care in time-pressured consultations.

A variety of methods can be used to elicit information about barriers impeding evidence-based practice such as informal discussions with professionals, purposeful qualitative research (individual interviews, focus groups), and representative surveys.[3, 6] Accurate assessment of barriers to evidence-based 'best practice' is key.[6] In general, implementation requires stakeholders (citizens, patients, healthcare professionals, managers, and policy makers) to change their behaviour. The theoretical domains framework is a useful behavioural framework summarizing key concepts from health and social psychology that can be used to identify barriers and enablers to implementation.[7, 8] Search the literature for pertinent methods.

Choosing strategies

An evidence base has emerged over the past several decades that, while less complete than ideal, is an essential first reference point from which strategies can be identified and selected for research transfer. Continual updates of evidence to inform how best to transfer research in different contexts are produced globally through the Cochrane Effective Practice and Organisation of Care Group[9] (Box 7.6.4).

There are no 'magic bullets' in research transfer: interventions might be effective in some circumstances and none are effective under all circumstances.[10] Thoroughly research your strategies, interrogating the extant evidence for their effectiveness just as a clinician might interrogate the evidence base for a new drug or treatment before using it. The risk of harm from poorly conceptualised research transfer is considerable.[2] Look at relevant journals such as *Implementation Science* and *Evidence & Policy* (see ➲ Further resources).

Myths, fashions, and fads plague research transfer. For these reasons, pay attention to taxonomies, descriptors, and standardized terms for strategies that might be used in getting research into practice.[11, 12] Be explicit in your implementation plan about your theoretical approach, your assumptions about the professional mind-set, and your choices (are they theoretically driven, pragmatically determined, or simply selected according to what is affordable at the time?). Your choice of strategy should reflect your analysis of barriers (see Box 7.6.3), the available evidence about the effectiveness of strategies if tested previously in circumstances comparable to your own, resources available to you, and other practical considerations.

Box 7.6.4 Cochrane Effective Practice and Organisation of Care (EPOC) group

This international group aims to undertake systematic reviews of the effects of:

- professional interventions (e.g. continuing medical education, quality assurance strategies, audit, and feedback)
- organizational interventions (e.g. multidisciplinary teams, practice systems)
- financial interventions (e.g. reimbursement mechanisms)
- regulatory interventions (e.g. statutory requirements).

Reviews and the specialized register are published in the Cochrane Library. Abstracts are open access.

Consider:

- Political and macro-policy interventions for reform may be necessary if barriers to research transfer stem from factors in the overarching healthcare system.
- Specific organizational interventions may be necessary if barriers relate to local healthcare organizations.
- Approaches involving social influence (local consensus processes, educational outreach, opinion leaders, marketing, etc.) may be useful when barriers relate to local professional peer groups.
- Audit and feedback may be useful when healthcare professionals are unaware of suboptimal practice and can respectfully reinforce change.
- Traditional educational approaches may be useful when barriers relate to healthcare professionals' knowledge, skills, and attitudes. In general, interactive educational activities are more likely to lead to research transfer.
- IT solutions, such as electronically generated reminders as tested in highly computerized academic health science centres, show promise in chronic disease management.
- Patient-mediated interventions when barriers relate to information processing within consultations (especially tools for sharing evidence such as patient decision aids).
- 'Push' strategies deliver to clinicians whereas 'pull' strategies are those whereby practitioners themselves seek out research. Long-term partnerships between practitioners and researchers have also been recommended as a platform for research transfer.[12]
- Strategies used to transfer research to public health practitioners and policy makers include evidence portals and 'knowledge brokers'.[12]
- Strategies can often be optimized by incorporating behaviour change techniques[13] addressing specific barriers and enablers and applying user-centred design approaches.

Getting research into practice requires adequate resources for the development of local evidence messages and implementation activities, so seek out others who share your goals, particularly those with authority to assign or redirect resources. Quality improvement units or departments within hospitals may include individuals with appropriate technical skills to support development and implementation of local guidelines. Regional health authorities can augment site-based research transfer within their jurisdiction. Performance management in large organizations can reinforce fundamental principles such as evidence-based practice. Document your choices, your reasons, and your trade-offs. Your implementation plan should be a succinct, engaging document from which roles and responsibilities can be tasked and activities monitored.

Evaluating impact and contributing to a better understanding of how to get research into practice

Metrics should include both process and outcome indicators. You might evaluate participation and activities; or intermediate outcomes such as practitioner knowledge or changes in clinical behaviour, like treatments, prescribing or counselling practices, in recognition of the longer-term, 'downstream' population outcome. Resources and access to large population datasets might readily permit relevant measures of 'downstream' population outcomes. This is especially useful if measures are unobtrusive and routinely collected.

Adopt a constructive, collaborative approach when developing the evaluation section of your implementation plan, explaining why you have selected specific outcomes for tracking and evaluation. Invest time to find or create sound instruments for evaluation. Explore academic partnerships to strengthen research transfer. Include quantitative and qualitative methods. Whenever possible, consider sophisticated evaluation designs such as cluster trials if ethical and logistic conditions permit.[14] Implementation research is the scientific study of methods and strategies to promote the uptake of research findings.[6] This body of scholarship must grow if population health is to improve and frustrations in achieving effective research transfer remedied. Evaluation design should reflect the interest in producing results that will be locally or generally applicable.[6] There are opportunities to create learning public health systems by embedding implementation science in research transfer.[15]

Key issues

Success in getting research into practice will ensure that patients and populations benefit from evidence-based best practice. While there is an increasing rigour with which to approach research transfer in healthcare settings, greater demand among those responsible for research transfer for a more scientifically sound knowledge base will further accelerate development of the discipline. There is greater recognition now that research transfer requires sophisticated, theoretically informed, and resolute effort.[11] Specialist expertise is growing. Healthcare leaders who seek to transfer evidence into routine practice must themselves adopt an evidence-based approach.

Further resources

Journals

Implementation Science. Available at: ℗ https://implementationscience.biomedcentral.com, (accessed 23 August 2019).

Evidence & Policy. Available at: ℗ http://policy.bristoluniversitypress.co.uk/journals/evidence-and-policy, (accessed 23 August 2019).

References

1 Grol R. (1997). Beliefs and evidence in changing clinical practice. *British Medical Journal*, **315**, 418–21.

2 Muir Gray J. (2009). *Evidence-based healthcare and public health: how to make decisions about health services and public health*, 3rd edn. Elsevier, London.

3 Grol R, Wensing M, Eccles M. (eds). (2005). *Improving patient care. The implementation of change in clinical practice*. Elsevier, London.

4 Grol R, Baker R, Moss F. (eds). (2004). *Quality improvement research: understanding the science of change in health care*. BMJ Publishing, London.

5 Nutley SM, Walter I, Davies HTO. (2007). *Using evidence: how research can inform public services*. Policy Press, Bristol:

6 Straus S, Tetroe J, Graham I. (2009). *Knowledge translation in health care: moving from evidence to practice*. Wiley-Blackwell, Oxford.

7 Cane J, O'Connor D, Michie S. (2012). Validation of the theoretical domains framework for use in behaviour change and implementation research. *Implementation Science*, **7**, 37.

8 Atkins L, Francis J, Islam R, et al. (2017). A guide to using the Theoretical Domains Framework of behaviour change to investigate implementation problems. *Implementation Science*, **12**(1), 77.

9 Cochrane Effective Clinical Practice and Organisation of Care Group. Available at: ℘ http://epoc.cochrane.org/ (accessed 23 August 2019).

10 Grimshaw JM, Eccles MP, Lavis JN, et al. (2012). Knowledge translation of research findings. *Implementation Science*, **7**(1), 50.

11 Leeman J, Birken SA, Powell BJ, et al. (2017). Beyond 'implementation strategies': classifying the full range of strategies used in implementation science and practice. *Implementation Science*, **12**(1), 125.

12 Lavis JN. (2006). Research, public policymaking, and knowledge-translation processes: Canadian efforts to build bridges. *Journal of Continuing Education in the Health Professions*, **26**(1), 37–45.

13 Michie S, Wood CE, Johnston M, et al. (2015). Behaviour change techniques: the development and evaluation of a taxonomic method for reporting and describing behaviour change interventions (a suite of five studies involving consensus methods, randomised controlled trials and analysis of qualitative data). *Health Technology Assessment*, **19**(99), 1–188.

14 Weijer C, Grimshaw JM, Eccles MP, et al. (2012). The Ottawa Statement on the ethical design and conduct of cluster randomized trials. *PloS Medicine*, **9**(11), e1001346.

15 Wolfenden L, Yoong SL, Williams CM, et al. (2017). Embedding researchers in health service organizations improves research translation and health service performance: the Australian Hunter New England Population Health example. *Journal of Clinical Epidemiology*, May, **85**, 3–11.

Chapter 7.7

Workforce

Felix Greaves and Charles Guest

Objectives

- To understand the internal and external influences on the public health workforce
- To help you identify practical steps you can take to improve the public health workforce in your area.

Why is this an important public health issue?

Public health depends on the public health workforce. An adequate supply of well-prepared public health professionals is essential for an effective public health system.

The workforce needs education, training, development, and motivation, and it needs to be sufficiently big. Maintaining and improving the workforce is an important role for public health practitioners—don't slip into the assumption that this is someone else's problem.

Definitions

The *public health workforce* is the body of people who work intentionally to improve a population's health. It is a diverse group of people with skills in health promotion, health protection, health systems management, information management, and many other disciplines. It requires expertise in everything from working with communities at the frontline through to influencing decision makers in boardrooms and the corridors of power.

Public health specialists have been through a specific training programme in relevant knowledge and skills, and are regulated. There is normally a formal public health body that sets standards for membership, often through a defined training curriculum and examinations.

Public health practitioner is a more inclusive term that also includes a wider range of workers. They may not be regulated or may have their regulation linked to their primary profession (e.g. as a nurse, doctor, or dietician). They are essential to the running of public health systems.

Professionalism is claimed by an increasing number of public health practitioners. It includes a responsibility for maintaining competence or skill, based on scientific knowledge. Claims of professionalism also bring expectations of honesty, confidentiality, the avoidance of conflicts of interest, commitment to improving practice, and the exercise of accountability.[1]

Credentialing refers to the accreditation of public health practitioners by a recognized body with appropriate jurisdiction. The precise mechanisms and bodies involved in credentialing vary around the world, but in most countries the aim is to increase focus on competencies that can measure work performance and educational achievement in content areas identified as central to public health practice.[2]

The *human resources function* is the part of an organization with responsibility for the management of the workforce. Its role is vital and wide-ranging, and an often-neglected part of an organization. Good public health practice requires optimizing our partnership with, and input into, this function. The human resources department is involved in:

- selection and recruitment
- training (see Box 7.7.1)
- monitoring staff performance
- organizational design, including managing change
- employee relations
- leadership development and succession planning
- workforce analysis and planning
- developing pay and performance policies.

Box 7.7.1 How does public health training in the UK work?

Public health registrars are recruited into a training programme from both medical and non-medical backgrounds. Trainees follow a defined curriculum and must demonstrate competence in a number of stated technical disciplines, as well as in particular behaviours and attitudes.

Training normally takes five years and includes an Master's in Public Health degree. Progression is by yearly assessment of competencies against a specified framework and by passing examinations, both set by the Faculty of Public Health. Training takes place in a range of institutions including local healthcare organizations, in health protection, in national organizations, and in academia.

What are the influences on the workforce in my organization?

- *Politics:* National and regional government have a role in determining the size of budgets, the degree of autonomy and, the organizational structures within the public health sector. Public health is concerned with making controversial decisions about scarce resources so that it attracts the attention of politicians.
- *The changing demography of the workforce:* Over time, the make-up and expectations of the workforce change. Social and educational influences, such as family and school, shape people's work and career expectations (see Box 7.7.2).
- *The changing demography of the population:* Populations are always changing—in some countries, there are changes in the urban–rural distribution and aging is a major challenge everywhere. The nature of the local population affects what the local public health workforce will need to do.
- *The changing expectations of the population:* the healthcare sector is seeing an increase in consumer behaviours, and less reverence for traditional professions. There are increasing expectations of customer service. There is also a trend towards increased transparency of

Box 7.7.2 Public health in England: a changing workforce context

In England, much of the public health workforce moved from the National Health Service to local government in 2013. People moved from a command-and-control, technocratic, and clinically led culture to a locally focused and politically responsive environment. As a result, public health practitioners have found it easier to influence wider determinants of health, including housing, urban planning, and licensing, but harder to influence the direct commissioning of health services. A Select Committee report identified that: 'The loss of advice on healthcare planning was identified as a threat to the effectiveness of commissioning.'[a] In addition, staff trained for one organizational culture have had to adapt to another, where the ability to influence elected members was an important new skill. The UK Faculty of Public Health updated its training curriculum in 2015, reflecting some of the new skills required.

a) House of Commons Health Committee (2016). Public health post-2013, HC 140. The Stationery Office, London. Available at: ℛ http://www.publications.parliament.uk/pa/cm201617/cmselect/cmhealth/140/140.pdf (accessed 23 August 2019).

information, including availability of knowledge around performance of health systems and decision-making processes.

- *Reorganizations:* As part of governments' attempts to grapple with the complex and rapidly changing public health demands, public health workforces and institutions are prone to frequent reorganizations and restructurings. The workforce may develop 'change fatigue' because of constant changes, and this can lead to a loss of motivation and innovation.
- *Internationalization:* In poor countries, valuable trained staff are often tempted abroad by the offer of salaries and better opportunities. Wealthy countries, aware that they do not have to pay the cost of training these individuals, may actively recruit and welcome staff from abroad (see ➲ Chapter 5.1).
- *The public and private sector divide:* The limited public health workforce faces competing demands from the public and private sectors and increasingly from non-governmental organizations. There are different levels of resources between sectors and therefore different working conditions. This may lead to a drain of valuable human resources from one sector to another, with the public sector most at risk.
- *Regulation:* There is a move towards stronger regulatory structures in healthcare in many countries. For public health workers, this may mean increased workforce assessment (e.g. revalidation) and requirements for continuing professional development.
- *Internal culture:* The internal culture of an organization, including the set of values, norms, and customs contributing to its unique character, has a profound effect on the workforce. Some of this culture may be explicit—for example, the expectations in a mission statement—but unwritten rules, language, and beliefs may be even more important (see Box 7.7.3).[3-5]

> **Box 7.7.3 The World Health Organization workforce practice code**
>
> There is considerable variation in the supply of trained medical personnel in different countries. There is one doctor per 55,000 people in Malawi; one doctor per 300 in Australia.
>
> In 2010, the World Health Organization (WHO) and its member states formally adopted a code on the international recruitment of health staff. It states:
>
>> Member States should strive, to the extent possible, to create a sustainable health workforce and work towards establishing effective health workforce planning, education and training, and retention strategies that will reduce their need to recruit migrant health personnel.
>>
>> (WHO Global Code of Practice on the International Recruitment of Health Personnel, May 2010)[a]
>
> The adoption of this code, with its collection of procedural and institutional mechanisms for monitoring a workforce, was described as a significant step forward towards improving international cooperation and maintaining the capacity of health systems, but evaluations of the code in practice have been equivocal.
>
> a) World Health Organization (2010). WHO Global Code of Practice on the International Recruitment of Health Personnel. WHO, Geneva. Available at: ◌ http://www.who.int/hrh/migration/code/practice/en (accessed 25 August 2019).

- *Models of care:* The delivery of healthcare services is changing. Increasing chronic disease prevalence and healthcare costs are leading to new models of care provision, including more treatment in the community. Technology offers opportunities for long-distance monitoring and improved communication. In many areas, there are changes in health insurance coverage and use, and other funding models for care are emerging. The public health workforce needs to respond to these changes and to build structures and skills that allows it to work across organizations and disciplines.

What can I do to improve the workforce in my organization?

Plan your workforce and think about succession

- Think ahead. Understand the age profile and where future shortages are likely. Coordinate your training programmes to fill these gaps.
- Plan succession. Continuity allows knowledge to be built up as to how things work. Large corporations carefully plan transfer of power when people leave important positions. If you know people are planning to leave, whatever their role, create a handover plan.

Ensure training and development

- People value training and opportunities to develop, and these things also improve retention and effectiveness. Training budgets are often limited and vulnerable: use them, protect them, and make sure that time is made available for training.
- Consider developing a mentoring scheme, matching a less experienced member of the team with a more experienced mentor. The development of a long-term, two-way relationship helps transfer skills and knowledge, and can benefit both parties.
- Coaching for team members can provide specific guidance around their skills and ways of working.
- Think about alternative ways to provide educational opportunities such as short courses, continuing education, or distance learning.
- Make sure training is relevant. Some professional training can be narrowly conceived, outdated, and unsuited to an increasingly multidisciplinary and independent world.

Allow new ways of working

- Think about how to enable flexible working. Allow your team members the freedom to manage how and where they work.
- New technology can make health workers more efficient. Consider holding meetings by teleconference or video call.

Create an attractive organizational climate

- People want to work somewhere pleasant. Do junior staff feel empowered enough to speak up at meetings? Are there unwritten rules about how people behave? Think about the positive attributes of your culture and enhance them. Think about the negative ones and how you can eliminate them.
- Work on your induction programme. Induction is an opportunity to promote the positive aspects of your organizational culture.

Think more widely about the pool of available people

- It may be necessary to look outside the usual pool of talent to find the people you need—there may be a 'hidden' workforce that you might otherwise miss.
- Try actively recruiting more mature candidates, or those returning to the workforce after a career break. Bring in people from other sectors with relevant experience. People now often have portfolio careers, so make the most of their experiences elsewhere—with suitable support for their transition to a new role.
- Engage mature staff in dialogue about best use of their skills and knowledge. Support them to plan their career path and retirement.
- Roles may need review and redesign to suit older people, such as reduced hours with more emphasis on training other staff.
- Volunteers present a potentially useful resource but need careful management and resources. They need proper administrative support, funds for continuing education, access to information, regular communication, and formal recognition programmes.

Inclusive management

- Ensure management involvement and support. Coordinated support from senior management and middle and line managers across an organization allows access, opportunity, and support to all workers.
- Communicate the aims and purpose of the organization consistently and effectively. Keep staff updated about changes or developments.
- Make sure your team is involved in the planning process. A participatory approach to project planning and implementation helps to create employer and worker ownership and longer-term success.

Promote staff health and wellbeing

- Think about workplace health promotion programmes. Can you change the workplace to encourage the ideas we promote to the population?
- Programmes that cover a variety of health-related issues address more behavioural risk factors and engage more workers.
- Work with occupational health and safety initiatives within your organization.
- Rowe and Kidd[6] set out useful ideas for resilience that would promote health and wellbeing for us all. For example:
  - make home a sanctuary
  - value strong relationships
  - have an annual preventive health assessment
  - control stress, not people
  - recognize conflict as an opportunity
  - manage bullying and violence assertively.

Motivation

Everybody is motivated by different things. There are theoretical models that may be useful in thinking about what you can do to encourage your staff and keep them motivated. It's not just pay (although that is important). Use these models to consider what other aspects of working life could become sources of enthusiasm in your team (see also ➔ Chapter 6.1).

Maslow's hierarchy of needs

This theory[7] suggests that there is a hierarchy of different needs that we seek to fulfil. These can be seen as a pyramid, with the most basic needs at the bottom, becoming increasingly complex as you approach the top. Once one set of needs is fulfilled, we then seek the next highest set of needs—see Table 7.7.1.

Herzberg's motivation hygiene hypothesis

Herzberg distinguished between positive factors that motivate people and hygiene factors that need to be present or people will be dissatisfied. It is also called the 'two-factor theory' of motivation.[8]

The *positive factors*, or motivators, might include responsibility, recognition, or the challenge of work. These may make people actively enjoy their role.

Hygiene factors do not necessarily create satisfaction but their absence will lead to dissatisfaction. Examples include wages and job security.

Table 7.7.1 Maslow's hierarchy of needs

Level of need	Example	What it might mean at work
Self-actualization (top of the pyramid)	Self-realization, personal growth	Being innovative and creative
Esteem	Social recognition, self-esteem and accomplishment	Receiving that cherished promotion
Social	Being part of a group, friendship, intimacy	Having a group of friends to talk to in the office
Security	Protection, security, law	Having a contract, getting paid regularly, and feeling safe at work
Physiological (bottom of the pyramid)	Food and shelter	Having an office that is warm and dry

In practice, an employer needs to think about getting both these right. You need to provide the basics, such as job security, a decent workplace, and payment. But that is not enough: you also need to challenge your staff, put them in a position where they feel they are respected, and validate their work in some way.

Working together

Public health practitioners rarely work in isolation. To do your job, you will need to work effectively in a team with the people around you. These may be formal teams working within or between organizations, or informal groups of people coming together to think about a problem. Either way, you will be part of a team—see ➲ Chapter 7.4.

Future challenges

The actions of individual public health practitioners in choosing how we work and with whom we work will remain critical in defining our workforce. There are significant future challenges, particularly in adapting the workforce to address future healthcare changes related to shifting demography, expectations, and technology.

It will be important to continue to demonstrate the value of the public health workforce to ensure a constant supply of people for the many and varied roles required.

The ongoing problem of global health workforce stability poses a challenge of sustainability. An increased awareness of the issues, and acceptance of the ethical and logistic complexity involved, has led to progress on the part of global institutions and this needs to continue.

Summary

The workforce presents a relatively neglected area in public health practice but the existence of an effective public health workforce is vital to the performance of the public health function. To create the public health workforce of the future, we must understand and work with our colleagues in human resources. Public health practitioners will need the skills of leaders, managers, planners, and team members to play a full part in delivering this workforce.

Further resources

Further reading

Beaglehole R, Dal Poz MR. (2003). Public health workforce: challenges and policy issues. *Human Resources for Health*, 1, 4.

Public Health England (2016). *Fit for the future – public health people: a review of the public health workforce*, Public Health England, London. Available at: ℘ https://www.gov.uk/government/uploads/system/uploads/attachment_data/file/524599/Fit_for_the_Future_Report.pdf (accessed 23 August 2019).

Royal Society for Public Health Vision, Voice and Practice (2015). Rethinking the public health workforce. Available at: ℘ https://www.rsph.org.uk/asset/B84C8AA9-7526-425E-B6F73BB1C7053BA0 (accessed 23 August 2019).

World Health Organization (2016). *Health workforce and services: draft global strategy on human resources for health: workforce 2030*. WHO, Geneva. Available at: ℘ http://apps.who.int/gb/ebwha/pdf_files/WHA69/A69_38-en.pdf (accessed 23 August 2019).

World Health Organization Global Health Workforce Network. Available at: ℘ http://www.who.int/hrh/network/en (accessed 25 August 2019).

References

1 Thistlethwaite JE, Spencer J. (2008). *Professionalism in medicine*. Radcliffe, Oxford.

2 Goldstein BD. (2008). Credentialing in public health: the time has come. *Journal of Public Health Management Practice*, 14(1), 1–2.

3 World Health Organization (2017). Global Health Observatory data repository. World Health Organization. Geneva.

4 Taylor A, Gostin L. (2010). International recruitment of health personnel. *Lancet*, 375(9727), 1673–5.

5 Tankwanchi A, Vermund S, Perkins D. (2014). Has the WHO Global Code of Practice on the International Recruitment of Health Personnel been effective? *Lancet Global Health*, 2(7), e390–1.

6 Rowe L, Kidd M, (2010). First *do no harm: being a resilient doctor in the 21st century*. McGraw Hill, Maidenhead.

7 Maslow AH. (1943). A theory of human motivation. *Psychological Review*, 50, 370–96.

8 Herzberg F, Mausner B, Snyderman BB. (1959). *The motivation to work*, 2nd edn. John Wiley & Sons, New York.

Index

Notes. Tables, figures and boxes are indicated by t, f and b following the page number vs. indicates a comparison or differential diagnosis